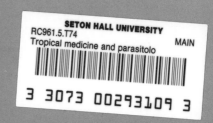

TROPICAL MEDICINE AND PARASITOLOGY

Classic Investigations ● Volume II

TROPICAL MEDICINE AND PARASITOLOGY

Classic Investigations • Volume II

EDITED BY

B. H. KEAN, M.D., Clinical Professor of Medicine (Tropical Medicine) and Clinical Professor of Public Health, Cornell University Medical College; Director, Parasitology Laboratory, The New York Hospital-Cornell Medical Center; Attending Physician, New York Hospital.

KENNETH E. MOTT, M.D., Assistant Professor of Tropical Public Health, Harvard School of Public Health.

AND

ADAIR J. RUSSELL, Medical Editor, Tropical Medicine Unit, Cornell University Medical College.

Cornell University Press   ITHACA AND LONDON

Copyright © 1978 by Cornell University

First published 1978 by Cornell University Press.
Published in the United Kingdom by Cornell University Press Ltd.,
2-4 Brook Street, London W1Y 1AA.

International Standard Book Number: 0-8014-0992-6
Library of Congress Catalog Card Number: 76-12908
Composition by Examiner Graphics, New York, N.Y.
Printed in the United States of America by LithoCrafters, Inc.
Librarians: Library of Congress cataloging information appears on the last page of this volume.

HELMINTHS—HELMINTHIC INFECTIONS

CHAPTER **14**

Hookworm

NEW WORM OF THE HUMAN INTESTINE
(AGCHYLOSTOMA DUODENALE)
CONSTITUTING A SIXTH GENUS OF
NEMATODES FOUND IN MAN

Nuovo verme intestinal umano (*Agchylostoma duodenale*) costituente un sesto genere dei nematoidei proprii dell 'uomo. Annali Universali di Medicina, 106: 5–13, 1843. Translated from the Italian.

Angelo Dubini
(1813–1902)

One of a brilliant group of nineteenth-century Italian clinicians and epidemiologists, Angelo Dubini had a distinguished career which finally led to his appointment to the chair at the University of Padua held some 300 years earlier by Bernardo Ramazzini, the father of occupational medicine. While Dubini is best known for his discovery of Ancylostoma duodenale, *which later was shown to be the causative agent of human hookworm disease, he made many other contributions to medicine, notably in the field of neurology.*

The first description of A. duodenale *is documented in this historic paper.*

In the order of nematodes native to man, five [sic] genera of worms are known: *Filaria, Spiroptera, Strongylus, Ascaris, Trichocephalus,* and *Oxyuris*; of these, only the last three live in the intestinal canal.

A sixth genus of cylindrical entozoa found in humans (or a fourth genus of those found in the intestines) consists of a little worm not longer than four and a half lines [1 line = 1/12 inch— Eds.] which lives in the duodenum and the beginning of the jejunum. Even though it has not hitherto been seen or described by others, nevertheless the worm was found in at least 20 cadavers out of 100 which were dissected with the aim of finding it.

History of the Discovery

Beginning in May 1838, while dissecting the cadaver of a peasant woman who had died on Ward No. 3 of the Maggiore Hospital of Milan of pulmonary infarction complicated by hepatic and splenic congestion, I encountered a little worm in the small intestine, in the midst of much gray mucus. When compared microscopically to *Oxyuris vermicularis* and *Trichocephalus dispar* and to smaller specimens of the *Ascaris lumbricoides,* this worm impressed me as having really distinct generic characteristics.

Four years later, on 9 November 1842, I happened to see it again in Ward No. 2 in the cadaver of an old woman who had been afflicted with hydrothorax combined with hydropericardium. After removing the worm from the yellowish mucus of the jejunum in which it was lying, I applied myself to studying its structure and to making a reasonably accurate picture of it, using a powerful Brunner microscope.

On 13 December of the same year, while opening the duodenum of a man who had died of jaundice (in order to examine the opening of the common bile duct), I discovered in the midst of a dense yellowish-red mucus, a third specimen of the same genus, which I recognized to be female like the other two, and which confirmed the accuracy of my previous observations.

I had yet to investigate the arrangement of the reproductive organs of a male specimen. On the 15th of the same month I was able to complete my studies on a dozen worms which were found at the beginning of the jejunum in a woman who had died of an abcess in the right chest; the abscess was accompanied by a large effusion of turbid serum. On 21 December, I found four more worms in the jejunum of a man with hydrothorax, in the midst of gray mucus.

287

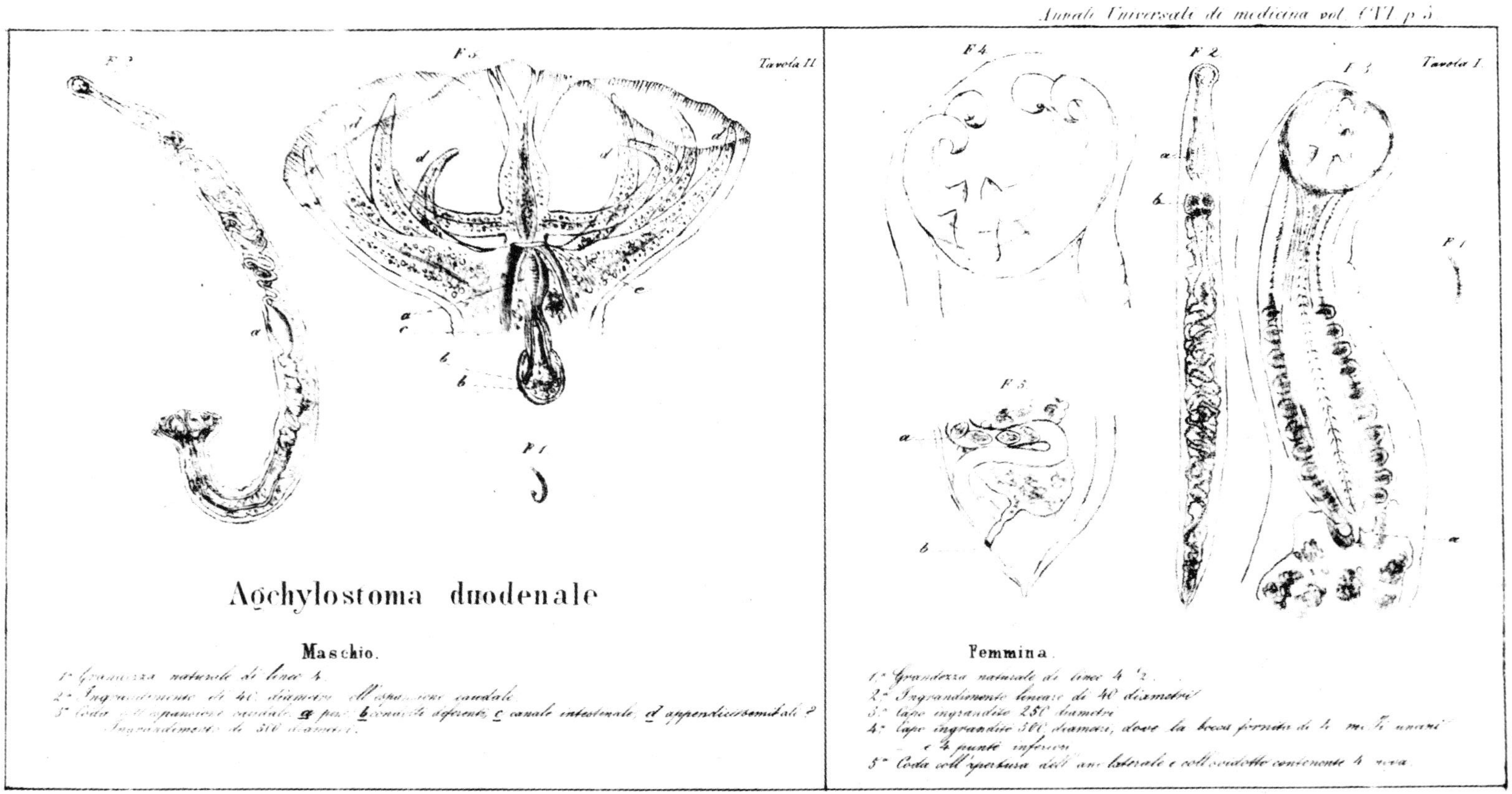

Plate 44. Sec. II Agchylostoma duodenale. Male. *Fig. 1.* Natural size 4 lines. *Fig. 2.* Magnification with the enlarged tail. *Fig. 3.* Cross-section of the tail. (a) penis; (b) vas deferens; (c) intestinal canal; (d) appendices.
Female. *Fig. 1.* Natural size 4½ lines. *Fig. 2.* Magnification. *Fig. 3.* Head magnified. *Fig. 4.* Head magnified. The mouth with four soft hooks and four lower points. *Fig. 5.* Cross-section of the lateral anus and oviduct containing four ova.

On 1 January 1845, I saw many of them scattered through a white mucus of the jejunum of a man who had died of double pneumonia and ulcerative colitis. Two of them were firmly attached by their heads to the mucosa, and the mucosa was specked with small red dots.

I did not fail to find them afterward, occasionally in great numbers, either in a free state or adhering by oral extremities to the mucosa, sometimes in individuals who had died of chronic diarrhea, with or without intestinal ulcerations, and sometimes in patients with anasarca or asthma. In the small intestine of these individuals, however, there was always a great deal of dense mucus, for the most part yellowish-red in color. In some of those who died of chronic diarrhea the mucosa was consistently characteristic—an infinite number of black dots strewn over the tips of the intestinal villi, as if they had been spattered by minute particles of charcoal powder. Many observations over a period of several years have led me to believe that the alteration of which I speak, although unusual and little-known, in many cases may cause chronic diarrhea.

Finally, in a woman who had died of spotted typhus and in whose intestines were many ulcers with a highly congested base, I found four of the same worms at the beginning of the jejunum; toward the end of the same intestine I found 20 or more *Ascaris,* and in the caecum hundreds of *Trichuris.* Five other lumbricoids were rolled up in the stomach.

By repeating the dissections and reiterating the appropriate observations I became fully convinced of the facts that I am about to expound, namely:

(1) That these new helminths are not rarely encountered when they are looked for. Their presence certainly cannot be inconsequential to the individual even though, like the tricepholids, they may not give rise to particular symptoms.

(2) That their exclusive habitat is the duodenum and the beginning of the jejunum.

(3) That a necessary condition for their existence is an unusual amount of mucus secreted by these two portions of the intestine; mucus which can vary, however, in its physical qualities, being sometimes whitish, sometimes gray, sometimes yellow, and sometimes yellow-red.

(4) That the mucosa, to which the worms sometimes adhere by their oral cavity, may appear to be normal or else slaty, greatly specked with black or red, or also simply hypervascular.

(5) That the variety of illnesses from which these people died does not permit us to establish a relationship between the affliction and the presence of the worms, I could only observe that it was among those with deteriorated constitutions —people who were weak, dysenteric, emaciated, or anasarcous—that they were most likely to be found.

(6) That their presence does not exclude that of other helminths; on the contrary, they are frequently associated with other helminths.

Afterward, thinking about the reasons which had delayed their discovery until now, it appears that I do not err in reducing them to the following:

A few years ago (starting with the most recently initiated pathologic studies of typhoid fever or of tuberculosis with intestinal ulcerations) people began to open the intestines to examine the mucosa. The ancients, who either looked at them intact or did not open them up regularly, could not have had any knowledge of a worm, which was, moreover, small enough so as not to be felt by chance by squeezing the intestine. However, let us say that the practice of the moderns was not the most favorable for finding the worms as they were accustomed to opening the intestines and washing them immediately with a great deal of water before examining the entire mucosa. In this way the mucus was washed clean and fell to the bottom of the water together with the helminths that had nested there. Finally, the abundant mucus (yellowish-red or gray and less than transparent) in which they are ordinarily enveloped, as well as their small size, provide great obstacles even to the most astute observers.

It is sufficient to separate the intestine little by little from the mesentery, about an arm's length at a time, thereby stretching it. Split it lengthwise with the enterotome, spread it out over one of the thighs of the cadaver, and examine carefully the mucus which it contains. In order to see the mucosa underneath, the mucus is then removed using the back of the knife without any need for washing it. When there exists a great deal of gray or reddish mucus in the duodenum or jejunum, it will not be difficult, if one looks closely, to see small worms embedded up in it. They are somewhat curved in on themselves, transparent in the anterior quarter of their length, yellowish or reddish or brown in the posterior three-quarters, and marked at the point in between by a little black sphere which is the stomach, ordinarily filled with blackish material.

Classification

Order: Because of the following characteristics the new helminth is placed in the natural order of the nematodes. *Cylindrical, elastic body; intestinal canal opening into the mouth at one extremity and into the anus at the other; genital organs distributed in two different individuals.*

Genus: It forms a distinct genus because of further characteristics that become sufficiently clear when one uses a magnification of 40, 250, or 500 diameters. *Head not distinct from body; round mouth furnished with four hooks folded back toward the center and situated above conical eminences which project from the interior of the pharynx; esophagus enlarged at the bottom like a club and distinct from the spherical blackish stomach; blunt tail in the female, spread out like a fan in the male; a single central penis in which are inserted two small vas deferens.*

Species: The only species in the genus I established (which will be indicated by the word Agchylostoma, from *agkylos,* curved, and *stoma,* mouth) is this little worm previously referred to, which is about four and one-half lines in length, transparent in the anterior, and marked by wavy yellow, brown, or red stripes in the posterior three-quarters. A black spherical dot marks the boundary between the transparent and colored parts. Posteriorly the female has a blunt tail which is slightly curved (Plate 44, Sec. I, fig. 1). The two words *Agchylostoma duodenale* can indicate the species which we shall now examine anatomically with the help of a microscope.

Microscopic Analysis

Viewing the worm with an enlargement of 40 diameters, it seems to be covered with a transparent derma furrowed laterally with minute grooves (Plate 44, Sec. I and II, fig. 2). The head shows at its extremity four little blue bodies which approximate when the mouth is closed. If the head of the worm is cut crosswise and placed on a glass slide with a drop of water, covered and slightly crushed by another thin piece of glass, and then studied under the microscope with an enlarge-

ment of 250 (or better, 500) diameters, it can be seen that these four little bodies are nothing more than four hooks turned inward toward the center of the mouth (Plate 44, Sec. I, fig. 4). Underneath these hooks, arising from the funnel-shaped pharynx, are four conical projections which are turned upward, two smaller than the others. The esophagus (Plate 44, Sec. I, fig. 2a) extends downward, getting larger and larger, and then contracts at the opening into the stomach. Here the opening of the cardia is surrounded by four soft papillary projections hanging down into the cavity of the ventriculum (Plate 44, Sec. I, fig. 3a). The stomach (Plate 44, Sec. I, fig. 2b), full of black matter, is prolonged into the intestine, which is marked by irregular swellings and leads to the worm's posterior extremity; it ends by opening, via a narrow channel, into a lateral slit at the apex of the tail (Plate 44, Sec. I, fig. 5b). In the female this central intestine is surrounded by the oviduct in which elliptical eggs can be seen (Plate 44, Sec. I, fig. 5a); in the male, on the other hand, it is surrounded by the flexible sperm duct which enlarges into a sort of seminal vesicle about halfway down the length of the worm (Plate 44, Sec. II, fig. 2), and then narrows again and goes on toward the genital organs of the tail. This (Plate 44, Sec. II, fig. 3) is composed of the last portion of the intestine (c), which opens up in its center into a circular hole (e); of the club-shaped penis (a) into which run the two little efferent ducts (bb); and finally of a membrane (ddd) which constitutes a sort of funnel whose transparent walls are reinforced by eleven stumplike appendices which, with some diffidence, I call seminal vesicles, not being able to guess their true functions (Plate 44, Sec. II, fig. 3dddd).

Differential Characteristics

The *Oxyuris vermicularis* (Brem.) which is not similar to *Agchylostoma* except possibly for its small size, is distinguished from every other cylindrical worm in humans by a transparent vesicle which swells its head and which appears in the form of two small ala at the sides of the esophagus. Moreover, it is not longer than a line and a half and is always a milk-white color. The male has a tail that does not expand fanlike but is blunt and spiraled; the female, on the other hand, has a tail that is straight and attenuates to a very sharp point. Their favorite site is the rectum.

The other genus which it might be suspected to resemble is the *Ascaris lumbricoides,* but even the smallest ascarids are never less than a few inches long. The head of *A. lumbricoides* is distinguished from the body by deep, circular furrows; its mouth exhibits three soft valves instead of four hooks; its body shows two marked longitudinal furrows; the penis of the male is double or bifid rather than single, and the tail ends in a blunt point, showing no expansion whatever.

The capillary prolongation which makes up the head of the *Trichocephalus dispar* makes it possible for me to dispense with further differences. The *Bothriocephalus* and the *Taenia,* which are the other two known inhabitants of the human intestine, are distinguished from the nematodes by their flat shape.

CLINICAL AND ANATOMICAL OBSERVATIONS ON THE DISEASES OF EGYPT

Klinische und anatomische beobachtungen über die krankheiten von Egypten. Archiv für Physiologie Heilkunde, 13: 528–575, 1854. Selections from pp. 554–561. Translated from the German.

Wilhelm Griesinger
(1817–1868)

Griesinger's greatest fame was achieved in the field of psychiatry, but his interest in that specialty developed through his earlier experiences in internal medicine. He was, indeed, one of the pioneers in linking medicine with psychiatry.

He started his studies at Tübingen, but had to leave that university because he was a member of a banned student corps. He therefore went to Zurich in 1837 and later to Paris for his medical training.

The relationship between anemia and hookworm disease was first established in this paper, but not accepted until Wucherer confirmed his work in 1866.

Everything which has been reported up to now, including the odd typhus forms of Egypt, has its counterpart in Europe, as well as in our German sphere of observation. We now come to several still poorly understood, extremely peculiar diseases which are common in Egypt.

The recent fortunate discoveries by my colleague Dr. Bilharz in Cairo of entozoas, about which there is still little understanding, are already the general property of science. I refer to his own reports for an excellent description of the anatomy and the life cycle of these organisms. I wish to discuss here the pathological conditions induced by two of these entozoas in the body. The reader will gain insight into a completely new field of pathology—the Egyptian one—the extent of which has not yet been determined.

Ancylostomiasis and Chlorosis

Ancylostoma duodenale, a 4–5-lines-long [1 line = 1/12 inch—Eds.] nematode discovered by Dubini in Milan, was first found in Egypt by Drs. Pruner and Bilharz in the spring of 1851 during our autopsies. The organism was found in the upper small intestine, sometimes in huge numbers; it adheres tightly to the mucosa, the resulting wound extending into the submucosa. Often the worm itself, engorged with blood, lies in a small blood-filled cavity in the submucosal layer. In the presence of many ancylostomas, the involved section of the intestine is often filled with blood from the numerous wounds.

We consider an abundance of these entozoa in the intestine to be the cause of a disease which anyone who has ever practiced in an Egyptian hospital learns to know in its most advanced, incurable form. Milder and less severe forms of the disease can be found everywhere in city and country, in the fellahee of the upper Egyptian villages as well as in the soldier; in the girls who fetch water from the river as well as in the writers of the Divan; at times, it is even found in persons of higher social standing. We have mentioned it occasionally in this journal as ''Egyptian chlorosis'' and will continue to use this designation.

In the records of our clinic in Cairo we find 71 cases designated as chlorosis (as already mentioned, all were men). But in at least three times as many cases the chlorotic condition was complicated by other diseases. We consider it only a very moderate estimate that one-fourth of the Egyptian population suffers to a greater or lesser degree from this disease. The enormity of the loss of manpower to the country, joy of life, and premature death through this disease can be appreciated by everyone.

The symptoms of this disease are simply those of anemia. The milder stages are characterized by pallor of the skin and the mucosa; other symptoms include venous murmur in the jugular veins, a tendency to palpitations, prolonged tachycardia, and slight fatigue on exertion. These patients are, as a rule, not emaciated but, on the contrary, are often rather fat; their appearance is frequently somewhat bloated, and, in some cases, slight intestinal disturbances are as frequent as in the true chlorosis. The Egyptian physician Broussaisist has therefore called this disease chronic gastroenteritis, and he is closer to the truth than he knows.

After several stages, the chronic form becomes a much more serious condition which is readily recognizable from a distance. The patients remain rather obese for a long time, but later most of them become emaciated. Often they develop edema in the lower extremities, the eyelids, and other parts; their skin, even when it has been heavily pigmented, always becomes a dirty, pale yellow, yellow, or green-white. Also, in Negroes the skin becomes paler and grayer. At the same time it becomes very withered, flabby, cool, dry, and scaly; the conjunctiva is blue-white, and the lips and all visible mucous membranes are deathly pale. Marked generalized weakness and fatigue, which increases with each movement, makes the patient very indolent and apathetic; there are frequently vague muscle pains in the extremities as well. Palpitations corresponding to the heart beat, the intensity of which we have never seen before, persist in many patients. If they cease on continued rest, they usually reoccur after only a few steps, not infrequently accompanied by more or less severe aching, precordially. The second heart sound can be heard readily at times when the patient is a few steps away from the examiner; auscultation reveals either loud sounds everywhere or the short, weak first sound and/or indistinct with a systolic, blowing, rushing murmur. The pulse is very rapid and weak. In all the larger arteries one hears a blowing sound, while in the jugular veins, loud rushing and roaring with vibrations can be felt. In a very few cases, all the signs of organic heart disease are found including hypertrophy, mitral and aortic insufficiency, and/or stenosis, and so on. Patients often suffer from vertigo, frontal and temporal headache, and ringing in the ears; respiration is rapid, short, and the breath sounds weak. Dyspnea occurs after a few steps; in several patients we noticed a moderate emphysematous curving of the thorax. The urine is ample,

very pale, and rarely contains albumin. The patients are constantly hungry and sometimes have strange cravings. At times a gastritislike state occurs with a fluctuating slight fever, coated tongue, and abdominal tenderness; the spleen is only moderately enlarged in exceptional cases; the liver is frequently diminished in size. The overall condition of the patient must be viewed as a state of advanced anemia or fluid retention.

If the patients are taken care of and well-nourished, they can remain in this condition of chlorotic marasmus for years; but in other cases, it runs a rather acute course. Occasionally someone will recover completely if he changes climate and living conditions—this we saw in some soldiers returned home on leave for six months—but the majority of individuals in whom the disease has reached the degree mentioned remain pale, chronically ill, and miserable in spite of excellent care; for them, slight, acute diseases are accompanied by prostration and life-threatening complications; most of them finally die from dysentery. It is obvious that they weaken more rapidly the more they are forced to do heavy labor or the more they are required to undergo the incapacitating treatment for chronic gastritis. But even without such evident adversities of intercurrent diseases, we have seen a few patients die of anemia in spite of treatment with iron, wine, and so on. They become slowly edematous (with infrequent traces of albumin in the urine), finally developing diarrhea without dysenteric changes of the intestinal mucosa.

The cadavers of the individuals who had suffered much for a long time from chlorosis, either by itself or in combination with other diseases, showed hydropic changes in various places including flabby, pale muscles and an extensive generalized anemia of the brain, lungs, stomach, and intestinal mucosa. The heart was generally, but not always, large, being hypertrophic, especially on the left side; it was usually very pale, especially the inner muscle layer and the endocardium and the valves were often dull and thickened (this *Archive,* Vol. 12, 1853, p. 557). The veins were empty; only in the heart were there small, soft, brown clots with some fibrin. In several cases, however, the heart and large veins contained a watery, light red, brothlike liquid with relatively very few large, pale blood corpuscles. Very frequently the spleen and kidneys would show a fatty, waxy consistency. The spleen, and even more often the liver, would show a greater or lesser degree of generalized atrophy. I am unable to estimate to what extent this anemia, as in the cadaver, is a complication of other diseases; even less so, since dysentery and bilious typhoid produce a similar picture of anemia, as mentioned above. I can assure you that the number of cases of anemia was relatively substantial and that in our country, with the exception of those who have bled to death, we almost never find anemic cadavers like those we see daily in Cairo.

From the very beginning I directed my attention to this disease. Having been called upon to direct the Health Service of Egypt, I found it necessary to try to find the source of this grave and widespread disease. For a time I believed that I would have to consider this disease a result of dysentery; later I connected it with syphilis, intermittent fever, and malarial diseases in general, poor nutrition, and the homesickness of soldiers. Nothing relating to these diseases, however, applied to all or even to the majority of cases; there were always cases which did not fit into any know pattern of disease. Nor was it possible to deduce something significant from the results of the treatment. The most potentially useful therapy proved ineffective on the whole. In addition to good nutrition, I tried three medicines— iron preparations, quinine (starting with the malaria hypothesis), and calcaria phosphorica. These medicines were never mixed, but were always used one at a time, continuously, and in a consistent fashion. All had the same result; the milder cases very frequently improved, some of them very significantly, but very few to the extent that I could consider them completely cured. The serious cases seldom showed improvement, but remained either the same or worsened. These patients, the great proportion of those found in military hospitals, who remained bedridden in the same condition for as long as six months, finally had to be sent home or discharged from the army as unfit for service.

I believed that I would have had to leave Egypt with these negative and sad results regarding the etiology and treatment of this important disease when suddenly, during one of my last autopsies in Cairo (17 April 1852), light was shed on this matter. The case was that of an obese 20-year-old soldier from the first military division; diarrhea was given as the clinical cause of death. All organs, but especially the brain and lungs, were highly anemic, the latter being markedly edematous. There was extensive dilitation with moderate hypertrophy of the left ventricle; the entire heart muscle, particularly the endocardium, was very pale and somewhat fatty; the valves were normal; a fibrin and blood clot was present in the heart. A few spoonsful of fatty effusion were present in the abdomen. The liver was reduced to about half its normal size but kept its proportions; it was flaccid, tough, light brown, and anemic; bile was abundant and dark brown; fibrin clots were found in the portal vein. The spleen was small, tough, and anemic; the kidneys were pale, solid, and fatty; the bladder was filled with clear urine. The stomach and intestinal mucosa were anemic throughout; in the large intestine solid feces with much blood were found. *The duodenum, the whole jejunum, and even the upper half of the ilium were completely filled with fresh, red, partly coagulated blood. Thousands of ancylostomas were hanging in the mucosa of the small intestine, each with its own small petechia resembling the bite of a leech.*

It was clear that in every respect the deceased belonged to the "chlorotics," and had bled to death. Since then I have become convinced that the "Egyptian chlorosis" is an entozoal disease, above all an ancylostomiasis. Thus I leave it to the reader if and to what extent the entozoa of the portal vein, which will be mentioned in another article, contribute to the production of the anemic condition. A short time after that autopsy I left Egypt. I was unable to get and never will get positive proof for my opinion by way of statistics and analysis. The testing of the same, which is of such far-reaching consequence for the health and life of the Egyptian people, will be in the hands of subsequent truth-loving investigators in that country.

With this hypothesis most of the questions relating to this disease, for which no general cause is otherwise found, are answered. The extent of the spread of the ancylostomas, which at times are found in almost every cadaver, corresponds to the frequency of the "chlorosis" in a given area. The amount of blood found in cadavers with many worms in the small intestine is often extraordinary. It is obvious that many different modifications of the (rapid or slow, abundant or sparse) leeching of blood by the worms are possible, just as we see the disease run its course sometimes in a slower, more chronic manner, while at other times it takes a more rapid course. The daily blood loss in the small intestine must naturally result in anemia. One should further remember that the condition described with violent palpitations and well-preserved panniculus corresponds primarily to an anemia caused by excessive blood loss, while anemic conditions caused by poor nutrition, malaria, or chronic diseases of various organs do not manifest themselves in just this way. With continued blood loss, the remaining blood becomes increasingly watery; the more watery the blood the more severe the hemorrhages; this vicious cycle seems to be at the bottom of the chlorotic marasmus. Neither improved nutrition nor tonic medicines restore the blood so long as the cause of the anemia persists. One would have thought that the intestinal bleeding caused by the ancylostomas would have attracted attention by the presence of bloody stools. However, the single bleeding is, as a rule, sparse; it only becomes harmful by repetition. Blood coming from the upper small intestine is not recognizable in the copious fecal mush of the Egyptian, which is caused by the heavy consumption of bread. Actually extensive bleeding is not necessary for the production of anemia; extraction of the amount of blood which hundreds or thousands of ancylostomas consume for years for their own sustenance would surely suffice for the development of a severe anemia. Blood found in the eliminations by an attentive doctor could be ascribed to hemorrhoids, chronic dysentery, and many other more common causes before thinking of the cause described here.

ON A DISEASE COMMONLY CALLED "OPPILAÇÃO" OR "CANÇAÇO"
[Pallor or Perpetual Fatigue—Eds.]

Sobre a molestia vulgarmente denominada oppilação ou cançaço. Gazeta Medica da Bahia, 1: No. 3, 27–29; No. 4, 39–41; No. 5, 52–54; No. 6, 63–64, 1866. Selections from pp. 27–28, 39–40, 63–64. Translated from the Portuguese.

Otto Edward Henry Wucherer
(1820–1873)

Though born in Pôrto, Portugal, Wucherer came with his father, a German merchant, to Salvador, Bahia, Brazil, where he spent his childhood. He was educated in Germany and received his M.D. degree from the University of Tübingen. In London he worked as an assistant at St. Bartholomew's Hospital.

Shortly after his return to Bahia in 1849, Wucherer and John Ligertwood Paterson, a Scottish physician, identified yellow fever there, a disease which had not been recognized in Brazil since 1686. The physicians of the city and the lay press rejected his diagnosis despite the yellow fever infirmary in his home, his wife's death from yellow fever, and his unselfish services to the community.

This remarkable physician was a well-known herpetologist and furnished specimens to the British Museum and London Zoological Garden. Wucherer's association with Paterson, and José Francisco Silva Lima brought mutual stimulation which resulted in classic descriptions of hookworm, filariasis, ainhum, and beriberi.

In response to criticism by the Imperial Academy of Medicine in Rio de Janeiro, Wucherer published a reply, "Questions on Cause and Effect Are Not Decided by Opinion or by Votes, But by Rigorous Appreciation of the Facts."

This paper confirms Griesinger's conclusion that the cause of tropical anemia is infection with hookworm.

An unfortunate case of this disease, which we saw a short time ago in our clinic, prompted us to carry out certain investigations whose results perhaps deserve the attention of the readers.

On 13 December last year (1865), we were called to the cloister of São Bento in this city to see a patient. He was a slave in the Inhatá sugar mill which is near the City of Santo Amaro, where he has lived for approximately one year; before that he used to live by the shore of the São Francisco River.

The patient was of the dark race, 30 years old, married, average height with a well-built and strong body. The skin was pale, but there was no notable emaciation; the face was swollen, mostly in the eyelids, and there was edema in the hands and feet. The skin was dry, and the body temperature was low, especially in the extremities. The patient was lying down, and his features expressed great anxiety since his respiration was exceedingly difficult, particularly when he made any movement. He could sit up for only a few minutes because he became dizzy when not in a supine position. The examination of the chest was negative except for some edema in the lower and posterior parts of the lungs.

He had no appetite, was thirsty, and had frequent nausea; the tongue, as well as all buccal mucosa and the palpebral conjunctiva, presented an extraordinary whiteness.

He was constipated; he had abdominal ascites and edema of the subcutaneous tissue of the abdomen. The urine was clear, with a strawlike color and almost without urine odor; the specific gravity was 1.007, and its temperature was 27.5° C. A systolic murmur could be heard over the precordium and a low continuous murmur over the jugular veins. The pulse was rapid and shallow. The liver and spleen were enlarged, but the abdomen did not present any tenderness. The patient stated that he had seizures in the past when he lived by the shore of the São Francisco River. He was never given to the use of alcohol, but his companions related that he had the habit of eating mud. In the beginning, he was healthy at the Inhatá sugar mill, but, a few months after his arrival and marriage, his present complaints began.

The drinking water at Inhatá comes from springs and is good. However, "fatigue" is frequent there among the slaves, whereas it is very rare on the shores of the São Francisco River. The nourishment of the slaves of the Order [slaves belonging to the Church—Eds.] is good, both at Inhatá sugar mill and on the shore of the São Francisco River, and it is unlikely that the nourishment of our patient became worse after his marriage. Thus, the anemia of this patient could not be attributed to poor nourishment, excessive work, or excessive use of alcoholic beverages.

His condition was grave, and no improvement could be expected with tonics, or with iron, which the patient had already used for some time (ferric wine with quinine). Besides, the effect of these treatments would be too slow for such a desperate case. We considered using the Gameleira milk (*Ficus doliaria Mart*) [Leche de huergon popular later for treatment of *Trichuris trichiura*—Eds.] whose excellent effects have been extolled, but it was not available to us. We know that drastic laxatives, like the cathartic tincture of LeRoy, and others, were frequently used in "fatigue" with success. Having heard that the Gameleira milk was a drastic laxative, we decided to substitute elaterium, and we prescribed two grains of this substance, divided into eight doses, to be given once every three hours. We left then, dissatisfied with this treatment. As soon as we had some time we tried to read about this disease which, during the more than 20 years that we have lived in this country, had appeared frequently to be unresponsive to various kinds of treatment.

The name "hypoemia," which was familiar to us because we had read some years ago the speech of Dr. Jobim in the *Revista-Medica Fluminense* of 1835, was the one which attracted our attention. It was mentioned in the *Journal Schmidts Iahrbücher*, Vol. 96, and in an article on geographic medicine by Dr. Hirsch which covered Dr. Griesinger's work on this disease. Dr. Griesinger was a physician at the Cairo Hospital from October 1851 until May 1852, and it was there that he performed special studies on intertropical hypoemia which is very frequent in Egypt. Dr. Griesinger worked very hard during that time trying to determine the cause of the disease. On the eve of his departure for Germany (17 April, 1852), while performing an autopsy on a patient who had died of hypoemia, he discovered in the duodenum, jejunum, and the first part of the ileum, in addition to hemorrhages in the mucosa, small ecchymoses similar to those produced by leeches; attached at these ecchymotic points were small white worms.

Examining them under the microscope, he recognized that these worms were of the species *Ancylostoma duodenale* which had been discovered first by Dubini in Milan in 1838. Back in Germany, Dr. Griesinger published the results of his observations on the entozoic diseases of Egypt, but it seemed that no one else continued the study of hypoemia as caused by *Ancylostoma*. Perhaps Dr. Hirsch contributed to this indifference because, having found no mention of the worms in the account of the autopsy described by Dr. Jobim, he advised caution in adopting that etiology.

Consulting Martius' booklet, *Systems materiae medicae vegetabilis brasiliensis*, we found that Gameleira was included among the anthelmintics, and this confirmed the parasitic origin of the disease with which we were dealing. We returned to the cloister the next day with the purpose of prescribing for our patient the milky juice of Gameleira; however, this was not possible because he had died at two o'clock in the morning after having several bowel movements. We insisted on performing an autopsy and were quite surprised when we found in the small intestines exactly what Dr. Griesinger had described.

Since the worms were very minute, it is not surprising that they went unnoticed for quite a time. We took some home, and upon examining them under the microscope, found that they corresponded to Copland's description of *A. duodenale* in his *Dictionary of Practical Medicine.* We were later convinced that there was no difference between our specimens and his description.

It seemed to us then that the continuous loss of blood caused by these worms, not only that which they needed for their sustenance, but also the amount lost after they finished their extraction, was enough to account for the anemia. By their presence and, even more, their continuous destruction of the mucosa, the worms had to be a constant source of irritation; this fact helped to explain other symptoms of the disease.

Now, however, it was necessary to verify the presence of *Ancylostoma* in cadavers of patients who had died of other diseases and to determine that their presence in cases of hypoemia was not merely a casual coincidence. With this aim, to date, we have performed autopsies on 12 cadavers of persons who died of other diseases; phthisis, organic heart disease, Bright's disease, cerebromalacia, injuries, and so on, without ever finding any *Ancylostoma.* . . .

We verified the presence of *Ancylostoma* in cadavers of five individuals all of whom had the symptoms of hypoemia in its more severe degree. In all of them, the anemia was of such a type that we could not account for its being produced by those circumstances which are classically blamed as causes of "fatigue." This was particularly true in our first patient, who did not present severe lesions in the hematopoietic organs and who did not live under very hygienic conditions. It seemed evident to us that the *Ancylostoma,* if not the sole cause of the anemia, had contributed greatly to its aggravation.

Indeed, although the presence of these worms in the intestine was always accompanied by anemia, it was still necessary to rule out the possibility of the anemia being caused by prior diseases and by so doing to determine whether it was an effect rather than a cause, or whether its presence was accidental.

Could it be that the *Ancylostomas,* so common in certain countries that they are almost always present in cadavers whether they died of hypoemia or some other disease, are, in this sense, similar to the *Ascaris* or *Trichocephalus?*

The answer is "No."

We opened 12 cadavers of individuals who had died of several other diseases and tried carefully to find the *Ancylostomas,* but we could not find them. Some of these cadavers were anemic and, owing to that, we inferred that the anemia per se, did not always necessarily bring about the presence of *Ancylostoma.*

There was no doubt that a large number of worms living off blood and actually causing numerous, small hemorrhages could produce within a certain time an excessive anemia like that found in cases of intertropical hypoemia. In the absence of other causes to which anemia might be traced, it seemed logical to conclude that the cause lay in the *Ancylostoma.*

Because they live on a more elaborate fluid, the blood, these worms must be much more harmful than those which subsist on gastric juice.

However, where do the *Ancylostoma* come from?

The spontaneous generation of the entozoa is not scientifically acknowledged today although some naturalists try to defend this hypothesis in order to explain the origin of creatures of a more simple organization, the infusoria or protozoa.

The entozoa germs are introduced into the animal from the outside. Thus, using the *Ascaris* and others as an example, we can prove that the incubation of their eggs or their procreation are dependent upon certain conditions and favorable circumstances which are present in many but not all individuals. These conditions are, in part, known to us, but many times one which seems to us very important is not known. The incidence of ascariasis in the inhabitants of Paris is lower than in those who live in the country; Davaine attributes this to the fact that the former use, almost exclusively, filtered drinking water which is devoid of the ova of those worms.

Nothing is known about the way in which the eggs or the embryos of *Ancylostoma* are introduced into the human body and under what conditions they exist outside it, but it is very probable that they were ingested either with solid food or drinking water. Judging from the frequency of "fatigue," the infestation should be even more common; however, the germs do not always form colonies. Colonization occurs only in individuals who are exposed to certain conditions, probably those mentioned hitherto as causing the disease.

The use of unsuitable food, of poor variety and excessively starchy, with the exclusion of certain stimulants and seasonings; slow digestion either because of excessive work or lack of exercise; the circumstances such as cold and humidity which generally deteriorate the functions of the body; and finally, carelessness about drinking water are conditions which facilitate the development of *Ancylostoma*.

Might there be a method of determining the presence of *Ancylostoma* and of distinguishing the anemia caused by them from malarial cachexia?

Thus far it has not been possible to find *Ancylostoma* in the feces of our patients even after we used strong anthelmintics. However, this diagostic tool, even if it were reliable, would not be used very frequently by our colleagues. We have reason to assume that the worms are present in those cases in which anemia is excessive and where the patients live under those conditions which favor the reproduction of the worms.

We have not collected enough facts to decide which of the two anthelmintics is more effective against the *Ancylostoma*. We can only state that patients seem to do better with the combined use of ferruginous preparations and anthelmintics than without them. . . .

Perhaps we may return to this important matter if new observations and studies . . . enable us to clarify some doubts left by the investigations which we have undertaken. Of particular importance is the fact that this disease which occurs with such frequency in Brazil does not respond to the usual therapeutic measures.

ON *ANCYLOSTOMA DUODENALE* (DUBINI)

Intorno all'anchilostoma duodenale (Dubini). Gazzetta Medica Italiana Lombardia, 38: 193–196, 1878. Translated from the Italian.

Giovanni Battista Grassi
(1854–1925)

A major contributor to the understanding of malaria, Grassi was also a student of the intestinal worms of man, particularly Ancylostoma duodenale. *He was born at Rovellasca in the Italian province of Como and studied medicine at the universities of Pavia and*

Catania. After further training in Heidelberg and Zurich, he was appointed to the post of professor of zoology and comparative anatomy at Catania and in 1895 was called to the chair of comparative anatomy at the University of Rome. He was the first to furnish experimental proof that only the Anopheles genus is a carrier of malaria. Grassi devoted the last years of his life primarily to malaria control in Italy.

Corrado Parona
(1848–1922)

Though a graduate in medicine from Pavia, he chose a career in natural science and zoology. Even before his graduation in medicine (1873) he was an assistant in the department of zoology and comparative anatomy. From 1875 to 1881 he was professor of natural history in the Technical Institute of Pavia. Eventually he became professor of zoology and comparative anatomy in Genoa, rising to rector in 1904.

Ernesto Parona
(1849–1902)

Ernesto Parona was a physician at the time of this publication.

The diagnosis of hookworm disease by stool examination was first reported in this article.

It is obvious as one studies this very interesting organism that much basic information, in both the zoological and clinical areas is still unknown. In fact, in Leuckart's erudite work regarding the history of its development, he mentions that mature *Ancylostoma* and segmenting ova are found in the small intestine of man. "Whatever then becomes of these ova," the author continues, "has not yet been observed. Neither do we know the way in which the parasite is introduced into man." Wucherer, in Brazil, has not probed the matter very deeply. He is reported to have seen *Ancylostoma* ova as well as the early stages of development taken from the duodenum of a cadaver. He is also reported to have observed that these stages correspond to those of *Dochmius trigonocephalus* (as Leuckart had already assumed); however, in his report on chlorosis in Brazil, he hints of these facts only briefly, almost in passing. He had also sought ova and larvae of *Ancylostoma* in stools, with no success.

The celebrated work of Heller states that the diagnosis should be etiologic: thus far no one has discovered either *Ancylostoma* or its ova in stools. Nothing further is found in the famous book by Cobbold, nor is anything instructive gained from the very recent work of Davaine. We note finally that all these classics lack an accurate description or even an accurate drawing of the ovum.

Today we are able to fill this gap partially; but for the present, we will restrict ourselves to publishing a general report on the conclusions of our investigation.

Embryologic Notes

(1) In the intestine (duodenum and jejunum) one consistently finds, with *Ancylostoma* in the mature state, ova in segmentation. All stages up to the morula are found, although ova in the first and second stages of segmentation are more abundant, and very often unsegmented ones are not found. However, one never finds either an embryo or a larva.

We have been able to verify all this in six cases; four of them were studied at Maggiore Hospital in Milan and two at the School of Pathological Anatomy in Pavia. In two cases in Milan we extended our investigations to include the stomach and found only ova in the process of segmentation, just as we had found in the intestine.

(2) The ova in segmentation (never at a stage beyond morula, as shown by observation) appear in recently evacuated feces. For over a month we found them there in great numbers in two individuals, but they were scarcely found in a third individual over a period of eight days. They are easily recognized as *Ancylostoma* eggs by their oval shape, very smooth surface, and thin, doubly outlined shell. At first, they may be confused with those of *Oxyuris*; however, differential diagnosis soon becomes obvious because *Oxyuris* ova although also oval, are proportionally longer than the *Ancylostoma* eggs and, in addition, are quite flat on one side. Finally, embryos are also found in recently evacuated feces.

Ascaris eggs undergoing segmentation, or as embryos, resemble *Ancylostoma* ova somewhat; however, segmentation still occurs in them a few weeks after they are evacuated, while the embryo will appear only after a few months. Prior to segmentation, they are completely different.

In vomitus (of an individual unknown to us) we encountered the same findings as in the stools of the above three cases.

(3) These ova will develop under suitable conditions; first, there is formation of an embryo similar to that of *D. trigonocephalus* and to those of many other nematodes; the embryo will lengthen and adapt itself to the ovum by doubling over; when it reaches approximately three times the maximum length of the ovum, it pierces its shell. A larva is thus born which in certain characteristics resembles that of *D. trigonocephalus* and, in others, is clearly differentiated from it. This larva will gradually increase in size, becoming quite long and undergoing at least two moults; that is, it will shed its skin at least twice. Soon afterward, it will change into another larva, in some characteristics still similar to that of *Dochmius,* which will then undergo another moult. However, as of today, we are unable to say what happens afterward.

Apparently, the embryo is already capable of locomotion and one can see it turn in various directions within its shell. The larvae make quite a number of different movements, principally in a spiral direction. Water will neither stop them nor slow them down; the action of glycerine, on the contrary, is fatal as early as a few minutes after exposure. The more developed the larva becomes, the more brisk the movements will be. Lukewarm water will enhance the movements while cold water and the chilled slide will slow them down; consequently, they are very sluggish on cold days. The so-called indifferent liquids are the suspensions which affect the appearance of the larvae very little (we usually used distilled water with 0.75 per cent sodium chloride). It is useful to know this if one wishes to study the anatomy of this organism. We would like to mention that the embryos do not go through the large head or tadpole stage.

It is possible to see from the very brief report presented above that the story of *Ancylostoma* development is very different from that of the other human helminths; on the other hand (as was expected), it resembles that of the similar *D. trigonocephalus.*

(4) Development takes place if pure feces is placed in a covered container, to which is added albumin, mixed with dirt or diluted with water. We have achieved the best results by preserving feces in a well-stoppered container.

(5) Temperature greatly influences the rate of development; when the vessel is kept in a vest pocket, embryos will appear in the eggs as early

as eight hours after the feces have been evacuated and, after only two days, will have deserted the eggshell. On the contrary, in a barely lukewarm environment, the same embryo formation will be delayed three or four days. As we mentioned, 15 days are required for the development of the larvae to the advanced stage.

(6) It is remarkable that, even after 15 days of culture, along with second-stage worms, ova with embryos or in segmentation can still be found, all of normal appearance.

(7) At the onset of the second stage, especially when the larva seems to be moulting and is moving actively in the microscopic field, its organs are not distinct, bringing to mind *Filaria sanguinis hominis*. Whether filaria is not, per chance, an *Ancylostoma* larva should be investigated.

Our thinking is supported primarily by the following facts: (a) filaria is an embryo and the mature organism is not known (Leuckart); (b) filaria is found in Brazil and Egypt where *Ancylostoma* is very frequently encountered; this *Ancylostoma* infestation causes a type of anemia called "intertropical" in Egypt and Brazil where hematuria also occurs; (c) in the duodenum and jejunum of individuals who died from intertropical anemia, bloody mucus and blood clots were found; a lentil-size ecchymosis was found on the mucosa. Bilharz has found in the intestine, particularly in the submucosal connective tissue, small cavities filled with blood and inside them at times a male, at other times a female *Ancylostoma*. It is not impossible for the larvae to pierce the vessels injured by mature *Ancylostoma* and to enter the circulation. This would seem to take place, by chance, only in exceptional cases. Other helminths, also in unusual cases, will make extraordinary migrations, as have been described many times.

(8) We shall not fail to mention that one of us (Grassi) swallowed a large pill loaded with *Ancylostoma* eggs undergoing segmentation. Forty-five days have already gone by and no symptoms attributable to the presence of this parasite have appeared and no eggs have been found in his feces. Another individual (who wishes to remain anonymous) has also swallowed recently some feces loaded with *Ancylostoma* larvae.

We fed a dog a large quantity of feces full of eggs undergoing segmentation for a few days; he ate them avidly. However, the following day, he eliminated many of the eggs unchanged or nearly unchanged, despite the fact that they were in the segmenting stage.

Clinical Notes

In our previous report, we had established the following facts:

(1) The diagnosis of *Ancylostoma* is very easy. To do this rapidly, it suffices to examine a little feces or vomit, diluted with any medium, at the microscopic magnification of at least 90 diameters. If the material is fresh, only *Ancylostoma* ova undergoing segmentation will be found; if it is stale, embryos and larvae will also be found.

(2) In spite of our painstaking efforts, we have never encountered, either in feces or in vomitus, *Ancylostoma* in the mature or larval state; we were also unable to find them in blood, either pure or contaminated, or in any other unusual matter.

(3) Although we examined the feces and vomitus from many persons varying in age, social condition, state of health, and so on, we found *Ancylostoma* eggs in only three cases.

Since these three were patients at the medical clinic of our university, the diagnosis was made by our esteemed teacher, Professor Orsi, who kindly authorized us to divulge to the public everything connected with this subject.

The first case (anemia) concerned a young lady of 22, a farm woman, in whom the other etiologic factors could not account for the very severe anemia; the second case (malarial cachexia, widespread atheroma) involved an alcoholic adult, a baker; in the third case (fecal impaction) the patient was old, atheromatous, and debilitated. In the latter case, the eggs were less abundant than in the two previous ones.

Since the publication of the previous report was delayed by circumstances beyond our control, we are now able to add further interesting statements on this subject.

A. By examining the feces of a considerable number of individuals, either healthy or afflicted with very different diseases, we were able to find *Ancylostoma* eggs in the following instances:

The first case was that of a 33-year-old farmer in the medical clinic, who presented a diagnosis of mitral insufficiency and early mitral stenosis. The patient, whose constitution originally had been strong, appeared to be more cachectic than his heart affliction alone would cause him to be. He had an abundance of *Ancylostoma* ova.

The second case concerned a steward, 40 years of age, a patient in the same clinic. Although not very debilitated, he was afflicted with colitis. He showed rare *Ancylostoma* ova in the frequent and abundant bowel movements.

The third patient was a 53-year-old laborer who had suffered repeated and resistant attacks of fever due to malaria and was admitted to our hospital with a right-sided pneumonia. He showed all the symptoms of a severe anemia and of unresolved pneumonia. (Some *Ancylostoma* eggs were found.)

The fourth case was a fruit peddler, age 22, admitted to the hospital for general weakness and stomach upsets. He had a slight splenic enlargement accompanied by severe anemia. He showed an extraordinary number of *Ancylostoma* eggs.

The fifth case concerned an eight-year-old girl, admitted to our clinic because of malarial cachexia. Examination revealed some *Ancylostoma* ova.

The sixth case was that of a 30-year-old woman, admitted to the hospital for an atypical intermittent fever which had begun two months earlier. The patient presented severe anemia and edema of the lower limbs with moderate ascites. Abundant *Ancylostoma* ova were seen.

B. With the exception of the second patient, none of the above patients had previous or present intestinal complaints; however, all of them, except the second, were constipated.

C. With repeated examination of the feces containing *Ancylostoma* eggs we were able to find fairly large nuclei which, because of the deeper brown color, stood out from the remaining fecal matter; in these, with the proper procedure, we were able to obtain the color characteristic of Heller's test for hematin.

D. In order to eliminate the *Ancylostoma,* an anthelmintic composed of santonin, calomel, jalap, and powered sugar was administered to the young lady in whom Professor Orsi had diagnosed anemia. A subsequent bowel movement weighing approximately 100 grams was loaded with eggs. In five grams, taken at random from the bulk, we counted 22 completely developed *Ancylostoma* uniformly scattered in the feces. Therefore, proportionately, it can be estimated that the patient eliminated 440 *Ancylostoma*. In

spite of the repeated administration of the anthelmintic, the feces on subsequent days still contained eggs although they were scarce; there were no fully developed *Ancylostoma*.

E. We also administered the aforementioned powder to the patient of the first case, and this resulted in the quick elimination of 15 *Ancylostoma* in a single bowel movement. During the following days, despite continued anthelmintic treatment, no additional parasites were expelled. However, the feces still abounded with eggs which, as usual, were undergoing segmentation.

We would not have understood why additional *Ancylostoma* were not excreted if we had not recalled that, during autopsies, some *Dochmius* and *Ancylostoma* were adherent to the intestine, and in part, others were free. Therefore, we assumed that the anthelmintic was effective against the free *Ancylostoma* and ineffective against those adherent to the intestine.

F. In very fresh feces from the third, fourth, and sixth cases, we found, together with many eggs in segmentation, larvae very similar to those of *Ancylostoma* in the first stage of development, except for the additional presence of rudimentary genital organs. In the feces of a 35-year-old beggar, also admitted to our hospital, who was convalescing from pneumonia and suffering with cachectic ecthyma, we found only the larvae mentioned above. It seems to us that they belong to *Ancylostoma*. This is inferred since neither larva such as these (according to Leuckart) nor the *Ancylostoma* exist in Germany.

The facts mentioned above, albeit inadequate to warrant practical deductions, seem to us not without significance, particularly since they concern cases of severe anemias, the etiology of which we found to be either obscure or uncertain. They are also significant because the anemia occurs with fair frequency, at least in our territory, and because the hope for effective medication is not unreasonable.

NOTES ON THE HELMINTHOLOGY OF EGYPT, I. THE LIFE HISTORY OF THE *ANCYLOSTOMA DUODENALE* (DUB.)

Notizen zur helminthologie Egyptens, I. Die lebensgeschichte des anchylostomum duodenale (Dub.). Centralblatt für Bakteriologie und Parasitenkunde, 20: 865–870, 1896. Translated from the German.

Arthur Looss
(1861–1923)

After preliminary education in the schools of his native Chemnitz, a city of Saxony, Looss went to the University of Leipzig, where he studied science from 1880 to 1884 under Leuckart. He received his degree in 1885 with a dissertation on the trematodes. In 1889, Looss joined the faculty at Leipzig, becoming professor in 1896.

In 1893 he went to Egypt to pursue research in the field of helminthology, and he returned to that country for further studies three years later. He was finally appointed professor of biology and parasitology at the University of Cairo, a chair especially created for him. During the 18 years of his tenure in that position, he did his most important research in tropical medicine.

At the outbreak of World War I, Looss was forced to flee Cairo within 24 hours, leaving his papers and his library behind. After serving in the war, he took an assistantship in the Zoological Institute at Giesse and in 1922 was made honorary professor at that institution, which had given him an honorary M.D. the previous year.

Looss elucidated the hookworm's entire life cycle and mode of transmission in an extensive series of papers, monographs, and books. From his works the editors have selected five separate segments which convey his thinking and substance of research.

At the end of September of this year [1896] a patient from the village of Saft-el-Melouk was admitted to the Government Hospital [Alexandria]. He was suffering from severe anemia, and in his feces numerous *Ancylostoma* eggs were demonstrated on the first examination. The case gave me a welcome opportunity to look more closely at this parasite which is so important to the general welfare of the Egyptian population, especially since, apart from Leuckart's investigations on the development of *Ancylostoma trigonocephalum*, we know very little about the life history of *Ancylostoma*. This lack of knowledge, however, refers only to the first stages of the worm's development which take place externally. From all the available literature and so far as I can recall, intermediate and transitional forms between larvae and mature parasites have never been found in man, in spite of much searching. I have succeeded in growing the latter artificially. Before I get to their description, however, a few words are necessary about the fate of free living larvae which have not yet been adequately clarified in spite of repeated investigations by

Perroncito, Parona, Grassi, Lutz, Leichtenstern, and others. Unfortunately, the pertinent literature is not available to me.

Eggs and Young Larvae

For the study of the processes of embryonic development in more detail, the egg of *A. duodenale* is a poor subject. Although its shell is thin and transparent, the ovum is small and its yolk is turbid and granular; its most unpleasant property, however, is that when fresh it is exceedingly difficult to alter its position by moving the cover glass, which is absolutely necessary if one wishes to get an accurate picture of the origin and positioning of the cells in the embryo. Since I was not interested in studying the finer processes of segmentation, I merely studied the first phases and convinced myself thereby that their development in principle is the same as that recently described by Strassen for *Ascaris megalocephala*. But when the number of segmented cells reached 16, it was hardly possible to keep the individual elements apart; later the embryo became smaller and more opaque. The forms which it assumes in this process are already extensively illustrated in the literature.

The development of the eggs is influenced by several factors. As older authors have already emphasized, the most favorable medium is actually formed feces, and the more solid, the better. In liquid stools development is not only retarded, but a large number of the eggs die. Of great influence, furthermore, is the chemical composition and reaction of the feces. I noted several times that in very liquid stools (as produced by administration of laxatives) as well as in strongly smelling ones, a large percentage of the embryos die. The results can be modified, if one mixes approximately equal quantities of feces and animal charcoal into a mush. Not only does the bad odor almost completely disappear, but all of the eggs grow rather rapidly. In contrast, the addition of water to the feces hinders the development of the eggs. In general, addition of a little water merely slows it down, but increasing quantities cause an increasing number of eggs to die before development is completed. A few, however, emerge even in almost pure water, provided that they are not submerged too deeply. The developing eggs need plenty of air. In a given portion of the feces the eggs lying at the periphery develop first. The ones lying in deeper layers develop more slowly; even after two weeks, if one removes the inner portion of the formed feces with care, one will find eggs in the four- and six-cell stage which evidently have not yet lost their capacity for development. This also applies to eggs in watery surroundings. If there is only a thin layer of water above them, the development takes place slowly, but if the water is deeper the eggs die quickly. This is true at least with water standing in vessels, as used in our laboratories. Finally, temperature greatly influences the development of eggs. In the Alexandrian summer the temperature is generally about 27° C both day and night. Under these conditions the peripheral layer of the feces is covered with emerged and emerging embryos 24 hours after its elimination. The effect of cooler nights (21–22° C), which are now beginning, so inhibits their development that the first embryos appear only after 36 to 40 hours. A temperature of 1° C acting for 24 to 48 hours kills the eggs without exception.

Under favorable conditions these embryos grow rather quickly to larvae. In this process they absorb very fine, solid particles in their intestine whose lumen, confined by a thin cuticle, then appears plainly as a 0.005 mm-wide cavity. The latter is even more apparent if one keeps the young worms in water or very dilute feces because the colorless intestinal content then contrasts with the granular intestinal wall. The absorbed food material is then deposited in the form of small, fatlike globules in the intestinal cells. The more solid the feces in which the larvae live, the more granular and opaque the intestine itself appears. In the beginning the increase in size of the body results from growth in both length and width; after approximately four to five days (at 27° C median temperature) the organisms are 0.48 mm long and 0.03 mm wide, rather plump and indolent worms whose inner morphology shows no changes from the earlier stage. However, during this time (about the second or third day) the outer membrane has been renewed and the animals have shed their skin. This evidently takes place quickly, and it is not often possible to observe the specimens during this process; it is most likely to be seen in cultures which are kept cool and develop more slowly. The process of

shedding is not remarkable and, as stated, leads to no change in the appearance of the parasites.

From the fifth day on, external changes again become noticeable, but these are slow and more obvious and are preliminary to a second shedding of the skin. The body membrane is seen to consist of two layers, the outer one of which begins to detach itself more and more from the rest of the body until it finally loses connection with it completely and covers it all around with an exceptionally thin and delicate chitinous coat.

Simultaneously the inner body begins to show changes. At the head end three indistinct small lips appear under the old skin, each of which evidently supports two very fine and delicate papillae. The cylindrical buccal cavity which was previously so clearly evident and provided with strong refractile walls, as well as the chitinous teeth in the esophageal bulb, disappear. The esophagus itself becomes more elongated and thinner; the three segments previously so clearly evident fade considerably but not completely, so that one can still recognize on the esophagus, even after shedding, a somewhat thickened upper part and, connected with this by means of a slender tube, a slim, cylindrical bulb. The rest of the inner organs show no recognizable changes. The tail is a little bit shorter and more rounded than before, and the anus lies about 0.06 mm in front of the new tail end.

While the outer skin gradually separates from the body, the latter becomes more slender; at the same time it seems to contract a little in length so that the old skin extends to a degree over head and tail. Moreover, the mobility of the worms now increases noticeably; they no longer move around lazily but rather are more lively within the surrounding medium; yet the body, as far as I have observed, never takes on more than a simple S-form. In the process the old outer skin forms the already described, regular folds on the curved sides.

On reaching this stage the external development of the young *Ancylostoma* is completed; the organisms are ripe for transfer. In the great majority of cases they do not cast off the outer chitinous skin, even if they are kept in water for a longer period of time; then, of course, they are deprived of the possibility of further intake of food from the outside. But along with them one always finds a varying number which have lost their chitin coat; and in these cases also further intake of food from the outside does not take place. In contrast to previous stages the organisms do not grow any further. From this it follows that the larvae of the *A. duodenale* undergo only one and, in exceptional cases, two sheddings during their external life cycle. Therefore, in this respect they are analogous to *A. trigonocephalum,* according to Leuckart's observations. It is also clear that the process last discussed, and designated by several older authors as "encystment," is nothing more than an ordinary shedding process, except that it does not necessarily at first lead to the casting off of the old coat.

In relation to their living conditions these mature larvae differ remarkably from the young ones. As already mentioned, solid feces are by far the most favorable medium for the latter, while water is detrimental or practically fatal for them. The mature "encysted" larvae not only are able to live in pure water but actually seem to prefer it. They keep themselves afloat in it for some time by means of their active, sinuous movements; gradually, however, they sink to the bottom and there, after some time, assume a rigid state which in turn leads to death. Thus far, I have not succeeded in keeping the parasites alive in water longer than 10-20 days. Within the unaltered feces, at the temperature prevailing here at the present time, however, death occurs more quickly. In this respect, my experiments are not yet concluded. I must emphasize that, as has been stated by older authors, neither eggs nor larvae of *A. duodenale* can stand complete desiccation. They remain alive, however, when the liquid present in their environment (mud or clay) is reduced to a minimum; but if this environment dries out completely, then the parasites perish without exception. To be sure, if they are moistened again after desiccation, movements seem to reappear; but not infrequently, these are only due to currents in the liquid resulting from the water's penetrating the desiccated worm. A short time later the latter disintegrates into those strongly shining granules and flakes which older authors considered to be a "calcification of the cyst," but which in reality represents the remains of the dead parasites.

From this report the following facts emerge as to the life history of *A. duodenale*. The eggs deposited with the feces of the host find the most favorable conditions for their development if the feces do not come in direct contact with water, that is, if they are excreted on dry ground accessible to air, and if water approaches them gradually and in very small quantities. Thus the larvae may be transported; they keep themselves afloat for a time but gradually sink to the bottom without immediately losing their vitality. The latter occurs only after some time elapses, if the environment remains moist, but immediately if it dries out completely. The larvae are transported only in running water or in moist, solid substances and never by means of dust or dry air. The reintroduction into the final host occurs through embryo-containing water or mud, as long as this is moist. . . .

NOTES ON THE HELMINTHOLOGY OF EGYPT, II. THE TRANSMISSION OF THE LARVAE (*Ancylostoma duodenale*)

Notizen zur helminthologie Egyptens, II, Die uebertragung der larven (*anchylostomum duodenale*), Centralblatt für Bakteriologie und Parasitenkunde, 21: 913–917, 1897. Translated from the German.

Arthur Looss
(1861–1923)

In this report, Looss records the negative experiments of oral feeding of Ancylostoma *larvae and the sexual forms of the free-living state.*

In order to transfer the mature larvae into an experimental animal it was necessary first to separate them as much as possible from their present environment. As already mentioned in the first report, a mixture of the egg-containing feces with approximately the same volume of animal charcoal has the advantage of bringing a considerable percentage of larvae to development and maturity, especially when the more or less thick and viscid mass is stirred occasionally, exposing the more deeply lying eggs. In order to isolate the mature larvae from this mass, the following process, after many futile attempts, has proved most successful. After the larvae have attained full maturity, one dries the feces-charcoal mass (I used the Petri dishes customary among bacteriologists for culture) in open air until a thin but solid crust forms. Then one fills the dish up to rim with pure water and lets this stand undisturbed for 10 to 20 minutes. If one then pours it into another vessel by a slight movement of the dish, examination with the magnifying glass shows, in addition to very fine particles of feces, countless *Ancylostoma* larvae which move sinuously in a lively way; these larvae had migrated from the solid mass into the water above them. The same process can be repeated with the same result six, seven, and eight times after the nutrient substratum has dried again and has formed its solid crust, as long as living and strong larvae are still present. A culture prepared in this way still provides, after two months and with every addition of water, numerous viable larvae. It is possible to obtain in this way, if not all, at least the greatest part of the larvae present.

The larvae which initially float in the water gradually sink to the bottom where, after 24 hours, all of them gather; with them, however, there is also the majority of the small particles which have been absorbed by the water from the feces. For further purification, I poured off the muddy water and replaced it with fresh, filtered water; however, even after five or more washings the larvae could not be entirely separated from the adhering stool particles.

The results of experiments with larvae which were prepared in this way were very dramatic, but unfavorable. Immediately following or not more than three to five minutes after the administration of only one or two cc of the liquid in milk or water, or with bread and fruit, all experimental animals retched severely and in the vast majority of cases the stomach was completely emptied, thus rendering the whole experiment negative.

It seemed obvious to search for the explanation of this phenomenon in the unremoved and transferred fine fecal particles which could possibly have caused a nauseating or toxic action in the animals; therefore, it meant removing these particles if possible. This was successfully accomplished in the following way. If the larva and foreign-body-containing liquid is filtered through ordinary, preferably somewhat solid filter paper, initially a liquid, somewhat muddy in the beginning but later entirely clear, flows through first; gradually, however, a few larvae which had bored actively through the paper, make their ap-

pearance in the filtrate. The number of these larvae which have passed through becomes greater in time and gets to be enormous if one lets the filter stand for some time (for instance overnight) after all the water has run off, and it is protected from drying out only by covering. If one now pours on fresh clear water, countless larvae which during the night have bored through the paper run off with it and are washed away. If one lets this stand again for a few hours, the process can be repeated until all larvae, that is, the ones that are still alive, have passed through. By gradual settling on the bottom, decanting, and adding fresh filtered water one can then continue the cleaning process until all chemical components of the feces have been removed and the larvae are contained in pure water without admixture of foreign material.

Strangely enough, even with the use of this cleaned infective material, symptoms were observed which were very similar to those described above. However, real vomiting did not occur as frequently; in most cases retching occurred and the animals were obviously sick, always immediately after feeding. Very often sudden attacks of diarrhea developed. These observations leave little else to do but to look for the cause for the above-mentioned symptoms in the parasites themselves and to assume that in some way these parasites irritate the host organism, especially when they are present in great numbers. First, there is the possibility that the young worms by their active movements work mechanically on the mucosa of the stomach to cause nausea. But then this should decrease as the amount of food with which a certain number of larvae are absorbed increases since the larvae contained therein are more dispersed, and not all can come in contact with the mucosa. I did not notice the slightest difference in the result, whether the larvae were administered in very little milk or in as much milk as the dog's stomach was able to hold. Another possible explanation of the dramatic vomiting is that the young *Ancylostoma* larvae themselves or the liquid in which they are contained is toxic to the experimental animals. That the liquid is not toxic is proved by repeated experiments. Many larvae were kept six or more days in a little water; this was then poured off carefully, mixed with milk and given to the dogs; there was never the trace of a reaction. Therefore, nothing remains but to ascribe to the parasites themselves a toxic influence on the host organism. The observations which we frequently make on patients suffering from ancylostomiasis lead to very similar conclusions. In some cases of severe anemia, in spite of repeated treatments, not more than a dozen worms can be eliminated or are found in the intestine after death. It is difficult to understand that the loss of blood alone and the damage to the intestinal wall which the parasites inflict upon their host are sufficient to cause such a serious disease. It is certainly quite significant from the outset whether the patient in question has a strong constitution or a sickly, weak one which can only offer slight resistance to the harmful effects of the parasite. Even after taking this into account, there remains in many cases an obvious disparity between the number of worms and the disease caused by them, a disproportion which points to the possibility that a previously not sufficiently observed factor may be contributing to the development of the *Ancylostoma* anemia. I do not consider it at all improbable (in fact it is probably certain) that the *Ancylostoma*, in addition to extracting blood and damaging the intestinal wall, exert a toxic action on their host, further, the assumption is obvious that the secretion of the large head glands, whose opening at the edge of the mouth, plays a role. Assuming that the worms have such a toxic action, some explanation is needed for the observation that *Ancylostoma* anemias are cured slowly and with difficulty, even when the parasites are eliminated completely and no new infection is possible. I expect to return to this question in the near future. [The need for iron obviously was not appreciated—Eds.].

Initially, I used monkeys as experimental animals, but since these are rather costly, I soon looked around for a possible substitute. The first experiment with young dogs, just weaned from their mother, succeeded immediately; from then on, I used mainly dogs as experimental animals. Young cats, too, are able to harbor the parasites for a time; whether this holds true for guinea pigs and rabbits is still uncertain; results with gray rats were negative in all cases. Experiments with young foxes were hopeless from the start because all of those which I received proved to be infected with an *Ancylostoma* which in the mature stage differs very little, albeit characteristically, from

that of man; in contrast, early forms of the fox *Ancylostoma* are absolutely indistinguishable from those of *Ancylostoma duodenale*.

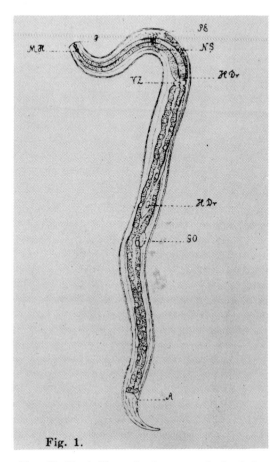

Fig. 1.

Plate 45. Fig. 1. Young *Ancylostoma* on the fourth day after transmission. P: papillae of the head; MH: buccal cavity; PE: excretory pore; NS: nervous system; H Dr: neck glands; VZ: closing cells of the esophagus against the intestine; GO: genital organs; A: anus.

Even if the *A. duodenale* possesses a rather remarkable ability to adapt to hosts other than the normal carrier, this adaptability is not unlimited. The infection of dogs and cats, for example, is accomplished with some expectation of success only in very young animals which have just been weaned. But even here a considerable percentage of young parasites still passes through the intestine without settling in it. This latter behavior becomes increasingly the rule as the experimental animals get older, and after perhaps three months it is hardly possible to cause one or the other larva to remain. In experimental animals something very similar occurs during the growth of the parasites transmitted in the first experiments. They are gradually eliminated from the intestine without reaching their complete development, and while still many specimens of the last transmitted worms are encountered, the older ones become more and more infrequent. In fact, I have not succeeded at all in having the parasites produce mature eggs in the dog. The largest worms that I

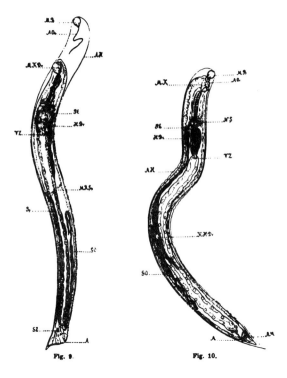

Fig. 9.   **Fig. 10.**

Plate 46. Fig. 9. Male before last shedding, 14–15 days old. The animal body has separated completely from the old skin (AH) and contracted slightly. MB: mouth cup; AOe: old esophagus lining, attached to mouth cup; Sp: spiculum; MRSp: retractor muscles of the spiculum showing an almost diagonal course here; GZ: large ganglion cell complex leading from the nerves to the ribs of the bursa. *Fig. 10.* Female at the same stage and of the same age. The animal has not contracted, and filled out the old skin almost completely. The old esophagus lining is also already loosened and folded together. KHDr: nucleus of the large neck glands; AM: muscles of the anus.

have obtained thus far measured around 8 mm, but they were normally formed. On the basis of these observations it seems a little doubtful whether Rathonyi who found work horses used in the mines of Brennberg near Oedenburg in Hungary massively infected with *Ancylostoma* actually had encountered the *Ancylostoma* of man. In any case, strict proof of the identity of both forms has not been offered. But since the personnel of the mines suffered from ancylostomiasis to an extraordinarily high degree, the horses in the mines could easily have been infected. On the other hand, a certain probability exists that the horses were infected with *A. duodenale*. Even in this case, however, Rathonyi's observations would only show the result, interesting though it may be, that under certain conditions *A. duodenale* affects the horse and can reach complete maturity. The horse in any case is not a necessary part of the life cycle of the parasite, as Rathonyi presumably points out.

[We have omitted the balance of the article in which Looss describes the male and female hookworm, see Plates 45 and 46—Eds.]

CONTRIBUTION TO THE LIFE CYCLE OF THE HOOKWORM
(A Reply to Professor Dr. Leichtenstern)

Zur lebensgeschichte des Ankylostoma duodenale. Centralblatt für Bakteriologie, 24: 441–449, 483–488, 1898. Translated from the German.

Arthur Looss
(1861–1923)

During a three-month vacation in Europe, I found here in Leipzig an article by Professor Dr. Leichtenstern on *Ancylostoma duodenale,* an article in which the author bitterly complains about "the curious ignorance of the literature" which I showed in my article about the life cycle of the hookworm. His accusations culminate in the statement: "One could almost assume" that it was "less a matter of ignorance than an intentional disregard of the same" (the literature). I will not concern myself further with the latter remark, but will excuse it with Professor Leichtenstern's state of irritation; however, regarding the other accusations of ignorance, that is, gross neglect of prior studies on *Ancylostoma* and its life cycle, I must offer a few words of explanation or defense. . . .

I wrote this report, as is seen at its beginning and its end, in Cairo. As rich as Egypt is in material for empirical research in the broad field of natural science, it is commensurately poor in all scientific aids to which the worker in Germany is accustomed and which are available to him elsewhere without any difficulty. Thus, at this time, there is no great medical-scientific library in Cairo such as there are in all universities and in many larger cities and institutes in Europe. True, the Anglo-Egyptian government has made laudable efforts to create one, but this requires time and considerable funds. As things stand now, any individual has difficulty procuring anything on his own, but it is even more difficult for the helminthologist who not only must keep in touch with the zoological but also with the extensive medical literature.

Thus, under the present circumstances, there are only two ways open to the research scientist who has to work in Egypt: either he works only by himself and for his own pleasure, keeping everything he observes and discovers buried in his bosom; or he makes his observations available to those who are interested, publishing regardless whether the form is perfect (as is rightfully expected in the centers of scientific life) or not. I chose the latter. It is my intention to contribute to the improvement of our knowledge as far as I am able, and it is my conviction that the merits of prior authors will prevail in any scientific question, regardless of whether they are or are not cited in every later work. . . .

When I was writing my report, I was not in any position to say that we had progressed splendidly in the knowledge of the life cycle of the *Ancylostoma*. Even after the publication of my report, I was still of the opinion that not everything had been clarified by it that required clarification. Time has not only confirmed my conviction but has also shown that I was right much more than I had anticipated. In further studies I became acquainted with other facts which I should like to consider as being of importance; whether they are significant in reality is up to Professor Leichtenstern to decide. Although the facts of which I am going to speak are established, the investigation of their significance has not terminated. I would not have proceeded with their publication if

Leichtenstern's attacks—which picture my observations as nothing more than warmed-over facts, accompanied possibly by an intentional denial of the merits of earlier *Ancylostoma* researchers—had not challenged me to prove that I could not only warm over well-known material but that, in spite of my brief eight-month experience and my scarcer material, I had advanced further than my predecessor with his many years of experience and his hundreds of cultures.

First, it has been found that the young *Ancylostoma* larvae immediately after their arrival in an animal display a strong impulse toward migration. In order to study more carefully the very first change of the worms after their transfer, I tried to introduce them into rats, guinea pigs, and other animals, some with food, some with drink, and some directly by dropping larvae-containing water into their mouths with a pipette. In all these cases the larvae did not settle in the intestine, but passed unchanged per anum. However, after careful examination of the experimental animals 24–48 hours following the infection, I found very lively and active larvae in the esophagus and in the larynx; that is, parts of their bodies were moving not on but in the upper layer of the mucosa. Even two weeks after feeding I found in one guinea pig (in the trachea but no longer in the esophagus) a number of living larvae which had grown, little but quite distinctly. Repetitions of the experiment always led to the same result; however, what becomes of these larvae I cannot say at this time, since I had to terminate the experiment. This fact of the migration of the young *Ancylostoma* larvae and their (partial) penetration into the mucosa is evidently related to their aforementioned behavior with respect to the filter paper. ITS SIGNIFICANCE BECAME CLEAR TO ME ONLY WHEN I DISCOVERED THAT THE MOUTH IS NOT THE ONLY WAY IN WHICH THE *ANCYLOSTOMA* LARVAE CAN ENTER THE HUMAN BODY. THEY ARE ALSO ABLE TO BORE THROUGH THE SKIN!

The experimental subject on whom I made the latter observation was myself. I must, however, go back to explain this. In association with my tests on *Ancylostoma* I made some with *Rhabdonema strongyloides (Anguillula intestinalis)*. Because I had no other subject I tried to infect myself with the filiform larvae; and, an examination of the feces after an appropriate period produced the highly surprising (to me) finding of the presence, not of rhabditites, but of significantly numerous *Ancylostoma* eggs! Up to this point I had had no idea that I was suffering from ancylostomiasis; although for weeks I had often felt rather exhausted and indisposed, I had nevertheless blamed this on the unusual heat of the Egyptian summer. A laboratory infection was not considered.

But how could the infection have occurred? True, considering *Ancylostoma* larvae harmless, I had had no misgivings about allowing the larvae-containing water to get on my hands as I filtrated them, particularly since the larvae were pure. However, the contaminated hands were carefully kept away from the mouth and were always thoroughly washed with soap and then disinfected with sublimate solution or 90 per cent alcohol before meals. However, an outside infection could have occurred: on the occasion of a hunting excursion into the interior, we were surprised by a *chamsin*, the hot desert wind; the mineral water taken along was quickly exhausted, and finally we had no alternative but to use the water of the Nile and of various canals in order to quench our burning thirst. An infection with *Ancylostoma* larvae could have taken place at this time, but as conditions on the whole were good, this was highly improbable. In Egypt, insofar as I know, distinct *Ancylostoma* foci do not exist, but also on the contrary, considering the general distribution of the worm among the country population, a uniform distribution of its embryos on the ground must be assumed. A severe infection from a single exposure was highly improbable; moreover, the lingering course of my sickness did not favor this particular assumption. As I see now, and as Leichtenstern already has pointed out, simultaneous massive absorption of *Ancylostoma* larvae leads to a very acute onset of anemia with violent symptoms. . . .

In my own case, it was thus practically out of the question that my illness, with its very slow course, was due to a single severe infection. The matter remained inexplicable to me until I had another experience. During one of the abovementioned tests with guinea pigs, a drop of water with high larva content fell on my hand one day and rolled off. I paid no attention to this moist spot which dried by itself after a few minutes. But at the same time I felt there an intense burn-

ing very similar to that produced by the touch of a *Pelagia noctiluca*, and the spot became extremely red. What was the meaning of this? The cause could only be the *Ancylostoma* larvae. A test with water alone had no success. Then, after the larvae had again settled on the bottom of the vessel in which I kept them in pure water, a drop of the larval sediment was sucked up by a pipette, applied to the back of the hand which had been cleaned previously, and were spread out lightly with the shaft of the scalpel. Even before the liquid had entirely dried up, the reddening of the skin and the burning sensation started exactly as before. I then scraped off the last moisture residue from the epidermis with the edge of a scalpel and put it under the microscope. The *Ancylostoma* larvae previously present in such abundance had disappeared except for a very few indolent ones; in their place among the scraped-off epidermal cells were found numerous empty worm skins! The larvae themselves could only have penetrated the skin. Immediate pricks with a disinfected needle into the formerly moist spot on the skin failed to indicate the whereabouts of the larvae; none could be detected in the blood which oozed out. A few minutes later no blood at all flowed from newly made punctures nor was it possible to squeeze out any blood by pressure. In areas away from the moistened place, blood escaped normally after pricking. Furthermore, the pricks in the infected area swelled almost immediately, like pustules, and the entire spot started to swell. The next day the hand was swollen so much that I thought it best to ask for medical help. After a three-day treatment with lead (Goulard) water applications the swelling subsided, but the pustules disappeared only after two weeks.

After what has been described, it can hardly be doubted that the *Ancylostoma* larvae had thus penetrated the skin. But what became of them within the body? One thing was clear immediately: if they had found their way into the intestine in any way, then my own ancylostomiasis was really understandable. As scrupulous as I had been about keeping the larvae away from my mouth, I had been careless about protecting my skin and especially my hands. If they found their way into the intestine, then a remarkably successful result of this experiment will be forthcoming in this field of research.

Naturally, immediately after I had established

the presence of *Ancylostoma* as the cause of my continuing indisposition, I undertook two expulsive cures within a week. The conditions did not permit me to examine the stool more accurately. However, an examination of the stools undertaken about four weeks after the last cure showed a significant reduction in the number of eggs. Besides, my general state of health had improved so much that I no longer felt any discomfort. About this time, an infection of my hand occurred. Soon after this, because of other investigations, I abandoned the experiments with *Ancylostoma* and from that time on I have had nothing more to do with living materials of this worm. As carefully as I watched my condition following the accident with my hand, I could not detect any sudden appearance of disease symptoms; my general state of health remained passible so that after about one month my vigilance declined. Only two to three months later a feeling of tiredness and depression recurred occasionally. An examination of the stools showed a very considerable number of *Ancylostoma* eggs. Expulsion cures repeated three times since then, supplemented by considerable doses of thymol (6 grams per day), have to this day not freed me entirely of the parasite. I wish to add that during the entire course of my illness a pronounced anemia did not appear.

This is the extent of my experiences; first the positive fact stands out that the *Ancylostoma* larvae are capable of penetrating the human body through the skin. Furthermore, although it is not yet certain, there is a great probability that the larvae absorbed in this way reach the intestine in a manner which at present is still unknown. There they grow to sexual maturity just as do those introduced directly per os. In this manner they must at least once bore through the intestinal wall. Presumably the darkness which has been shrouding the investigation of the submucously encysted worms described by Bilharz and Griesinger will now be dispelled. Highly interesting—and for me, almost positive proof that these "encysted" organisms in the mucosa are those which have penetrated the skin—is a case reported by Grassi. It is not a question here, according to my interpretation, of either "strayed specimens" or those that have bitten down to the mucosa or "those retarded in their development," but rather one of very normal, young *Ancylostoma* which on penetrating the intestinal wall, normally occurring when they are a much

smaller size, remained behind for some reason. However, these are only speculations. What we need here first of all are observations; it will now be my task to determine on experimental animals the location of the larvae in the body and to see whether and how they reach the intestine from the skin and how they behave there. Unfinished as my experiments are at this point and since they are only published by requests, as I already mentioned, I will refrain at this time from adding to them further conclusions and observations.

When I wrote down my "derogatory" remark, that we still know very little about the life cycle of *Ancylostoma,* I did not intend to detract from the merits of my predecessors, but it has been a source of satisfaction to me to see this assertion amply justified by what has followed. And yet does not the statement hold true, even today, in the face of a number of new questions which have again arisen and await solution? Nature goes along its own hidden ways and does not tie itself to hypotheses and formulas; I still would not like to claim even today that we know the "life cycle" of *Ancylostoma.* . . .

ON THE PENETRATION OF ANCYLOSTOMA LARVAE INTO THE HUMAN SKIN

Ueber das eindringen der ankylostomalarven in die menschliche haut. Centralblatt für Bakteriologie and Parasitenkunde, 29: 733–739, 1901. Selections from pp. 733, 736–739. Translated from the German.

Arthur Looss
(1861–1923)

Some time ago I claimed that the larvae of the *Ancylostoma* had the ability actively to penetrate the human skin and, after introduction, to develop in the digestive tract of their bearers, reaching the intestines in an unknown manner to reach maturity. I admit that this claim might arouse doubts as to its correctness since it is an event which, until then, was without analogy in the history of parasites. Not only did it appear improbable after all our experiences that the same parasite could reach its destination in two different ways, active and passive, but there was no known case at that time in which intestinal worms were able to penetrate into the bowel from the skin of the host. On the other hand, I believe that the history of our knowledge of the life cycle of parasites has taught us enough never to be surprised that the parasites, perhaps more than any other animals, reject formulas and schemata set up by us when they are attempting to attain their special purposes and aims. While I have admitted that there might be intelligent doubts as to the correctness of my statements, I will say again that they are correct to a certain degree. I would have hoped that doubts would have been expressed less vehemently and in a somewhat less foolish manner. . . .

In order to secure the most definitive results, the experiments were performed on humans; in fact, I tried it first on a fresh cadaver. A piece of the skin of the thigh was excised and warmed in a vessel at 37°C and one drop of larvae-containing water was dripped upon it. With this, the isolated piece of skin shrank so much that the test was unsuccessful; a part that had been scraped off still showed fluid, and under the microscope there were some live and some more or less shrunken and dried larvae. Therefore, it appeared best and safest to use a living person for further experiments. Colleague Madden, F.R.C.S., professor of surgery at the Medical School at Kasr-el-Aini Hospital, was kind enough to offer me amputated limbs for my work. I have availed myself of his offer only once. This is the way the test was done:

One hour prior to the scheduled amputation of the lower leg of an 18-year-old boy I had the skin scrubbed thoroughly with soap and water and dried completely. Then, as in the former experiments, the drop of water, heavily infected with larvae, was dripped onto the skin and left absolutely undisturbed. It gradually spread a little and dried completely in about ten minutes. Redness of the infected skin could not be seen. I abstained from asking the patient whether he had been aware of anything, as in his condition a reliable answer was unlikely. After the operation, about one hour after infection, the piece of skin which had been circled for recognition was excised, stretched tightly with needles, and, in this condition, gradually hardened in alcohol and finally embedded and cut.

The examination of the sections first yielded the fact that the main entrance spot for the larvae was the hair follicles. As far as the drop had covered there was practically not a single follicle found which was entirely free of young *Ancylo-*

stoma. In a few, only solitary ones were found; in others, however, namely in the larger ones, masses of larvae had collected.

Commonly, the larvae were in the most diverse phases of penetration, their tails still projected freely to the exterior while the head bored between hair surface and the bordering upper epidermal laminae. Inside the hair follicles the larvae crowded toward the hair papilla. When particularly numerous in the same follicle, they completely destroyed the outer root sheath. Having reached the hair papilla they left the follicles to penetrate the adjacent tissue of the cutis vera. I have observed in a few of my preparations a number of penetrating larva with their heads already outside the hair follicle while a large part of the body still remained in it (see Plate 47, Fig. 3). This shows that about one hour after infection the first larvae bypass the skin freely. I have never seen a larva in a follicular gland opening into a hair follicle. As far as the results of this first experiment are concerned, the hair follicles form the main entrance for the young *Ancylostoma* and the cause of this should not be too difficult to appreciate. Because of the lack of prehensile organs and surrounded (in the present test) by clean water they evidently lack the strength to make a primary opening in the surface of the skin; therefore, they use the delicate fissures between hair and the interior surface of the hair follicles into which they can penetrate easily. Arriving in a fissure of this kind, their bodies find enough support to allow the head to push forward.

It is obvious that the larvae look for fissures that are delicate (on the free skin without other support) and this explains why they are found in great masses under the upper, most horny, and somewhat loosened epidermal layers. Here also they evidently push themselves forward as soon as they have found support for their bodies; in some rare cases they appear in sections caught at the moment when, after penetration of the stratum mucosum, their upper bodies are in the peripheral part of the corium (see Plate 47, Fig. 2). They make little use of the openings and passages of the sweat glands or the follicle glands. Of the many hundred larvae that had penetrated, not a single one was found in the gland ducts.

In short, these are the results of my first attempt. That actual penetration of *Ancylostoma* larvae into the skin does occur can now be looked upon as unassailable. Further tests under diversely modified conditions, as well as others,

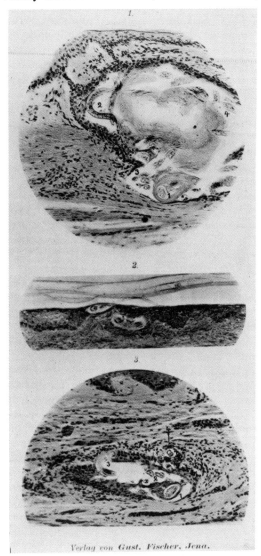

Plate 47. Fig. 1. Section of a hair follicle with penetrated larvae. In (1) cross-section of a hair, in (2) a larva caught in a larger cross-section, in (3) and (4) numerous transverse sections through other larvae. *Fig. 2.* Larva among the uppermost detached epidermis pushed forward and moved over into the lower skin. Found twice. *Fig. 3.* Larva moved from hair follicle into the surrounding tissue. In (1) cross-section of a hair, in (2) cross-sections of larvae still in the hair follicle, in (3) the head of the moved larva. (This one has only been tangentially taken, the rest is located on the following section which, however, is somewhat pushed together so that it is not quite suited for photography.) In (4) cross-section of a larva totally penetrated into the connective tissue.

for the possible confirmation of the paths of the larvae in the body, are in preparation.

In addition, I must point out that in Egypt skin penetration as a route of infection acquires a great significance when compared with eating and drinking. It cannot be denied that in eating unwashed vegetables, isolated larvae occasionally will be ingested. The same can happen in drinking, but I would like to deny that infection occurs in this way as the rule in the population of Egypt because of the simple fact that the larvae, even in high temperature when their movements are liveliest, cannot subsist in water and sink in a few hours. In cooler water this sinking occurs very fast; in a glass cylinder about 20 cm in height, for instance, one half-hour suffices. The larvae can only be brought to the surface with the shaking of the vessel. Under such circumstances they can be swallowed by drinking running water in which they are near the surface. However, running water destroys them so that the possibility of infection is always trifling.

In drinking stagnant water an ingestion of worms can only occur when the water is stirred up and the entire deposit is raised. A custom such as this, however, is not the fashion in Egypt or elsewhere.

When the earth is recovering from floods, one can observe the workers in the fields standing for hours in mud up to their knees. They also work in it with their hands. They wash in it when there is no water to wash in and let it dry on their skin. Thus it is unquestionably clear that in this mud *Ancylostoma* larvae would have the most superb opportunity and the time to invade the skin. As the local natives are not particular as to their bodily functions, the mud is always renewed with worm eggs, and the larvae can, in their long life span, assemble in sufficient quantities to induce severe new infections. I am convinced that this mode of infection, through the skin, is a simpler explanation for infection of the Egyptian population than the ingesting of worms in food and drink. Furthermore, in the plowed fields like the ones in Cologne, in the rice fields of Italy and other countries, conditions in tunnel building or ditch digging, and so on, the conditions for outdoor laborers are essentially the same as those described for the Egyptians. I am convinced, therefore, that both the active penetration of the *Ancylostoma* larvae and the passive deposition, respectively, play important roles, especially when the laborers do not wear shoes as is the custom in southern countries.

For the illumination of my statements on the behavior of the larvae while penetrating the skin I will add some photographs which Colleague Bitter was kind enough to produce.

Cairo, February 1901

THE LARVAE IN THE LYMPHATIC VESSELS

The Anatomy and Life History of *Agchylostoma duodenale* Dub.—A Monograph. II. The Development in the Free State. Records of the Egyptian Government Medical School, Vol. 4, 631 pp. and 10 plates, 1911. Selections from pp. 521–524.

Arthur Looss
(1861–1923)

When the larvae have penetrated the skin it is evidently the lymphatic system into which they first seek to find their way: in the lymphatics, at any rate, particularly in the superficial network of capillaries, they are often found in considerable quantities shortly after infection. But having once reached a lymphatic vessel they apparently continue their journey without delay, as I conclude from the fact that even a few hours after their entrance the superficial lymphatics are in the main again found empty and only in places show a few delayed specimens. By the route of the lymphatics and through the ductus thoracicus, or the smaller main lymphatic trunk of the right side, the larvae finally reach the right side of the heart. Before doing so, however, they have to pass through certain lymphatic glands, above all the groin and shoulder glands; here their behaviour is very interesting. I have studied it in a number of experiments in fresh preparations and have observed the following:—

If thin pieces of the glands are examined in a slightly compressed state at a time when the first larvae have just arrived in them, these larvae may be seen wandering about between the cells in characteristic serpentine movements exactly similar to those observable in the subcutaneous connective tissue. The only difference is that in the glands the movements are slightly slower, as though the larvae found it more difficult to advance. As time goes on, the number of larvae arriving in the glands becomes greater, and among them some may now be observed which have a small number of lymphatic cells, sometimes only three or four, sometimes twelve or more, adhering to their skin so firmly that the larvae carry them along in their movements. The number of these lymphatic cells steadily increases; they commence to form a mantle which becomes ever more continuous all round the body of the individual larva and, as is easily comprehensible, accordingly hinders its movements. The larva now advances only very slowly and its movements, which were first lively and progressive, gradually change into stationary writhings which constantly decrease in intensity. Finally, even these movements cease, and the internal organisation of the larva, which was previously clear and distinctly perceptible, becomes indistinct, granular and cloudy. At the end of the process, a dead larva, the internal organs of which have completely crumbled away into an opaque granular mass, is found enclosed in a thick pad of granular leucocytes. The later stages of this process may be easily recognised in sections through the lymphatic glands owing to the considerably intensified staining capacity of the cells which have accumulated round the larvae.

The process here described seems to go on fairly rapidly, for the "captured" larvae, as we might term them, may be found in greater or less numbers as early as two days after infection. I have also had the impression as though a strong single infection stimulated the activity of the glands; at any rate, the captured larvae are found in such cases in distinctly greater numbers than in others where fewer larvae had been administered. On the whole, however, the number of larvae rendered harmless in the lymphatic glands is small in comparison to those which pass through them unharmed. From the different observations I have made it seems as though the larvae are able to withstand the attacks of the lymphatic cells for a certain length of time; or possibly, also, the lymphatic cells do not at once commence their attacks; if the larvae succeed in escaping from the glands within this time they are saved; if they do not succeed, then they fall a prey to the lymphatic cells. Thus as in bacterial invasions the lymphatic glands act to a certain extent as protective organs against the penetrating larvae.

While on their journey through the lymphatic system I have actually observed the larvae in the lymphatics of the skin, in the vessels leading to and from the glands of the groins and shoulders, in the ductus thoracicus and one of its contributories, and finally rather often in the lymphatics of the lung. Since it is not necessary for them to pass through the latter on their way from the skin, it is not at first clear how they get there; a possible way of explaining this phenomenon will be discussed presently.

The Larvae in the Blood Vessels

At first, as we have seen, the larvae chiefly enter the lymphatics and only later the blood-vessels. Consequently, if sections are examined from experimental animals preserved two or three hours after infection, it is very seldom that a larva is seen in a blood-vessel. Afterwards the number of such larvae increases, but so far as I have observed, it never reaches even approximately that of the larvae which penetrate the lymphatic ducts. Further, it is at first exclusively the veins which the larvae enter; but later they are found—sometimes in great numbers—in the arteries also; this fact will receive detailed discussion later. The larvae once they have entered a vein seem to travel fairly rapidly with the blood to the heart; it is at any rate not easy, and often requires much time, to find one in sections through the blood-vessels. I have actually seen them in the various veins of the skin, in veins from the neighbourhood of the axillary and inguinal glands and in the vena azygos.

In the innominate vein the larvae arriving with the blood meet those arriving through the lymphatics, and are carried by the blood stream through the right part of the heart and the pulmonary arteries into the lungs. In these vessels it is less difficult to find the larvae in sections, since the part of the circulatory system in question must be traversed by all the larvae. In the case of the dog mentioned above, which was infected three times with the larvae of *Agchylostoma duodenale*, the whole of the right chamber of the heart was cut into sections, and in these 34 larvae were found free in the coagulated blood.

The Larvae in the Air Passages

In the lungs the larvae are carried by the arterial blood-stream into the finer ramifications of the pulmonary artery, where I have actually found them in vessels only 0.02 mm in diameter.

On the other hand, I have not succeeded in seeing a larva precisely in the act of its escape from the vessels; sometimes, it is true, appearances seem strongly to indicate that certain larvae are with the hind part of their body still lying in the vessels, with the forepart in the adjacent tissue; but it is difficult to determine with certainty whether this is really the case or not. In the parenchyma of the lungs larvae are not seldom met with; but as a rule they seem to pass quickly into the alveoli, whence they begin the active part of their migration. Their behaviour in the bronchi, so far as I have observed it, presents nothing remarkable; they always lie free upon the epithelium. In the trachea, on the other hand, larvae are not seldom observed which lie wholly or partly in the epithelium; moreover from this point onwards an interesting difference becomes apparent between the behaviour of the larvae of *Agchylostoma duodenale* and those of *Agchylostoma caninum*. I may here point out at once that the reason for this divergence lies in the essentially different conditions under which the larvae of the two species are placed in the dog. For *Agchylostoma caninum*, the dog is the normal host, and the conditions, in particular the nourishment, it finds in him are such as it is accustomed to. For *Agchylostoma duodenale*, on the contrary, the dog is an abnormal and, as we have seen, a comparatively poor host; the conditions, above all the nourishment, it finds in him are such as it is not accustomed to. If due attention is paid to this difference the divergence in the behaviour of the larvae in the dog will be easy to understand.

Turning first to those of *Agch. caninum*, they creep upwards in the trachea of the dog, partly upon and partly in the mucous membrane. Occasionally, a larva may be found which has penetrated more deeply into the wall and wanders about in its connective tissue portions, or lies in a gland; but by far the greater number travel straight up through the larynx into the oesophagus. In the larynx also some may be seen in the glands and the connective tissue parts, now and then even free in Morgagni's pouches, etc. Those which have reached the oesophagus, so far as I have observed, travel exclusively upon its mucous membrane; it should, however, be stated that on the whole it is not frequently possible to actually apprehend larvae in sections through the oesophagus. This becomes fairly comprehensible if we remember that any larvae lying free on the oesophageal mucous membrane will be passively swept away by every act of swallowing, and so despatched to the stomach. As a rule it is thus a matter of chance for the individual larva whether it is sent down passively, or has to perform active migration—for some part at least—to the stomach.

Another important fact, easily to be verified by observation, is that the larvae commence to grow with their arrival in the air passages. Among those which have reached the upper portions of the trachea—not, however, among those still wandering about in the lower part—there are nearly always some with a provisional mouth-capsule more or less completely formed and the skin detached around the body, in other words, ready for the third ecdysis. The ecdysis itself, however, never takes place before the respective larvae have reached the intestine; for among the very large numbers I have observed in the stage and position mentioned I have never seen one which had already cast its skin. For their growth, the larvae of course require food which they obtain from the mucous membrane of the trachea. Since I have at this stage never distinctly seen formed elements in their intestine, it must consist of liquid matter. This food is their normal food, and hence the larvae also develop normally. When they arrive in the intestine they are more or less ready to undergo the third ecdysis by which they acquire the provisional mouth-capsule. Their food thenceforward consists of the epithelium cells of the mucous membrane, as was already pointed out, for *Agchylostoma duodenale,* in the first part of this work.

The larvae of *Agchylostoma duodenale* are not in equally favourable conditions. They also feed while creeping up the trachea, and grow distinctly; but the whole process is much less rapid and, so far as I have observed, never leads even to the first traces in the formation of the provisional mouth-capsule. I have not the slightest doubt that the unsuitable nature of the food is the cause of this retardation, as it is the cause of another very suggestive phenomenon. The larvae, perceiving, as it were, that they are not in their right surrounding, try to escape by making their way into the tissues of the tracheal wall. The fact is still little pronounced in the lower region of the organ, but becomes very marked in the

upper end and the larynx, varying of course additionally with the age of the experimental animal. The larvae thus deviate from their normal path, and but comparatively few reach the intestine by the oesophagus.

On comparing the microscopical pictures which the larvae of the two *Agchylostoma* species thus offer in the trachea of the dog, it is impossible to escape the conviction that the cause of the divergence lies indeed in the fact above given. Both kinds of larvae, owing to their thigmotropic tendencies, enter the skin and the lymph or blood vessels whence they are passively carried to the finest ramifications of the pulmonary artery. There, for the first time after having left the skin, they can again make use of their boring capacities; but as soon as they are free and commence to grow, these capacities seem to become gradually lost. I have already mentioned that in the wider bronchi and the lower portions of the trachea the movements of the larvae are markedly different in character from those they are seen to make while still in the free state, or in the subcutaneous tissue and in the lymph glands. The larvae now feed as parasites and grow, but from this juncture onwards the particular nature of the environment makes itself felt. The result is that the larvae of *Agchylostoma caninum* can develop without hindrance, while those of *Agchylostoma duodenale,* in their—according to its age—more or less unsuitable host, have to fight against more or less unfavourable conditions, trying to escape so far this is possible. The fact is a good illustration of what I endeavoured to show, namely, that the various species of parasites are not able to adapt themselves without delay to all sorts of changes in their surroundings. . . .

ANKYLOSTOMIASIS IN PUERTO RICO

New York Medical Journal, 71: 552–556, 1900.

Bailey Kelly Ashford
(1873–1934)

Soon after receiving his M.D. from Georgetown University, Ashford went to Puerto Rico for service during the Spanish-American War. After the war, he returned to the island, where he discovered the presence of hookworm and launched a campaign for its extermination. He spent some time working in Brazil, studying other tropical diseases, including sprue. In 1906,

Ashford first envisioned Puerto Rico as a center of tropical research, and in 1926, when the island's School of Tropical Medicine was completed, he was appointed professor of mycology and tropical medicine, a post which he filled until his death.

This is the first of Ashford's important contributions to our knowledge of hookworm disease.

I have the honor to report upon 20 cases of the severe anaemia commonly seen among the poor of this island. One of the first observations made by professional men here is the prevalence of anaemia, especially among the poor. This is at first attributed usually to starvation or poor food, then to malaria, and then to the "climate." Through the kindness of the physicians of Ponce I am able to state something as to the mode of treatment adopted up to this time. Some have observed that the ignorant peon treated himself by purging, with beneficial effects for a time and a relapse to previous conditions soon afterward. Iron and arsenic have been prescribed largely, but with little benefit. Some physicians have frankly declared it beyond their power to cope with the disease, which they regarded as a pernicious progressive anaemia of obscure origin. The stools had been examined, but, no worms being evident, this, as a cause, was dismissed. I was led to examine the faeces for the ova of *Ankylostoma duodenale*, and found them in great numbers. Soon after, a large dose of thymol brought away the parasites, male and female. No sooner had I stated my results to the physicians of this city than they agreed as to the diagnosis and verified the parasite and its eggs. Their testimony is as follows:

(1) This disease is the most destructive and general disease of Puerto Rico.

(2) It is found typically and very frequently among the poor and badly fed.

(3) Most cases are similar.

(4) Bad food and bad hygiene are responsible for much of its power for evil.

(5) Blood foods have never exercised more than a temporary influence on the course of this disease.

(6) Improvement follows purgation.

(7) Up to this time the existence of this parasite had not been proved on this island, or, if proved, not within their knowledge.

In studying this disease I have taken 20 cases which I considered typical of "Puerto Rican anaemia," or "tropical chlorosis." These cases were selected from the provisional field hospital for indigent and sick Puerto Ricans, established after the flood of August 10, 1899, in this city. Although the histories of these cases are inclosed, I should like to refer to such points as seem to me interesting and of frequent occurrence in this disease.

1. *The Family History.*—Most patients give a history of deaths in the family from a like disease. At times this history is truly appalling and casts a light on the extent of the infection among the people. Many claim the deaths to have been due to "malaria" or "diarrhoea" or "obscure fever." Of course, this matter is problematical, but it is fair to suppose, inasmuch as the disease is often marked by irregular fever, with intermissions, that their diagnoses may be questioned, and to recollect that our own physicians have in the past placed on malaria responsibilities which do not belong to it. But questions as to chills are extremely unsatisfactory. I know there is much malaria here in the lowlands. I have followed such cases through their course, but the testimony of local physicians coincides with mine, that malarial organisms in the blood are not so often seen as would be supposed. Chills, then, are not so frequent; there are few "ague cakes;" the pallor is not that of malaria, and the sclerae are not icteric. The most suggestive fact outside of blood examination is that the cases come from the mountains and the valleys; some of the very worst cases I have seen came from highly salubrious mountain districts. Nevertheless, I hesitate to affirm that many cases of malarial cachexias do not exist to swell the sum of anaemics here.

2. *The Previous History of the Patient.*—The diet is a powerful factor in turning the scale against the unhappy victim of ankylostomiasis. Rightly the physicians here quote its influence. Personally, I have eaten and slept in all parts of this island, not alone on the frequented roads, but in those rarely visited by strangers, and can submit my testimony to that quoted in support of this influence. The relation of the daily life among the working classes has been confirmed in talking with many owners of sugar and coffee plantations and their employees. They rise at from 4 to 6 A.M. Some take a little black coffee, some boiled water and sugar, some nothing. They work till 11, when they breakfast on about four ounces of

codfish and a few pieces of plantain. They return to work at 1 and continue till 5 P.M. Dinner is composed of rice and beans; some have only boiled rice with lard, and some boiled rice alone. It may be mentioned that they get plenty of bad rum and some bad wine. This seems a slight enough diet, but the hurricane deprived them of even this, and the sick poor came drifting down on Ponce. I believe it not probable that those degraded to the level of people whose life is bounded by a tropical plantation, enjoying little beyond the cutting of cane and picking of coffee, can have a high standard of personal cleanliness, and, as a fact, bathing is not often practised. Faeces are distributed over the earth wherever the individual happens to be while at work, or in a little shack when at home, but directly on the ground always. Indeed, faeces pollute their very houses. Ponce is a town of perhaps 40,000 inhabitants, yet it has no sewerage and is in the lowlands near the sea. Closets and kitchens are in conjunction in many houses. The water soon takes up its quota of whatever is noxious. Those who are clean in their habits, and the educated classes are a most cleanly people, are polluted by the filth of the poor and ignorant. The configuration of this island is one of steep mountains and deep ravines, with broad plains near the sea. Heavy rains wash the larvae from each faecal deposit into these watercourses, and this muddy water is probably one source of contamination. Contaminated earth on the hands of laborers is another; fouled garden is another. The larvae have not yet been demonstrated in the water or mud. The drinking water of nearly all well-to-do people is filtered, and in this class we do not find so great a preponderance of this disease.

3. *The Subjective Symptoms.*—It is difficult to obtain a history of the disease from its inception, for many have it from infancy. Generally it is possible to obtain some such history as this: A variable appetite, some nausea and vomiting, pain in epigastrium, either constipation or diarrhoea (or these may alternate), sometimes dysentery; swellings of the feet and ankles, no loss of weight, sleeplessness, restlessness, tinnitus aurium, giddiness, faintness, severe headache, palpitation of the heart, progressive debility; little perspiration, but kidneys active; fever sometimes, but not chills. I have not been able to get a history of geophagism nor of intesti-

nal haemorrhage described by some authors. Sometimes the patients improve for a time after medication, but not permanently.

4. *Objective Symptoms.*—Pallor: This is divided into three classes by a prominent physician, but I can not see that it has reference to more than the individual color of the patient, whatever that may be, irrespective of the disease. The conjunctivae, lips, tongue, gums, nails, and cheeks are in some cases perfectly pallid, the mucous membranes especially being of a deathly white. The skin is generally a pasty yellow, a dirty brownish-gray, or a grayish-white. Expression: A passive expression is often seen, and its peculiar character is heightened by puffiness of the eyes and bloating of the face. Oedema: This is simply the usual accompaniment of severe anaemia. Practically every variety is seen, the chief being, in order of importance—oedema of the feet and ankles, oedema of the face, ascites, and oedema of the scrotum. Hypostatic congestion of the lungs exists often. The important point is that with this disease there may be emaciation. This has not been present often in my cases; on the contrary, the patients are apparently well nourished. Anaemic ulcers are sometimes seen on the legs and an incorrect accusation of syphilis may be made. Corneal ulcers are at times seen. One of my cases presented corneal ulcers of both eyes. Respiratory symptoms: Generally none from this disease save in increased rapidity of breathing from anaemia, serious accumulations, or hypostatic congestions. Liver: No constant symptom. Spleen: No constant symptom. Heart: These symptoms are very aggravated; signs of a pernicious secondary anaemia. Pulsating vessels: Both jugulars, superficial veins of the arm, and vessels about the root of the neck and heart in severe cases, with greatly dilated heart; pulsating suprasternal and supraclavicular regions and diffused pulsations in the anterior thoracic wall. All kinds of deductions might be made by a careless observer. Haemic murmurs are almost constantly present, and are in many cases heard in the veins of the neck.

The urine: No albumin is found and the specific gravity is constantly low. The pulse is weak, rapid, soft, and compressible.

The blood: Attention is invited to the accompanying summary of blood examinations. The following deductions are drawn:

(1) A severe anaemia, falling as low as that of Addison's anaemia in count of red cells in some cases.

(2) A very low haemoglobin average and a very low color index.

(3) A marked eosinophilia in some cases. Forty per cent reached in one case. This follows the observation of Neusser.

(4) No leucocytosis common to the disease itself. Leucocytosis recorded is always apparently due to complications, as noted.

(5) Frequent presence of normoblasts, and in some cases megaloblasts, but never a majority of megaloblasts.

(6) Poikilocytosis common. Manson denies this.

(7) Utter unreliability of blood foods without removal of the cause, the *Ankylostoma*. This blood examination was the first line of research taken up, and, as soon as anaemia was proved, the patient was given blood tonics, with temporary supporting treatment suited to the individual case, with the idea that the patient might be carried along until the true cause could be discovered. Of course, now, all treatment has been substituted by anthelminthics, chiefly male fern and thymol, and the blood and heart tonics will be again tried when the eggs have disappeared from the faeces. I was led to examine the stools carefully from the high eosinophile count, and it is certainly evident that trichinosis has a rival for high counts in ankylostomiasis.

The *Ankylostoma* was found in all cases save one, a case of tuberculosis pure and simple. This patient was chosen to represent a contrast, and I think he does. There is true leucocytosis, and the eosinophiles are not much in evidence. Moreover, the red cell count is much higher than all the others, as is the haemoglobin record. In calling attention to this infection we enter upon a large field. The histories of this disease have been made up to show what percentage of the people have the disease in certain countries: 25 per cent in Egypt, 20 per cent in Maitland, 52 per cent in Madras; 13 per cent in Kioto, Japan; but no percentage can be cited as yet for this island. Dr. B. Scheube, of Greiz, speaks in his work of its existing in the Antilles, but no island is specified, nor is the extent of the disease stated. From my own observation, and from the opinions of the resident physicians of the island, I believe it to be widespread and destructive. Only 20 cases have been examined, yet all, save one, have given me the ova of this parasite in large numbers. As the 20 cases were chosen at random from hundreds more just like them clinically, and as the one exception noted was chosen only for contrast, I am convinced that further investigation will show that the disease has killed its hundreds, and that it is curable and preventable. The proof of its prevalence lies naturally in the hands of all scientific physicians of this island. I can not further judge than from a short experience and the positive evidence of 19 cases submitted.

Manson states that 75 per cent of the people of India in certain localities are infected. Williams quotes 52 per cent in Madras. Griesinger, in Egypt, quotes 25 per cent. B. Scheube, 13 per cent in Kioto, Japan. A glance at its geographical distribution is appalling. Egypt is so full of it that it is known as Egyptian chlorosis and forms the great basis for rejection of recruits for the army. The French, of the French Antilles, call it *cachexie aqueuse* and recognize its full importance; and literature is full of its ravages in South America. Thornhill regards it as of greater importance in Ceylon than cholera.

There is in Puerto Rico a dense population in a small country. In a space of about 100 miles by 60 we have probably over 1,000,000 people. Of the working class it cannot be denied that a large percentage have anaemia, and, should the future verify my suspicion, means are at hand to increase not only the well-being of those now suffering, but to insure to the owner of large haciendas of coffee and sugar a better class of labor; to insure to the army protection from the invaliding from anaemia of such troops as are enlisted here; to insure protection against the disease to our American troops; to relieve the State and the hospitals here from the expense of caring for a large number of anaemics who are now slowly dragging on to a fatal end. Perhaps our own sick reports will unfold some additional facts. I mention here only such possibilities as have occurred to my mind; but it is a significant fact that, though it is present in Germany, Scheube notes that it is confined to a few cases. In other words, it appears to assume only such proportions as a country will allow it to assume. I repeat, I have no certain knowledge of the proportions it has assumed here. I have been able only to call atten-

tion to what I consider to be its extensive prevalence, and I cannot quote any full experience
from treatment. I have given thymol in several
cases with the always easily demonstrated presence of the parasite. From the exceeding kindness and the scientific spirit shown by the local
doctors, I cannot doubt that it will be but a short
time before measures will be taken, if there is
sufficient extent of the disease found, to alleviate
the conditions. . . . I shall not lengthen this
paper by any description of a parasite so well
known and so fully described by the professor of
helminthology at the Army Medical School, nor
shall I make further remark on the history of the
disease, its evident prophylaxis and simple cure,
until I can call to my aid a more extensive famil-
iarity with it.

ON THE CAUSAL RELATIONSHIP BETWEEN "GROUND ITCH," OR "PANI-GHAO," AND THE PRESENCE OF THE LARVAE OF THE *ANKYLOSTOMA DUODENALE* IN THE SOIL

British Medical Journal, 1: 190–193, 1902.

Charles Albert Bentley
(1873–1949)

*An English physician educated in Liverpool and Edin-
burgh where he received his M.B., Bentley spent most
of his life in southwest Asia. He also worked in Liverpool and Egypt prior to going to Bengal as director of
public health and medical officer of the Ceylon Tea
Company in Assam from 1900 to 1907.*

*The relationship between the mode of entry of An-
cylostoma duodenale and clinical disease is found in
Bentley's report.*

In the *Journal of Tropical Medicine* for March
1st, 1901, an article appeared under the heading
"Water-itch; or Sore-feet of Coolies," describing a disease with which all tea garden medical
officers in Assam, Cachar and Sylhet, are familiar. Apparently a similar affection is very prevalent on the sugar plantations of the West Indies;
for in the annual report, by the Surgeon-General
of Trinidad, for the year 1900, it is mentioned
that "ground-itch is very prevalent during the
rainy season on the sugar plantations, amongst
the East Indian labourers." It is further remarked
in this report, that although the disease is not a

serious one, it is a matter of great importance to
the planters, on account of the number of labourers it incapacitates from work.

The disease has been defined by Dr. Dalgetty
(Sylhet), one of the writers referred to, as: "A
superficial vesicular dermatitis, which occurs
epidemically among the coolies working on tea
gardens during the wet months of the year, which
solely attacks the feet, and which has a considerable resemblance to ordinary scabies." In place
of this definition, I substitute one which I think is
perhaps more suited to the condition.

Definitions

Ground-itch (synonyms: pani-ghao, water-
itch, water-pox, water-sores, sore feet of coolies)
is an affection of the skin confined entirely to the
lower extremities, and probably always associated with the presence of the larvae of the
Ankylostoma duodenale in the soil of the affected
areas; endemic in Assam and the West Indies,
and possibly present in other parts of the tropics;
characterised by its periodical epidemic appearance in the infected areas, coincident with the
onset of the rainy season; with typical lesion consisting in a primary erythema, followed by a vesicular eruption which frequently becomes pustular, and in severe cases may result in obstinate
ulceration or even in gangrene.

Prevalence

In Assam the disease is almost universally
known by the name "pani-ghao" (literally,
water-sore), a term which has been applied to it
probably because it only occurs during the seasonal rains when the earth is saturated with moisture. On tea gardens, where the disease has once
appeared, it becomes a yearly recurring
epidemic. Sporadic cases may occur as early as
May, but the general outbreak does not usually
appear until a month or six weeks later, and does
not disappear until about the end of October,
when the ground has become comparatively dry
again. People of all classes are liable to contract
the disease, although it is rare for a European to
be attacked.

The disease may generally be said to attack the
different individuals in a community with a frequency directly proportionate to their exposure to
the source of infection. All observations point to
the earth as being the infecting medium, and

faecal contamination of the soil as being the most active agency in the propagation of the disease, which in over 90 per cent of cases is contracted in the immediate neighbourhood of the coolie lines, as the collection of coolie houses is termed.

Etiology

As previous observers have pointed out, this disease is one of great importance to the employer of coolie labour; for during the seasonal epidemic more than 5 per cent of a labour force may be temporarily invalided by its attacks.

Until recently nothing was known as to the cause of the affection, although various suggestions have been made from time to time. Dr. Seheult (Trinidad) has stated that the condition is probably due to some chemical irritant present in the soil, either natural or due to manure used in cultivation. Dr. Dalgetty (South Sylhet), led astray by the superficial resemblance which the lesions of the disease bear to ordinary scabies, has described an acarus as the cause. His article in the *Journal of Tropical Medicine* was mainly devoted to an account of the anatomical characters and life-history of this mite, which certainly occurs as an accidental infection of neglected water-sores, and may almost constantly be found in the scab or crust round the edges of any untreated ulcer in this part of India.

I have been familiar with this disease in its clinical aspects for the past three years, have frequently met with it in tea-garden practice both in Cachar and Assam; but until this present season I have had no opportunities for investigating the nature of the condition.

I had been engaged in investigatory work for some two months before my attention was called to Dr. Dalgetty's article. After reading it, I felt greatly surprised that my observations appeared to be entirely at variance with those recorded by him. As a result, I repeated my experiments and observations, in order to satisfy myself as to their accuracy.

A few simple experiments served to show conclusively that the condition, although possessing a superficial resemblance to scabies, is in no sense an analogous disease. Dr. Dalgetty's methods of investigation are open to sources of grave error; thus he says: "If care be taken to evacuate the pustule completely, and to remove at the same time any crust that may happen to surround the spot, then in a certain percentage of cases the ova of an acarus may be seen." He adds that he has frequently found living acari in this way, which is hardly surprising, seeing that they may be found by the score on any dry dead animal matter which is exposed to the air. If, however, he does not find the mite in this way, "he lays the pus or crust aside for a day or two, covered up and moistened with sterilised water, but not covered with a cover slip."

It naturally follows that very soon some mite in search of food finds its way to the specimen put aside for future inspection. I first found the acarus on the scab taken from an old water-sore, but on the same day I was fortunate to come across a colony of the same acari feasting upon the body of an *Anopheles* mosquito that I had put aside on a slide about a week before. Since then I have found the mite on all sorts of decaying animal matter, such as dry faecal matter, dead flies, etc., and recently I bred about a hundred of them for experimental purposes upon the dead body of an *Ankylostoma*.

It may here be remarked that the acarus described by Dr. Dalgetty seems to prefer dry to moist surroundings, and certainly appears to breed very much more readily in the former.

In order to prove, however, whether or not the mite could produce the lesions of the disease, the following experiments were tried:

Experiment No. 1.—A small quantity of soil was taken from a known infected area near to some coolie lines, and after being moistened was applied to the arm, where it was kept in contact with the skin for a period of six hours, with the result that typical water-sores followed. The soil that had thus been utilised, as well as the unused portion, was then carefully examined with the microscope, but no sign of any acari could be found.

This experiment showed that the cause of the disease must be sought for in the soil from areas near the coolie lines. This soil, as has already been mentioned, is contaminated with faecal matter in a very marked degree. Careful microscopic examination of samples of the soil from different areas was undertaken. The following list of living objects which were found present in these samples were noted down for future reference:

(a) Rhabditiform larvae of the *Ankylostoma duodenale* (recognised by comparison with special cultures of larvae) were present in great numbers.

(b) Minute leeches.

(c) Minute earth worms recognised by their setae.

(d) Several species of rotiferae.

(e) Several different species of infusoriae, both amoeboid and ciliated.

(f) The spores and hyphae of several microscopic fungi.

(g) Bacteria, rod shaped, curved, spiral (?) and micrococci.

While making these observations several further experiments were performed in order to show whether or not some chemical irritant in the soil might be regarded as the cause of the condition under consideration.

Experiment No. 2 — A small portion of the same earth that was obtained for previous experiments, and had been proved to contain the cause of the disease, was sterilized by being baked for a considerable time. Some of it was then moistened and applied to the arm, as described previously. It failed, however, to produce any irritation, and thus completely negatived the idea that a chemical irritant in the soil was the cause of the disease.

It is a well-known fact that the Indian coolie is not very particular in regard to the disposal of human refuse. He will not adopt any proper conservancy system, and latrines, if erected on tea gardens, are never used by the labour force. The coolie walks but a few yards from his dwelling in order to relieve himself. In this way the cultivated areas for some distance round the lines in most tea gardens is constantly being contaminated with faecal matter. The coolies themselves recognise that this accumulation of filth is the cause of the disease, and as far as possible they try to avoid exposure to infection by shirking work in the parts of the garden in close proximity to the lines. When obliged to walk over the infected soil they almost invariably protect their feet by wearing "kurrams," a kind of wooden sandal.

In this part of Assam the disease appears chiefly among the labourers who are engaged in hoeing; it affects the strong and healthy quite as frequently as the weakly and anaemic. Cases occurring among hoeing people almost always show the eruption on the instep and ankle. This is no doubt due to the nature of their work, which necessitates their remaining near the same spot for a considerable time, and ensures that their feet are in contact with the soil, while a constant shower of moist earth falls from the hoe upon their feet and ankles. Of the total cases 75 per cent occur among men. This is explained by the fact that during the time when the disease is prevalent, the strong men are engaged in hoeing while the more weakly men, the women, and children are at work plucking.

Among pluckers, the disease is very much more frequently seen on weakly individuals and those whose caste customs forbid a high standard of personal cleanliness. Among this class of coolie the lesion is almost always confined to the underside of the foot or to the clefts between the toes, and can generally be traced to neglect to wear kurrams, or to want of sufficient care in cleansing the feet after return from work. Want of cleanliness may certainly be regarded as a strongly predisposing cause of infection, and this fact rather than any inherent susceptibility must be looked upon as the reason why anaemic and debilitated coolies so frequently suffer from the disease. The reason that so few robust plucking people are subject to the affection is no doubt to be sought in the almost universal adoption of kurrams by the better coolies, combined with careful washing of the feet immediately on leaving work. The weakly coolie is always dirty and negligent in matters of this kind. He often eats his food without washing his hands, and it is probably quite exceptional for him to wash his feet at night.

Symptoms

The first symptom is an intense itching and burning at the spot where afterwards the eruption appears. This is sometimes so distressing as to cause the sufferer to rub his feet on the ground or some other hard rough surface in order to obtain relief. A faint papular eruption may be distinguished at this time, although sometimes a slight erythema is all that can be detected. This may occur within a few hours of infection, or may be deferred for 24 hours.

Later, usually about the second day, a distinctly vesicular eruption appears, which may be confined to the skin between the toes, or be found under the arch of the foot, or as in a large number of cases be chiefly seen in isolated patches over the dorsum of the foot, reaching sometimes several inches above the ankle. Apparently the affection is confined entirely to the lower extremities, no cases having been reported as occurring on any other part of the body, except as the result of experiment.

If early treatment is adopted the disease may be aborted, the vesicles drying up, and the patient becoming fit for work again in two or three days; more frequently the vesicles become pustules, or they burst, discharging a watery fluid, and then becoming open sores. If pustules have formed, unless they are speedily opened, the process may extend, the pus appearing to burrow under the surrounding healthy skin, and so forming large bullae. In this way an area of several square inches may be denuded of skin.

In a large number of cases very severe inflammation occurs associated with acute pain and great swelling, preventing the sufferer from walking; sometimes also extensive ulceration or even sloughing or gangrene takes place.

Microscopic examination of the soil in parts of the garden where the disease was never contracted showed that earth worms and minute leeches were present in greater number there than in the faecal-infected places. Infusoria were to be found in pretty nearly as great numbers where decaying vegetable matter was present, and certainly could not be looked upon as a likely cause of the disease. Of the probable causes, some bacterium, some species of fungus, or the rhabdoid larvae of the *Ankylostoma*, has to be considered.

Meanwhile a large number of cases of watersore had been carefully examined. In the earliest stage, when only a slight erythema showed where the vesicular eruption would shortly appear, blood films were prepared from the part affected. Nothing definite was derived from this procedure, although a few micrococci were seen once or twice. Scraping a patch of erythema showed on several occasions objects which at first were taken to be fibres of cotton or the shrivelled hyphae of fungi, but when at last an intact and easily recognisable specimen of an *Ankylostoma* larva was found, these objects were more carefully examined under a higher power, when they proved in a number of cases to be undoubtedly the empty sheaths of similar larvae. In the vesicular stage bacteria of certain kinds, lymph cells, a few blood cells, and once or twice a small amoeboid organism were discovered. The pustular form of the disease showed staphylococci and streptococci, together with a few rod-shaped

bacilli. Not having a microtome or other apparatus necessary for preparing sections, it was impossible to make this part of the investigation as complete as could have been wished.

Failing to find any definite cause for the disease by microscopic preparations for the lesions themselves, I once more turned my attention to the search for the cause in external Nature, and to this end the following experiments were undertaken:

(a) Some ordinary soil was sterilised by heat, and after being moistened with sterilised water was infected with a small quantity of faecal matter, containing numerous ova of the *Ankylostoma duodenale*.

(b) A similar preparation of soil was infected with a small quantity of faeces, which on examination were found to be free from ankylostomal infection.

These two preparations were incubated at the ordinary temperature of the air for about a week. At the end of this time sample "*a*" was swarming with larval *Ankylostoma* and various forms of bacteria and fungi, and sample "*b*," but for the absence of the dochmii, presented a similar appearance. Of "*a*" and "*b*" respectively two small quantities were taken, the first portions of which were kept moist, while the second were gently dried at the temperature of the air for a period of eight hours. Previous experiments with cultivations of the larvae of the *Ankylostoma* had shown that gentle drying at ordinary temperatures for a period of six hours was sufficient to kill the larvae. The four preparations were then applied (after remoistening the two desiccated samples with sterilized water) to the wrists of the subjects of experiment, who retained them in a position for a period of about eight to nine hours. At the expiration of that time the bandages were removed. Fifteen hours after the first application of the earth, however, considerable erythema with a minute papular eruption appeared over the spot to which the earth containing embryo *Ankylostoma* had been applied. Within 24 hours a distinctly vesicular eruption had developed, followed by pustules exactly resembling those found in the lesions of ground-itch. In the other cases a faint reddening of the skin was produced, which shortly afterwards entirely disappeared.

The small portions of soil which had been applied to the skin were then re-examined under the microscope. The sample which had been known to be swarming with the active embryos was found to contain no living larvae, one or two dead specimens being all that could be detected. The sample that had contained dead embryos was seen to be full of their shrivelled bodies. Apparently, therefore, the living larvae had entered the skin, and their entry had been followed by lesions similar in every particular to those found associated with the condition known as water-sore.

It now remains to review the fact which various observers have recorded with reference to the clinical nature of the disease, and see whether or not they appear to agree with the theory deduced from the results of the experiments and microscopical investigation described above. The disease only occurs when the atmospheric temperature is fairly high and the earth is saturated with moisture; moreover it only occurs in areas in which, as has been already shown, there is constantly increasing faecal infection of the soil. Where the disease is prevalent ankylostomal infection is extremely common. Giles, Dobson, Rogers, and others, have shown that upwards of 75 per cent of tea garden coolies are the subjects of ankylostomal infection, and my own observations point to an even more general infection in certain districts. Thus recently among some 300 coolies, in all conditions as regards health, whose stools I examined microscopically, only one individual showed freedom from ankylostomal infection. It may thus be readily imagined what an enormous number of larvae of this parasite may be set free in the soil when the conditions are favourable to their development.

As I have previously shown desiccation at comparatively low temperatures is sufficient to kill the larval *Ankylostoma* this is a simple explanation of the fact that water-sores are never seen during the dry season. At this time the ground is hard, and on tea gardens, owing to pruning and other processes of cultivation, is also denuded of the vegetation which affords protection from the rays of the sun during the rains.

The result is that the embryo *Ankylostoma* — which hatches out from the ova within the first two or three days after they have been expelled from the host, in the faeces — perishes almost immediately.

The very rare occurrence of the disease among the rural population is explained by the different methods adopted in the bushes for the disposal of human filth. It appears probable that the acuteness of the inflammation attending an attack of ground-itch is largely governed by the nature of the organisms which accompany or follow the larval *Ankylostoma* in its passage through the skin. That this entry through the epidermis can and does occur has been recently demonstrated by Dr. Looss and Professor Sandwith, of Cairo; but I believe that I am the first to identify this entry of the parasite as the cause of the distinct and well-known skin affection so prevalent in this and other parts of the world.

A NEW SPECIES OF HOOKWORM (*UNCINARIA AMERICANA*) PARASITIC IN MAN

American Medicine, 3: 777–778, 1902.

Charles Wardell Stiles
(1867–1941)

During his student years, Stiles studied at Wesleyan University in Connecticut, at the College of France, and at the Universities of Berlin and Leipzig. In the last of these institutions he studied under Leuckart and received the A.M. and in 1890 the Ph.D. He then did postgraduate work at the Trieste Zoological Station, at the Pasteur Institute, and at the College of France.

After a period as zoologist for the Bureau of Animal Industry of the United States Department of Agriculture, he was appointed professor of medical zoology at Georgetown University and concurrently served as special lecturer in medical zoology at Johns Hopkins. In 1902, Stiles joined the United States Public Health Service, ultimately becoming its medical director in 1930. Upon retiring from government service, he became honorary associate of the Smithsonian Institution.

An indefatigable worker on almost all aspects of parasitic disease, Stiles served as secretary of the International Commission on Medical Zoology from 1910 to 1927. Stiles stimulated the campaign for the eradication of hookworm in the southern states of the United States of America.

As noted by Siqueira (Revista Brasilieira de Malariologia, 17: 83, 1965), Lutz described differences between the Brazilian hookworm and the European hookworm in 1888, but failed to classify it as a new species.

Stiles' original description of Necator americanus as a new species causing human disease follows.

Engaged upon a study of hookworms (genus *Uncinaria*), I requested Dr. Thomas A. Claytor, of Washington, D. C., and Dr. Allyn J. Smith, of

Galveston, Texas, to furnish me with some specimens from their recent cases of uncinariasis in man. Dr. Smith kindly sent me some material (B. A. I., No. 3,310) which I promptly examined, and noticing that the worms did not agree with the common form, *Uncinaria duodenalis,* but were much more closely related to *Uncinaria stenocephala* of the dog, I communicated with him again to inquire whether the parasites in question were actually from a man or from a dog. He has replied that they were from a man.

In connection with Dr. Claytor's case, which occurred in this city last summer, I had made a microscopic examination of the feces and had called Dr. Claytor's attention to the fact that the eggs did not agree with the measurements usually given for *U. duodenalis,* but it did not occur to me on a superficial examination of the parasites in question that they might represent a new species. Dr. Claytor has recently very kindly furnished me with some adult worms (B. A. I., No. 6,612), and I find that these agree with the specimens forwarded by Dr. Smith, and also with hookworms of man collected by Dr. Bailey K. Ashford in Porto Rico.

These parasites differ from all of the members of the genus *Uncinaria* which I can find recorded, and on that account I propose to base a new species, *Uncinaria americana,* upon them.

In order to determine the frequency of this species in man, I would request physicians who treat cases of uncinariasis to forward to me specimens of the parasites for determination. The characters of the two species which occur in man may be seen from the following diagnoses:

Genus *Uncinaria* Frölich, 1789.

Generic Diagnosis. —Sclerostominae with anterior extremity curved dorsally; mouth round to oval, opening obliquely, limited by a transparent border and followed by a chitinous buccal capsule; the dorsal portion of the capsule is shorter than the ventral, and is supported by a conical structure, the point of which sometimes extends into the cavity; at the base of the buccal capsule are found two ventral teeth; toward the inner free border the ventral wall bears on each side of the median line chitinous structures or teeth, often recurved in shape of hooks; the inner dorsal wall may also bear teeth.

Type Species. —*Uncinaria vulpis* Frölich, 1789, in *Canis vulpes.*

Old-world hookworm, *U. duodenalis* (Dubini, 1843) Railliet, 1885, of man.

Specific Diagnosis. —Body cylindric, somewhat attenuated anteriorly. Buccal cavity with two pairs of ventral teeth curved like hooks; and one pair of dorsal teeth directed forward; dorsal conical tooth not projecting into the capsule.

Male: Eight to 11 mm long; caudal bursa with dorsomedian lobe, and prominent lateral lobes united by a ventral lobe; dorsal ray divides at a point two-thirds its length from its base, each branch being tridigitate; spicules long and slender.

Female: Ten to 18 mm long; vulva at or near posterior third of body.

Eggs: Ellipsoid, 52 by 32μ, laid in segmentation. Development direct without intermediate host.

Habitat. —In small intestines, chiefly in upper part, of man (*Homo sapiens*).

New-world hookworm, *U.* (*Monodontus*) *americana* Stiles, 1902, of man.

Specific Diagnosis.—Differs from *U. duodenalis* chiefly in the following characteristics: Ventral recurved hook-like teeth are absent from the mouth, their place being taken by a pair of semilunar plates, somewhat similar to *U. stenocephala.* Dorsal conical tooth projects prominently into the buccal capsule.

Male: Dorsal ray of caudal bursa divided to its base, each branch being bipartite at its tip.

Female: Vulva in anterior half of body, but near the equator.

Eggs: Slightly larger, 64 to 72μ by 36 to 40μ, in some cases partially segmented, in others containing fully-developed embryo when oviposited.

Type Host. —Man (*Homo sapiens*), at Galveston, Texas.

Type Specimen. —No. 3,310 B. A. I., U. S. Department of Agriculture.

A more complete description of this species will appear in a later paper, but the above is sufficient to distinguish *U. americana* from any other form of this group thus far described. It will be seen to differ radically from *U. duodenalis,* and to approach *U. stenocephala* of dogs in some characters and *U. cernua* of sheep in others.

From the above discussion it is clear that at least two species of hookworms (*U. duodenalis* and *U. americana*) contribute to the disease uncinariasis in man. *U. duodenalis* is known to be an old-world form, and the indications are that it has been introduced into this country. *U. americana* is known to occur in Texas, in Virginia, and in Porto Rico, and this wide geographic separation shows very clearly that in the new world we have a special, heretofore undescribed parasite which causes uncinariasis. This further indicates very strongly the correctness of the view that uncinariasis is endemic in the southern states, although it is rarely recognized.

The new parasite of man appears to be a member of the group for which Molin proposed the generic name *Monodontus*. Railliet has recently recognized several genera to hold the representatives of the generally recognized genus *Uncinaria*, but I am inclined to reserve opinion for the present upon their validity.

OBSERVATIONS ON THE ETIOLOGY AND TREATMENT OF THE ANEMIA OF HOOKWORM DISEASE IN PORTO RICO

Journal of Clinical Investigation, 11: 809, 1932 (Abstract from 24th annual meeting).

Cornelius Packard Rhoads
(1898–1959)

During a surgical residency at Peter Bent Brigham Hospital under Harvey Cushing, Rhoads developed pulmonary tuberculosis. After convalescence at the Trudeau Sanatorium, he decided to study pathology and returned to the Boston City Hospital. In 1929 he was invited to work under Simon Flexner at the Rockefeller Institute and was appointed pathologist to its hospital in 1931. He continued at Rockefeller until 1940, when he succeeded James Ewing as director of the Memorial Hospital and also became professor of pathology at Cornell Medical College. His personal dedication and zeal were responsible for the formation of the Sloan-Kettering Institute.

William Bosworth Castle
(1897–   )

The discoverer of the relationship between vitamin B12 deficiency and pernicious anemia, Castle was a native of Cambridge, Massachusetts, and a 1921 graduate of Harvard Medical School. After 18 months as a medical house pupil at Massachusetts General Hospital he joined the Department of Physiology at Harvard Medical School. In 1925 he went to the Thorndike Memorial Laboratory at Boston City Hospital under Dr. Francis Peabody and later Dr. George Minot. For eight months, in 1931 and 1932, Castle was the director of the Rockefeller Foundation Commission for study of anemia in Puerto Rico. He returned to Harvard Medical School and held several distinguished chairs. In 1968 he became faculty professor emeritus of Harvard University.

Ashford felt that iron was ineffective in the treatment of hookworm anemia. Castle had recently elucidated the role of achlorhydria and intrinsic factor in pernicious anemia, and George C. Shattuck at the Harvard Medical School encouraged Castle to focus his attention on the anemia of hookworm in Puerto Rico. Rhoads and Castle collaborated in this study of the role of iron deficiency in hookworm infection.

Study of over 150 cases of hypochromic anemia associated with hookworm infestation demonstrated that the morphological and physiological characteristics of this anemia are similar to those of other hypochromic anemias without hookworm infection encountered both in Porto Rico and elsewhere, and regarded as mainly due to defective blood formation. No evidence for the presence of substances due to the activity of the hookworm capable of acting either as depressors of blood production or as hemolytic agents was found. Since it was demonstrated that the intramuscular injection of red blood cells into these patients produced increased blood formation, it is logical to assume that the effect of blood loss produced by the hookworm may be significant as a loss of potential hematopoietic factors leading to defective blood formation.

No significant effect upon the anemia was produced during periods of from two to three weeks and frequently for longer periods either by the elimination of the hookworms or by the administration of a diet enriched by 300 grams of meat and 1500 cc of milk daily or by a combination of these. On the other hand, the daily administration of 6 grams of iron ammonium citrate was almost invariably followed by promptly increased blood formation indicated by reticulocyte crises followed by rapid increases of red blood cell and hemoglobin values and general clinical improvement, despite the persistence of heavy hookworm infestation and the original deficient diet. Substances containing the extract of liver described by Whipple and his associates as of value in hemorrhagic-dietary anemias in the dog were somewhat effective but never as effective as iron in the dosage employed; the liver extract described by Cohn, Minot and their associates as effective in pernicious anemia was found to be without effect. Since in studying these cases of hookworm anemia deficient diets were found to be the rule and gastric anacidity a frequent finding, as is the case in hypochromic anemias not associated with the hookworm, it is suggested that dietary deficiency and gastro-intestinal changes are of major etiological significance.

CHAPTER **15**

Strongyloidiasis

ON A DISEASE CALLED "DIARRHEA OF
COCHIN CHINA"

Sur la maladie dite diarrhée de Cochinchine. Comptes Rendus
Hebdomadaires des Seances de l'Academie des Sciences, 83:
316–318, 1876. Translated from the French.

Louis Alexis Normand
(1834–1885?)

*The son of a music teacher in Clermont, Normand
enrolled in the Naval Medical School and became surgeon first class in 1865. He completed his examinations at the national faculty in Paris in 1869. He
traveled extensively, especially to Indochina, where he
made his observations on strongyloidiasis. In 1870 he
was appointed port physician in Toulon and retired
there in 1880. It is presumed that he died there in
1885.*

*The relationship between Cochin China diarrhea
and infection with* Strongyloides stercoralis *is recorded
in this paper.*

[The following are excerpts from a letter addres-
sed to the President (presumably of the Academy
of Sciences) by Vice-Admiral Jurien de la
Gravière; his direct quotations from Normand appear in italics—Eds.]

Dr. Normand, physician first class in the
Navy, presented to the academy toward the end
of June a confidential report which summarized
the discovery of a frightening disease which
causes great damage to our troops and crews in
Cochin China. On 3 July, a new group of patients
arrived at Toulon, making it possible for Dr.
Normand, with the assistance of Dr. Bavay, professor of pharmacy in the Navy, to conduct investigations to confirm his first impressions about
the disease.

*"Today, in regard to the disease called diar-
rhea of Cochin China, I can prove that from time
to time and most often in serious cases, a parasite
is found which has never been found before under
similar circumstances. I searched in vain for this
parasite in other patients afflicted with analogous
symptoms but their afflictions apparently came
from other sources."*

It is of great importance to make known the
nature of this disease which afflicts about one
thousand people every year and to clarify its
diagnosis.

The parasite, about 1/4 mm in length, was discovered and classified under a new order by Dr.
Normand, and was named *Anguillula stercoralis*
by Dr. Bavay. It is visible to the unaided eye. If a
prepared slide is examined under the microscope
at a magnification of 50x to 60x, a considerable
number of these worms are seen squirming and
moving about violently inside the more or less
transparent mass in which they are imprisoned.
The parasite lives in the intestinal tissue; it is
possible that the glands of the intestine are its first
host. Normand frequently saw the animal thrust
itself against the capsule from which it was trying
to escape. This covering appeared to be an
agglomeration of nucleated bodies forming irregular cylinders; it is longer than the worm and
larger in diameter because in its search for an
opening, the parasite could fold over to the opposite side of the capsule only to encounter again
the object that opposed its exit; as its attempts
were futile, it would resume its previous position.
The nuclei which had accumulated around the
covering disappeared gradually in small masses
as though they had been shaken off by the worm.
The covering seemed to be made of a totally
transparent substance; by looking through it
sideways, one could distinguish the internal organs of the parasite. After a successful effort, the
animal escaped from the shell which subsequently assumed the appearance of a flexible,

transparent tube that had suffered some folding. Meanwhile, the worm moved about with great vigor. The internal organs appeared extremely clear and empty, significantly different from the tube from which the worm had been liberated earlier.

"*Among other observations which I made frequently,*" Dr. Normand added, "*is the following: A worm having the cephalic end caught in a mass of epithelial cells was shaking its head vigorously in all directions in order to free itself. This spectacle which I observed for ten minutes or so can be likened to a dog caught in a net trying furiously to get out.*"

Some patients who are afflicted with diarrhea of Cochin China suffer a less intense infection; the causal agent disappears quickly, the destructive lesions are less serious, less extensive; recovery comes quickly if the patient follows a rational diet. Milk is very helpful in this disease since it suppresses the mucus rapidly. Symptoms of this illness do not persist if the patient follows this treatment and specific diet.

Other patients, more heavily infected, relapse easily, even after the diarrhea has been arrested. The worm is still present and continues its devastation, with new "hatchings" [sic] occurring each day.

The intestine cannot function physiologically; it becomes impossible to continue the milk diet; the feces indicate lientery which contributes to general weakness; occasionally protein foods are completely undigested. After some time, more than a year after infection, the patient may recover. The diarrhea sometimes ceases suddenly and, little by little, if the patient lives in sanitary conditions, he recovers a degree of vigor and weight. At other times, the disease evolves progressively into a terminal condition. This third group of patients develops enterocolitis, either after an intense infection or after a long period of alternating recovery and relapse. An abuse of liquids or foods, a variation in the temperature of the intestine, causes an increase in mucus throughout the intestine; thus inflammation develops analogous to that which accompanies a serious dysenteric infection; and in a few hours, the patient is dead.

At other times the process is less rapid and may become entirely chronic. The patient, having fought for a long time against the effects of diarrhea, develops an extreme marasmus and suc-

cumbs, due to anemia. More often, respiration ceases after a few hours of struggle.

Does this abridged paper offer a therapeutic treatment? Until now, milk has been the only reputedly efficacious agent. Twenty times Dr. Normand produced rapid cure of cases which had been subjected to an unwise regimen; however, in those cases in which the symptoms were severe and intense, there was greater resistance.

The microscope revealed immediately whether it was a matter of persistent infection or the effect of parasitism. If the patient does not have any more parasites, therapy is based exclusively on alleviating the irritation and relieving the patient of his discomfort. If the parasitic infection persists, other agents will have to be used.

"*I hope,*" said Normand in conclusion, "*that the facts which I have accumulated will be disseminated rapidly and that some other colleague, more fortunate than I will find a parasiticide which can be employed in these rebellious cases. I would like to try mineral waters; at the moment I am experimenting with santonin, mercury, and arsenic; I expect to try next the essential oils, the sulfurs, and quinine without neglecting hygienic and dietary considerations which will enable the individual, exhausted by the fight to expel the parasite and later to repair the damage that it caused.*"

ON THE TYPE AND PURPOSE OF THE INVASION OF *ANGUILLULA INTESTINALIS* INTO THE INTESTINAL WALL

Ueber art und zweck der invasion der *Anguillula intestinalis* in die darmwand. Centralblatt für Bakteriologie und Parasitenkunde und Infektionskrankheiten, Abteilung I. Originale, 27: 569–578, 1900. Selections from pp. 569–571, 573–578. Translated from the German.

Max Askanazy
(1865–1940)

Born in Stallrpönen, Germany, Askanazy studied medicine at Königsberg. After a distinguished career as the occupant of the chair of pathology at the University of Königsberg, Askanazy became director of the Institute of Pathology at Geneva in 1905, a post he held for 35 years. In addition to his contributions to the knowledge of Strongyloides, *he pursued investigations in such disparate areas as diseases of the blood, of the parathyroid gland, and of the teeth.*

The pathologic changes of the small intestine in strongyloidiasis are superbly documented in this article.

In various scientific fields, a preconceived idea often becomes an established dogma which, being difficult to trace to its source, can impede the advancement of knowledge. The view that insignificant plant microorganisms are capable of penetrating the living tissue of highly organized mammals, even that of man, and utilizing such a complicated organism, intended for the most delicate biological achievements as a simple culture medium, did not find easy acceptance. Did one not harbor, along with other doubts, a certain reluctance to recognize generically related microbes of saprophytes vegetating on dead organic matter as active intruders into the living animal body? Today it has been established about many infections that certain bacteria do not proliferate on specific disease products as well as on other organic material, but rather that the disease products themselves are formed because the particular bacteria proliferate in the body. This same reluctance to ascribe to lower forms of life the capability of active invasion into animal and human tissues still holds true for the most part in the case of parasites. The hypothesis that intestinal parasites live exclusively in the intestinal lumen and feed on feces is so old that many do not even ask for proof any more. One could see exceptions to this rule in cases such as *Echinorhynchus* and *Ancylostoma duodenale* which obviously penetrate the parenchyma of the intestinal wall. My own investigations have led me to the conclusion that the female intestinal trichinae also migrate into the intestinal mucosa and submucosa, subsequently depositing their young there, particularly in the associated lymphatic vessels; the young are then carried away from the intestine by the lymph. The possibility that female intestinal trichinae absorb at least some juices from the tissues for their nourishment naturally cannot be excluded. These observations concerning intestinal trichinosis then suggested the following question: What is the relationship of the other entozoas of the intestinal tract to its wall? My thoughts went first to the whipworm whose relationship to the wall of the cecum has become the object of a lengthy discussion. With the help of serial sections I was able to prove that the trichocephali, males and females, can pene-

trate into the upper layer of the mucosa of the appendix. The impetus for this invasion into the living tissue of the host is, in all probability, their need for nourishment. This was substantiated by the fact of the constant presence of iron-containing pigment in their intestinal epithelia— as well as the red-yellow diffuse coloring of their body, which is noticed at times and which resembles the color of hemoglobin—as a result of the nourishing of the whipworm by the absorption of blood, or at least blood pigment, from the intestinal wall. That blood-sucking round worms store such iron-containing pigment in their intestinal epithelium can be demonstrated in the case of lung parasites of the frog and toad (*Angiostomum nigrovenosum* and *rubrovenosum*). These experiments prompted my statement and warning: "The relationship of the other intestinal parasites to the intestinal wall will have to be kept in mind." A favorable opportunity to pursue this question so important for an understanding of the biology of entozoas and their parasitic activity in the intestine was provided by a case of infection with *Anguillula* (strongyloides) *intestinalis*.

In June of 1899 a sick forester was treated in the local Medical Clinic of Privy Councilor Lichtheim; during his careful examination the presence of large numbers of larvae of *A. intestinalis* was detected in the stool. The patient, a drinker, had been suffering for a long time from diarrhea which was reported to have been occasionally bloody. In the autopsy performed on 19 June, four and a half hours after death, I discovered a left lateral bronchial cancer with metastases to the liver and left adrenals, a chronic interstitial inflammation of the kidney, hypertrophy of the left ventricle, and bronchopneumonic foci in the right lung. The following observations were made with regard to the gastrointestinal tract: Under the microscope, young, motile *Anguillulae* could still be recognized in the bile-stained contents of the stomach. The mucosa was, on the whole, slightly thickened, somewhat uneven, and contained several small hemorrhages, especially at the fundus. The contents of the small intestine consisted of bile-stained pulpy mucus and showed, on microscopic examination, large, mature specimens of the parasite as well as numerous young, active *Anguillulae*. In the duodenum (in which a finger-sized diverticulum was found on the posterior wall) and in the jejunum, where several small-to-lentil-sized,

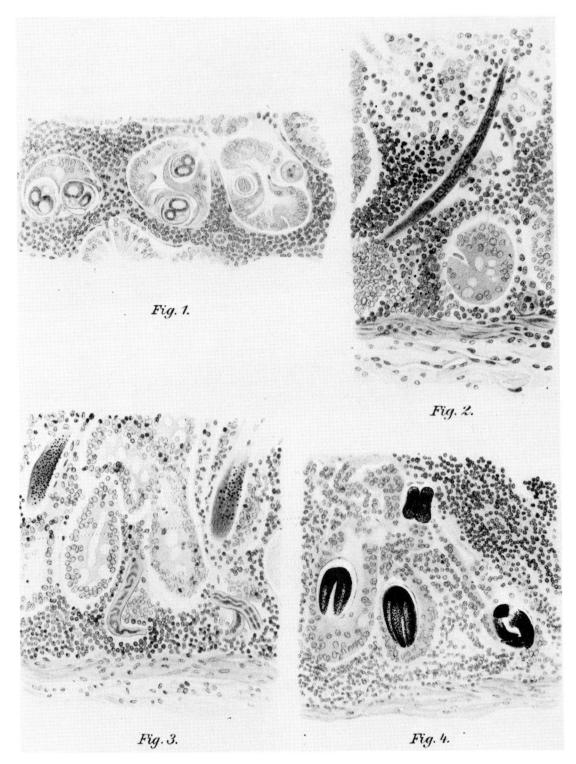

Fig. 1.

Fig. 2.

Fig. 3.

Fig. 4.

white chylangiomata were observed, the mucosa appeared unchanged and pale. In the ileum, the mucosa, except for slight congestion, was free of changes. The mucosa on the ileocoecal valve appeared pseudomelanotically pigmented; similarly, in the colon ascendens the mucosa was gray and a few, very small, almost black round polyps were present in the folds of the mucosa. In the rest of the colon the mucosa showed only slight hyperemia while in the rectum it again was a pseudomelanotic gray, and three pea-size polyps were found. The brown content of the large intestine contained numerous moving *Anguillula* larvae.

A more careful examination of the morphology of the *A.* (strongyloides) *intestinalis* has been made by Professor Braun in conjunction with this case and reported on in this journal (Vol. 26, No. 20/21, p. 612) with the inclusion of characteristic drawings. I concentrated only on the investigation of the following question: What relationship does *A. intestinalis* have to the intestinal wall? For this purpose the intestine was opened, as usual, lengthwise along the root of the mesentery. Then, before the surface of the mucosa was touched in any way, 14 pieces were cut and removed from various sections of the intestinal tract together with the adhering intestinal mucus and carefully placed in a solution of Flemming's chromosmium acetic acid containing 4 per cent formaldehyde. This method, used in earlier analogous studies, has proved very satisfactory to me. The pieces were hardened in alcohol, thoroughly saturated with celloidin, and cut. Flemming safranine was used for staining the fixed specimens; for those specimens treated with formaldehyde, hematoxylin, and hemalum were used. . . .

What is the relationship between the tissue of the mucosa and the position of the parasites? First it must be emphasized that the whole area of the mucosa can be attacked by parasites and that it is possible to encounter the worms in large numbers from the tip of the villi to the base of the mucosa, up to the muscularis. Naturally, they are observed most frequently in the region of the Lieberkühn glands from which form the main mass of the mucosa. Some of them settle in the lumen of the crypts; however, remarkably, the majority seem to make their way, from the very beginning, through the epithelial gland walls. Hence, even though Golgi and Monti have already found the parasites under discussion in the lumen of the crypts of Lieberkühn, this finding is not of decisive importance for an understanding of the active progress of *Anguillula* into the tissues of the intestinal wall, since these lumina represent only a direct continuation of the intestinal cavity itself. In my opinion, the uniqueness of the invasion process relates to the fact that the animals do not choose the apparently easy way into the open portion of the glands but instead crawl with remarkable skill and pronounced predilection through the structures of the gland epithelia. This observation has been consistently repeated at various points along the intestinal canal, and it is strange when, on longitudinal section, one sees the body of the worm threaded right through the middle of the epithelial seam or where, as in Plate 48, Fig. 1, the transversely pictured body of the parasite is covered or surrounded like a capsule by the epithelia. . . .

In addition, the parasites, especially the young ones, are sometimes encountered between the gland epithelium and the stroma, that is, the tunica propria; finally they are encountered at times in the stroma itself, either between the glands or directly above the muscularis mucosae (Plate 48, Fig. 3) which is in direct contact with the parasites at a few points. Also there is no lack of worms which lie stretched transversely or obliquely across the middle of the gland. Naturally, exact distinction cannot always be expected of the boundary between gland epithelium and connective tissue. Occasionally, small groups of young worms were found in an otherwise empty, rounded cavity in the floor of the mucosa which resembled the cross-section of a lymph vessel. After observing large numbers of *Anguillula* in the tissues of the mucosa on prepared sections, I

Plate 48. Fig. 1. Cross-section of *Anguillula* mother worm in the epithelium of Lieberkühn glands, lying on the right between epithelium and stroma. *Fig. 2.* A young larva lies in part already embedded in the mucosa, with the posterior portion of the body protruding into the intestinal lumen. *Fig. 3.* In the upper layer of the mucosa lie two fat droplets containing mother worms in glands; in the lower region of the mucosa are young animals above the muscularis mucosae. Plentiful aggregates of lymphoid round cells on the floor of the mucosa. *Fig. 4.* Four worms, because of their content of chyle fat stained deep black, lie predominantly in the epithelium of Lieberkühn crypts. Infiltration of the mucosa with small round cells.

found that, as a rule, the muscularis mucosae seemed to check further penetration of the parasite. Only once did I see a young larva which had reached the submucosa. It was encountered fully stretched out, with its body in the mucosa reaching down to an engorged blood vessel lying under the mucosa. The intestinal parasites invading the mucosa can occasionally penetrate into the submucosa as has already been proven. Bilharz, Griesinger, Grassi, and Prowe found *Ancylostoma duodenale* in submucous cysts of the intestinal wall, and I have also found an intestinal trichina in a submucous lymph vessel. With regard to *Anguillula,* O. Leichtenstern, after hearing of my findings, kindly informed me that in 1885, in the first autopsy of a pertinent case, he not only encountered *Anguillula* mother worms free in the intestinal mucus and in the crypts of Lieberkühn, but also in the submucosa; these findings have not been published. On the basis of my numerous preparations, however, I would consider penetration into the submucosa as a rare occurrence, as compared to the invasion of other intestinal parasites. The worms primarily occupy the mucosa.

Is the invasion of living intestinal wall tissue by *A. intestinalis,* as just described, a vital process, or is it perhaps a purely post-mortem phenomenon? We may refute the notion that invasion of the parasites occurred only after death on the basis of the following considerations. First, let it be remembered that the examination was carried out on material prepared a few hours after death; further that I demonstrated strikingly similar pathology of intestinal trichinosis in the intestine obtained from live animals under ether anesthesia. Our experiences concerning the relationship of the whipworm to the mucosa demonstrate that these parasites would rather leave than reside in or penetrate the intestinal wall of their dead host. Finally, it is important to note that the parasites did not wander aimlessly through the tissues but were found only within certain limits and that the mucosa of the lower small intestine and particularly the large intestine, in the lumina of which there was truly no lack of *Anguillula* larvae, were completely free of invading parasites post-mortem (and probably also *intra vitam*).

Therefore, if we conceive of the process of invasion into the living intestinal tissue as an active penetration by *Anguillula,* the following question arises: For what purpose do the animals undertake such an attack on the intestinal walls of their host? A favorable incidental observation in our case puts us in a position to give a definite answer. The osmic acid of the Flemming acid mixture has shown on the microscopic sections of the intestinal wall a pronounced lymph stasis in which the chyle stood out significantly by black staining from the central villus vessel and the villus stroma up to the submucosa. However, an unexpected and at first extraordinarily striking effect of the osmic acid appeared on the parasites themselves in the intestinal wall. The animals were stained deep black in large numbers so that even at very weak magnifications they were readily apparent in the region of the mucosa (Fig. 4). Often the cross-sections of the worms were almost as black as ink, stained as deeply black as the occasional fat cells lying in the submucosa. On somewhat stronger magnifications there remained no doubt that the deep black stained forms in the mucosa corresponded to the body of the worm which was often rolled together and wound up. Worms were also found whose body had first taken on a gray stain, and while the rosy ground tone of the parasite body tinted by safranine faded more and more, the black stain became more and more profound. On viewing with high power and immersion lenses it could be ascertained clearly that the black color was due to a layer of very fine, black granules. Undoubtedly this black staining can be explained by an intake of chyle by the invading parasites. This simultaneous demonstration of chyle in the tissue and the lymph vessels of the intestinal tract by osmic acid permitted the easiest comparison and identification with the fine fat granules in the worm body. That it was not a question of fatty degeneration in a great number of worms was further evidenced by the lack of any other decomposition in the black-stained worms. This is also important because the first fat droplets were seen repeatedly in the intestinal epithelium of the mother worms at a time when the rest of the body did not include any fat droplets. Thus a purpose for the invasion by the *Anguillula* into the intestinal wall can be deduced immediately from our preparations. The animals penetrate the tissues of the intestinal wall in order to partake of the prepared food juices of man, the chyle. Perhaps their propensity for remaining in the upper small intestine is influenced by this consideration for their nourishment. One probably cannot consider the *A. intestinalis* as very benign for that reason. No positive data has been obtained so far as to whether the animals absorb blood; several iron stains made gave a negative result.

That the animals are not stationary in the mucosa but migrate within the mucosa is probably consonant with this tendency to look for a food source in the intestinal wall. This supposition is suggested by two observations. The first is more or less a negative one; namely, the lack of any kind of connective tissue proliferation which one might expect in the surroundings of a parasite embedded in living tissue. The second phenomenon is the presence of empty, abandoned, round bore holes or passages in the mucous membrane. One frequently notices round, sharply outlined gaps in the mucosa which correspond completely to the circumference of the bore passages filled with parasites. Some of the empty bore holes can probably be explained because in cross-sections the worms may have artificially fallen out from their position. Even with good celloidin saturation this cannot always be avoided and is evidenced by the presence of the displaced worm cross-sections above the area of the cut. But there are also many empty bore holes in places where such a subsequent falling out is not probable, and these indicate that a worm moved out from there a short time ago.

In these otherwise empty bore holes there are interesting formations which, since they do not belong to the tissues of the intestinal wall, must come from parasites. There are oval bodies which on comparison with the longitudinal sections of the mother worm are in complete conformity with respect to their size, shape, and color with the eggs lying in the mother's body. In Flemming preparations they appear brown, strongly granulated, also filled with individual fat droplets and then black granules; in formaldehyde sections they have a light, pale look and seem likewise granulated. Within the interior of these eggs no further components of the mother worms can be demonstrated, neither the covering of the genital tube nor the otherwise always plainly appearing body cuticula. In individual sections (serial sections especially) one recognizes the free position of the eggs in the mucosa. It is interesting that a

number of eggs are in the segmentation stage; one notices cross-sections of eggs which have segmented into two, four, and then into about a half dozen cells and finally changed into a convolution of numerous small cells with distinct, but palely stained nuclei and mulberry-shaped surface; in this the further arrangement in form of an embryonic body likewise is observed. In this way all stages from the yet unsegmented egg to the development of the grown embryo can be followed. The process of segmentation of the eggs suggests, by the way, their further free development in the mucosa, since the eggs in the genital organs of the mother animals showed no evidence of segmentation. There is no lack of young worms in the mucosa, but it is hard to decide whether they are embryos freed in the mucosa or penetrated young larvae, yet most of them probably emerged in the mucosa.

The thought that the embryo used the glands of the digestive canal as a nest was already held by Normand, who occasionally saw the embryo surrounded by epithelium. Golgi and Monti obtained further results; their work, which appeared in Italy, became known to me only after finishing my investigations. These authors report, as already mentioned, the presence of the *Anguillula* mother worms in the lumen of the Lieberkühn glands, in which just the worm part with the genital opening was seen to be embedded. They further saw, "*a ridosso delle cellule epiteliali*" in the floor of the glands many eggs, isolated, or in groups of 2–6 and were thus able to observe the segmentation phenomena up to the development of the larvae. That this report, as far as I know, has attracted no further notice is probably due to the fact that one cannot with certainty determine from this presentation whether the eggs really lie embedded in the middle of living tissue. If they are present, how do they get there if the mother worms stay only in the gland lumen? According to my investigations, it is clear that the *Anguillula* mother proceeds actively into the living tissue and that she leaves her eggs where the clear traces of the bore passages betray her. From the somewhat schematic illustration of Golgi and Monti I conclude that the eggs in their case were likewise present primarily in the epithelium since the eggs are drawn in place of missing epithelium in the gland wall. Yet the close relation of parasitic existence of the *Anguillula* to the epithelium and to the living tissue of the intestinal wall has not been recognized and appreciated by the authors at all—perhaps under the spell of old ideas.

The deposition of the eggs in the mucous membrane, by the way, explains the finding that occasionally very young worms (up to three adjacent) appear embedded free in the mucosa in wider, round bore passages having the circumference of the mother animal.

We can summarize the results of our investigations in the following way. The *A. intestinalis* bores into the intestinal wall, primarily into the mucosa and often into the epithelium of its glands, in order to absorb food, as is proven by the chyle ingestion of the worms. But in this connection the mother animals perform still another function, in that they deposit their eggs in the tissue of the mucous membrane. These eggs change into embryos which then emerge toward the intestinal lumen. If we pursue this concept a little further, it must first be emphasized that we have recognized in the *Anguillula* another nematode which is not afraid to penetrate actively into the living tissue of the human intestinal mucosa in order, like the whipworm, to seek its food and, like the intestinal trichina, to harbor its young appropriately. But while the intestinal trichina releases a good part of its living young into the lymph stream and thus directly into the inner part of the body, the *Anguillula* only deposits eggs; the young emerging therefrom migrate into the intestinal lumen where they are found massively in contrast to the young trichinae. . . .

The question at issue, whether the *A. intestinalis* can be counted among the real parasites, can easily be answered in the affirmative for the worm feeds on the juices of the human intestinal wall and deposits its offspring in the midst of living tissue. As I have explained, furthermore, trichinae which penetrate into the intestinal mucosa (or at times even into deeper intestinal wall layers) are rarely found in the stool; this holds true in the analogous way also for the mother worms of the *A. intestinalis* which also are not found in the stool. As I interpreted the extremely rare presence of young trichinae in the intestinal mucus and in the feces by their place of birth in the intestinal mucosa, the sparse occurrence of *Anguillula* eggs in the intestinal content agrees extremely well with their deposit in the parenchyma of the intestinal wall.

Thus it has been proved that the nematodes of man like *Ancylostoma duodenale,* whipworm, intestinal trichina, and *Anguillula intestinalis* represent not only intestinal, but also intestinal wall parasites, whereby their parasitologic position is characterized more precisely. It must not be forgotten in this connection that the *Ascaridae* are by no means above suspicion; that is, they also undertake excursions into the living intestinal wall. In an earlier article, I have already pointed out that there is iron-containing pigment in their intestinal epithelia and that there is a marked adaptation of their head for boring and gnawing activity. A few isolated reports are already at hand on defects found in the mucosa caused by *Ascaridae* in man, dog, and dolphin [sic]; in the latter, Guiart found in one of the defects, a complete head of a worm.

SOME OBSERVATIONS ON THE LARVAE OF *STRONGYLOIDES INTESTINALIS* AND THEIR PENETRATION THROUGH THE SKIN

Quelques notes sur les embryons de "Strongyloides intestinalis" et leur pénétration par la peau. Thompson Yates Laboratories Report, 4: 471–474, 1901–1902. Translated from the French.

Paul Van Durme
(1877–1947)

A native of Ghent, Van Durme received his medical degree with honors at the University of Ghent in 1901. He was working at the Liverpool School of Tropical Medicine at the time of this publication and received the diploma in 1902. He subsequently studied at the other centers of tropical medicine in London, Hamburg, and Marseilles before spending a year in the Läennec Clinic in Paris.

Nominated as professor of legal medicine in 1910, he became ordinary professor (including tropical disease) in 1919. A popular lecturer, he became emeritus professor in 1934 and retired.

The penetration of the skin by Strongyloides stercoralis *is beautifully reported in this paper.*

One of the most interesting questions in parasitology has recently been raised. We know that intestinal parasites enter the body of the host via the gastrointestinal tract, the eggs or embryos being swallowed with food and drink. This was the only mode of penetration known until the observations made by Dr. A. Looss in Cairo and by

Dr. C. A. Bentley in Assam alerted us to the possibility of another path of infection. . . .

Before demonstrating this fact, I think it might be useful to indicate briefly how I have obtained the larvae with which I did my experiments. The feces containing the eggs of *Strongyloides* came from a chimpanzee imported from Africa four months ago. Let us emphasize here a point worthy of note; the authors who studied *Anguillula* in man always found the embryos already hatched in the fresh stools, to which they attached diagnostic significance: that is, the eggs of *Uncinaria,* which could easily be confused with those of *Anguillula,* are always immature when evacuated. However, in my chimpanzee, as well as in four other infected monkeys, I have never found any embryos in the fresh excrement, but only unhatched eggs at various stages of segmentation. Nevertheless, all the other characteristics, form, dimensions, and evolution, were identical to those of the human parasite. To study the subsequent development of the eggs and embryos, I placed the feces, spread out on previously sterilized humid earth, in a Petri dish and maintained them at a temperature of about 25°C. The rhabditoid forms developed rapidly into male and female embryos which in turn gave birth to a new generation. This stage soon lost its rhabditoid character, each embryo being transformed into a strongyloid larva. Without dwelling for the moment on the life cycle of *Strongyloides intestinales,* let us say that, at different intervals, from the third day on, we could see some strongyloid larvae. This seems to confirm the observations of Grassi, Golgi, and Monti who affirm that this form can arise directly from the first rhabditoid embryo, without the intermediary of sexed individuals. The strongyloid larva is probably the final stage of extraparasitic life; indeed, from the seventh day on, one observes no more transformations. In some of my samples which were particularly well developed the number of larvae was enormous. Thus I had the opportunity several times to observe a curious phenomenon; one morning, I found contrasted against the dark bottom of one of my cultures about 30 whitish buds or sprigs, one to four mm in length. On examining them closely, one could detect undulating or gyratory movements; I can compare them only to minute feelers trying to catch hold of something along the way. They attached to rough surfaces especially, became immobile, and disappeared,

only to reappear a little later. The microscopic examination showed us that we were dealing with compact bundles of strongyloid larvae (Plate 49, Figs. 1 and 2). Transferred on the point of a needle to a drop of water, one of these buds dispersed into a milky cloud, a pure culture of larvae. The phenomenon became so intense for several days that all the crests and projections were covered by a creamy rim. The embryos at this stage are endowed with great activity: they rapidly traverse the microscopic field, displacing particles of every kind which surround them. Their power of resistance to external agents is far greater than that of rhabditiform embryos. Whereas the latter resist a weak solution of hydrochloric acid (two per cent) for only a few minutes, the strongyloid larvae preserve their motility for half a day. Placed in blood serum, they survive for several hours.

All of this suggested to us the idea of studying the actions of the embryos on the skin. The phenomenon described above greatly simplified the technique to follow; in effect, we did not have to isolate the larvae by complicated manipulations, at the risk of weakening their vitality. The abdominal region of a series of guinea pigs was washed and shaved, and a drop of pure culture was placed on the surface of the skin. For about ten minutes, one could follow with the lens the swarming mass scattering in different directions. We were careful to keep the skin damp for about a half hour. At the end of this time, a light erythema was visible at the point of inoculation. No more embryos could be found in epidermal scrapings under the microscope. Some hours later, the vascularization of the skin was very apparent. By the end of 24 hours, an oozing vesicular pustule had formed; at the same time, a desquamation of the epidermis appeared which lasted several days. We draw attention to the fact that the reaction occurs only at the spot where the emulsion has been placed; the rest of the surface remains intact. The phenomena described cannot be blamed on foreign mechanical irritations. One will note that the symptoms correspond to the disease state described by Bentley, under the name of "Pani-Ghao."

Strips of skin were excised and fixed after 30 minutes, one hour, and 20 hours. After a half-hour, the larvae are found already deeply engaged in the dermis. One encounters them most often in the areas surrounding the hair follicle, at

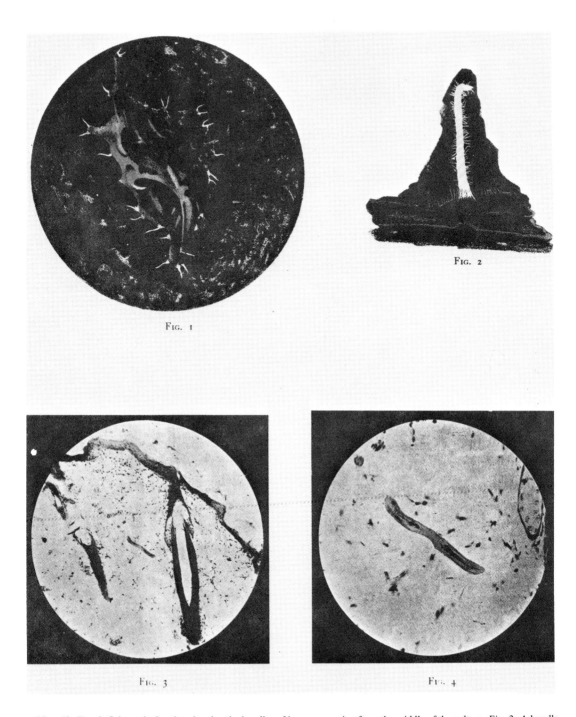

Fig. 1

Fig. 2

Fig. 3

Fig. 4

Plate 49. Fig. 1. Schematic drawing showing the bundles of larvae emerging from the middle of the culture. *Fig. 2.* A bundle magnified. *Fig. 3.* Cephalic extremity of an embryo engaged in the dermis. *Fig. 4.* The same view at a more powerful magnification.

the level of the sebaceous glands. We have not been able to find a whole embryo in these sections, but several times we have found the cephalic and caudal extremities, whose characteristic form leaves no doubt as to the nature of the foreign bodies (Plate 49, Figs. 3 and 4). The sections cut the larvae transversely, obliquely, and longitudinally. All the figures indicate that the cuticle is not perfectly smooth; four parallel folds, notably, run the length of the body of the embryo.

The fixed skin sections, after an hour, present fragments of larvae down to the subcutaneous areolar tissue.

Twenty hours after inoculation, all the larvae have not disappeared; although less numerous, they can be seen at different levels in the dermis. This fact is not astonishing: the embryos travel capriciously, sometimes retracing their route; thus one understands why all do not penetrate deeply.

Our preparations do not permit us to follow the worm's course during its peregrinations in the tissues; these tissues do not seem to be notably injured by its passage. Looss affirms that larvae penetrate through the hair follicles, having often found them there beside the hair. I have never found a single larva at this spot. Nevertheless, the mechanism indicated by Looss appears the most reasonable. While it must be admitted that the embryos actively force a path in the tissues, it is difficult to understand their buccal armature's being powerful enough to pierce the horny epidermal layer.

Can they arrive by this route in the intestine and there transform themselves into adult worms? The question is most interesting: its importance from the prophylactic point of view is inescapable. I would like to have completed my research on this subject, but being obliged to interrupt it, I thought it useful to add a second parasite to the list begun by Looss with *Uncinaria*. . . .

STUDIES OF THE ROUTE OF INFECTION OF *STRONGYLOIDES* AND *ANCYLOSTOMA* AND THE BIOLOGY OF THESE PARASITES

Untersuchungen über den infektionsweg bei strongyloides und ankylostomum und die biologie dieser parasiten. Archiv für Schiffs und Tropenhygiene, 18: 26–80, 1914. Selections from pp. 49–53, 55–62. Translated from the German.

Friedrich Fülleborn
(1866–1933)

Fülleborn received his doctorates in medicine as well as in philosophy and natural sciences from the University of Berlin. During and after his student days, he worked in the laboratory of Rudolf Virchow. He was interested in many phases of science, including ornithology, geology, and anthropology. In 1894 he spent some time studying the fauna of North America.

From 1896 to 1900 he served as a military surgeon in German East Africa and thus had the opportunity to study the natural history of that continent and the diseases of the region.

In 1901 he returned to Germany and began a lifelong association with the Institute for Naval and Tropical Diseases in Hamburg. He was also appointed extraordinary professor at the newly established University of Hamburg. Although he was an inspired and dedicated teacher, he finally decided that his educational activities were occupying time and draining energies that might better be devoted to research. His investigations in the field took him to China, India, and the entire Western Hemisphere. In 1930, Fülleborn became director of the Hamburg Institute and full professor at the University of Hamburg, and he held these posts until his death.

Fülleborn used the basic discoveries of Grassi, Askanazy, Looss, and Ransom to complete his work. The demonstration of the life cycle of Strongyloides *and the speculation about external autoinfection is found in this classic paper. His clinical acumen is evident in the description of external autoinfection in his second paper.*

Research on the Migration of the *Strongyloides* and *Ancylostoma* Larvae in the Body of the Host

The route of migration of *Ancylostoma* and *Strongyloides* larvae from cutaneous penetration to the lung has been clarified by Looss and is universally accepted so that repetition can be spared. . . .

Looss, accordingly, in his last paper, based on Lambinet and Schaudinn, maintained that 90 per cent of the larvae reach the intestine by the tracheo-esophageal route; at the same time he refused to exclude the possibility that *Ancylostoma* larvae, after traversing the entire lung, can enter the greater circulation, reaching their natural destination in one way or another (he found larvae in the pulmonary veins as well as the arteries of the trachea and peritracheal tissue).

A quantitative answer to the question of how many of the larvae applied to the skin migrate through the tracheo-esophageal route cannot be computed exactly. From our experience only a portion of the larvae applied to the skin survive the prolonged migration to the lung and then, somehow, eventually reach the intestine.

On the other hand, another experimental approach was possible; namely, the disruption of the tracheo-intestinal route through surgical intervention and the comparison of such animals after infection with normal animals who were similarly infected. The numerous investigations utilizing proximal fistulas of the small bowel failed because of the early death of the dog, while the trachea or esophagus could be sectioned surgically without difficulty.

If the route of infection occurred exclusively by tracheo-esophageal passage, then intestinal infection should fail to appear after tracheal or esophageal resection; if, however, it did occur, then infection might take place by another route.

The experiments have shown that after division of the tracheo-esophageal passage a slight intestinal infection developed. In all probability this occurred by entrance into the greater circulation via the pulmonary vessels, especially in severe *Strongyloides* infections which are always associated with the presence of filariform larvae in the kidney; they evidently, on the basis of pathologic findings, reached this location embolically. Nevertheless, it must be demonstrated that larvae reaching the intestinal wall embolically are capable of penetrating into the lumen. . . . That larvae, which were embolized to the intestinal vessels, penetrated and infected the intestine, was demonstrated in an experiment in which tracheal mucus from both a percutaneously infected dog and a tracheotomized dog was injected into a duodenal artery with the subsequent production of a massive *Strongyloides* infection.

The route of infection after cutaneous penetration by the larvae, as described by Looss, has been confirmed since I, as well as others, followed the *Ancylostoma* and *Strongyloides* larvae through their entire course from the trachea to the intestine. A small proportion of the larvae evidently (according to Sambon) reached the small intestine from the lung via the pulmonary veins, left heart, and intestinal arteries.

In *Strongyloides* this result was surprising, since previous experiments had shown that the excess filariform larvae often smothered in the stomach lumen while those which penetrated the

walls survived. Why, then, don't filariform larvae die when they descend to the intestine via the esophagus and stomach after percutaneous infection? Parallel tests in tracheotomized dogs showed different results if the dogs were fed with filariform larvae directly extracted from fecal cultures or with lung material from other dogs previously infected percutaneously. In the first instance, the resulting infection was minimal; in the latter, a severe intestinal infection occurred. Therefore, in spite of only a slight morphological difference, the filariform larvae of the lung are already altered biologically; this is evident not only by their tolerance to stomach passage but also by the change in their penetrating ability. . . .

Experiments Regarding the Migration of *Strongyloides* and *Ancylostoma* Larvae After Percutaneous Infection

Percutaneous Infection after Tracheotomy

4 July 1911. A dog free of *Ancylostoma* and *Strongyloides,* as determined by culture of its feces, underwent tracheotomy. Both proximal and distal ends were closed so that between the laryngeal and pulmonary sections a gap was produced which was several centimeters wide; a double cannula (as used in human tracheotomies) was used, with the outer discs sutured to the skin.

On the same day between 3:00 and 4:00 P.M. the shaved neck skin which the dog's tongue could not reach was infected percutaneously with large numbers of *Strongyloides* larvae and a few *Ancylostoma* larvae. After penetration of the larvae, the skin was first cleaned with cotton and water and then with alcohol and ether and finally was covered with collodion.

5 July 1911. At 10:00 A.M. no larvae were found in the tracheal mucus. To test the short-necked dog's inability to reach the tracheal wound—a drop of dilute hydrochloric acid on the wound caused restlessness; however, the dog did not even attempt to lick the wound—he was given a muzzle which was removed only at feeding times.

6 July 1911. Today one *Ancylostoma* larva was found in the tracheotomy mucus.

7 July 1911. The viscid tracheotomy mucus contained a large number of *Strongyloides,* some of which were molting.

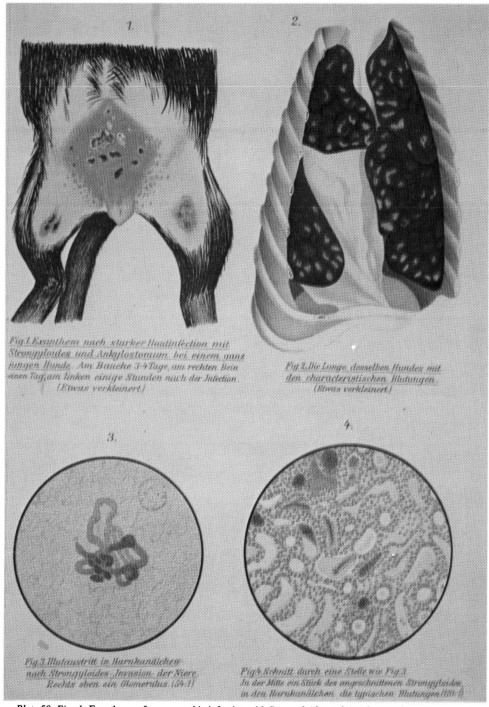

Fig.1.Exanthem nach starker Hautinfection mit
Strongyloides und Ankylostomum bei einem ganz
jungen Hunde. Am Bauche 3-4 Tage, am rechten Bein
einen Tag, am linken einige Stunden nach der Infection.
(Etwas verkleinert)

Fig.2.Die Lunge desselben Hundes mit
den characteristischen Blutungen.
(Etwas verkleinert)

Fig.3.Blutaustritt in Harnkanälchen
nach Strongyloides Invasion der Niere.
Rechts oben ein Glomerulus. (54:1)

Fig.4.Schnitt durch eine Stelle wie Fig.3.
In der Mitte ein Stück des angeschnittenen Strongyloides,
in den Harnkanälchen die typischen Blutungen (176:1)

Plate 50. Fig. 1. Exanthema after severe skin infection with *Strongyloides* and *Ancylostoma* in a very young dog. On the abdomen 3–4 days, on the right leg one day, on the left a few hours after infection. *Fig. 2.* The lung of the same dog with the characteristic hemorrhages. *Fig. 3.* Blood extravasation in tubules after *Strongyloides* invasion of the kidney. A glomerulus in the upper right. *Fig. 4.* Section through an area like Fig. 3. In the middle, a piece of the cut *Strongyloides;* in the tubules, typical hemorrhages.

The *Strongyloides* larvae in the tracheotomy tube had almost all died; however, active live larvae were seen at the lower end of the trachea while none was present at the upper end. . . .

The landmarks of this experiment are:

Between the second and third to the fifth and sixth days after percutaneous infection, gradually decreasing numbers of *Strongyloides* and *Ancylostoma* larvae were found in the tracheotomy tube mucus; the *Strongyloides* were numerous, and the *Ancylostoma* were sparse.

In spite of the fact that the trachea was incised, *Strongyloides* rhabditiform larvae were found in the feces from the eighth day after infection (a few *Ancylostoma* eggs were found in the feces as seen in the continuation of this protocol on the 28th day after infection).

In the trachea, *Strongyloides* developed to the filariform female stage. They were numerous ten days after percutaneous infection and diminished gradually thereafter. (On the 23rd day after percutaneous infection the trachea was opened and only three filariform females were found).

Percutaneous Infection after Esophageal Section

8 July 1911. A terrier in whose feces no *Ancylostoma* or *Strongyloides* were found on culture was operated on in the afternoon to create an esophageal fistula by total incision of the esophagus. Then the dog was infected in the neck with copious amounts of *Strongyloides* and some *Ancylostoma*.

9 July 1911. In the saliva of the upper fistula opening there were no larvae.

10 July 1911. The dog was given water to drink which naturally emanated from the fistula. Numerous *Strongyloides* larvae were present in this water, but *Ancylostoma* larvae were not to be found. . . .

11 July 1911. Mucus from the upper esophageal fistula contains many *Strongyloides*.

12 July 1911. Like the previous day.

13 July 1911. In the mucus from the upper esophageal fistula there still are *Strongyloides*.

14 July 1911. In the mucus from the upper esophageal fistula no *Strongyloides* are found in ten preparations.

15 July 1911. In the mucus of the upper esophageal fistula there are no *Strongyloides;* feces, there are no rhabditic spawn (cultures of

feces of the 15 and 16 July are also negative). . . .

The findings in the esophageal fistula dog are quite analogous to that of the percutaneously infected tracheotomized dog; except for stragglers, *Strongyloides* filariforms emptied out from the third to the sixth day from the upper esophageal fistula opening while the sparser *Ancylostoma* larvae could not be found. On the eighth day post infection rhabditiform larvae originating from filariform females were found in the trachea; these decreased in number or were not detectable as of the 12th day. . . .

Even though the penetration of larvae from the upper to the lower esophageal section cannot be completely excluded in these experiments, they all show again and again that the majority of *Strongyloides* and *Ancylostoma* larvae are eliminated after interruption of the tracheo-esophageal tract but even so, a slight infection occurs.

The Path of the Larvae to the Intestine in Subacute Infection after Elimination of the Tracheoesophageal Tract

. . .To determine whether *Strongyloides* filariforms reached the intestinal vessels embolically after lung passage and were capable of developing to maturity, the following experiment was done.

9 August 1911. A dog whose feces proved to be free of *Strongyloides* and *Ancylostoma* by culture had a tracheotomy. Into a duodenal artery was then injected tracheal mucus containing copious *Strongyloides* and fewer *Ancylostoma* of another dog, previously infected percutaneously, which priorly had been carefully washed with NaCl.

13 and 14 August 1911. No rhabditiform larvae were seen in the feces. There was slight diarrhea.

15 August 1911. The dog which had an intestinal attack last night was killed; during the narcosis the intestines emptied themselves spontaneously and several rhabditiform larvae were found which continued to develop in the cultures. The lung was normal. The trachea contained much mucus, but even after thorough examination no worms were found in it. The small intestine contained copious mature filariform females at the spot where the duodenum was injected. In many

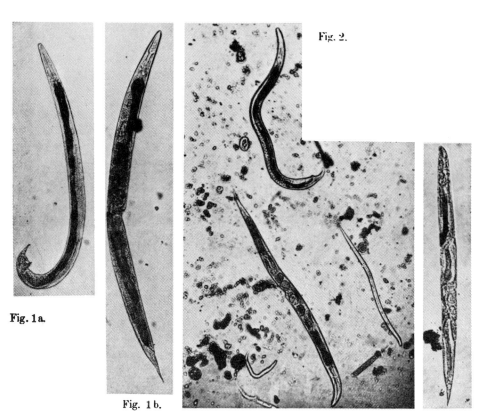

Fig. 1a.

Fig. 1b.

Fig. 2.

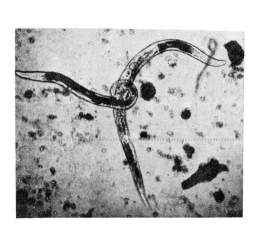

Fig. 3.

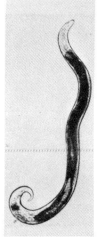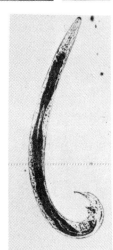

Fig. 4.

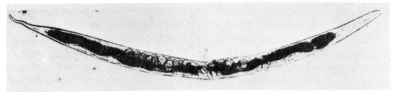

Fig. 5.

preparations there were four or five parasites, while the first portion of the duodenum (which as a rule is most infected) seemed to contain fewer larvae. . . .

This test proves that *Ancylostoma* or *Strongyloides* which reach the stomach embolically via the lung can become sexually mature *in loco*. . . .

Chief Results of the Series of Experiments on Percutaneous Infection

These proved that the normal route of infection of percutaneously penetrating *Ancylostoma* and *Strongyloides* was from lung to the intestine via trachea and esophagus. A small number of parasites, according to the experiments with *Strongyloides*, may pass from the lung veins and the left heart and reach the intestine by embolism via the intestinal arteries. Plates 50 and 51.

SKIN URTICARIA AND AUTOINFECTION IN *STRONGYLOIDES* CARRIERS

Hautquaddeln und ''Autoinfektion'' bei Strongyloidesträgern. Archive für Schiffs und Tropenhygiene, 30: 721–732, 1926. Selections from pp. 727–729. Translated from the German.

Friedrich Fülleborn
(1866–1933)

Fülleborn's biography appears with the preceding article.

Spontaneous Urticaria at the Buttocks in *Strongyloides* Carriers and Its Possible Association With New Infection

Of my ten most frequently observed *Strongyloides* carriers, eight state that occasionally they felt pruritus in the buttock area. The appearance was so characteristic that I was able to diagnose *Strongyloides* infection on this basis. According to the personal experiences of F. [Fülleborn referred to his patients by initials—Eds.], an irritating pruritus accompanying the urticaria occurs, intermittently, any time during the day

but especially during the night in bed. With rubbing and scratching of the skin the urticarial patches become so large that on F.'s very sensitive skin areas the size of a hand, at the buttocks, are indurated ''hard as a board'' with urticaria; at times, the urticaria extends to the waistline in bands one or two fingers wide.

Since urticaria appeared in the buttock regions in all eight cases, it was feasible to associate them with the presence in feces of the *Strongyloides* (not, to be sure, the rhabditiform phases, since they are incapable of penetrating the skin, but rather of the filariform larvae). But it is entirely possible that, after defecation, rhabditiform phases can develop into filariform larvae in the anal folds in residual fecal matter, particularly since I ascertained that at hatching oven temperature, as well as in the ''natural hatching oven'' of the anal folds, the filariform stage of *Strongyloides* larvae can be found after less than 24 hours. Thus, the continued development to filariform larvae can occur even in fastidious persons who bathe daily.

As a matter of fact, the very same appearance which was observed spontaneously on the buttocks of *Strongyloides* carriers can be produced experimentally in them with a small piece of damp gauze edged into the anal cleft. On the other hand, it appeared that precise cleanliness after each defecation and thorough washing of the anal area would lessen the frequency of the appearance of the urticaria. In a colleague returning from the tropics, these appeared only after he no longer had the opportunity of taking daily baths; in another of my cases, an unusually severe urticaria resulted following an appendix operation when the patient was prevented, because of the surgical dressing, from his daily anal washing. The penetration into the surrounding skin of filariform *Strongyloides* larvae, which developed in the anal cleft, not only causes urticaria but also must be a cause for permanent new infection of the *Strongyloides* carrier. It could also, as I presumed in 1914, perpetuate a *Strongyloides* infection of the intestine of humans. The case of Mr. Horr, which has been followed by me for 24

Plate 51. Fig. 1. Strongyloides from the dog; free-living rhabditoid male (a) and female (b). *Fig. 2. Strongyloides* from the dog. Rhabditoid male and female with brood, and a filariform larva. Next to this, from the same cultures (about 2 days old), a female with brood hatched inside. The animals of these cultures are strikingly small. *Fig. 3.* From culture like Fig. 2. Copulating animals. *Fig. 4. Strongyloides stercoralis* from man, rhabditoid male. *Fig. 5. Strongyloides stercoralis* from man, rhabditoid female.

years, probably represents the "welt-rekord" in this regard.

. . .We must not forget that it is possible for *Strongyloides* infection to persist within the intestine for ten years without a new infection; the long life of the filaria makes this possible.

ON VARIOUS FACTORS INFLUENCING THE DEVELOPMENT OF *STRONGYLOIDES STERCORALIS* AND AUTOINFECTION

Taiwan Igakkai Zassi, 27: 1–56, 1928. Translated from the Japanese (Extracted).

Masao Nishigori
(?–1940)

A graduate of the Taihoku Medical College in Taipai, he worked with Professor Sadamu Yokogawa in the Department of Pathology. There he studied the life cycles of Strongyloides *and* Heterophyes. *Later he became a general practitioner in Gunma Prefecture near Tokyo, where he died.*

On Various Factors Influencing Autoinfection in a Shift from Rhabditiform Larvae Directly to Filariform Larvae in the Intestines of the Host.

One problem in explaining autoinfection with this parasite is the difficulty of determining the factors involved in the direct development of rhabditiform larvae into filariform larvae in the host's intestines. Ōhira says that due to some unknown factor the larvae that have not yet left the intestine become filariform larvae and induce autoinfection. According to Shimura, the larvae remain for a long time in the intestines of the host, become well developed, and change into filariform larvae; or the rhabditiform larvae, having gained an ability to invade the intestinal walls of the host, bring about autoinfection by their invasion. However, the processes involved in autoinfection have not yet been studied sufficiently.

Relationship between Duration of Rhabditiform Larvae's Presence in the Intestines of the Host and Autoinfection

When larvae excreted by the host were placed in an incubator at the same temperature as prevailed in the host (from 37 to 40° C), the larvae all developed directly into filariforms in from nine to ten hours, as had been reported previ-

ously. When the oxygen or air surrounding the culture media was replaced by other gases during cultivation of larvae, these larvae developed directly into filariform larvae. If they were not quickly excreted and remained in the host's intestines for a long time, rhabditiform larvae were considered to have developed into filariform larvae. I assumed that when a dog who had been heavily infected, experimentally, and who had continuously evacuated many rhabditiform larvae became constipated, many filariform larvae would be found in the feces.

A morphologic study was made of the larvae in the infected dog's feces after the animal had been given injections of one per cent morphine hydrochloride, Pantopon, Pabinal, or a similar preparation which caused constipation for from one to several days. Among the ten larvae excreted in feces after 24 hours of constipation in a dog who had been given 1 ml of morphine hydrochloride, and then 1.5 gr of bismuth subnitrate, two of the larvae had very much elongated esophagi; the first 0.167 mm and the latter 0.143 mm, forming 42 per cent of the body length. Although they had not shed their skins, they could be clearly identified as filariform larvae and moved more livelily than the other larvae. Another larva had an esophagus that had not yet reached the middle of the body, being 38 per cent of the length, but it was obviously in the process of changing into a filariform larva. In the rest of the larvae, comparison of the length of the esophagus with those in larvae (all of them rhabditiform larvae) found in the soft feces of an ordinarily infected dog showed them to be much elongated. A moderately infected dog who received daily for three days from 1 to 1.5 gr of bismuth subnitrate produced a solid fecal excretion. After discontinuance of the medication there was one excretion daily, and in examining the feces for larvae, a comparison with the previous results showed that because of prolonged constipation there were many more filariform larvae. Larvae Nos. 2, 3, 5, 7, 8, and 9 were filariforms which had either shed their skins or were in the process of doing so. The other rhabditiform larvae had elongated esophagi (from 27 to 36 per cent of the body length) and indications of a gradual change to filariform larvae. These phenomena, caused by constipation in infected dogs (that is to say, a long sojourn of the larvae in the intestines, occasioning their prolonged exposure to an unsuitable temperature), can cause the direct development of rhabditiform larvae into filariform larvae.

It may be that the same process takes place in humans infected with *Strongyloides stercoralis*. A soldier whose disease had not yet reached the stage of diarrhea had a solid bowel movement every morning; upon immediate examination of the feces there were found many rhabditiform larvae with elongated esophagi, as well as completely transformed filariform larvae. In an examination for larvae in the stool, the average body length of the rhabditiform larvae was 0.352 mm, esophagus length, 0.095 mm, 27 per cent of the body length. In an examination of solid feces excreted once daily, since the larvae's sojourn in the intestines was longer than in the previous instance, their development was more advanced, with an average body length of 0.392 mm. Here, however, larvae Nos. 1 and 18 had long esophagi (32 to 37 per cent of the body length), and were the so-called filariform larvae. Nos. 4, 5, and 19 were likewise completely developed filariform larvae, with esophagi respectively 39, 42, and 41 per cent of body length. Subsequently, this same patient received 2.5 gr of bismuth subnitrate three times daily for two days. Immediate examination of the feces after 48 hours of constipation revealed a great number of active filariform larvae, ten of which were measured. Only four larvae, Nos. 1, 2, 4, and 8 were still rhabditiform larvae; the other six had increased body length and elongated esophagi and were filariform larvae.

These filariform larvae, found in the feces of dogs and humans, bored into the mucosa of the dogs' intestines and were able to cause autoinfection; this was shown very clearly in the examination of the dogs that were sacrificed in the experiments. It is known that when such rhabditiform larvae remain a long time in the intestinal tract of the host, they develop into filariform larvae and induce continued autoinfection as their number increases. Thus, we know that constipation is one factor in inducing autoinfection with these larvae.

Other Factors in Autoinfection

When unsuitable gases are used in culturing the larvae outside the host, when the culture medium is acid, or when various chemicals inappropriate for the development of the larvae are used, some of them disregard the environment and directly become filariform larvae. When the contents of the host's intestines become unsuitable (through putrefaction or fermentation) for the survival of the larvae, some of them become filariform larvae and are able to induce autoinfection. When a high degree of constipation was induced experimentally in dogs by the administration of bismuth subnitrate, a great number of filariform larvae were mingled with the first feces excreted after constipation; as explained previously, this was due to their long sojourn in the intestines. Because of the high degree of constipation, various changes occur in the intestines causing the rhabditiform larvae to develop into the filariform larvae. Therefore, when the medicine was stopped, although as a reaction there was much diarrhea, it was not unusual to see filariform larvae. Experimental dog No. 52 had a bowel movement once or twice daily, and his feces were strongly acid (he suffered from a skin disease over his whole body either because of severe dermatitis or intestinal fermentation). Microscopic examination showed many dead larvae. Nevertheless, a detailed study occasionally showed one or two filariform larvae which were either in the process of developing or completely developed. An examination after the dog was sacrificed very clearly indicated autoinfection. In other words, inappropriate intestinal contents in the host will cause some of the larvae to change directly to filariform larvae, known to be one of the factors promoting autoinfection.

Morphologic Studies on the Larvae of *Strongyloides stercoralis* in Various Parts of the Body Due to Autoinfection

The larvae appearing in various parts of the host's body because of autoinfection might be one of the three forms: directly developed filariform larvae, a small number of rhabditiform larvae, and larvae in the process of development. However, as stated above, after the rhabditiform larvae and the larvae in the process of development have caused ulceration, they are able for the first time to penetrate those sites. They are found in comparatively large numbers on the edge of ulcers and in the lymphatic spaces in submucosal tissue, but they have not yet been observed boring into or invading a healthy intestinal wall. On the other hand, those larvae that have developed directly into filariform larvae easily penetrate a healthy intestinal wall and appear in various parts of the host's body. Because of this autoinfection, there appeared in the body of the host filariform larvae measuring in length from 0.345 mm to 0.565 mm, with an average of 0.436 mm. This size is in agreement with the direct development into filariform larvae in an external environment. In the sputum of a patient with autoinfection, Shimura found larvae measuring an average of 0.400 mm to 0.479 mm (it was rare to find one measuring over 0.5 mm), in contrast with larvae cultivated under ordinary external circumstances. In his experiments, Fülleborn used filariform larvae collected from ordinary culture media. When infection was established, the larvae traveled through the host and appeared in tissues, lungs, and trachea; their length in tissues was comparatively shorter than at the time of infection. Shimura had said that the larvae in sputum were the same as in the tissues in autoinfection; however, we cannot explain the matter as simply as that.

By infecting dogs orally with filariform larvae of indirect development, it was found that larvae move around in the body to the abdomen, to the thorax, and to other parts. These were measured and were found to have an average body length of from 0.527 mm to 0.621 mm, the smallest being 0.562 mm and the largest 0.655 mm. The difference of body length between these larvae and those apparently due to autoinfection was 0.126 mm to 0.133 mm, on the average. The latter were the filariform larvae which developed directly in the body of the host and moved on from there; they can be distinguished clearly from the indirectly developed filariform larvae causing infection.

It was stated above that in autoinfection the larvae normally migrate not only through all the tissues of the body but sometimes also via the systemic circulation. In Teissier's case, although he reported their appearance in the peripheral blood in three days, it was not clear whether they were filariform or rhabditiform larvae. In dog No. 60, in my experiments, the three larvae obtained from the femoral vein were filariform larvae.

Shimura, in a case in which autoinfection was occurring, searched the peripheral blood, like Teissier, but could not find any larvae and expressed doubt about the possibility of rhabditiform larvae existing in the peripheral blood. I have done little investigation along this line, having had one experimental case in which, I regret to say, I cannot state positively whether or not rhabditiform larvae could be detected in the peripheral blood. However, in cases of autoinfection, I have examined larvae found in the abdomen, the thorax, the liver, and the lungs, but I have not yet found a rhabditiform larva. In the lungs, especially, all the larvae found were well-developed filariform larvae, and no transitional stage was observed. Since those entering the systemic circulation pass through the lungs, the appearance of rhabditiform larvae in the peripheral blood seems very illogical to me.

Now a word of caution: the filariform larvae, in autoinfection, obtained from the feces of the dog immediately after defecation, were shorter than those obtained from the human feces; and again, the filariform larvae obtained from the feces of the same dog(s) were sometimes long and sometimes very short. The above facts may be considered proof of the biological necessity of those rhabditiform larvae to adapt themselves rapidly to new conditions during their development when they encounter an unsuitable environment and to transform immediately into filariform larvae.

The human intestinal tract is longer than the dog's. Therefore, after their regular development in the small intestine the rhabditiform larvae pass into the large intestine and, under the influence of varying environmental conditions, develop directly into filariform larvae. However, since the intestinal tract of the dog is shorter, the not-yet-fully-developed rhabditiform larvae pass comparatively more rapidly into the large intestine and, when the environment is unsuitable for them, they become filariform larvae capable of inducing autoinfection.

The rhabditiform larvae from the feces of the dog have an average body length of 0.327 mm; those from human feces 0.426 mm, a difference of 0.099 mm. In the transition from rhabditiform larvae to filariform larvae, the development of the two sizes of larvae, large and small, is easy to understand. In the same way, it is easy to understand the presence of the large and small varieties of filariform larvae in the human patient and in the above-mentioned dog. That is, when the not-yet-fully-developed larvae descend into the large intestine and are subjected to various unsuitable environments, they immediately become filariform larvae and are usually smaller than the well-developed filariform larvae.

I observed that when I administered bismuth subnitrate for a long time, thus causing conditions in the intestines unsuitable for the presence of the larvae, the filariform larvae in the feces were only 0.310 mm long (with an elongated esophagus of 0.130 mm, 42 per cent of the body length). Moreover, not infrequently did I see filariform larvae from 0.320 mm to 0.374 mm in length. In order to prove that I was not mistaken, after washing in physiologic saline rhabditiform larvae collected from feces, I injected them into the femoral veins of two dogs in whose lungs I subsequently observed the appearance of exceedingly short filariform larvae. I also made this additional experiment: after washing in physiologic saline many rhabditiform larvae collected from the cecum of a dog, I injected them into the abdominal cavity of another dog and let them develop directly into filariform larvae. After 17 hours, the dog was sacrificed and the filariform larvae were collected from the abdominal cavity and the lungs and measured. The results indicate that the filariform larvae were exceedingly short. Furthermore, the filariform larvae developing directly from rhabditoid larvae and causing autoinfection can be identified by a large genital primordium which is composed of more than ten already divided cells.

Etiologic Significance of Autoinfection with This Parasite, and Instructions Regarding Its Prevention

There has already been a thorough discussion of the pathogenicity of this parasite. In regard to the significance of the parasitism by the female worms, if they are not present in great numbers, they will be harmless. On the contrary, when the larvae of this parasite move down in the intestinal tract and develop there, irritating the intestinal wall by their constant activity, chronic diarrhea develops; also, due to autoinfection, the larvae penetrate deep into the intestinal wall and form small ulcers about the size of flax seeds on the surface of the mucosa of the large intestine. From the surface of the ulcers the filariform larvae as well as the rhabditiform larvae penetrate in great numbers and destroy the tissues, causing severe diarrhea. Also, due to autoinfection, the migrat-

ing larvae induce chronic peritonitis and pleurisy and, with invasion of the lungs, chronic bronchitis. They invade the spleen, the kidneys, and other important organs by way of the systemic circulation, and, as a result, they severely damage the patients. Many Japanese scholars, especially Yokogawa, Ōhira, and Shimura studied the facts of autoinfection, paying attention to the etiology of strongyloidiasis mentioned above. Fortunately, I have had success with my animal experiments on autoinfection and have described all the cases in detail from the standpoint of anatomy and histology.

Changes in the Intestinal Wall

Before severe diarrhea begins, the mucosa of the large intestine is comparatively little changed and there are not many rhabditiform larvae found among the villi, as in the upper part of the small intestine; but when diarrhea occurs, they infiltrate the small cells of the mucosa. When there is much irritation because of large numbers of larvae, catarrhal changes in the mucosa can be seen plainly and, in addition to a general increase of goblet-shaped cells, there are occasional indications of mucosal atrophy and of ulceration with exfoliation of the mucosal epithelium. The larvae collect fairly heavily in these places, and there is marked evidence of congestion of the blood vessels. It is not unusual to find the filariform larvae penetrating the mucosa and muscle layers even if the mucosal surface is healthy. As the pathologic changes develop, small ulcers are formed in the mucosa, and the destructive process is carried deep into the submucosal tissues until eventually the lamina propria is involved. Rhabditiform larvae or filariform larvae invade these places in the greatest numbers, and infiltrates of leukocytes are also seen. Even with small numbers of larvae in the submucosal tissues and the mucosa, their presence was generally easy to detect because of accompanying pathologic changes. Here and there, one found infiltrations of leukocytes around the larvae; that is, the formation of parasitic nodules. In addition, great numbers of parasites were found in the lymphatic spaces causing marked swelling of the lymphatics and the capillaries. Due to the invasion by the larvae of the individual lymph nodes or groups of nodes, there was lymph node destruction. The changes in the muscle layers were, in general, not serious, but there were occasional nodular changes caused by the bodies of the parasites. There were many larvae in the connective tissue around the blood vessels, the lymphatics, and the nerves of the muscle layers; sometimes parasites were found between the muscle fibers. Muscle fiber degeneration and cellular infiltration were not rare. Many larvae had penetrated the surface of the serosa, causing inflammation and forming nodules in some places. It was not uncommon to find generalized edematous swelling, especially in the lymph glands.

The Mesentery and the Mesenteric Lymph Glands

Larvae were often detected in the mesenteric tissue adjacent to the cecum and the large intestine, especially in the lymphatic vessels. Many were often found successively penetrating a single lymphatic channel. Larvae in the surrounding fatty tissue and in connective tissue also caused cellular infiltration. In regard to the mesenteric lymph nodes, especially in the ileocecal region, many larvae were observed in the afferent lymphatics; others were about to enter either the nodes or the parenchyma under the capsule. There were many larvae in the lymph nodes which, by their activity, had destroyed the cells of the comparatively soft parenchyma and had so damaged the cells that only the stroma remained. Many larvae infiltrated successively; in one place they were found by the score in bunches, blocking off lymphatic vessels. Thus, the larvae do great damage to the lymph nodes; this can be seen on the surface with the naked eye. Finally, damage is done to the lymphatic channels. The dilation of the mesenteric lymphatic vessels extends distally, and the enlarged vessels often can be observed in the intestinal wall. Even though no pathologic changes are evident in the liver, Shimura asserts that, in a human case, he saw penetration of liver parenchyma by larvae and resultant small necrotic foci. In the lungs . . . hemorrhagic spots were plainly visible macroscopically, and many larvae could be detected in the tissues.

In a detailed examination of sections, the larvae were mainly in the walls and within the alveoli. The lung capillaries were markedly congested, with scattered hemorrhagic foci. There was a high degree of cellular infiltration in places of old pathologic changes, exfoliation of epithelial cells, and collections of epithelial-like cells and polymorphonuclear leukocytes. Many of the small bronchioles and the somewhat larger ones were filled with polymorphonuclear leukocytes and exfoliated epithelial cells of the bronchi. In many places the epithelial cells of the bronchioles were mostly exfoliated and the bronchioles were filled with larvae, pus, and products of cell exudation. Interalveolar walls were infiltrated by small round cells and were thickened; the capillaries were congested. There were occasional nodes formed of epithelioid cells and young connective tissue cells. These lesions closely resembled those that would be left by the passage of *Ascaris* through the lungs.

As described above, in addition to these larvae causing chronic diarrhea by their irritation of the intestinal tract, they cause damage to various organs through autoinfection. And now, still a more important word of caution: numerous case reports up to the present have shown chronic peritonitis and stubborn bronchial catarrh. Their serious clinical significance must not be overlooked.

Measures for Preventing Autoinfection with These Parasites

Over 50 years have elapsed since the discovery of *Strongyloides stercoralis,* and, although its pathogenic significance is clear, as described above, there is as yet no adequate treatment for it. The prevalence of autoinfection cannot be overlooked. Leichtenstern had experience with a case that extended over 14 years, with an extraordinary course of disease; also, Fülleborn reported another instance of parasitism in which the illness lasted 24 years. Such cases indicate how stubborn the disease can be in humans who develop autoinfection and how difficult is the cure. This parasite, differing from other nematode parasites, penetrates deeply into the intestinal mucosa, and therefore, is exceedingly difficult to eradicate. Not only that, but it is common knowledge that no specific remedy has yet been found for its destruction. Consequently, therapy up to the present has pertained to treatment of symptoms; in chronic diarrhea, administration of astringents to suppress it; in bronchial catarrh, a cough medicine. Doctors have been satisfied with such treatment and have not considered methods of preventing the dreaded autoinfection. This method of treatment is certainly regrettable, although little has been known about autoinfection. According to my experiments, the chief factors causing autoinfection by these parasites are: (1) the length of the larvae's sojourn in the intestinal tract after they have undergone a certain development; (2) the unfavorable nature of the contents of the intestines affecting the larvae.

In addition to being an astringent, bismuth subnitrate seems to effect changes in the intestinal contents, thus creating an unfavorable environment for the larvae, encouraging autoinfection by them. . . . The use of bismuth subnitrate and other astringents in cases of strongyloides, therefore, is not only meaningless, but furthers autoinfection, with exacerbation of the patient's symptoms. In order to prevent autoinfection with these parasites, patients should have two or three bowel movements daily; this would avoid a long sojourn of the larvae in the intestinal tract. In patients in whom there are already many ulcers in the mucosa of the large intestine, the penetration by the larvae is much easier and the prevention of autoinfection difficult. In these patients, by avoiding astringents orally and by administering astringents per anum after enemas about three times daily there is a chance of preventing autoinfection, and it may be possible to heal the ulcers. If autoinfection can be prevented in the early stages of infection, the short-lived female parasites will die, and I believe that healing will occur spontaneously. This should be proved clinically in the future.

Conclusions

In the course of autoinfection, these larvae follow three main courses in the host's body:

(1) They enter the lymphatic space or vessels in the mucosa of the large intestine; they leave the intestinal wall in the flow of lymph; they then enter the lymph nodes in the ileocecal region and in the upper part of the large intestine; then, through the thoracic duct, by way of the heart, they reach the lungs.

(2) Actively piercing the intestinal wall, they reach the abdominal cavity. Some of them immediately penetrate through the diaphragm into the thoracic cavity; afterward, from the surface of the pulmonary pleura, they invade the parenchyma (lung); others penetrate through the capsule of the liver, entering the parenchyma; afterward, they reach the lungs by way of the heart.

(3) From the surface of the mucosa of the large intestine the invading larvae enter the blood capillaries; they then pass through the portal system to the liver and the heart and so reach the lungs.

CHAPTER **16**

Ascariasis

LUMBRICUS TERES, OR SOME ANATOMICAL
OBSERVATIONS ON THE ROUND WORM
BRED IN HUMAN BODIES

Philosophical Transactions, 13, 153–161, 1683.

Edward Tyson
(1650–1708)

*After receiving the A.B. in 1670 and the A.M. in 1673
from Magdalen Hall, Oxford, Tyson embarked upon
the study of medicine and was granted his degree in
1677. In that same year he made the acquaintance of
Robert Hooke, who influenced him greatly and proposed him for Fellowship in the Royal Society in 1679.
The following year, Cambridge awarded him the M.D.*

*His first paper dealt with the scent bags in polecats,
and soon thereafter he published a treatise on abscess
of the liver in which he presented the classic account of
cholelithiasis and suppurative cholangitis. After many
additional studies in anatomy and comparative
anatomy, he published a number of papers on various
types of* Lumbricus *and, in 1691, a discourse in which
he demonstrated that hydatids are living organisms.*

Tyson's anatomy of Ascaris lumbricoides *antedates
Redi's description by one year. This is Tyson's original
description.*

Having been so large in my former instance, in
my Discourse on the Joynted-worm, I intend to
contract my self in this. Not that our present subject is scanty, or does not afford a sufficient
plenty of remarkable observations; but I chose
rather to select what most suites our design. For
to be exact and nice in all particulars, would require a just treatise, and exceeds the bounds I
have at present set my self.

I shall therefore here give the anatomy of the
Lumbricus teres, that common round worm
which children usually are troubled with: and in
this more particularly make my remarks upon the
organs of generation in both sexes, and herein

show how vastly different they are from those
parts in the common earth worms, and it may be,
most others. And withall I had designed, together
with this, to have given the anatomy of the earth
worm, but since have altered my intentions: and
at present shall refer to the account given of it by
the famous Dr. Willis reserving my farther observations of it to another opportunity. This sort
of worm . . . is usually about a foot long, or
something more, or less; but I have hitherto observed that the male is generally lesser than the
female: so that by their bigness in the same body I
have before dissection been able to distinguish
the sex. They are about the bigness of a wheat
straw, or a goose quill; their colour white; but
being subjects so generally known to all, I shall
forbear a further description of their outward
parts; only as I remember I did not observe those
feet, or asperities on the annuli, as in the earth
worm. At both extremes they grow narrow. Their
mouth is composed of three lips as in our figure
(Plate 52, Fig. 1a). So the leech hath three cartilaginous teeth set in a triangle, by which they
make the wound in the skin in suction. The anus
is a transverse slit a little before the extreme point
of the tail.

In opening the body I found I cut thorow a
large muscle under the skin: which muscle in
earth worms I find is spiral; as in a good measure
is their motion likewise; so that by this means,
like the worm of an awger, they can the better
bore their passage into the earth. Their reptile
motion also may be explained by a wire wound
on a cylinder; which when flipped off, and one
end extended and held fast, will bring the other
nearer it. So the earth worm having shot out or
extended its body, (which is with a wreathing) it
takes hold by those small feet it hath, and so
contracts the hinder part of its body.

Likewise I observed that dividing this part there issued out a copious ichor [sic]; which is naturally discharged by some pores or small vents in the skin; which in the earth worm is of great use, by rendering the surface of the body slippery, that so it might the easierly glide into the earth. And in these other worms of the intestines this humor (as in leeches) makes a covering to the body, which is often cast off, and observed as a mucus, in the stools of those troubled with them.

In these . . . animal bodies I never observed those transverse diaphragms which are so numerous in earth worms, and do intersect or rather so deeply depress the intestine. But the cavity chiefly seems to be filled with the genital parts, which I shall now describe: Onely shall first remark that the passage from the mouth was some what straightened for a short space, and was distinguished, as in our figure, from the following ductus; which was a strait intestine continued to the end of the body without any winding or other distinction of a stomach that I could observe.

As to the genital parts of the male I could here observe a penis, a vesicula feminalis, and a testis: in the female a pudendum, vagina uteri, cornua uteri, and spermatick vessels. The penis in the male was placed at the tail or opposite extreme to the head; and seemed to be able to exert itself almost the length of a barley corn, or proportionably to the length of the vagina in the female.

At the root of the penis was inserted the neck of the vesicula seminalis, which gradually grew larger as it ascended in the body, and usually did reach almost half way. 'Twas filled and turgid with a milkie juice; which it received from a slender vessel of the same colour inserted into it. Which after one turning, the latter was afterwards very much convoluted; and being so, forms that body I call the testis.

Altho this part be so loosely contexed, as even to the naked eye, it appears but a continued vessel, and may easily be unravelled its whole length, which I measured was above a yard: yet I make no difficulty of giving it the name of a testis; since 'tis now sufficiently known, that the testes in more compleat animals are onely a congeries of vessels. And a rat, besides this worm, is not the only subject wherein I have found them thus loose and easily separable.

In the female worm, almost about the middle of the body, but more towards the head, I observed an orifice or pudendum, which led into the vagina uteri; which soon divided into the two cornua which were large, and remarkable. For descending something winding towards the tail, they were then reflected again, and did each of them terminate in slender vessels, white, as they were, but much smaller; and did lye in several convolutions and windings amongst them. These I take for spermatic vessels. Having taken those vessels, with the cornua uteri and vagina, out of the body, and laid them on a paper to dry; I found from each cornu, to the end of the spermatic vessels which I had preserved, that they measured about one foot.

I opened the cornua uteri and found them turgid with a milky juice, having placed a little of it upon a small microscope, I plainly perceived 'twas nothing else but an infinite number of small eggs; tho to the naked eye it appeared onely as a fluid body. These eggs when fresh, appeared, as is represented in our fourth figure (Plate 52) covered with abundance of small asperities; but as they grew dry their surface appeared smooth.

By comparing that small quantity I did observe, in which I could distinguish so many eggs, with the whole substance contained in both the cornua, I cannot guess there can be so few as 1,000 eggs in each female worm.

How far different this worm is from common earth worms as to these parts, I need only to refer to Dr. Willis's . . . account of it, to show. And I am yet to learn what worm out of the body has these organs thus formed. Whence once there, the case is plain how they propagate themselves. And Menjotius, and all before him, that were of that opinion, are mistaken; who say that these worms do not generate; nor have any distinction of sexes. . . . And I think nothing can be plainer then this distinction of sexes in them.

But I find on the other hand, there are many who do not only allow them to generate, but do make them viviparous too.

Thus P. Borellus tells us, "I have seen an enormous worm drawn forth from the body of a man infested with a countless number of worms, and I have seen a large worm extracted from this man's feet." So Amatus Lusitanus tells much such a story; that a girl voiding a large worm, and the father treading on it, "and from the innards of this worm, other worms came forth." Foelix Platerus gives an observation of a boy that was

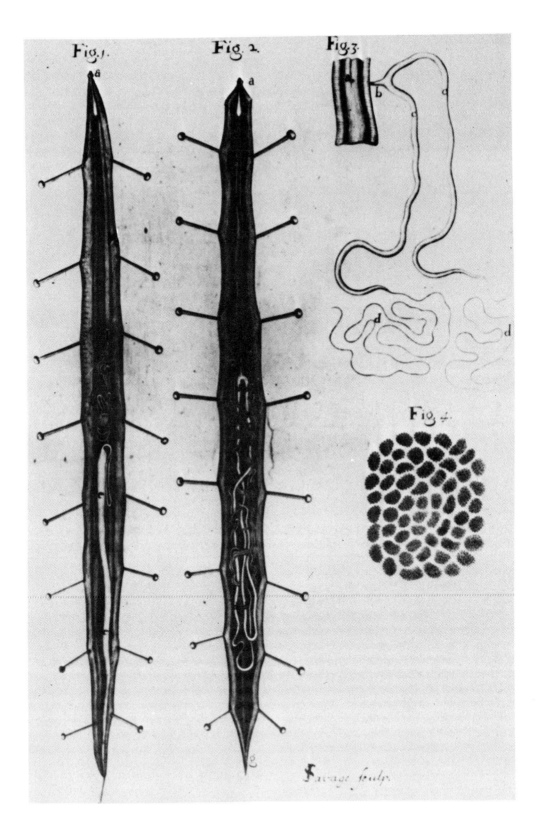

hydropical, and voided all his excrements upwards who dying in the hospital, and they observing a motion and palpitation in his belly, were afraid to bury him till they had sent for the doctor. He opening [the boy] found the intestines in some places swelled as big as his thigh, in others so convoluted, intorted, and twisted, that hindred any passage downwards, either of excrements or wind. "In fact, the boy's intestines were stuffed with a very great number of living worms; these worms were, in turn, filled with other smaller worm." Dominicus Panarolus is very express, and tells us he observed it thus in two several persons. "In both persons, flesh-colored worms about 16 inches long were expelled. These worms bore many little worms in them and the little worms looked like so many tiny sticks of wood. These small worms were innumerable; they were slender and white, being about six inches long, and on being born they slithered like so many tiny serpents." But whatever is related of this nature I cannot but think it is a mistake; and that they were imposed upon by the genital parts of this worm; which not warily examined, might easily make them to think they are so many small worms. For they are not viviparous but oviparous, as I have shewn; and their containing so vast a number of eggs in the cornua uteri, as I have expressed, does sufficiently account for that prodigious quantity, that are sometimes observed to be bred in animal bodies.

Panarolus tells us he once saw the stomack and guts stuffed with them so that they ascended up to the throat. Baricellus by the use of crude mercury brought away from a patient above a hundred. Weckerus did the like with the use of tansy seed and syrup of violets. Gabucinus saw voided by stool 177. Benivenius saw voided by a child 7 years old 152 worms. And Hollerius, out of Musa, gives us an history of a man 82 years old, who voided above 500. And Petrus Paulus Pereda saw a nobleman's child in a few days void almost a thousand, and she voided 40 in four hours' time.

Those animals are usually the most multiparous, whose young are the most exposed to danger, and were it not so here that the greatest part of the litter of this worm is usually carried forth by the faeces, it could not be avoided but we should be devoured by an enemy we breed in our own bowels. That caution therefore of Heers I think is necessary: to avoid the giving the powder of these worms for expelling others, since we cannot be secure but that at the same time we may sow the seed for propagating more.

NEW INVESTIGATIONS ON THE DEVELOPMENT AND PROPAGATION OF *ASCARIS LUMBRICOIDES* AND *TRICHOCEPHALUS* OF MAN

Nouvelles recherches sur le développement et la propagation de l'ascaride lombricoide et du trichocéphale de l'homme. Comptes Rendus Hebdomadaires des Seances de l'Academie des Sciences. Memoires, 3 ser. 4: 261–265, 1862. Translated from the French.

Casimir Joseph Davaine (1812–1882)

Another of the great scientists of the last century who had neither his own laboratory nor an official academic appointment, Davaine began his studies in St. Amand-les Eaux. He later studied in Lille and then began his medical studies in Paris, presenting his thesis for the M.D. in 1837. From 1838 until his death he practiced medicine in Paris and carried on research in microbiology and parasitology, collaborating with his former professor Pierre Rayer and with Claude Bernard.

His genius is reflected in his description of phagocytosis by human macrophages 14 years prior to Metchnikoff. In this paper, Davaine demonstrates that the site of "excystation" of Ascaris and Trichuris is the small intestine.

By the previous communications I was led to believe that the egg of the *Ascaris lumbricoides* and of the *Trichocephalus dispar* is expelled from the intestines before having acquired any degree of development. The development usually starts several months after egg laying and the embryo remains confined in the egg shell for a long time, long enough at the time of my last communica-

Plate 52. Fig. 1. The male worm, opened. (a) the three lips of the worm; (b) the esophagus (or gullet); (ccc) the large intestine; (d) the penis; (ee) the vesicula seminalis; (f) the testis. *Fig. 2.* The female worm, opened. (a) the mouth; (b) the gullet; (ccc) the intestine (or gut); (ddd) the vagina uteri; (e) the two cornua uteri; (fff) the spermatic vessels; (g) the anus. *Fig. 3.* The genital parts of the female. (a) the pudendum or foramen as it appears on the outside of the skin; (b) the vagina uteri; (cc) the two cornua uteri; (dd) the spermatic vessels. *Fig. 4.* The eggs of this worm as they appear under the microscope.

tion that one could say that the embryonic life of these two entozoa is the longest that has been reported in any animal. Three years have passed since then and life continues in most of these embryos. I will give an account of the experiences by which this fact has been established in an exceptional way.

First, I will speak of a few other investigations with which I have not yet entertained the Society. The eggs that I preserved in water since 8 October 1857 and since the end of September of the same year were useful to me in my work. Having ascertained that the embryos stay alive latently when the temperature is lower than that of the human body and that the sojourn in the gastric juice is insufficient to dissolve the egg shell, I was forced to presume that this shell could not be dissolved or softened except by the action of intestinal juices and that the embryo would not leave the egg except at the usual temperature of mammals. In order to determine whether these presumptions were true, I made the following test in June 1859. *Ascaris* eggs containing an embryo and other eggs which had not yet undergone cell division were put together in about equal numbers in very small flasks whose openings were closed with a simple fabric. These flasks introduced into the stomach of a dog were collected two days later in the feces of the dog, and their contents were carefully examined under the microscope. In these flasks I found undivided eggs, but those which contained an embryo could not be found. A certain number of embryos were free in the flask. The same experience repeated with some modifications gave the same results (See *Le Journal de Physiologie* of Dr. Brown-Séquard, II, No. 6, 1859).

One can conclude from these facts that the egg shell is not dissolved by the intestinal juices because undivided eggs were found intact in the flasks but the egg shell is sufficiently softened so that the embryos within, activated by the heat of the intestines, could pierce it and escape.

In October 1861, the *Ascaris* eggs preserved since October 1857 appeared not to have undergone any alteration. Wishing to assure myself that the embryos were still alive and not wanting to attempt an experiment on man, I tried to transmit them to a cow. I chose the cow because I believed that the *Ascaris lumbricoides* inhabited this animal as well as man.

Three or four hundred eggs of the *Ascaris* were given with suitable precautions to a one-year-old cow. Four months later she was slaughtered, but in spite of meticulous investigations, no type of worms could be found in her intestines.

What is to be concluded from this experience? That the embryos were no longer alive? But we will see in a later experiment that they were still very much alive. We concluded that the *A. lumbricoides* does not develop in the cow. Indeed, the *Ascaris* of this ruminant was not considered specific in the era when the *Ascaris megalocephalus* of the horse and the *Ascaris* of the pig were confused with the *A. lumbricoides* of man. But one knows today that there are three distinct species; it may be that the *Ascaris* of the cow is the fourth species.

The 8th of October of this year (1862) I again examined carefully and with great interest the *Ascaris* eggs preserved since 8 October 1857; that is, for five years. The embryos in a certain number of these eggs, estimated to be one-third, were found to be inactive, but the others were evidently intact.

I maintained a certain number of these eggs for several hours at a temperature of 30° to 40° C. Then, I let the embryo out by crushing the shell carefully; I saw several move actively, evidently alive. However, in order not to harbor any doubts on this subject, I performed the following experiments.

A rat was starved for 24 hours so that its bowel would be empty. I gave it some milk containing a great number of these *Ascaris* eggs preserved for five years. Twelve hours later the rat was killed. The milk filled the entire gastrointestinal tract from the stomach to the cecum. In the stomach and the first part of the small intestine, I found all the eggs intact. In the second half of the small intestine, but almost exclusively in its terminal portion, I found embryos outside the eggs and quite alive and others that were only emerging from the shell. One of these which I examined for a while under the microscope emerged under my eyes. Many eggs were still intact. I ascertained clearly that the shell was not dissolved. The embryos emerge at one end of the egg where it seemed to me a small operculum existed; they turn back outside the shell and use it as a support to complete their exit. An obvious question is what has happened to the embryos which remained alive in the rat's intestine. One can foresee that these worms, incapable of development in the rat, must be expelled in the rat's feces. This is indeed what happened in the following experiment:

A rat was fed for a week, exclusively on milk containing *A. lumbricoides* eggs; the feces were collected every day. Microscopic examination showed that these embryos were expelled in the feces and that they arrived alive externally.

This experiment yielded yet another interesting result; many eggs are expelled before the embryo has left the shell or while it is on its way out. Thus, it can be concluded that if the eggs remained longer in the rat's intestine or if the rat's intestine were longer, all the eggs would have hatched in the intestine of this animal. This reflection will find its application apropos *Trichocephalus dispar* which we will discuss.

The same tests were made with the eggs of *T. dispar* preserved since September 1857, that is, for five years like the preceding ones. Having but a small number of these eggs at my disposition, I found very few in the intestinal contents and in the feces. I did not see a single free embryo or any emerging from the shell but by attentive examination after crushing the egg there was no doubt as to the integrity and the viability of these embryos.

In accordance with the observed facts about the *A. lumbricoides* it can be assumed that if experiments were done on an animal whose intestine might be very long and with a larger number of *Trichocephalus* eggs, one would observe the embryo of this latter worm being hatched. It is remarkable indeed that the *A. lumbricoides* egg does not hatch in the stomach or in the first part of the intestine of the rat but in a part of the intestine which corresponds to the course and the duration of the stay in the small intestine of man which is the natural habitat of the *Ascaris*. One can judge by analogy that in man the *Trichocephalus* egg hatches when it has reached the terminal portion of the small intestine or in the cecum which is the natural habitat of this worm. The intestine of the rat is too short to supply the needed length, and this is without a doubt the reason I found eggs that were still intact in the feces.

The facts mentioned above show that the eggs of the *T. dispar* and of the *A. lumbricoides* develop outside the body of man, but the embryo only hatches when it is brought into the intestine by food or drink. Two conditions are doubtless necessary for this hatching: the softening of the shell by intestinal juices and the activity of the embryo under the influence of heat of about 40° C. In whichever animal supplies these conditions, the egg hatches if it remains in the intestine long enough; however, the embryo does not linger to be expelled, and dies if the animal is not of the kind where the worm cannot acquire its final form. The length of the latent life of the egg of the *Ascaris* and the *Trichocephalus* of man is five years. So I can repeat here even more strongly what I said in a communication at the Academy of Sciences in June 1858: "In this long interval of time the eggs of the *Trichocephalus* and of the *Ascaris lumbricoides*, without any doubt, can be carried away by rain into streams, rivers, and ditches whose water is used for drinking or for the preparation of foods. By this route, these fully developed eggs can reach the intestine of man where the embryos will undergo mature and complete development."

ON THE LIFE HISTORY OF *ASCARIS LUMBRICOIDES*

British Medical Journal, 2: 5–7, 1916.

Francis Hugh Stewart
(1879–1951)

Stewart received his undergraduate education at St. Andrew's University and his medical education at the University of Edinburgh. In addition, he held the degree of D.P.M. from Cambridge. Immediately upon taking his M.B. and Ch.B. in 1904, he joined the Indian Medical Service and was successively assigned as medical officer to various distinguished regiments. He saw active wartime duty both on the north eastern frontier from 1911 to 1912 and during World War I on a number of Asiatic and African fronts. A few months before his retirement in 1921, he was named Officer Commanding the Indian Station Hospital in Quetta.

This is the first demonstration of the route of migration of Ascaris *larvae, although Leuckart's influence led to the erroneous conclusion that two hosts were involved in the cycle.*

Preliminary Note

The development of *Ascaris lumbricoides* is at present almost universally considered to be direct. It is well known that the eggs passed in the faeces of man undergo development in the outer world up to the formation of a motile vermiform embryo. The egg containing this embryo may readily reach the alimentary canal of man, and it is supposed that it there hatches, and that the larva, having escaped, develops in this site into the adult. This theory is based on the work of Davaine, Grassi, Calandruccio, Lutz, Epstein, Jammes and Martin, Martin, and Wharton. I have not at present access to the works of these authors in the original with the exception of the articles of Jammes and Martin and of Wharton. Summaries sufficient for the present purpose are, however, available in the textbooks of Leukart as regards Davaine, of Railliet, Manson, Clifford Allbutt, and Castellani, as regards the later writers.

Davaine administered ripe eggs to rats, and found that after 12 hours free live larvae were to be found in the lower part of the small intestine. He also introduced ripe and unripe eggs in glass capsules closed with linen into the alimentary canal of the dog and found that after the lapse of a certain period the ripe eggs had disappeared, whereas the unripe eggs remained. He concluded that hatching and development occurred in the alimentary canal of the definitive host.

Grassi administered ripe eggs to himself, and two months later found eggs in his stools. Calandruccio infected a child of 10 which had previously suffered from worms, but had been relieved of these parasites by anthelmintics. Lutz fed an adult on ripe eggs, and found evidence of the subsequent appearance of adult worms. Epstein's work is unfortunately not available even in summary, but from the context of the references it is clear that he successfully infected man.

Jammes and Martin worked on the line of experimental hatching of ripe eggs in artificial and natural solutions, and found that hatching took place readily and *en masse* in 0.8 per cent salt solution (which they consider to be an alkaline solution) at 37° to 40° C. Martin found that the embryos of the ascarids from the calf, pig, horse and dog hatched best in alkaline solutions, and that when developed eggs were introduced into the alimentary canal of an animal they passed through the stomach unaffected and only hatched after they had been subjected to the action of the alkaline juices of the intestine (Ext. quoted from Wharton).

Wharton states that direct infection can take place, but that the embryos must be ''completely developed.'' He does not give the period necessary to secure this complete development.

In spite of the general acceptance of the theory there is a considerable bulk of evidence against it.

Davaine administered three to four hundred ripe eggs to an ox—an animal which is stated to harbour *A. lumbricoides*—and found that after four months no worms were present in the intestine. Küchenmeister experimented with a dog, which, however, escaped from his observation. Leukart fed a rabbit on ripe eggs, and found no worms after 10 days; a dog was also treated, and was equally unresponsive after 14 days. This very experienced helminthologist also fed a pig for three weeks on several thousand ripe eggs, and did not find any worms on section. An experiment on man was arranged in 1857, but it is not clear that it was carried out. He also administered to a horse the eggs of *Ascaris megalocephala*; to a dog those of *Ascaris marginata*; to a cat those of *Ascaris mystax,* with invariably negative results.

Leukart, therefore, maintained that the life history of *A. lumbricoides* would be found to be completed by an alternation of hosts. He supported this opinion by the facts known with regard to (1) *Ascaris acus,* which is found as an encysted larva in *Leuciscus alburnus,* and in the adult form in the pike, and (2) a larval *Ascaris* found encysted in the muscles of the mole, which, when administered to the buzzard, continues to develop, although it does not yet become adult. He considered that Davaine's rat experiment, if correctly described, did not point to the direct development of the worm, but to the fact that the rat was an intermediate host. He pointed out the case with which the larvae liberated in the faeces of the rat could be conveyed to the intestine of the definitive host—man. He attempted to confirm the experiment, but employed a mouse in place of a rat, and found that the eggs were passed unaltered in the faeces of the mouse. He therefore abandoned this line of research. He attempted to find the intermediate host among invertebrate animals, experimenting with a number of insects, snails, and earthworms, but without success. Von Linstow suggested that *Julus guttulatus* might be the intermediate host.

Ascariasis, both in man and the pig, is of extraordinary frequency in the colony of Hong Kong and in South China generally. I therefore, while stationed in this colony, had an unusual opportunity of studying the subject. I commenced experiments in the spring of 1915. Two young pigs were obtained aged two months. The faeces of both were examined and found to be free of *Ascaris* eggs.

Pig A was fed throughout the course of the experiment on tinned milk and rice flour. Large quantities of ripe eggs from the *Ascaris* of the pig were administered to it on 13 occasions between September 20th and December 6th, 1915. The age of the eggs employed varied from 26 to 64 days, and they invariably contained well-developed motile embryos. They had been incubated at a temperature between 25° and 30° C. in a damp atmosphere. They were administered under varying conditions, after food and after 12 hours' starvation, with and without the addition of sodium bicarbonate. The total number of eggs used must have greatly exceeded several thousand. This pig was killed on December 15th, 1915. One small *Ascaris* only was found in its intestine.

Pig B was fed between September and December, 1915, in the same manner as Pig A, on tinned milk and rice flour; from January, 1916, onward he was fed on boiled rice and vegetables. Between September 27th and December 2nd, 1915, large quantities of ripe eggs from the *Ascaris* of man were administered to him on nine occasions. The age of the eggs varied from 22 to 106 days. They also had been kept during the colder months in an incubator between 25° and 30° C. in a damp atmosphere. The faeces of the pig were repeatedly examined for *Ascaris* eggs but none were found. Between January 5th and February 27th, 1916, large quantities of eggs from the *Ascaris* of the pig were administered, the age of the eggs varying between 17 and 73 days. The faeces of this animal were again examined repeatedly, but up to April 17th no eggs of *Ascaris* were found.

These two series of experiments thus strongly confirmed the negative finding of Leukart's experiment with the pig.

On April 6th, 1916, I took up Davaine's experiment with the rat. Four specimens of *Mus decumanus* albino had been obtained. Their faeces had been repeatedly examined and no eggs of nematodes had been found.

At 2 p.m. on April 6th ripe eggs of *A. lumbricoides* from man were administered to all four rats. The faeces passed between 8 p.m. on the 6th and midday on the 7th were found to contain free larvae of *Ascaris lumbricoides*. These larvae moved in a languid manner in normal salt solution. Eggs of the *Ascaris* of the pig were administered to all four rats on April 7th and 9th, and to Rats A, B, and D on April 10th. Eggs of the *Ascaris* of man were again given to Rat C on April 10th. The faeces continued to contain free *Ascaris* larvae. Specimens of the faeces were preserved in an incubator between the temperatures of 25° and 30° C. Live larvae were found in these specimens after the lapse of three days. The experiment of Davaine was therefore fully confirmed.

On April 12th a further development of the experiment took place. Rat C died, but I was prevented from examining this rat or observing the remaining three until April 15th. Rat C was preserved during the interval in an ice chest. On April 15th it was examined. A small quantity of blood had escaped from its nostrils. No nematodes, larval or adult, were found in the stomach or intestines. The lungs were found to be congested. Portions were removed and teased out in normal salt solution. Numerous nematode larvae in active movement escaped from the tissue. The liver was also examined and a small number of larvae found. No larvae were found in the spleen or kidneys.

The Rats A, B, and D were on this day obviously suffering from the pneumonia. A small quantity of blood was issuing from the nostrils of B and D, and all three were breathing in a rapid and exaggerated manner.

On April 16th Rat D was killed. The same nematode larvae were found abundant in the lungs. No larvae were found in the trachea, liver, heart, spleen, kidneys, stomach, intestine, or in the masseter and lumbar muscles.

Rat A had apparently recovered from its illness on April 17th, Rat B on April 18th.

The organs of C and D were examined by serial sections. In the lungs the greater part of the air vesicles were found to be filled with red blood corpuscles. Larvae were found in the air vesicles and in the bronchi of D. No larvae were found in the other organs examined, namely, liver, kidneys, and spleen.

As a control another specimen of *Mus decumanus* albino (E) obtained from the same source as A, B, C, and D, and five specimens of the wild *Mus decumanus* and two of *Mus rattus* obtained from the town of Victoria were examined. No larvae were found in their lungs.

The Rat B was killed on April 22nd. The lungs, trachea, nasal cavities, liver, heart, spleen, stomach, and intestines were examined. No larvae or other worms were found. The lungs appeared slightly fibrosed but otherwise normal. The rat had therefore freed itself from the parasites 16 days after the date of the first infection and 12 days after the date of the last infection.

Further experiments were made to confirm the results obtained.

On April 22nd two white rats, F and G, were given large quantities of mature eggs. Rat F was treated with the eggs of an *Ascaris* of the pig, which were 80 days old. On April 25th the treatment was repeated. On the 27th the rat was obviously ill and breathing at the rate of 134 per minute. It has continued alive, although very seriously ill, up to the date of writing—May 3rd.

Rat G was fed with eggs of the human *Ascaris* 54 days old. The doses were repeated on the 24th and 25th. On the 26th it was extremely ill, and breathing at the rate of 160 per minute. On the 27th it died. *Ascaris* larvae were found in the lungs and liver.

A piebald mouse said to be one year old was treated with the same culture as the Rat G on April 24th, 25th, and 26th. On the 28th it was seriously ill, with respirations at the rate of 120 per minute. It died on that day. Lungs and liver were richly infected with larvae. (Sections showed that the larvae in the lungs were situated in the air vesicles, in the liver in dilated blood capillaries.)

It is interesting to compare the last experiments with Leukart's experiment with the mouse. Leukart asserted that the eggs were passed in the faeces unaltered. I found in addition to a few unaltered eggs a small number of free but dead larvae. It is probable that Leukart did not give sufficiently large doses of eggs to cause the death of the animal, and thus failed to observe the larval stages of the parasite.

Having traced the infection to the air vesicles and bronchi of the rat and mouse, it became necessary to ascertain whether the larvae in these situations were capable of further development in the definitive host.

Portions of the lungs of Rat D were administered on April 16th to the Pig B, which had been used in the experiments on direct infection described above. This animal was killed on April 30th, and stomach and intestines, heart, lungs, and liver were examined. No ascarids were found in any of these organs.

Several factors may have been responsible for this failure: (1) The larvae may require to undergo further development either in the outer world or in a second intermediate host; (2) the larvae in the lung of Rat D may have originated only from the first dose of eggs administered to it, and may therefore have belonged to the *Ascaris* of man. It is a point in debate whether the *Ascaris* of man (*A. lumbricoides*, L.) is or is not specifically identical with that of the pig (*A. suilla,* Dujardin). Infection experiments only will be able to decide this point. (3) The Pig B may have been rendered immune to *Ascaris* infection by the large doses of eggs administered to it previously. The eosinophile index of the blood was observed to rise after several of these administrations.

Summary of Results

The life history of *A. lumbricoides* presents an alternation of hosts. Eggs develop mature embryos in the outer world in a damp atmosphere, preferably at a temperature of from 25° to 30° C. When ripe eggs reach the alimentary canal of the rat (*Mus decumanus*) or mouse (*Mus musculus*) they hatch. The larvae liberated enter the bodies of their host, a few only escaping in the faeces. Between four and six days after infection they are found in the blood vessels of the lungs, liver, and spleen. The host is seriously ill with symptoms of pneumonia. On the sixth day they have passed from the blood vessels into the air vesicles of the lung, causing haemorrhage into them. On the tenth day they are found only in the air vesicles of the lung and in the bronchi. If the disease does not prove fatal the host recovers on the eleventh or twelfth day. On the sixteenth day the host is free from parasites.

The further course of the life-history requires further experiments for its elucidation. I have commenced experiments with this object, but among the uncertainties of military service it may not be possible to bring them to a conclusion. I therefore consider it advisable to publish the results obtained. It is obvious that the transfer of the parasite from the bronchi of the rat and mouse to the intestine of man and of the pig could be readily effected. The intermediate host might readily contaminate the food of the definitive host or the dust and earth of his surroundings.

LIFE HISTORY OF
ASCARIS LUMBRICOIDES
AND RELATED FORMS

Journal of Agricultural Research 11: 395–398, 1917. Selections from pp. 396–398.

Brayton Howard Ransom
(1879–1925)

Born in Iowa, educated at the University of Nebraska, he received his Ph.D. in 1908. He went to George Washington Medical School in 1902 and was an assistant in the division of zoology of the hygienic laboratory, Public Health and Nursing Hospital Service, 1902–1903, when he became assistant in charge of the Zoology Division, Bureau of Animal Industry, United States Department of Agriculture. He became its chief in 1906.

Winthrop Davenport Foster
(1880–1918)

At the time of this publication, he was employed at the United States Department of Agriculture, Bureau of Animal Industry, Zoology Division, as a junior zoologist.

The complete life cycle as worked out by Ransom and Foster is recorded here. Few details have been added since.

Repetition of Stewart's experiments in feeding rats and mice with Ascaris eggs gave results agreeing very closely with those which he has recorded. We have noted wider variations as to the time at which the larvae may be found in various organs and have observed them in several locations in addition to those in which they were seen by Stewart, but the results of our experiments were essentially the same as his, and point to a migration of the larvae to the liver, lungs, spleen, and other organs, and finally from the lungs to the alimentary tract by way of the air passages through the trachea and into the esophagus, during which migrations they undergo considerable development and structural change and increase to a size of 1.5 mm or more in length. In most of our experiments the eggs of the pig Ascaris were used, as Ascaris from pigs was more easily obtainable than parasites from human beings. In addition to our experiments on rats and mice we made further attempts, with negative results, to infect pigs.

Our unsuccessful attempts to infect pigs by feeding Ascaris eggs were made on animals several months old. It is noteworthy that Epstein, in his carefully controlled experiments with *A. lumbricoides* used very young subjects and that the positive results which he obtained can scarcely be explained upon any other assumption than that a direct development of the parasites occurred following feeding of the eggs—that is, development without an intermediate host. The experience of one of us (B. H. R.) in certain investigations on the life history of *Syngamus trachealis,* our failures, and the failures of others to infect pigs with Ascaris, the failures of various investigators to infect adult human beings, and Epstein's positive results in the case of young subjects, suggested the possibility that age is an important factor influencing the susceptibility of human beings and pigs to infection with Ascaris, and that many of the failures to bring about experimental infections would not have occurred if younger animals had been used as subjects. Our belief in this possibility was strengthened by the discovery of an Ascaris larva in a fragment of lung from a pig about six weeks old which had died from unknown causes in May, 1917, a finding which indicated a migration of larvae like that which occurs in rats and mice. The intestine of this pig contained numerous immature ascarids, the largest about 5 cm long. In order to test the possibility of infecting very young pigs, after several disappointments because certain sows reserved for the purpose of providing young pigs for experimental use either failed to farrow or devoured their newborn offspring, we finally succeeded in obtaining two young pigs from a sow which was found by fecal examination to be free from egg-producing ascarids. In the latter part of September, at the age of about two weeks, one of these pigs was given a large number of Ascaris eggs containing motile vermiform embryos. The number of eggs given was not determined, but there must have been at least several thousand. One week after feeding the pig which had been fed with Ascaris eggs was brought into the laboratory dead; death had occurred either the same day or late the day before; in any event, approximately one week had elapsed since the animal had been given a heavy dose of Ascaris eggs. The other pig continued in good health. Examination of the dead pig revealed a pneumonia, with numerous petechial hemorrhages in the lung tissue. Numerous ascarid larvae, varying in length from 0.7 to 1.2 mm in length, were found in the lungs, trachea, and pharynx; none in the liver, spleen, esophagus, small intestine or large intestine.

It is of interest to note in this connection that when rats or mice are fed large numbers of Ascaris eggs they commonly die of pneumonia about a week later, at a time when numerous larvae are present in the lungs, exactly as in the case of this pig. These findings are interpreted by us as clearly demonstrating that Ascaris larvae in young pigs, presumably also in children, behave in much the same way as in rats or mice, and strongly support the hypothesis that the migrations and development of the parasites are very similar in the two cases, the only important difference being that in rats or mice the worms are unable to continue their development to maturity.

Stewart's very important discoveries concerning the behavior of Ascaris larvae in rats and mice, the various contributions of other investigators toward the solution of the problem of the life history of *A. lumbricoides* and related parasites, and our own experiences outlined above, appear to justify certain conclusions, some of which in anticipation of a more extended statement in a future paper, may be briefly given as follows:

The development of *A. lumbricoides* and closely related forms is direct, and no intermediate host is required.

The eggs, when swallowed, hatch out in the alimentary tract; the embryos, however, do not at once settle down in the intestine, but migrate to various other organs, including the liver, spleen, and lungs.

Within a week, in the case of the pig Ascaris, the migrating larvae may be found in the lungs and have meanwhile undergone considerable development and growth.

From the lungs the larvae migrate up the trachea and into the esophagus by way of the pharynx, and this migration up the trachea may already become established in pigs, as well as in artificially infected rats and mice, as early as a week after infection.

Upon reaching the alimentary tract a second time after their passage through the lungs, the larvae, if in a suitable host, presumably settle down in the intestine and complete their development to maturity; if in an unsuitable host, such as rats and mice, they soon pass out of the body in the feces.

Heavy invasions of the lungs by the larvae of Ascaris produce a serious pneumonia which is frequently fatal in rats and mice and apparently caused the death of a young pig one week after it had been fed with numerous Ascaris eggs.

It is not improbable that ascarids are frequently responsible for lung troubles in children, pigs, and other young animals. The fact that the larvae invade the lungs as well as other organs beyond the alimentary tract and can cause a serious or even fatal pneumonia indicates that these parasites are endowed with greater capacity for harm than has heretofore been supposed.

Age is a highly important factor in determining susceptibility to infection with Ascaris, and susceptibility to infection greatly decreases as the host animal becomes older. This, of course, is in harmony with the well-known fact that it is particularly children and young pigs among which infestations with Ascaris is common, and that Ascaris is relatively of rare occurrence in adult human beings and in old hogs.

EXPERIMENTAL INFECTIONS ON HUMAN BODY WITH ASCARIDES

Japanese Medical World, 2: 317–320, 1922. (This is the English translation of a Japanese article which appeared in Tokyo Iji Shinshi [Tokyoer Medizinische Wochenschrift] No. 2299, 1971–1978, 7 October 1922; a summary was published in Japanese Medical World, 3: 30, 1923.)

Shimesu Koino
(1897–1971)

Koino was born at Tomiyama-cho, Awagun, Chiba Prefecture, near Tokyo. After graduating from the Faculty of Medicine, University of Manchuria in 1920, he worked for a while on plague in Dairen Hospital. He returned to Tokyo to study in the Department of Parasitology at Keio University Medical School under Professor Mikinosuke Miyajima. In 1927, he transferred to the Department of Pediatrics in Keio University Hospital and worked under Professor Mitsutoku Karasawa. He opened a private office for the practice of pediatrics in Tokyo two years later. In addition to his research on ascarides, Koino studied the route of infection of Trichostrongylus orientalis *and its treatment.*

Stewart in 1916 and Yoshida in 1917 reported on the routes of infection of ascarides, and said that the larvae of ascarides do not become adults in the intestine, but they pass through the intestinal wall once into the lungs and thence down the esophagus return to the intestine and become adult there. Since these facts were reported many more have been reported to clarify the route of ascarides infection. There were not a few investigators who attempted experimental infection in humans. Among them are Grassi and his student Calandruccio, Lutz and Epstein. But their purpose was to determine how the infection took place, whether or not it was direct or indirect infection, and they did not make clinical observations. Lutz, however, reported in 1888, that after seven feedings to a man who was 37 years old with eggs of ascarides, the man had fever, pulmonary infiltration, respiratory difficulties with complication of bronchitis. Aside Lutz's report there have been no detail observations on the symptoms and course produced by the movements of the ascarides larvae in the human body.

In the artificially infected animals, I observed hemorrhages in the liver or lung or pneumonia in limited areas in the lungs. From these observations it came to me that the same changes might take place in the liver and lung of infected man and that a certain symptom might be produced by a certain number of larvae. Since ascarides infection in young man is not serious and it can be cleaned easily by anthelmintics, I fed my younger brother, who had no natural ascarides infection with a large number of ascarides eggs and made close observations following the test feeding. Several days later I myself fed with still a larger number of ascarides eggs. The clinical symptoms in both cases were the same and I came to a conclusion that the clinical pictures were produced by ascarides infection.

The First Experimental Feeding

A healthy man of 21 years of age showed no ascarides eggs in stool. He was fed on August 4th with 500 mature eggs of pig ascarides, *Ascaris suum*. The following description is the clinical symptoms observed after the test feeding.

The body temperature on the third day was 37.4, then up to the eighth day it was in the morning from 36.4 to 36.9 and in the evening from 37. to 37.5. On the ninth day the temperature went up to 39.1 following a severe chill. He had sharp headaches, coughs, pains in chest, anorexia, general fatigue and difficult breathing. The following three days the temperature remained between 37.3 and 39 and the next day it came down to 37 and on the seventh days after the onset of the fever it came down to the normal.

The cough gradually became worse. The sputum increased with the cough; it was waterly mucous, containing no blood. The patient complained of pains in the front, side and back of the chest radiating some time toward the apeces. He complained of heavy feelings over the chest.

The number of respiration increased with the onset of the disease up to 27 to 32 per minute and came down to the normal on the thirteenth day after the test feeding or fifth day after the onset of fever. The pulse was regular, the expansion was medium and slightly increased with the rise of temperature.

There were no marked objective changes either in lungs or in heart; on the first day of the onset except the second pulmonary arterial sound was somewhat increased. On the evening of the second day there were dry rales and crepitations and occasional moist rales over the front, side and back. But there was no area of dullness to the percussion. Rales were heard all over the chest the next day. They were mainly dry, but there were occasional whistling rales. On the fourth day the rales in the front disappeared and they were gradually disappeared from the side and the back and on the sixth day they were entirely gone. On the eighth day after the onset of the symptoms, the symptoms completely disappeared and the patient recovered.

The liver and spleen were not palpated. There was no albumen in the urine. No ascaris larvae were found in the sputum.

The Second Experimental Feeding

The first experiment showed that Ascaris larvae migrate around in the human body and cause pathological changes in the viscera. It suggested that when larvae enter the lungs they cause ascaris pneumonia. But this single case could not exclude accidental complications, therefore on August 28th I myself took 2000 mature eggs of *Ascaris lumbricoides*, and carefully noted symptoms following the test feeding.

There were no marked prodromal symptoms. Only the next day there were slight headaches and decrease of appetite.

On the third day the temperature rose to 37.2, then gradually became higher. On the sixth day after the test feeding there was fever following chills, headache was severe and respiration and pulse were increased. The face was flushed and I was thirsty. There was heavy feeling over the chest. The cough was frequent with large amount of sputum.

The temperature on the second day after the onset rose up to 39.8 and remained between 38.7 and 40.2. It began to come down by crisis on the seventh day and on the ninth day it was normal. Respiration increased and became shallow. On the fifth and sixth days there was severe respiratory difficulty and the face was cyanotic. The number of respiration was from 56 to 58 per minute. From the seventh day on the number of respiration decreased with lowering of the temperature and on the ninth day it came down to 24 per minute, and on the sixteenth it became about normal, but it was increased by slight walking or work.

The number of pulse beats also was increased with the rise of temperature. It was from 90 to 120 per minute. On the fifth to sixth day, the expansion was very weak and became thready. The cough increased with the rise of temperature. Sleep was very much disturbed by it on the fifth to seventh days. It came in paroxysms with intervals of two to five minutes at the height of the attacks. The cough was less in the morning when the temperature was lower, but more frequent in the afternoon when the fever rose. The positions of the body materially influenced the frequency. The frequency of cough ran in parallel with the changes in the temperature. The cough subside on the eleventh day.

The amount of sputum increased with the increase of coughs. There was 35 cc. of sputum on the first day. On the fifth day up to 7 P.M. it was 155 cc. There was large amount of output for the following few days. A noticeable thing was that the sputum of the fifth and sixth day contained well-mixed blood. The eighth day on it decreased with the decrease of cough and on the twelfth day it was only 15 cc.

There was heavy feeling over the chest on the first day and dull spontaneous pain in the front of the chest. But it disappeared the next day. There was, however, slight pain over the chest with severe coughing.

Appetite decreased from the very beginning, but it was entirely lost with the rise of temperature and when the general symptoms became serious. It came back when the temperature was lowered and on the ninth day after the onset of the fever the appetite was almost normal.

There was severe lumbago on the third and fourth days and pains in the gastrocnemious muscles on the fourth and fifth days. It was felt as tense feeling on walking and as pressure pain when palpated.

The olfactory nerve became very sensitive. The dislike to the smells of beddings, towels and soaps and even perfumes was marked. The smell of peppermint was, however, acceptable.

As to the objective symptoms there was no dullness or rales in the lungs on the first day. The next day the respiratory sound in the right lung was impure and weak. There were dullness and increased vocal fremitus in the apex and the lower part of the back. On the third day there was dullness in the left apex, subclavicular region and the seventh rib on the axillary line. There was a tympanic area around the left mammary region. Rales, however, could not be heard anywhere. There was only a bronchial sound in an area around the 9th and 10th ribs below the scapula region. On the fourth day the dullness in the right lung became somewhat more marked. The interscapula region was slightly tympanic. In the left lung there was a distinct dullness in the interscapula region and also it was noticeable more or less all over the left lung. Rales were heard all over the lung. Here and there were heard dry, moist rales and also crepitations. The moist rales were fewer than whistling rales. On the fifth day rales were heard everywhere.

Thus the rales and dullness increased day after day until breathing became difficult and weak. But when the crisis had begun the rales and dullness gradually decreased and on the ninth day a few dry rales were heard only at the right back, and the next day no rales were heard and the breath sounds were entirely clear.

There were no marked heart disturbances. On the fifth, sixth and seventh days the apex beat was somewhat accentuated and the second pulmonary artery sound was impure.

The liver was palpable on the fourth day. It was enlarged to two finger breadth below the costal margin on the right mammary line and the edges were dull. It kept at this size until the tenth day when it was one finger breadth below the costal margin and on the twelfth day it was scarcely palpable and on the fifteenth day it hid behind the costal margin. The spleen was not palpable throughout the course. The output of urine was decreased, but no albumen was found.

The most interesting and important findings were that number of the larvae were found in the sputum as shown in the table below.

No. of days after the onset of fever	Amount of sputum	No. of larvae
1	35 cc.	0
2	50 "	0
3	60 "	1
4	100 "	5
5 till 7 P.M.	155 "	178
6	Not collected on account of the	
7	serious condition of patient.	
8	100 cc.	16
9	60 "	7
10	35 "	5
11	20 "	0
12	15 "	0
13	Small amount	0
14	"	0
15	"	0
16	"	0

As the table shows there was one larvae in the sputum collected on the third day, and the number of the larvae increased with the increase in the amount of sputum. On the fifth day up to 7 P.M. there were 178 larvae in 155 cc. of sputum. The condition of the patient became so serious that the collection of sputum was interrupted for the next two days. On the eighth day the number of the larvae decreased to 16 with the decrease in the amount of sputum. Thereafter the number of larvae decreased and on the eleventh day there was none found. At any rate the number of larvae spitted out in the sputum ran in parallel with the condition of the patient and the amount of sputum. There were a few larvae which were casting their skin.

The patella reflex was slightly accentuated, and the cornea and throat were congested.

Fifty days after the test feeding of the eggs of *Ascaris suum* the patient was given anthelmintics, but no worm was recovered. However, from the second patient who had been fed *Ascaris lumbricoides* eggs, 667 worms were recovered 50 days after the feeding by the use of anthelmintics. The sizes of the recovered worms were from three cm to eight cm. They were all immature.

Considerations

The foregoing infection experiments in human body show that the larvae of pig Ascaris move in the body as in human ascaris, and at the lung they cause pneumonia, headaches, fever, difficulty of breathing, pain in the chest, infiltration of lungs and bronchitis. The second experiment confirmed the first and the symptoms agreed with each other. The fact that the larvae were recovered in the sputum indicates that the Ascaris larvae migrate in the body and cause certain pathological changes on the route, and in the lung they cause a sort of Ascaris pneumonia. The larvae during the migration discard their skin.

Conclusions

(1) In the human infection experiments with ascaris of human and pig types, their larvae migrate in the human body as in an experimentally infected animal.

(2) The Ascaris larvae on migration in the human body cause pathological changes in the viscera.

(3) The liver is enlarged during the migration of the larvae.

(4) Ascaris pneumonia is produced during the migration of the larvae.

(5) Ascaris pneumonia is produced on the sixth to ninth days after the test feeding with initial symptoms of chills. There are headaches, fever, respiratory difficulty, coughs, sputum, pain in chest and bronchitis. There may be lumbago, pains in gastrocnemius muscles, olfactory hypersensibility.

(6) The Ascaris pneumonia is recovered in three days to eight days. The seriousness depends on the number of larvae.

(7) Hemoptysis may be present in Ascaris pneumonia.

(8) Larvae are found in the sputum during the Ascaris pneumonia.

(9) The amount of urine is reduced, but no albumen is found.

(10) Spleen does not appear to be enlarged by migration of larvae in the body.

(11) The larvae cast their skin while migrating in the body.

(12) The migrating larvae pass down the esophagus and through the stomach to the intestine where they grow and mature.

(13) The sizes of Ascaris worms in the body in fifty days after the test feeding are from three cm. to eight cm. long and they are immature.

(14) The pig Ascaris can not parasitise till adult worms in human. Therefore although morphologically they are the same, they are entirely different. If there is a strain of pig Ascaris which can parasitise in human it must be a deviated strain. Human body is not a good host for pig Ascaris.

CHAPTER **17**

Trichuriasis

ANATOMICAL LETTER XIV

Epistolarum Anatomicarum Duodeviginti ad Scripta Pertinentium Celeberrimi viri Antonii Marie Valsalvae pars Altera. Venice: Apud Franciscum Pitteri, 1740. Selection from Epistola Anatomica XIV, paragraph 42, p. 45. Translated from the Latin.

Giovanni Battista Morgagni
(1682–1771)

Morgagni was one of that remarkable group of men who made Padua one of the greatest of all centers of medical learning in the seventeenth and eighteenth centuries. Born in Forli, he was a pupil of Valsalva at Padua and served as professor at that university from 1715 until his death. Although he worked steadily and productively throughout his professional life, it was not until his 79th year that the results of his labors were published in five books of 70 letters. These constitute the true foundation of modern pathologic anatomy, correlating for the first time the records of autopsy findings with those of clinical observations.

The localization of Trichuris trichiura *in the cecum, as reported in the following letter, is one of his early observations.*

That you may be able to compare these worms with those to which that worthy man C. L., [indubitably Carl Linneas—Eds.] compared them: those that he saw were no thicker than a hair and hardly longer than a finger's breadth; he definitely judged them to be of the class of Teretes (round worms). Be assured of this: I dissected 11 cadavers consecutively, and in six of them— these being cadavers of men almost all of whom had died suddenly of blows, wounds, suffocation, or apoplexy—I definitely found worms. The first three or four that I saw were white, very thin, and at most a thumb's breadth in length. They lay hidden inside feces at the base of the appendix. Then I saw one inside the appendix of

the second corpse, almost in the middle; it was white, round, pointed at both ends, and so short that it hardly equaled in length half the tip of the little finger.

Nineteen hours after the man's death, I saw in the same appendix, which was empty because of an opening, two or three others just as tiny as the last worms. These were then still alive, of the same shape (if you exclude the tail which I shall describe presently), and somewhat less than the width of two thumbs in length. Lastly, in another corpse I found several, all longer than those mentioned, but equal in length to the last two joints of the little finger; these indeed were not inside the appendix (in which there were merely some rather hard particles of excrement), but in the part of the caecum which adjoined the appendix. So, too, at other times I discovered three at the ends of the caecum and the colon, about at the entrance of the ileum; there were none in the proximal part of the ileum or colon, and one in the entirely empty appendix not far from its opening. I observed that the first three were three fingers' breadth in length, but the last somewhat less; therefore, it is easy to suspect that when they have attained a fixed limit of length they move on to the opening of the appendix. When they have grown larger, they go out into the caecum; however, the extreme thinness of the tail might be an objection to such suspicion. They were very pointed at one end and gradually became a little thickened, turning from white to somewhat dark at the tail which comprised half their length; otherwise, they were totally white and thin as a hair. I noticed that the extremity of one of those that I had found at the orifice of the appendix terminated into something like a long thread, while the rest of the body was indeed a little longer but less slender, and throughout its length an inner line shone through. This line, or canal, as in those a little larger, had visibly translucent transverse tracts. I believe this canal had not been visible in the smaller ones because of their thinness; nor had it appeared in the tail (in the form of a thread or a hair and very long) that I observed among some of the larger worms that I later found inside a woman's appendix.

A REPORT ON THE TRICHURIS TO THE ACADEMY OF SCIENCE AT GÖTTINGEN

Nachricten von der trichuriden, der Societät der Wissenschaften in Goettingen. Göttingische Anzeigen von Gelehrten Sachen: Unter der Aufsicht der Konigliche Gesellschaft der Wissenschaften, Part 25, pp. 243–245, 10 October 1761. Translated from the German.

Johannes George Roederer
(1726–1763)

Born and educated in Strasbourg, Roederer completed his medical studies in Paris, where he graduated in 1750, and later studied in England and Holland. He became a well-known obstetrician in Strasbourg and was invited by Haller to be professor of obstetrics at the University of Göttingen in 1754. While his contributions to parasitology are significant, his reputation rests primarily upon his great work in both the theory and the practice of obstetrics. He subsequently returned to Strasbourg because of poor health.

The following article is among the first recognizable descriptions of Trichuris trichiura.

At this meeting, Dr. Roederer, physician in ordinary and now prosector, read a dissertation which concerns a certain type of worm in the human body not previously described. It is to be added to the three known worms—the round worm, the tapeworm, and *Ascaris lumbricoides*—and is called "trichuris" (hairtailed) by Dr. Roederer because of its shape. A high fever and mucoid diarrhea which was epidemic last winter killed many inhabitants and soldiers stationed here in Göttingen. On dissection of the cadavers, the first two species of worm were found in the small intestines, the third and fourth in the large intestine. Many of the fourth kind, trichuris, were found alone in the excrements, sometimes with the *A. lumbricoides*; sometimes they were passed by the patients. Dr. Roederer reports here his microscopic observations of the same; unfortunately, he was never

able to obtain living specimens. The worm is round and cylindrical and at one end has a blunted point; at the other end it elongates into a thin, threadlike tail. The greatest thickness amounts to about one-third of a line (the 12th part of a Rhenish inch); the length of the body is seven lines and the tail 15 lines. Dr. Roederer found some rolled together like spirals; others were less bent. The former are males, the latter females. In all of them the tail is bent. Body and tail are transparent, shiny, and white, and the body has a white, curved canal. The straight ones (females) have snakelike genital canals throughout the whole body which are oddly curved and contain a

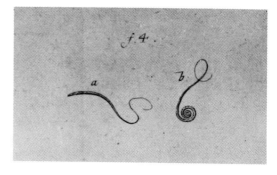

Plate 53. (a) the straight type of worm, not dissimilar to *Ascaris;* (b) the curving type of worm twisted into a coil.

white, transparent organ. The winding of the canals are constituted almost as in the testicles of other animals and similar to the procreative vessels of the rainworm. Dr. Roederer described these canals as well as the digestive canal in more detail and assured himself in this way that they pertained to reproduction because the white organ in them consists of small eggs which adhere together with mucus and which can be pressed out through the birth organ (recognizable from an opening not far from the tail). In the curved worm there are no eggs, and there is no special container other than the seminal canal. The wide, sinuous seminal canal starts at the tail with a closed end; it divides into two parts at the rounded end and unites again. From the blunted end, the birth organ extends like a very delicate thread. As the microscope revealed, it is contained in a sheath which arises from the continuation of the seminal canal. The seminal canal contains a tough, spermatic mucus which consists of very small vesicles and which emerges by itself from the worm if it decomposes. The digestive canal runs along the hollow edge of the worm without bending and is surrounded by the reproductive vessels. A simple canal seems to go through the tail; this contains a mass composed of irregular pieces. Dr. Roederer suspects that the worm searches through its dirty surroundings with its tail, like a proboscis, and with its point sucks up nourishment therefrom. Its composition is like a kind of jelly which runs easily when one cuts into it. The membrane is strong, hard, almost horny, and resists putrefaction for a long time; its smooth surface, as well as the surface of the proboscis, is covered with granules. If the worm dries a little, transverse stripes appear along its whole length, being without a doubt signs of the muscles which pull the animal together. This new kind of intestinal worm could be described according to the Linnean order as: *corpus teres, longa proboscis filiformis, genitale curuarum, eminens, rectarum, apertura lateralis.* [Plate 53 is from an article written by Roederer in collaboration with Carolus Gottlieb Wagler (Der morbo mucoso. Göttingen: Apud Victorinum Bossigelium, 1762. 211 pp.). Legends translated from the Latin—Eds.]

CHAPTER **18**

Enterobiasis

OXYURIS VERMICULARIS

Oxyure vermiculaire. Traité Zoologique et Physiologique sur les Vers Intestinaux de l'Homme. Paris: C. L. F. Panckoucke, 1824. Pp. 149–157. Selections from pp. 149, 153–157. Translated from the French version of the original German.

Johann Gottfried Bremser
(1767–1827)

While curator of the Museum of Natural History in Vienna, Bremser published his monumental work, Lebende Wurmer im Lebenden Menschen. A zoologist, he studied at Jena, where he received his doctorate. In addition to his interest in parasitology he published numerous papers on scarlet fever, cowpox, and measles.

Though pinworm has been known since antiquity, this is the first exact classification of Oxyuris vermicularis (Enterobius vermicularis).

The *Oxyuris vermicularis* lives in the large intestine, principally in the rectum. . . . During the winter of 1809, I found a great number of species of this worm in the large intestines of many wild rabbits, and I did not hesitate for an instant to rank them in this genus, although at the time I knew the oxyurids of the horse only from the drawings of Goeze and Rudolphi. Later, when I had these worms drawn to a scale larger than life size, I was struck by their similarity to those found in the rectum of man. I compared them more carefully and became convinced that the latter (the oxyurids) should no longer be ranked with the lumbricoids. The lumbricoids are always thinned out toward the two extremities and, furthermore, are very clearly distinguished from other nematodes by three papillae or buttons at the anterior end. The oxyurids are equally tapered toward their anterior extremity, but they are terminated at the other end by a point (this is espe-

cially true of the females); furthermore, they lack the three papillae at the beginning of the head. The interior structure of these two species of worm does not differ very much. I communicated my observations to Rudolphi, and this wise observer shared my opinion. His supplementary volume spoke of many new species of this type, but despite all this, I had not yet achieved the degree of certainty that I desired.

Goeze has drawn a worm of this type which he regards as a male, probably because he was unable to find any eggs. The males of all the nematodes are, in general, smaller than the females by one-half to one-third, and the termination of their tails is completely different. In Goeze's figures copied by Joerdens and Brera, one sees that the length is the same and that the termination of the tail is absolutely the same, but one sees no eggs. These may be females that have laid their eggs, or perhaps the eggs are either not yet completely developed or not yet fertilized. Finally, perhaps these individuals are deprived of sexual organs, as are the bees and ants. I am unable to decide. The oxyurids that Rudolphi found in the horse contained eggs, as did mine; therefore, all were females. Among the worms from the wild rabbits, there were many that had the end of the tail blunted and that were rolled in a spiral. I also noted on many a little spiculum; in general, however, these were smaller than are the females ordinarily. I concluded that the male oxyurids of man ought to be formed in the same manner, but among all the worms that I had at my disposal, I could not find one that had the same characteristics. This was true for a long time of the oxyurids of domestic rabbits and of a number of different mice. This circumstance almost made me believe that the development of the oxyurids was analogous to that of the lice which, in general, are viviparous and only produce females in the summer when nourishment is in abundance but which, contrariwise, lay eggs in autumn which, in spring, develop into both males and females. The males then fertilize the entire generation for the coming year. But while making the observation that domestic rabbits, horses, and men usually receive nourishment in sufficient quantity and that, consequently, the worms that they carry inside them are never in want, I began to presume, perhaps because of this, that the female oxyurids were able to multiply their species without the intervention of males. There are, by contrast, the wild rabbits and their worms lacking nourishment in the winter, and it's just in that season that I found male oxyurids. Famine does not have an advantageous influence, as we know, on the faculty of reproduction. It seemed to me that, conforming to the wise dispositions of nature which loves only to reproduce and conserve life, the generative faculty was divided between two individuals so that each of them would have less difficulty preserving the species and that the worms coming from a primitive form would be entirely destroyed. While I abandoned myself to these conjectures, feeling a sort of satisfaction at having perceived what I believed to be the reason one finds no male oxyurids in certain animals, leaving others to judge the probability of these conjectures, I communicated my opinions to Soemmerring. Shortly thereafter, he was kind enough to send me a small jar full of oxyurids preserved in wine. These worms came from his own son, who passed them after having taken an olive oil enema. Soemmerring suggested that I might find among them some worms that had the characteristics of males. I had searched for such a specimen for some time. I examined them and did find some. I later received from the same physician and from Hermann, additional samples which Rudolphi did not hesitate to characterize as males; he probably will find some more himself.

The result of these observations is that the worms known under the name of *Ascaris vermicularis* henceforth ought to be classed in the genus oxyuris and not in the genus ascaris and that the sexes of these oxyurids can be distinguished by the characteristics that we have reported.

CHAPTER 19

Toxocariasis

CHRONIC EOSINOPHILIA
REPORT OF A CASE WITH NECROSIS OF THE LIVER, PULMONARY INFILTRATIONS, ANEMIA AND ASCARIS INFESTATION.

American Journal of Diseases of Children, 73: 34–43, 1947.
Selections from pp. 34–39.

Josephine G. Perlingiero (Randall)
(1918–   )

Dr. Perlingiero was a pediatric fellow at the University of Pennsylvania at the time this article was published.

Paul György
(1893–1976)

A Hungarian educated at the University of Budapest, he was emeritus professor of pediatrics and formerly director of pediatrics, Philadelphia General Hospital. His area of major interest was nutrition.

Within recent years three "syndromes" centering around eosinophilia and pulmonary changes have been described in the literature; namely, Loeffler's syndrome, tropical eosinophilia or "eosinophilic lung" and pulmonary acariasis.

Since the description of these syndromes many cases of eosinophilic leukocytosis with pulmonary changes have been reported. Most of these cases have been found to occur in foreign countries, and only a relatively few in this country. It is primarily for this reason that the following case of eosinophilia with pulmonary infiltrations is being reported; a further reason is that it was found to be associated with necrosis of the liver in the presence of ascaris infestation.

Report of a Case

A two-year-old Negro boy was admitted to the Children's Medical Ward of the University Hospital on Oct. 12, 1944, because of fever, loss of weight, cough, vomiting and diarrhea. He had been well until two weeks before admission, at which time he became feverish and listless and began to have five to six loose green stools per day. The diarrhea lasted for several days and was then followed by constipation and vomiting after meals. About five days before admission he began to have a productive cough, mostly nocturnal, and was given ammonium chloride, acetanalid and compound mixture of opium and glycyrrhiza.

The significant facts in his past medical history included eczema beginning at two weeks of age and lasting several months, "asthmatic bronchitis" and bronchopneumonia at one month and possible pertussis at 18 months. He lived in Florida from his twelfth to his eighteenth month and is said to have ingested large quantities of "dirt" during that time. He was immunized against smallpox and diphtheria before he was seven months of age.

The family history was noncontributory, although the father was alleged to have had a positive Wassermann reaction.

The physical examination on admission showed a pallid, sallow, irritable, light-haired colored boy, in acute distress, with a temperature of 104 F, a pulse rate of 132, a respiratory rate of 40, pale lips and conjunctivas, thin mucopurulent nasal discharge, injected pharynx, shotty inguinal and axillary lymph nodes, an enlarged liver which was palpable four cm. below the costal margin in the midclavicular line and transient rales in the area of the lower lobe of the right lung posteriorly. The spleen was not palpable and the heart was normal. An initial blood count showed a hemoglobin value of 35 per cent and white blood cell count of 40,000, with 37 per cent eosinophils.

The child's subsequent clinical course was characterized by septic fever for several weeks (his temperature rising to 103 to 104 F each evening), by nocturnal cough, vomiting and distention, listlessness and anorexia. An early roentgenogram of the chest revealed "definite increase in the prominence of the pulmonary markings in both lung fields, which could be due in part to hypoventilation, but in addition to this showed some increased prominence of the pulmonary markings in the peritruncal region, particularly in the trunks in the lower lobe, roentgenologic observations which could support a diagnosis of Loeffler's syndrome in view of the high eosinophilia and the allergic history'' (Dr. E.R. Pendergrass). The child was given a short course of penicillin but showed no demonstrable response. He was also given several small transfusions in an effort to correct this anemia, which together with the eosinophilia remained unexplained in spite of the studies done.

The vomiting and distention did not seem to be relieved by conservative measures, and on October 21 an abdominal laparotomy was done to rule out an obstructive lesion in the right upper quadrant. At the operation the liver was found to be enlarged and to have small, gray-white lesions scattered over the smooth surface of all lobes. A biopsy was made; there were focal necrotic lesions with numerous polymorphonuclear neutrophils and eosinophilic leukocytes, and also numerous multinucleated giant cells. Shortly after the operation, in an effort to protect the liver, administration of methionine was started (3 Gm three times a day). He was also given a high caloric, high protein diet, vitamin K, stable ferrous sulfate and the usual supplementary vitamins.

After the laparotomy the child began to improve. His cough subsided gradually, and the daily rise in temperature was somewhat lower than had been previously noted. On two occasions (October 22 and November 22) edema of the lips developed, each time lasting several days and not associated with edema elsewhere. By the end of November there was also a peculiar odor and hypertrichosis of the legs and arms. About this time his temperature became normal, and it remained entirely normal, except for an occasional infrequent rise to 101 F, until he was discharged in April 1945.

On Dec. 23, 1944, the child vomited a single male adult ascaris, after which he improved remarkably, as evidenced by favorable changes in his behavior, activity, and appetite. Administration of methionine was temporarily discontinued; it was started again on Jan 23, 1945, and the drug was then given continuously throughout the rest of his hospital stay. Just prior to his discharge he was given the accepted treatment of hexylresorcinol for ascariasis.

On April 7 a second biopsy of the liver was made; the hepatic tissue was found to be essentially normal, with few remaining necrotic lesions encapsulated by fibrous tissue. The roentgenogram of the chest at this time showed only a slight increase in the pulmonary markings. The child was discharged on April 28 in good condition, his hemoglobin having remained above 60 per cent since the time of his operation. His eosinophilia however, persisted, his total white cell count at discharge being 28,000, with 75 per cent

eosinophils. His cough had not recurred. At the last visit, on Jan. 11, 1946, the child was in excellent condition, had been gaining weight steadily and was asymptomatic. His liver was barely palpable 1 cm. below the costal margin, the only abnormal finding being his moderate eosinophilia.

The other studies done during hospitalization and after discharge did not reveal any essential abnormality, and included the following: biopsies of bone marrow, lymph node and muscle; repeated cultures of urine, feces, blood, duodenal drainage, pharyngeal and bronchial secretions, abdominal fluid and material aspirated from the liver; tuberculin tests in all dilutions; agglutination tests for typhoid, paratyphoid and *Brucella abortus*; intradermal tests for trichinosis, lymphogranuloma inguinale and echinococcosis; repeated examination of stool for ova and parasites; tests of swallowing function; roentgenograms of the long bones; repeated van den Bergh tests; fragility tests; platelet counts, and sickling tests. Blood counts and serologic tests for one sibling showed nothing abnormal. A bronchoscopic examination after the cough had subsided (on November 22) showed a hyperemic bronchial tree, and the secretions obtained at this time contained no ova or parasites, no eosinophils, lipoid material or tubercle bacilli. A cutaneous test with ascaris extract elicited a strongly positive reaction. . . .

NEMATODE ENDOPHTHALMITIS

Transactions American Academy of Ophthalmology and Otolaryngology: 99–109, Nov.-Dec. 1950. Selections from pp. 99–104, 107–109.

Helenor Campbell Wilder
(1895–   )

A native of Baltimore, Helenor Wilder labored for 30 years in the section for ophthalmic pathology of the Armed Forces Institute of Pathology, where she was chief at the time of her retirement in 1953. Although she did not have an M.D. degree, her contributions to the eye pathology of neoplasms, radiation, and toxoplasmosis earned her honorary membership in the American Academy of Ophthalmology and Otolaryngology. In 1953 she was voted Woman of the Year in Science.

The significance of ectopic helminthiasis, especially as it effects the eye, came as a shock to ophthalmologists, and preceded the work on the more general aspects of larva migrans.

Routine examination of eyes at the Armed Forces Institute of Pathology disclosed a well-defined group in which the clinical histories and pathologic lesions were strikingly uniform. The eyes, with few exceptions, were from children. In most instances observation of a white pupillary reflex by the parents was the first evidence of ocular disease. On ophthalmoscopic examination there was seen behind the lens a pale mass with blood vessels coursing over it, and a diagnosis of retinoblastoma led to enucleation.

Eosinophilic abscesses, sometimes surrounded by epithelioid and giant cells, presented a pathologic picture not accounted for by the more commonly recognized granulomatous lesions of the eye. Special stains failed to demonstrate bacteria, fungi, inclusion bodies, or organisms of any kind. As the lesions resembled those seen in helminth infections elsewhere in the body and those described in the eyes of experimental animals, it was decided to reexamine specimens exhibiting a suggestive inflammatory reaction in the hope of finding the responsible organism. Forty-six eyes, each from a different patient, were selected for this investigation. On the basis of previous microscopic examination, diagnoses of endophthalmitis, pseudoglioma, and Coats's disease, i.e., external exudative or hemorrhagic retinitis, had been made. Serial sections were prepared on all available material, which in no case was complete since the specimens had been sectioned previously. Notwithstanding this handicap, nematode larvae (Plate 54) or their residual hyaline capsules were found in 24 eyes. In one case examination of over 2300 sections resulted in the discovery of a single larva, the entire worm being contained within 12 sections. In another eye, three larvae were found.

In nine eyes the larvae were exceptionally well preserved. These were examined by Dr. B. G. Chitwood, who gave the following report:

So far as can be determined on the basis of the material at hand, the specimens are third stage hookworm larvae. No information as to species has been obtained. However, Ancylostoma sp., Necator sp. and Uncinaria sp. are possibilities These specimens are the same stage but differ very slightly from Oesophagostomum larvae 24 hours after infection, as seen in sections of a pig's esophagus shown to us by Dr. D. A. Shark, Zoological Division, Bureau of Animal Industry. Furthermore, we are unable to distinguish between this specimen and a nematode seen in a pathologic section of a dog kidney.

The fact that the larvae in these cases have been recognized as hookworm does not rule out other nematodes (Strongyloides, Ascaris, etc.) as possible causative agents in endophthalmitis.

During the course of this study an unusual coincidence led for a time to the incrimination of a nematode larva which had nothing to do with the ocular lesion. In those eyes which were sectioned in paraffin, filariform larvae, very different in appearance from the larvae within the abscesses, were found apparently within the globe. They were all complete, unsectioned larvae and were not surrounded by cellular exudate. As in a fourth case the larva lay on top of the section, it was decided without question that they were contaminants, probably deposited by a parasitized fly on the slides while they were drying on the warm plate.

Clinical Data

The 24 eyes in which the presence of larvae was established were all from children. The youngest was three years of age, the oldest 13, and the majority were of preschool and early school age: three through five years, 12 patients; six through nine years, nine; 10 through 13 years, two.

Fourteen of the eyes were from girls, 10 from boys. Twenty-one of the patients were white and three colored. The specimens included 16 right eyes, six left and two with side unspecified. In two instances lesions in the remaining eye indicated bilateral involvement. Although the majority of the patients were from the southeastern United States, they were by no means limited to this region. It must be taken into consideration, however, that the children from northern and western states may have lived in or visited other localities. A preoperative diagnosis of retinoblastoma had been made in 20 instances, pseudoglioma in three, and in one in which the inflammatory reaction was particularly fulminating the clinical diagnosis was panophthalmitis. Anderson observed that glioma (retinoblastoma) was the usual clinical diagnosis in ophthalmomyiasis when the larvae were located subretinally. Neither helminth infection nor any systemic disease was mentioned in the records of 20 patients. One had a history of old nematode infection. One child was cachectic, one had frontal headaches at the time of onset of ocular symptoms, and another, continued ocular pain and visual loss following meningitis eight years before enucleation. Usually there were no clinical signs of local inflammation. In addition to the 24 proved cases, there were 22 which were believed, on the basis of a similar pathologic picture, to be probable nematode endophthalmitis although larvae were not found. In general the clinical pattern and geographic distribution closely paralleled those of the proved cases, although three patients were adults and one was from as far west as the state of Washington.

The most characteristic lesion was the eosinophilic abscess with a center in which the cytoplasmic granules tended to become basophilic as a result of necrosis. Surrounding the abscesses were epithelioid cells, occasionally with giant cells, and inflammatory granulation tissue infiltrated by eosinophils, lymphocytes, and plasma cells which frequently were multinucleated, some having as many as five or six nuclei.

There was considerable variation in the relative number of these cells in different lesions, apparently depending on duration and on the stage of disintegration of the larvae. Polymorphonuclear leukocytes were not conspicuous except in very early cases.

In nematode endophthalmitis as seen in the cases from the Institute the location of the lesion indicates blood-borne infection. The larval parasites gain entry to the host by one of two possible routes—through the skin or through the mouth. If they enter through the skin, they reach the right heart by way of the venous circulation whence they are carried through the lung to the left heart and so through the carotid, ophthalmic and ciliary arteries into the eye. If they enter by the mouth, they are probably transported directly to the intestine. They may then penetrate the intestinal wall and be carried by the venous circulation to the

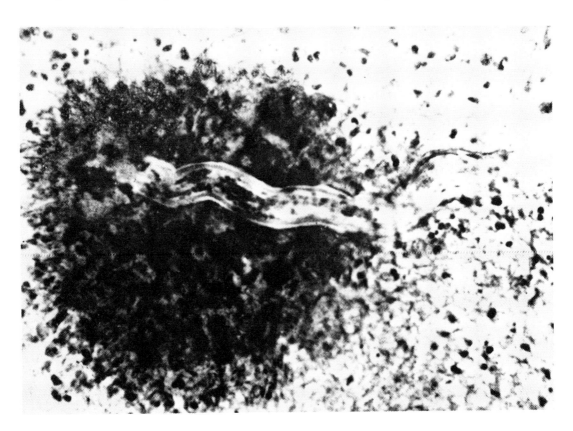

Plate 54. Nematode larva in eosinophilic abscess in vitreous membrane.

right heart and thence reach the eye by the same route as if they had entered through the skin. In either case migration through the lung, demonstrated by Fülleborn and others, readily accounts for their presence in the eye. Choroidal lesions indicate that the metastases are generally to the choroid, as in neoplasms, rather than to the retina, and that the larvae reach the retina and vitreous by direct invasion. Further proof of this was the case of Heath in which a larva was seen leaving a choroidal vessel by perforating its wall. Cataract associated with hookworm disease has been accredited to anemia, toxemia, or a combination of the two by Calhoun. He did not observe intraocular larvae clinically, and the eyes did not come to microscopic examination. He regarded retinal hemorrhages as the result of toxins, whereas Fülleborn thought it possible that they resulted from larval emboli.

Summary

Forty-six cases which had been diagnosed pathologically as pseudoglioma, Coats's disease, and endophthalmitis, and which showed similar inflammatory reactions, were the subject of special study. With few exceptions the 46 patients were children, the greatest number from the southeastern United States. In most cases a clinical diagnosis of retinoblastoma had preceded enucleation. Nematode larvae or their residual hyaline capsules were found in 24 eyes. In 22 others the characteristic reaction justified a tentative diagnosis of nematode endophthalmitis. In no instance was a parasite found in the original routine sections. Serial sections were necessary to demonstrate the larvae in every case. In nine eyes the larvae were exceptionally well preserved and were identified by Dr. B. G. Chitwood as those of hookworm. The exact species remains to be identified.

Conclusion

The finding of intraocular larvae by serial sectioning and the identification of the specific pathologic reaction that they evoke has led to the conclusion that nematodes play an important and hitherto unrecognized role in blindness in children, and particularly in the production of pseudoglioma and Coats's disease in the United States of America.

CHRONIC EOSINOPHILIA DUE TO VISCERAL LARVA MIGRANS

Pediatrics, 9: 7–18, 1952. Selections from pp. 7–8, 10–12, 14–15, 17–18.

Paul C. Beaver
(1905–   )

Born in Indiana, educated at Wabash College, Beaver obtained his M.S. and Ph.D. at the University of Illinois. He has taught parasitology since 1945 at the School of Medicine, Tulane University, where he is now emeritus professor of parasitology.

The following article describes the role of Toxocara canis *in visceral larva migrans.*

His co-authors on this paper were C. H. Snyder, G. M. Carrera, J. H. Dent, and J. W. Lafferty.

Among the causes of eosinophilia are the helminthiases. In the absence of demonstrable evidence of suspected helminth parasites, their presence in prepatent stages may sometimes tentatively be presumed. However, eosinophilia sometimes persists for periods far beyond known prepatency for all likely helminths. Then, depending upon geographic location, degree of eosinophilia, pulmonary signs and other related clinical observations, terms such as Weingarten's disease, Frimodt-Möller's syndrome, familial eosinophilia and eosinophilic pseudoleukemia have been employed to denote chronic eosinophilia of ill-defined etiology.

Four recent reports have described, in young children, chronic extreme eosinophilia accompanied by eosinophilic granulomatous lesions in an enlarged liver together with some degree of pulmonary infiltration, fever, cough and hyperglobulinemia. Typical lesions in hepatic tissue sections were described by Zuelzer and Apt, Perlingiero and György, Mercer et al. and Behrer. Parasites were not reported in the cases described by Zuelzer and Apt. The patient of Perlingiero and György vomited a male ascaris, but worms were not associated with the hepatic lesions and additional worms in the intestine could not be demonstrated either then or at subsequent examinations. In the cases reported by Mercer et al. and by Behrer the patients were found to have intestinal ascariasis along with nematode larvae which they identified as *Ascaris lumbricoides* in the lesions of the liver.

The present authors have studied three cases [only two have been included—Eds.] all of which are strikingly similar to the foregoing ones. However, these studies suggest a different etiology for this syndrome, which shall be designated as visceral larva migrans to distinguish it from cutaneous larva migrans (creeping eruption) to which it apparently is closely related. In both conditions there is prolonged migration of infective nematode larvae through the tissues, involving primarily the skin in cutaneous larva migrans and the internal organs in visceral larva migrans. Moreover, in both forms the invading larvae generally are of species naturally adapted to hosts other than man, remain immature and eventually perish in the tissues.

Report of Cases

Case 1. M. M., a white boy 16 months of age, was referred for study of eosinophilia. He had always been considered well until a few weeks earlier when anemia with eosinophilia was recognized during routine laboratory studies preceding a proposed elective herniorrhaphy at another hospital. The only symptom was questionable anorexia of less than two months' duration. The child had a pet dog, and had been seen to eat dirt.

Physical examination revealed an irritable and pale child. Liver was palpable 3 cm below the right costal margin, and the spleen 3 cm below the left costal margin.

Hgb. was 5.8 gm/100 cc and WBC count was 45 thousand/cmm with 70% eosinophils. There were 4.4% reticulocytes and platelets appeared normal in smears. Sternal bone marrow was considered normal except for eosinophilia. The serum protein level was 6.9gm/100 cc. (A/G=4.2/2.7). Results of the Wassermann, tuberculin and cephalin flocculation tests were negative. The level of serum bilirubin was normal and roentgenograms of the lungs showed nothing unusual.

Examination of fecal specimens obtained after purgation revealed no evidence of parasites. Examination of duodenal juice and cultures for strongyloides yielded negative results. Results of skin tests for trichinosis were negative.

At laparotomy, after correction of the anemia, the liver was studded with white plaques measuring 5 to 10 mm in diameter over the entire visible surface. Biopsy showed numerous areas of necrosis and extensive focal infiltration with eosinophilic leukocytes. Around some of the necrotic areas, in addition to eosinophils, there were numerous epithelioid cells and giant cells of the foreign body type. Eosinophils were also seen in some of the portal spaces. Except for the absence of parasites the lesions resembled closely those observed in Case 3 (vide infra). Cultures from the biopsy revealed no bacteria or fungi.

Patient was then discharged. When last seen at the age of 2½ years, he was in vigorous health. Liver and spleen were no longer palpable. Hgb. was 11.7 gm/100 cc and WBC count 18.6 thousand/cmm with 35% eosinophils. Hemograms of the patient's mother and his older sister revealed no abnormalities.

Case 3. J. G., a white girl, age 2½ years, had seemed to thrive until the age of 12 months when she apparently had mild transient jaundice. When she was about 15 months old, she began to look pale, lose weight, and become cross in distinct contrast to her previous sunny disposition.

From that time until admission she had frequent infections of the upper respiratory tract, once with pyoderma. Throughout the autumn of 1949 she showed daily elevations of temperature, at times reaching 41.1°C. Frequent courses of antibiotics and numerous symptomatic measures had provided only slight or transient benefit.

When it was discovered that she had severe eosinophilia (50 thousand WBC/cmm with 50% eosinophils), she was admitted June 5, 1950, for further study. She did not appear sick, weighed 13.6 kg and was 90 cm tall. The liver, which was 3 cm below the right costal margin, was smooth and not tender; the spleen was not felt. Hgb. level was 10.4 gm/100 cc and WBC count was 14.2 thousand/cmm with 50% eosinophils. All the other usual laboratory studies, including Wassermann, tuberculin and trichinella tests, yielded negative results. Repeated examination of stools and duodenal contents failed to reveal the presence of parasites.

Laparotomy disclosed an enlarged liver studded with white plaques. Section showed extensive areas of focal necrosis and pronounced inflammatory reaction around the necrotic foci and in the portal spaces. The necrotic areas were of irregular shape and measured as much as 0.5 mm in greatest width. In serial section reconstruction, the shape of these lesions was seen to be irregular and tortuous. Although in some regions there was total necrosis of all cellular elements, in whose place there was amorphous acidophilic material, in other areas the necrotic hepatic cells has been replaced almost exclusively by eosinophilic leukocytes and a few foreign body giant cells. Eosinophilic leukocytes were also present in large numbers around the areas of advanced necrosis mentioned above and in the portal spaces at some distance from these foci of necrosis. Occasionally, necrotic areas were surrounded by epithelioid cells and prominent giant cells of the foreign body type, even though no foreign body was seen within them. In five sections, portions of a parasitic organism were observed. The parasite, which from its general characteristics was obviously a larval nematode (Plate 55, Figs 1–3), was well preserved and showed no evidence of autolysis or degeneration. No bacteria were seen in the neighborhood of the parasite or in the necrotic areas. Around the larva there was a loose mantle of eosinophils, in some regions not over 30 μ in thick-

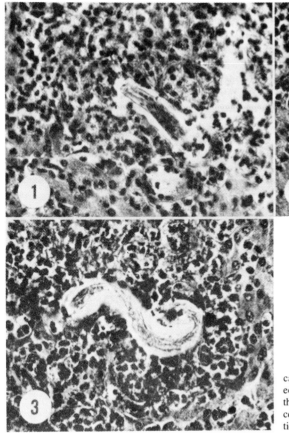

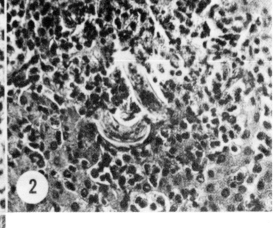

Plate 55. Fig. 1. Anterior end of Toxocara larva in liver of case 3. Note moderate inflammatory reaction, mostly eosinophilic. *Fig. 2.* Same larva as in Fig. 1 sectioned through lower level. Note close proximity of normal hepatic cells. *Fig. 3.* Same larva as in Figs. 1 and 2 showing midportion of body and character of reaction.

ness. Hepatic cells immediately adjacent to this zone of inflammatory reaction were well preserved. In some areas (Fig. 2) only 30 μ separated the larva from normal parenchyma.

Soon after laparotomy the patient was discharged. She continued to have recurrent febrile bouts and six months later the WBC count was still elevated—16.5 thousand/cmm with 34% eosinophils.

Cortisone therapy was then tried, and over a period of 21 days she received a total of 515 mg intramuscularly. There was some subjective improvement, and the eosinophilia of the blood receded to 28% of 8 thousand WBC/cmm then returned to higher levels. At this time it was learned that the family had a pet dog which had died of heart worms soon after the child was hospitalized. As a baby, the patient had had a habit of reaching out from the playpen to grasp handfuls of dirt, part of which she usually swallowed.

Two months after the cortisone therapy, she was given Hetrazan®, 100 mg three times daily for four days, and the same course was repeated twice thereafter at 10 day intervals. The eosinophilia increased from 28% to 40% following the first course, then receded to

10% and remained at that level for one month. One year after admission the patient was free of symptoms and physical examination showed no abnormalities.

The Parasite

The larva observed in the biopsy specimen was contained in five sections that were cut at a thickness of 7 μ. From these sections it was possible to reconstruct almost the entire worm; only the tip of the tail and a small portion of the body wall were not visualized. It was approximately 0.35 mm in length and 20 μ in diameter in the midportion. As situated in the tissues, the head end was viewed slightly obliquely and in all evident details resembled the infective stage of *Toxocara canis* or *T. cati*. It differed from the larva of *Ascaris lumbricoides* by its greater size and the form of its head.

For comparison of larvae in tissues, white mice were given infective eggs of *Toxocara canis* and

T. cati. On the eleventh day after 5,000 eggs had been fed, the larvae of *T. canis* were found in the liver, brain, kidneys, spinal cord and diaphragm. Excepting the lungs, other tissues were not searched. In pressed preparations of the various organs the larvae appeared to be free in the tissues and were actively motile. Progress among muscle fibers of the diaphragm was made with ease and was mostly backwards. Encapsulation was not observed in any organ although lesions were grossly visible in the liver, kidneys and lungs, especially the latter. Two months after feeding 10,000 eggs, active larvae were found in the liver and kidneys but dead encapsulated ones were also numerous. One was observed actively moving within a dense capsule in the kidney. They were most abundant in the brain, however, there being 40 of them actively moving about in a pressed preparation of 8 to 10 cmm of cerebellum. After two months and five months in the mouse, *Toxocara cati* larvae also were found most abundantly in the brain. Each of two mice were given relatively light infections of only 200 *T. canis* eggs. After three and a half and six months, respectively, 60 and 47 larvae, all living and active, were found in pressed preparations of the entire brain. Fewer, some of which were unencapsulated, were found in the liver, and one encapsulated but active larva was observed in the kidney of the mouse with the older infection. Microscopic studies of infected brain tissues have not been made; sections of liver showed lesions essentially as described by Hoeppli et al.

Morphologically the larvae of *Toxocara canis* were the same in all organs examined and even after three and a half months did not differ notably in size or structure from the infective stage in the egg. The length varied around 375 μ and the diameter in the mid-region was 18 to 22 μ in heat-killed specimens. The mouth was slightly subterminal and dorsal to a hood-like thickening of the cuticula over the anterior tip. Viewed from the side this process was a conspicuous feature, giving the appearance of a low spine or angular tuberosity. The tip of the tail was spinelike, bent slightly dorsad. Internal structures were poorly differentiated. A nonmuscular clear esophagus in the anterior third of the body joined an opaque granular intestine which could be traced with some difficulty to the region of the anus 30 to 40 μ from the posterior end.

The adult stage of *T. canis* is described in standard texts on veterinary and general parasitology. Its morphology has been reported more fully by Taylor. It is cosmopolitan in distribution and is the commonest large roundworm of dogs. In morphology and life cycle it closely resembles the human ascarid, *Ascaris lumbricoides*. Although it can be distinguished from human ascaris by its spearpoint-shaped head, this difference might be overlooked by the casual observer. This species, possibly incorrectly identified, has been reported only once from man, although the corresponding species in cats, *Toxocara cati,* has been observed in the adult stage 10 or 11 times in man.

Discussion

The authors' observations indicate that larvae of *Toxocara canis* were responsible for the symptoms and lesions in at least one and possibly all of the three patients. It is further suggested by these observations, along with earlier reports of similar cases, that the type of parasitism which the authors have called visceral larva migrans probably is common, especially among young children. Presumably, infective-stage eggs, when taken into the human intestine, hatch and the larvae migrate through the intestinal wall as they would in their normal host, the dog. In man and other abnormal hosts to which they are not adapted, however, instead of migrating through the liver via the blood stream, or through the lymphatics, to the heart, the lungs, the pharynx, and back to the intestine, a large proportion of them remain in the tissues. They migrate, or are carried, into various organs, especially the liver where they are able to survive for relatively long periods, wandering through the tissues, leaving in their wake lesions similar to those produced by hookworm and other types of skin-penetrating larvae which are responsible for cutaneous larva migrans.

It is not unlikely that larvae of *Toxocara cati* and other nematode species also may cause visceral larva migrans, although *Toxocara canis* probably is the commonest offender among the parasites of animals associated with man. *T. canis* eggs are known to be common in dooryard soil. Headlee found them in soil samples from 45% of 74 dooryards of New Orleans families in which one or more members had ascariasis. In a similar study they were found in four of 17 dooryards in southern Georgia; eggs of *Ascaris lumbricoides* were found in 74% and 82% of these same areas. *T. canis* being common, widespread in distribution, and carried by a host that lives intimately with children, it is not surprising that such an association should exist.

Other facts are of interest regarding dog ascarid larvae. Hocppli et al. found that, whereas larvae of human, pig and horse ascarids live only about two weeks in the liver of white mice, those of the dog ascarid remain alive and active for at least six weeks, and may be present though encapsulated after two months. Furthermore, a high percentage of dog ascarid larvae remain in the liver, whereas other species tend to become encapsulated early and die, or to escape from the liver to reach the lungs. Hoeppli remarked on the larger size and more active movements of *T. canis* as compared with other species.

Immune responses to helminthic infections are primarily caused by and operate against larval migration stages in tissues. In experimental animals, ascaris larvae are screened out and destroyed principally in the liver and lungs, although some are trapped in other organs. Sprent and Chen found that immunity to ascaris in white mice can be measured by the number of larvae that remain in the liver as compared with those that succeed in reaching the lungs. Lesions produced by various nematode larvae in tissues of immune hosts are strikingly similar in different hosts and different tissues, being eosinophilic granulomas like those seen in liver biopsies from children with chronic high eosinophilia. Also, the tissue reactions, including peripheral eosinophilia, are proportional in both intensity and promptness to the immune state and to the abnormality of the host.

Although reactions to parasites of man in abnormal hosts (experimental animals) have been extensively studied, knowledge of the reverse situation in which man himself is the abnormal host for parasites of other animals is limited mostly to cutaneous larva migrans. In this instance larvae spend variable lengths of time migrating through the superficial layers of the skin, producing tortuous linear lesions with infiltration of eosinophils into adjacent deeper tissues. As is well known, this condition in its severest forms is caused by larvae of the cat and dog hookworms, *Ancylostoma braziliense*, *Uncinaria stenocephala* and *Ancylostoma caninum*. Similar reactions of less severity and shorter duration may be caused by the cattle hookworm, *Bunostomum phlebotomum* and perhaps by a number of other species that normally enter their usual hosts percutaneously. Reactions in all instances appear to be proportional to the degree of sensitization. Dog or cat hookworms in some individuals, for example, may not produce the usual severe reactions and even the larvae of human hookworms, *Ancylostoma duodenale* and *Necator americanus,* may produce in individuals with a high degree of sensitization typical creeping eruption that persists for several days. Thus, it becomes apparent that in sensitized or hyperimmune normal hosts, and in abnormal ones, various nematode larvae behave similarly in man and in other animals. Although the conclusive demonstration of visceral larva migrans in the human host is inherently difficult, this condition may be as common as its cutaneous counterpart.

Conclusions and Summary

Three cases of chronic extreme eosinophilia with granulomatous lesions in the liver have been studied. A larval nematode observed in sections from the liver of one patient has been identified either as *Toxocara canis* or *Toxocara cati*, common cosmopolitan ascarids of dogs and cats; available evidence favors the former.

The term visceral larva migrans is proposed for this type of parasitism, known in animals but not previously described in humans. It is related to better known cutaneous larva migrans, in that both are usually caused by infective stage larvae of nematode parasites of other animals. Man being an abnormal host, either has unfavorable tissue reactions or otherwise fails to provide stimuli for usual tissue migration and development of the parasite. As a result, larvae remain active for variable periods in various tissues. Similar but less severe and less prolonged reactions occur when the larvae of normal nematode parasites of man invade the tissues of a hyperimmune individual.

Visceral larva migrans is usually a relatively benign disease, characterized chiefly by sustained eosinophilia, pneumonitis and heptaomegaly and probably is due both to direct tissue damage by migrating larvae and to allergic responses to their products. Its severity varies with the number of larvae in the tissues and the immune or allergic state of the infected individual.

CHAPTER 20

Filariasis Bancrofti

HELMINTHOLOGY

Helminthologie. Gazette Medicale de Paris, 18: 665–667, 1863. Translated from the French.

Jean-Nicolas Demarquay
(1814–1875)

The son of a farmer in Longueval, a village in the Somme district, Jean-Nicolas Demarquay struggled to earn the preliminary education which permitted him to study medicine and finally to receive a doctorate in medicine in 1847. In addition to making notable contributions in his own specialty, surgery, he published papers in a variety of fields, including hypnosis and pharmacology. He was an active participant in the military-political events of his time and received, for bravery, the Cross of Commander of the Legion of Honor.

During one of his operations, Demarquay discovered a microfilaria whose presence, although he did not understand its nature, he duly recorded in the following article.

Note on a Tumor of the Scrotal Sac Containing a Milky Fluid (Galactocele of Vidal) and Enclosing Small Wormlike Beings That Can be Considered as Hematoid Helminthes in the Embryo Stage

On 24 July 1862, I was operating at the hospital on a young man to rid him of a tumor occupying the left side of his scrotal sac. An aspiration with a trocar produced a whitish-yellow fluid, similar to milk. I reported this new observation of galactocele of the scrotal sac with the analysis of the fluid. (See the reports of the Society of Surgery and Medical Union, 1862.) We found no spermatic elements in this fluid. This young man left, completely cured, but he came back to us one year later with a tumor of the scrotal sac on the right side. A tap gave us, as the year before, a fluid quite similar to creamy milk. This time we made a microscopic study of the still warm fluid,

and we found some distinct elements which we illustrate in the drawing further on. This fact struck us vividly. The students of the service and several of my colleagues of the same hospital could verify the viability of these beings, which ceased with the cooling of the fluid. We thought it useful to publish this fact with the desiderata which accompanies it, and we did not want to change anything in the notes which have been submitted to me by Messrs. Flurin and Lemoine, internes of the service, any more than the notes of Mr. Davaine. If we were mistaken, this fact would thus remain useless; but if, as we think, it relates a new fact, subsequent observations will not fail to provide all its scientific value. From the clinical point of view, it already is interesting, since it demonstrates that one can encounter, within one year's time, a bilateral tumor of the scrotal sac containing a fluid similar to milk. This fact, plus those already published, will establish the natural history of this little-known disease improperly known under the name of galactocele of the sacs.

Observation—Mr. X., nineteen and a half years of age, originally from Havana, entered the Municipal Hospital 28 August 1863, to be treated for a tumor located in the right part of the scrotum.

While questioning the patient regarding the causes to which he attributed his disease, as well as about his past history, we learned that already in the past year, in the month of July, he was treated by Mr. Demarquay for an almost identical affliction on the left side.

The observation was presented at the Society of Surgery on 27 August 1862 and published in the Medical Union (11 November 1862). I refer to this very curious observation from the point of view of the nature of the fluid; in it one will find the details concerning the background of our patients.

Since his discharge, which took place 6 August 1862, this young man continued with his occupation; he went through an entire year without feeling any pain. At the beginning of last June he contracted blennorrhagia. The flow, quite abundant at the beginning, diminished very rapidly; but ever since he always had a slight discharge through the meatus. It was from the moment when he saw the discharge diminishing that the patient noticed the enlargement of the right scrotal region.

Upon examination we noticed that the skin of his scrotum was taut, however, without being too smooth; besides this, it was red. Upon palpation, the patient did not complain of acute pain; a tumor of the size of a large chicken egg and oval in form was palpated. A very marked fluctuation was noticeable. The mass could not be transilluminated; also the position of the testicle could only be determined by palpation. When pressing forcefully, the patient complained of pain in the posterior superior of the scrotum. Because he was uncertain about the location of the tumor, Mr. Demarquay tapped with an exploratory trocar. A thick bluish-white fluid came flowing out. The catheter was not removed, and about 100 grams of this fluid were extracted. Before it was replaced with an injection of iodine, the examination revealed a completely healthy testicle presenting only a few small irregularities. It was thus not a cyst of the testicle. The epididymis was enlarged in size especially in the head; but the persistence of this enlargement after the evacuation of the fluid removed any doubt that it was not a tumor of the epididymis. It was thus in the tunica vaginalis that the fluid was located. The irregularities noticed on the surface of the testicle, particularly a rubbing sound, which doubtless were the product of false membranes [sic], did not leave any doubt as to the diagnosis.

The patient did not have any complications following the iodine injection, and he was discharged as cured the eighth of September.

The extracted fluid was examined by Mr. Lemoine: A. the small parasite.—B. fat globules.—C. pus cells.—D. an egg.—E. structure formed by filaments of fibrin, containing fat globules (Plate 56).

The fluid extracted weighed a hundred grams. White, without a particular odor, it separated immediately into two portions, one fluid, the other flocculated, but which remained in suspension in the first portion.

The coagulated mass became more and more homogeneous as it diminished in size. When the fluid was examined under the microscope it was possible to recognize a very large number of fat globules of all sizes which undoubtedly gave it its whitish color. In the middle of these globules pus cells were encountered. The coagulated portion presented as well some irregular fibrin filaments.

Attention was drawn above all to a little elongated and cylindrical creature. The anterior four-fifths of the body had almost a uniform diameter; the posterior fifth became thinner and thinner and terminated in a fine point. This worm had extremely rapid movement of coiling and uncoiling in its different parts, especially its terminal extremity. Unusually transparent, its contour outlined by a fine distinct edge, it presented, when viewed longitudinally, a very thin circular line. It had no mouth or perceptible anus. The worm was completely transparent and did not show anything which resembled the digestive system or the genital system. Besides this little creature an oval egg was found whose granular content was separated from the wall by a clear space. The size of this egg was disproportionate to that of the parasite [sic].

These peculiar creatures were found in five successive preparations. Messrs. Lewis and Lecomte wished to examine them. The different preparations and the fluid were sent to Mr. Davaine, in accordance with their instructions.

Mr. Davaine was good enough to devote almost an hour and a half to the search for these little creatures; but it was impossible for him to distinguish any, even on preparations very incompletely dried out.

According to the drawing that was made, Mr. Davaine believed he could conclude that, considering the disproportion between the size of the egg and that of the parasite, and considering especially the total absence of organs visible within this worm, it must be immature and at the embryonic stage. It did not resemble, moreover, by its shape, anything already described.

Where did it come from? Let us consider this subject, with all the possible reservations. On seeing this parasite, our first idea was that it was introduced from the outside. One cannot deny the similarity to the *anguillule* of vinegar. It was only

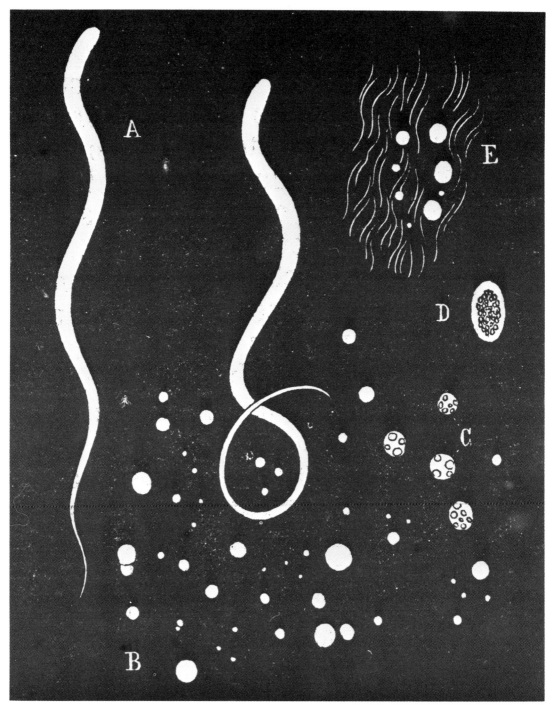

Plate 56. (A) The small parasite. (B) Fat globules. (C) Pus cells. (D) An egg. (E) Structure formed by fibrin filaments containing fat globules.

its persistence in showing up five times consecutively which especially attracted our attention. Let us say that there was only an analogy of shape with the *anguillule* of vinegar and that this infusoria is completely different by the presence, very easily verified, of its mouth, genital, and digestive organs. If the parasite were introduced from the outside, it could hardly have been by means of the trocar employed for the first time, nor by the tin basin which had served to collect the fluid and which could only have contained a little dust. There was no mixture of foreign fluid.

How to explain the impossibility of finding the little creature again in such a small preparation, especially when above all, the research was performed by an observer as experienced as Mr. Davaine? If the parasite was a simple *anguillule* introduced from outside, it should have continued to live and to move in spite of the cooling of the fluid. One could hardly assign the difficulty of seeing it again to its immobility and complete transparency. If the parasite perished following the cooling of the fluid, its death, according to Mr. Davaine, implied its essentially parasitic nature and its origin within the system; because all the entozoa are warm-blooded they die as soon as the temperature of the fluid containing them drops.

Let us add finally that the patient came from Havana, which would contribute to explaining the completely unique aspects of the extracted fluid.

These reflections, moreover, and the description of the parasite are presented with all due reservations and merely serve to attract the attention of the observers, if a similar case were to appear.

PRELIMINARY REPORT ON A SPECIES OF WORM, AS YET UNDESCRIBED, FOUND IN THE URINE OF PATIENTS WITH TROPICAL HEMATURIA IN BRAZIL

Noticia preliminar sobre vermes de uma especie ainda não descripta, encontrados na urina de doentes de hematuria intertropical no Brazil. Gazeta Medica de Bahia, 3: 97–99, 1868. Translated from the Portuguese.

Otto Edward Henry Wucherer
(1820–1873)

Wucherer's biography will be found in the chapter on Hookworm.

This is the first description of microfilaria in the urine of man.

Two years ago the late Dr. Griesinger of Berlin invited me by letter to examine the urine of patients affected with tropical hematuria for the eggs of *Distoma haematobium,* or *Bilharzia haematobia,* a nematode which, according to the investigations of Bilharz (its discoverer), Dr. Griesinger himself, and others, had been observed in the autopsies of people who had died with hematuria, or chylous urine, in Egypt.

Accepting this invitation, I carefully examined the urine of a considerable number of hematuric patients here in Bahia, but I never found the eggs. I do not believe that they could have existed without being noticed by me in these cases. On the contrary, I am convinced that the hematuria of Egypt, the Cape of Good Hope, and the Isle of France is caused by *Distoma haematobium* while the hematuria of Brazil has a different etiology.

The symptoms of the disease, as it manifests itself in Africa, are very similar on the whole to those of the hematuria observed in Brazil; nevertheless, there are some circumstances in which they differ. In Africa, the disease is very frequently found in children; however, I am not aware of a single case of chylous urine [sic] among children in Brazil. In Africa, the condition is very often accompanied by frank hemorrhage and, in many cases, by sand in the urine specimens; I am unaware of this having been observed in Brazil.

The symptomatology of both forms of the disease has been very well described in Rayer's work. There, in the medical history of a young Brazilian who, going to Europe, was examined and cared for by Messrs. Caffe, Orfila, Rayer, Astley Cooper, Marshall Hall, Clark, and others, the reader will find a faithful picture of the disease as it occurs here in Bahia.

Although I am forced to confess that the symptomatology of tropical hematuria as observed in Africa and Brazil is very similar, I must insist on the fact that it has been impossible for me, in spite of many investigations performed with utmost care, to find eggs of *Distoma haematobium* in the urine of hematuria patients I have examined. These eggs are of such dimensions and special configuration that I consider it impossible for them to have escaped my notice.

However, I must now report an unexpected result of my examinations. On 4 August 1866, I had to examine the urine of a woman, a patient of my friend Dr. Silva Lima [who gave the first description of ainhum—Eds.], who was in the Hospital da Santa Casa da Misericordia in this city. The urine had a milky appearance and contained some red, strawberry-colored clots; its specific gravity was 1.005 to 1.012, and its temperature was 25.5° C. When filtered, it remained milky almost to the same degree. Neither boiling nor nitric acid caused the formation of new clots. By examining a clot particle under the microscope, I found, besides many crystals of triphosphate, epithelial cells, red blood corpuscles, fat globules, mucus globules, vibriones, and so forth, some threadlike worms which were very thin at one end and blunt at the other.

In the blunt end a small point was visible which could not be identified as an opening. The body was transparent and seemed to contain a granular mass; however, it was not possible to distinguish its internal structure. At the time of the examination, suspecting that these worms had entered the urine casually, I had the patient urinate into a scrupulously clean glass container. However, in the urine thus obtained I found the same worms. As I examined the urine of so many hematuric patients without finding anything similar, I did not attribute the proper value to my discovery.

I was frustrated in my efforts to find eggs of haematobium, and some time went by without my examining the urine of other hematuric patients. On 9 October of that year [1866], Mr. Santos Pereira, a student (today a medical doctor), asked me to examine the urine of a lady whom he was treating for hematuria, and I was quite surprised to find in it the same worms that I had observed previously in the above-mentioned case of Dr. Silva Lima.

The circumstance of my having found these worms both times in the urine of women made me think that they might originate in the vagina, despite the fact that they did not have the slightest resemblance to the worms [sic] which are frequently found there, *Trichomonas vaginalis.* However, it was not long until a man appeared who was suffering with the same condition. My colleague Dr. Silva Lima kindly referred to me a patient who had been suffering with hematuria for two months. The first examination of this patient's urine was made with Dr. Silva Lima himself, in the presence of some other colleagues and students.

In our presence the patient urinated into a glass container which was put aside to allow the urine to settle. It was a little turbid and greatly resembled almost clear milk serum; it had a slight urine odor and did not seem to contain any blood. After a half-hour, a transparent clot had formed which was seen only when I wanted to pour the urine. I removed a fragment of this clot with a pair of tongs, and drained the liquid; as it fell the clot became very opaque, until finally there remained only a ragged scum similar to the film which forms on the surface of milk.

Examining, microscopically, a particle the size of a pinhead, I promptly discovered the worms that I had seen in the other two instances. They were alive and were making very brisk, wavy motions; so I had observed them also, in 1866, in the urine of Dr. Silva Lima's female patient. Even with a combination which produced a magnifying power of 400 diameters, it was not possible for us to learn the organization of these worms. They had the diameter of a white blood corpuscle, and their length exceeded that of the latter, 60 or 70 times. The urine did not contain red blood corpuscles, but had many white corpuscles which looked like leukocytes and many fat globules. During the following days, however, I had the opportunity of examining the urine of Dr. Santos Pereira's woman patient and of the man; both had improved. The worms had become gradually very rare, so that it was difficult to find any of them.

Because of the suspension of his treatment, the man had a relapse. His urine again became milky and it clotted; however, it did not contain the abundance of worms it did previously.

Many times during the past few years I have had the opportunity of examining microscopically the urine of patients—some from my clinic and others from my colleagues—with various diseases, and I have never found those worms except in the three reported cases of hematuria. Undoubtedly the reason I did not discover them much earlier is that, in the beginning, I had always neglected to examine the clots, looking for the eggs of the distoma in the sediment of urine; however, the clots are precisely where they are found in abundance.

Unfortunately I did not have in my possession

the latter part of Leuckart's work on the parasites of man which deals with nematodes; however, we do not find included in a list of human entozoa which is found in this work any worms resembling the ones I observed, not even in the list of Dr. Spencer Cobbold nor in the works of Küchenmeister and Davaine.

It seems rash to hazard conjectures on the occurrence of these worms in cases of hematuria and on their etiologic significance; therefore, I will refrain from doing so until I have made new investigations and have examined the cadaver of a hematuric patient which, thus far, I have been unable to obtain.

In the meantime I hope that this communication will serve as an incentive for some of my colleagues, better qualified and more fortunate than I, to attempt to shed light on a disease, the etiology of which is still enigmatic today.

ON A HEMATOZOON INHABITING HUMAN BLOOD, ITS RELATION TO CHYLURIA AND OTHER DISEASES

Appendix to the Eighth Annual Report of the Sanitary Commissioner with the Government of India, pp. 1–50, 1872. Selections from pp. 3–6, 8–12, 18–21, 33–35, 46–50.

Timothy Richards Lewis
(1841–1886)

Lewis entered the profession of medicine at the age of 15, when he was apprenticed to an apothecary in his native Pembrokeshire (Wales). After a few years he went to London for more formal studies, first at a dispensary in Streatham, then when he was 19 at the German Hospital at Dalston, and finally from 1863 to 1866 at University College. He then concluded his medical education at the University of Aberdeen, where he took the M.B. and the C.M. in 1867.

The year following his graduation, he entered the Army Medical Service as an assistant surgeon and was soon sent with Cunningham to study cholera in India after a preliminary period during which both men went to the Continent to familiarize themselves with the work being done in mycology and bacteriology.

Reaching Calcutta in 1869, Lewis and Cunningham spent some 12 years studying cholera and other Indian diseases and writing a number of important reports. Lewis was promoted to surgeon in 1873 and to surgeon-major in 1880. Three years later he returned to England permanently upon his appointment

as assistant professor of pathology at the Army Medical School in Netley, a post he held until his death.

Lewis' encounter with filaria described in the following article marks the first documentation of a micro-organism in the peripheral blood of man.

The Belief in the Existence of Human Haematozoa Long Entertained

For many generations writers on medical subjects have maintained that the human blood during certain diseased conditions is invaded by parasites. The opinion most in favour has been, that these in all probability were in the form of worms; but, so far as I have been able to ascertain, it has never yet been satisfactorily demonstrated that this condition really existed.

The Distomata Hitherto Discovered Are Too Large To Pass Through the Capillaries

That certain limited areas of the circulatory tract may become invaded by Entozoa has long been known: the portal vein, and the vessels in more or less direct relation with the intestinal canal, are the channels which have usually been thus affected; but the parasites found in these situations, such as the *Distoma haematobium*, discovered by Bilharz in 1851, and a few other imperfectly described distomata, are far too large to pass through any but comparatively capacious blood vessels. The instances on record in which they have been found in vessels beyond these limits are few, and evidently accidental occurrences. None of these, therefore, can, I think, be justly described as 'Haematozoa' in the strict sense of the term.

So Likewise Are Echinococci

The same remarks apply, with only very slight modifications, to the presence of Echinococci in the blood-vessels, a few young specimens of which, have, on rare occasions, been discovered (by Klencke and others) in the general circulation, but then only in vessels of considerable calibre.

Probability of Some Parasites Having Reached the Tissues in Which They Are Found, by Means of the Blood-Vessels.

It has also been inferred that the progeny of some Entozoa must be carried by the blood-current, as otherwise they could have not reached their destination so rapidly in the various distant parts of the body in which they have been found. That the *Trichina spiralis,* for example, during its earlier migrations, may be conveyed in this way, is, although strongly denied, I think not improbable. As their presence in the blood has not, however, been recognized, either in man or in animals, their sojourn in such channels, must, at all events, be of very short duration.

The Discovery of Microscopic Worms in Great Numbers in Human Blood

But that a condition should exist in which human blood should be infested by living active worms in either an embryo [sic] or mature state, to the extent hereafter to be described, had, I presume, scarcely been surmised—a condition in which they are persistently so ubiquitous as to be obtained day after day in numbers, by simply pricking any portion of the body, even to the tips of the fingers and toes of both hands and both feet of one and the same person with a finely pointed needle. On one occasion six excellent specimens were obtained in a single drop of blood, by merely pricking the lobule of the ear.

Date of Their Discovery in the Blood, and of Their Discovery in the Urine

Towards the beginning of July of the present year, whilst examining the blood of a native suffering from diarrhoea, a patient at the Medical College Hospital under Dr. Chuckerbutty's care, I observed nine minute Nematoid worms in a state of great activity, on a single slide. On drawing the attention of my colleague, Dr. Douglas Cunningham, to the preparation, he fully coincided in my opinion that they were precisely the same kind as those observed by me more than two years previously (in March 1870), as being constantly present in Chylous urine.

A Synopsis of the First Case Published

In a report on the microscopic characters of choleraic dejecta published at the time, . . . I had occasion to allude to this condition of the urine in connection with some cells observed in it, which closely corresponded in appearance with cells constantly present in choleraic discharges, and the opportunity was taken of drawing attention to the Entozoon. . . .

For the sake of convenience it may be well to refer to this case again. The patient was a deaf and emaciated East Indian, about 25 years of age, under the care of Mr. R. T. Lyons at the General Hospital, and was kept under observation for a period of two months, during which time his urine continued to present a white, milky appearance, and yellowish-white coagula rapidly formed in the vessel into which it had been voided. When a small portion of the gelatinised substance was teased with needles on a slide, and placed under the microscope, delicate filaments were seen, partly hidden by the fibro-albuminous matter in which they were embedded, and which I at first considered to be scattered filaments of a growing fungus. After being watched for some time, however, they were seen to coil and uncoil themselves, so that all doubt as to their nature was at an end. I had opportunities of showing them on various occasions to several persons; and having perfectly satisfied myself that their occurrence was not accidental, nor yet the result of subsequent development in the urine, after the manner of the Anguillulae which are so well known to develop in vinegar or starch-paste, I did not hesitate to draw attention to them as being the probable cause of the obscure disease known as "Chyluria."

Particulars Concerning the Patient in Whom the Haematozoa Were First Discovered

I regret that I lost the opportunity of fully ascertaining the previous history of the case in which the Haematozoa were first detected. Having satisfied myself of the identity of the worms previously observed in the urine and now in the blood, by careful comparison of their form, structure and measurement, I returned on the following morning to the Medical College for this purpose, but to my great disappointment found that the man had been discharged, at his own request, an hour before my arrival. He had, it appears, suffered from diarrhoea for about a fortnight, which had become greatly aggravated a few days before his admission into the hospital; but nothing further could be learnt of the state of his health beyond that he had complained of deafness, especially of one ear.[1]

He had left no address, except that he was a blacksmith living in a large bazaar in the neighbourhood; but as some three or four thousand persons are crowded into this bazaar, a great proportion of whom are smiths in some form or another, those acquainted with the intricate geography of such places in the East will not be surprised to learn that I spent a whole afternoon searching for him in vain. I then enlisted the friendly aid of the Police, but this also proved fruitless.

A Second Case of Filariae in the Blood, Associated with Chyluria

A few days after this occurrence, Dr. D. B. Smith informed me that there was a native woman in one of his wards suffering from haematuria, combined with a chylous condition of the urine, and very kindly forwarded a specimen of it on the following morning; this urine, as usual under such circumstances, contained the worms in abundance.

First and Second Attack

I saw the woman on the evening of the same day, and learnt that the complaint from which she was suffering had first made its appearance during the third month of her last pregnancy, but that it had apparently passed off in about five or six weeks. After the birth of this child, which was now five months old, the disease came on again: She was unable to suckle her infant, the lacteal secretion being altogether absent.

On pricking her finger with a needle, and distributing a drop of blood over several slides, I found that the Filariae were present in it also.

Other Symptoms and Progress of Disease

She remained under observation for a period of about two months, but there was no marked change in her general condition; her face, however, became swollen on one or two occasions, and appeared puffy, as also did the upper and lower extremities. The urine slightly improved in appearance, and the numbers of the Filariae in it as well as in the blood diminished; in the latter especially, at all events, the numbers obtainable by pricking the fingers or toes certainly decreased; and eventually, out of half a dozen or more slides, not more than one or two Haematozoa could be detected; on a few occasions several slides were examined without any being found.

The patient, however, could not be persuaded to remain longer in hospital: indeed, all patients thus affected soon get tired of being treated for their complaint, as there is seldom any great suffering which the patient can directly connect with this condition, and often no other very well marked symptom beyond general debility.

A Third Case of Filariae in the Blood, Associated with Chyluria

The most remarkable case which has come under my notice, in which the blood was affected in this manner, was that of a patient in one of Dr. Ewart's wards, whom he kindly placed at my disposal for observation and treatment. The man was an East Indian (with more of the habits of the native than of the European), about 22 years of age; he had been for about five years employed as cook on board one of the light-ships lying at the entrance of the Hooghly [river], spending only about three months of the year with his family on shore.

The prominent symptoms in this case were, extreme and persistent milkiness of the urine, which coagulated with great rapidity after being voided. On being heated the smell given off at first corresponded exactly with that of warm milk, but when the heat was continued for some time, was gradually replaced by the ordinary smell of urine. This condition came on suddenly about two months previous to his admission into the General Hospital. . . .

Extreme Extent of Infection

This is not surprising when the amount of fibro-albuminous matter which is constantly being drained from his system, as evidenced by the state of the urinary secretion, is taken into consideration; but when to this is added the fact that no matter at what portion of his body the circulation is tapped with the point of a needle, numerous active, well-developed Haematozoa are invariably obtained: on one occasion I obtained as many as 12 of these creatures on a single slide. As the drop of blood from which this slide had been prepared sufficed for the preparation of two or three other slides (which, however, between them did not contain more than half a dozen Filariae), the number infesting his whole body may be imagined. . . .

Haematozoa Even When Present Not Always Readily Detected

It must not be supposed that the Filariae are to be detected by taking a mere peep through the microscope; sometimes, certainly, I have observed one, or two even, in the first field examined; but this is by no means usual, and their detection often demands considerable patience. Each slide will require about a quarter of an hour before it can be satisfactorily explored; any one who imagines that they can be detected with the same ease as a white-blood corpuscle had better not make the attempt.

A Possible Cause of This Difficulty

Several slides may have to be examined, and it may be necessary to make a fresh puncture, for I have found the Haematozoa to be absent in several slides obtained from one finger, but present in all the slides obtained from another at the same time; whereas on making a fresh puncture in the finger where none had been found at first, it was ascertained that they were equally numerous in both. This is possibly accounted for by the little orifice made having become plugged by fat, etc., so that the blood squeezed through had to some extent been filtered, for although this microscopic Filaria can pass through any channel permeable to a red-blood corpuscle, still, when it is considered that the length of the former is nearly 50 times its diameter, the wonder is that they are not more completely prevented from escaping through so fine an orifice even when perfectly patent.

The Magnifying Powers Advisable To Employ

The search should not be undertaken with too high a magnifying power, but it should be sufficiently high to define the outline of a red-blood corpuscle quite distinctly. I have found that a good two-thirds of an inch objective answers the purpose of a searcher admirably; it embraces a tolerably large area, so that the preparation can be examined in a comparatively short time; but care should be taken to keep the fine-adjustment screw constantly moving, so as to examine the deeper as well as the superficial layer of fluid in each field as it passes under observation. Should anything unusual be observed, the low power must be replaced by a one-quarter inch or, better, a one-eighth inch objective.[2]

In order to keep the active Haematozoon under observation for some hours, a camel-hair pencil dipped in a solution of Canada-balsam or mastic in chloroform, should be passed along the edges of the covering glass, so as to prevent evaporation, and the formation of air spaces in the preparation.

The General Aspect of the Haematozoon During Life

The appearance presented by the Haematozoon when first seen among the blood corpuscles, in the living state, will not readily be forgotten and cannot possibly be mistaken for anything else. The remark made by a young Bengalee student on my requesting him to look into the microscope and tell me what he saw—"He is an incompletely developed snake, evidently very young, though very active"—so aptly describes the object as thus witnessed, that I feel sure that any one seeing the Haematozoon alive will not fail to be struck with the accuracy of the quaint reply (Plate 57).

During the first few hours after removal from the body the Filaria is in constant motion, coiling and uncoiling itself unceasingly, lashing the blood corpuscles about in all directions, and insinuating itself between them. It is not at rest for a single moment, and yet on the slide it appears to make but little progress, as it may frequently be watched for an hour in the same field without once giving occasion to shift the stage of the microscope. No sooner has it insinuated its "head" amongst a group of corpuscles than it is retracted, and probably the next instant the "tail" will be darted forth and retracted in a similar way.

The part which the Haematozoon appears to take in the production of disease will become still more evident when the condition of the kidneys and suprarenal capsules . . . obtained from a patient who died of Chyluria, has been described.

Tallowy Appearance Presented by Some of the Pyramids of the Kidney

To the naked eye none of these organs presented any marked deviation from the normal standard, except that the kidneys were more than usually lobulated, and, that on section several of the pyramids, especially near their apices, presented a smooth, tallowy appearance, suggestive of amyloid disease. No approach to the characteristic iodine reaction could, however, be obtained; but when longitudinal sections were subjected to microscopic examination, numerous translucent oil-like tubules of a somewhat varicose appearance could be observed running alongside the uriniferous tubes as if the lymphatics or minute blood vessels of the part had become plugged. These sections when placed in boiling ether, and afterwards subjected to prolonged maceration in it, did not appear to be materially affected by the process—the translucent oil-like tubules being quite as evident as before.

The Kidneys and Suprarenal Capsules Contained Numerous Haematozoa

No other morbid changes could be detected as having taken place in either the tubular or cortical tissue of the kidneys, but in every fragment, no matter from what part of the kidneys removed, numerous microscopic Filariae were invariably obtained, if the tissue had been properly teased, precisely analogous to those which had been detected in the blood and in the urine during life. Teased fragments of the suprarenal capsules

yielded similar specimens. On slitting open any portion of the renal artery, from its entrance into the kidney as far inwards as I was able to follow its ramifications, and gently scraping its inner surface with a scalpel, numerous Haematozoa could always be obtained. The renal vein when similarly examined also yielded specimens of the Filariae, but they did not seem to be so numerous in it.

The vessels themselves did not appear to be diseased, and such of the branches as could be seen with the naked eye did not strike me as being abnormally large. But whether the microscopic ramifications and the capillaries were distended or otherwise (in the absence of properly injected preparations of the organs) could not well be ascertained. . . .

The Filariae Detected in the Blood of a Man in Whose Urine They Existed More Than Two and a Half Years Previously

The foregoing account had just been transcribed from my notes, when I had occasion to visit the Government Printing Establishment, where, to my utter surprise, I saw, busily putting

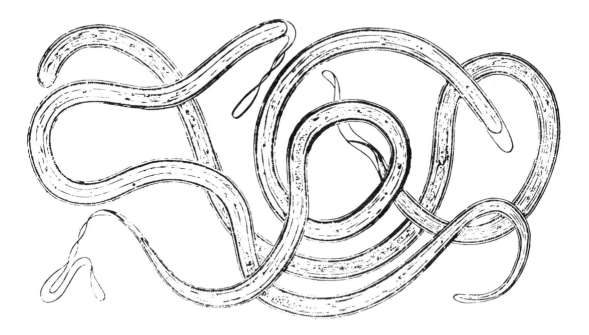

Plate 57. Various appearances presented by a single hematozoon, as observed under a one-eighth-inch immersion object glass.

into type a portion of the foregoing pages, the very man in whose urine these Filariae were first detected—more than two and a half years ago! Being rather below the average intelligence, he had not the remotest idea to what the manuscript referred.

At my request he called upon me in the afternoon, and I learnt from him then, that his urine had been perfectly healthy ever since he left the hospital, about April, 1870. It certainly looks healthy now, and is quite free from albumin. I prepared seven slides from blood obtained by pricking the middle finger of one hand, and three slides from the same finger of the other hand. On seeing me do this, the man enquired why I had made so many preparations, as on a former occasion I had only taken one slide; a circumstance, by the way, which I had quite forgotten; certainly I had not discovered Haematozoa. This little incident also conveys its lesson; had I taken a dozen slides on the first occasion instead of one, the date of the detection of Filaria in the blood would probably have been simultaneous with their detection in the urine. In the first four or five preparations examined nothing could be observed; in the two next taken up, one belonging to each hand, Haematozoa were detected, very active, but in no way differing from the excellent live specimens which I had obtained in his urine long ago, and in no way differing from the Filariae since detected in the urine and blood of so many persons. The measurements of two specimens were taken on the following morning after their activity had subsided; one was 1/76th of an inch in length by 1/3500th″ in breadth, and the other 1/80th of an inch by 1/3500th″.

The Prolonged Existence of Haematozoa Sufficient to Account for Recurrence of the Malady

Here is, therefore, definite information more satisfactory than that to be obtained by instituting comparisons between the Haematozoa of man and of animals, that, not only may those found in man live for a period of more than two and a half years, for certain, but that there is no evidence that they have any tendency to develop beyond a certain stage so long as they remain in the circulation. For aught we know to the contrary, these Filariae may live for many years, and thus, at any moment, no matter how long after a previous attack, nor in what country the person may re-side, he may be surprised by the sudden accession of Chyluria or any other obscure disease, such as will readily be understood by the physician when he becomes aware of the state of the blood.

If after the first brood of young Filariae, there be no provision for other broods to follow, then every attack would be a step towards permanent recovery, but of this I know nothing at present, although some of the cases recorded appear to warrant such an inference. Nor have I any definite knowledge as to how the blood originally becomes infected; to hint that it is possible if not probable that the Filaria may eventually be traced to the tank—either to its water or its fish—is the utmost that can be done.

Many other interesting questions suggest themselves as matters for future enquiry; such for example as to whether the foetus in utero is infected by the mother's blood: cases have been recorded which seem to favour such a supposition; such instances, however, may have been due to the particular localities in which the persons resided—parents and children having for generations been subject alike to the same influences. On one occasion, I attempted to solve this question, but the mother, who herself was very averse to having her finger pricked, peremptorily refused to submit the child to a similar trivial operation.

A Summary of the Principal Facts and Inferences Recorded

This paper having considerably exceeded the limits originally intended, it may be that the leading facts referred to have become obscured by the digressions that have been necessarily made, so that, before concluding, a short summary of the observations and of the inferences which have been deduced therefrom may be advantageous:

(1) The blood of persons who have lived in a tropical country is occasionally invaded by living microscopic Filariae, hitherto not identified with any known species, which may continue in the system for months or years without any marked evil consequences being observed; but which may, on the contrary, give rise to serious disease, and ultimately be the cause of death.

(2) The phenomena which may be induced by the blood being thus affected are probably due to the mechanical interruption offered (by the acci-

dental aggregation, perhaps, of the Haematozoa), to the flow of the nutritive fluids of the body in various channels, giving rise to the obstruction of the current within them, or to rupture of their extremely delicate walls, and thus causing the contents of the lacteals, lymphatics or capillaries, to escape into the most convenient excretory channel. Such escaped fluid, as has been demonstrated in the case of the urinary and lachrymal or Meibomian secretion, may be the means of carrying some of the Filariae with it out of the circulation. These occurrences are liable to return after long intervals—so long in fact as the Filariae continue to dwell in the blood.

(3) As a rule, a Chylous condition of the urine is only one of the *symptoms* of this state of the circulation, although it appears to be the most characteristic symptom which we are at present aware of.

(4) Lastly, it appears probable that some of the hitherto inexplicable phenomena, by which certain tropical diseases are characterised, may eventually be traced to the same, or to an allied condition.

The importance of a careful microscopical examination of the blood of persons suffering from obscure diseases, in tropical countries especially, is therefore more than ever evident, and opens up a new and most important field of enquiry—referring as it does to a hitherto unknown diseased condition.

Calcutta
October, 1872

----

[1] One of the patients brought to my notice, who had suffered from Chyluria for several months, had been in hospital for another complaint, and had actually left the hospital without having mentioned a word about the condition of his urine. He stated afterward that he did not like to do so, as it was no great inconvenience to him, and he imagined it was the temporary result of an "indiscretion."

[2] It may seem superfluous to draw attention to the similarity which exists between some vegetable fibres and some of the microscopic 'Filariae,' when the latter are not alive; nevertheless a very good objective is frequently required to distinguish them with certainty, as any one may prove for himself by subjecting the torn fluffy edges of a piece of blotting-paper to microscopic examination. Filaria-like fibrils will frequently be found.

A mistake of this kind is referred to by Leuckart as having occurred quite recently. A paper was published announcing the discovery of a filaria-like nematode in the intestines, blood, and tissues of a patient, which was expected to prove

as dangerous to life as the *Trichina spiralis*. These parasites subsequently proved to be nothing more than vegetable hairs!

FILARIA SANGUINIS HOMINIS

Medical Reports, China Imperial Maritime Customs, Shanghai (or China: Inspectorate General of Customs, Medical Reports, according to Union Serials list), No. 13, pp. 30–38, Oct. 1876—March 1877 (published in 1877). Selections are from pp. 31–34, 36–37.

Patrick Manson
(1844–1922)

Manson's biography will be found in the chapter on Malaria.

In the first paper, Manson confirmed his hypothesis that microfilaria of Filaria sanguinis hominis *was associated with elephantiasis. The next paper confirms his theory that the mosquito is the vector of* Filaria sanguinis hominis *and describes the development of filaria within the mosquito.*

. . . *Confirmation of the conjecture that Elephantiasis Arabum is a Parasitic Disease.*—I have lately found in the blood of a patient who came to me for the removal of an elephantiasis scroti, numerous specimens of embryo filariae. I am thus enabled to state positively that elephantiasis Arabum is a parasitic disease, and to establish on solid and incontrovertible grounds, what in a former report I conjectured was the true pathology of this puzzling affection. Much, of course, remains to be done in working out the details of the exact operation of the cause, but the cue having been given, these will follow in time. A substantial basis, at any rate, is laid, to guide us in searching for means to prevent and cure a hideous and often fatal disease, afflicting a large proportion of the inhabitants of tropical and subtropical countries.

Since what precedes was written I have met with the filaria sanguinis hominis in the human blood no less than fifteen times.

With the practice I had acquired in the detection of haematozoa in the blood of the dog, I commenced some time ago the systematic examination of human blood. To help me in the work, which is excessively tedious and laborious, I familiarised two Chinese assistants with the appearance of the canine haematozoon, and showed them how to manipulate for the detection of similar organisms in man. No selection is made of cases, but the first patient or healthy person who presents and is willing to have his finger pricked, is examined; six slides of blood, at least, being carefully searched. In this way we have got over 190 cases, with the rather unexpected result of finding haematozoa in 15 instances, or in about 8 per cent. To prevent mistakes or imposition, when the parasite is found by my assistants, I take care to verify the observation for myself from a fresh specimen of blood, which I see drawn. I failed to find haematozoa in four instances in which they were reported, but I believe my assistants' observations were correct; they were confirmed by the persons who supplied the blood. Their horror at the snake-like animal they had given birth to was conclusive. As my re-examination was made some days after the first detection of the parasites, it is likely that these had disappeared temporarily. This has happened in several instances I have myself closely watched.

The filaria sanguinis hominis resembles very closely in general appearance and movements the canine haematozoon described above. Accurate measurements are difficult to make on account of the restlessness of the animal when alive and the contraction which its body undergoes when fixed in desiccated blood. The short time when the blood is thickening, previous to thorough inspissation, is the most favourable for examining the animal; then, its movements are languid and admit of details being studied. From a number of observations, I conclude that it measures slightly less than 1/3000 of an inch in breadth, by about 1/90 of an inch in length, or thereabouts; on the whole its dimensions are rather under those of the canine variety. There are two or three points in which distinct and characteristic differences can be made out in the two species, when seen through a high power. The canine variety appears to be naked and structureless; the human, on the contrary, is provided with a very delicate noncontractile integument, within which the body of the animal is incessantly shortened and elongated. This, I believe, is the explanation of the appearance of a lash of extreme tenuity at the head and tail being sometimes visible, and sometimes not, and the occasional thickening of the extremity of the tail. The lash is the collapsed integument from which the head or tail has been withdrawn, and into which they are again projected. It seems

to have no elasticity or spring, but follows like a limp string the movements of the body of the animal. Unlike the canine haematozoon, in many specimens of the human variety, though not in all, there is about the centre of the body an elongated yellow patch, the structure of which with the microscopic power at my command I cannot make out. I believe it appertains to an alimentary canal. On close examination with a high power, distinct movements as of a mouth can be made out at the extremity of the head. They resemble the breathing movements of a fish's mouth. the aperture, if aperture exists, is not simple, but, I think, is provided with several lips.

In a future report I hope to give details of all the cases I have examined for haematozoa; at present I will confine myself to short notes of the cases only in which they were found.

Case 1. *Haematozoa and Elephantiasis Scroti*— ANGKHI, male, aet. 58; from Changchiu, Liauho-sia; cake baker; in comfortable circumstances. Father died long ago, he does not know of what disease; mother died from fever and dysentery; two brothers are alive and well, one brother died from fever and dysentery. He states that when 28 years of age, in the spring of the year, he had an attack of what he calls ague, accompanied by inflammation of the scrotum; the fever lasted for but one day, but it was two months before the scrotum recovered its original size; before doing so it desquamated. Since that time he has had attacks of fever every year from four to eight times, each attack being accompanied by inflammation of the scrotum. Two years ago the scrotum did not as formerly recover after the fever, but remained swollen, and has grown steadily ever since. Formerly he was strong and stout, but for the last ten years he has lost flesh. Has never had chyluria.

His scrotum presents the usual appearance of elephantiasis. I suppose it to weigh about eight pounds. On its under surface there is a solitary vesicle about the size of a split pea, and near this a bunch of dilated lymphatics: pricking these places gives vent to a drachm or two of coagulable milky lymph.

Blood from his finger or scrotum contained numerous specimens of filaria sanguinis hominis; nearly every slide contained one or two. On the second day of his stay in hospital, filariae could easily be found, though they had manifestly diminished in number. On the third day, though thirty slides were examined, not one specimen could be obtained, and during the five subsequent days, though frequent examinations were made, there was no reappearance of filariae.

I was anxious to keep this man under observation for

some time before operating on his scrotum, but the frequent examination of his blood seems to have alarmed his friends, and he was in consequence removed from the hospital unrelieved.

Case 2. *Haematozoa without concomitant disease*—SIN-TO, male, aet. 21; born in Tintai; came to Amoy about five years ago and became a pupil in the English Presbyterian Mission school. Does not remember to have suffered from any particular disease, except an attack of jaundice about four years ago, succeeding a smart fever (calls it ague) of one day's duration: his urine continued dark for about a month. He says he has been short-sighted ever since the jaundice. Never had abscess, boils, enlarged glands or anything resembling elephantiasis, lymph scrotum or chyluria, but has always been strong and healthy.

Being at the hospital one day, not as a patient, he saw a student examining the blood of a sick man; out of curiosity he submitted his own for examination. In six slides three filariae were found in full activity. A week afterwards I found them in nearly every slide. A fortnight afterwards, I searched six full slides very carefully, but could find none.

Case 3. *Haematozoa and Lymph scrotum.*—SIAH, male, aet. 45; a field labourer, lives in Lamoa, Choanchia. This man is intellectually very dull and his memory appears to be very imperfect, so that a reliable account of his early history is difficult to obtain. One fact he dwells on with great obstinacy, perpetually recurring to it during his examination; viz., that for twelve years he has suffered from feelings of discomfort and pain in his bowels, grinding of his teeth at night, and frequent seminal discharges. When 16 years of age, and again at 28, he had attacks of fever. Three years ago he had frequent fits of what he calls ague, the fever never continuing for more than one day at a time, but recurring every week or two. But before this occurred he noticed that his scrotum was itchy and covered with vesicles, which, when broken, would exude fluid in great abundance for seven or eight days. The scrotum and inguinal glands gradually enlarged, but it was not until they had attained considerable size that he became liable to fever. Last year he had a course of quinine at the hospital; since then he has had only one attack of fever, four months ago, and of three days' duration, and his scrotum he says has diminished very much. During the attack of fever, he says that the scrotum was not affected, but that the glands were inflamed.

The scrotum is not very large, but it is a characteristic "lymph scrotum." The left inguinal glands are slightly swollen; the right inguinal and right upper femoral glands are very much enlarged, feel soft and doughy to the touch, and are evidently varicose.

During a residence of about a week in hospital, this man's blood was daily examined, and on no occasion were filariae absent, varying in number from two to five in six slides. . . . [Manson proceeds to describe 12 more cases—Eds.]

From these observations I think the following deductions are justifiable:

(1) That a large ratio of the population of this province, and probably of other parts of China, is infested with the Filaria sanguinis hominis. The exact ratio cannot yet be stated, but if my observations are a fair guide, one in thirteen is near it.

(2) That the Filaria sanguinis hominis may be present in the blood, and yet the host be in good health, and exhibit no other morbid phenomena.

(3) That in the same person it may be present at one time and absent at another.

(4) That at one time or another it is very generally associated with elephantoid disease, and is almost certainly connected with the cause of such affections.

(5) That it is sometimes associated with a diseased condition characterised by frequently recurring attacks of fever, accompanied by general anasarca unconnected with heart or kidney disease. . . .

FURTHER OBSERVATIONS ON *FILARIA SANGUINIS HOMINIS*

Medical Reports, China Imperial Maritime Customs, Shanghai (or China: Inspectorate General of Customs, Medical Reports, according to Union Serials list), No. 14, pp. 1–26, April-Sept. 1877 (published in 1878). Selections are from pp. 1–2, 5–7, 9–11, 14.

Patrick Manson
(1844–1922)

Manson's biography will be found in the chapter on Malaria.
Manson definitely described the microfilaria and conjectured that the mosquito is the vector.

Before giving the results of my observations I will premise that, with the exception of cases of elephantiasis and allied diseases, the selection of subjects for examination was made without reference to their physical or social condition. Most were patients at the Chinese Hospital suffering from a variety of miscellaneous diseases, but many were relatives or friends in charge of patients and not themselves diseased; others again were students at the hospital, or their relatives or acquaintances.

The method of examination employed I have already described. In some instances, instead of dividing the drop of blood into six slides, I have latterly been in the habit of placing the entire drop between two slides, using one as covering glass for the other. By so doing I think the chance of the haematozoon escaping from under the covering glass is diminished, and there is a considerable saving of time effected.

The degree in which the general population of this district is affected with Filaria Sanguinis Hominis.

Number examined:	670
Filiaria Found in:	62
Percentage:	9.25
Proportion:	1 in 10.8

A certain proportion of these cases came to hospital and were examined because they were affected by what I shall hereafter show was filaria disease—elephantiasis. To arrive therefore at a correct idea of the degree of infection of the general population these must not be included in the calculation. Slighter degrees of filaria disease, viz. varicose lymphatic glands and mild cases of lymph scrotum, do not apply at the hospital on account of these affections, which as a rule, are discovered only when searched for, the patient coming to be treated for some other complaint. I will therefore include all cases of enlarged groin glands and half the cases of lymph scrotum as fairly representative of the general population.

A correction must also be made for temporary absence of embryos in the blood in individuals who at another time might be found to possess them. As most of my cases were examined once only, it might so happen that just at the time the examination was made embryos were absent. To arrive at this correction I collected the results of a considerable number of examinations in persons all known to have filaria embryos in their blood at some time, and found from this the proportion of times in which embryos were absent and present. In an aggregate of 89 such examinations they were found 55 times, not found 34 times. That is to say, if a certain number of persons are

examined once for filaria embryos and these are found in 55 instances we may infer that they are temporarily absent in a certain number of others, the proportion of present to temporarily absent being as 55 to 34. . . .

From these figures we may conclude that in Amoy and the surrounding districts on an average about one person in every eight is affected with Filaria sanguinis hominis, and that in searching for embryos they will be found about once in every 13 examinations. . . .

Elephantiasis and allied diseases are much more frequently associated with the parasite than any other morbid condition. To bring this out more clearly I have arranged the cases as follows:

Disease	Number Examined	Total	Number of Filaria cases	Total Filaria cases	Corrected for Temporary Absence	Proportion Affected	Percentage Contributed
Elephantiasis of Leg	10		1				
Elephantiasis of Scrotum .	15		4				
Lymph Scrotum	13	63	10	36	58.25	1 in 1.1	58
Lymph Scrotum and Chyluria	2		2				
Enlarged and varicose groin glands	23		19				
Inflamed Scrotum and Fever	2		2				
Hydrocele		412	3	16	25.81	1 in 16	25.8
Other Diseases	410		11				
Healthy	195	195	10	10	16.18	1 in 12	16.2
	670	670	62	62	. . .	. . .	100

I have elsewhere shown that varicose groin glands, lymph scrotum, elephantiasis and chyluria are pathologically the same disease, and if additional evidence were required to prove this it may be found in abundance in the cases now published and in those given in the last *Reports*. In the same paper I ventured to attribute these diseases to the parent of the embryos that Dr. Lewis had discovered in the blood and urine of chyluria cases; and I think I have now brought sufficient evidence together to prove my conjecture, although the tests of experiment and postmortem examination are still wanting. Mere coincidence will not account for the frequent, and in some forms of the disease almost invariable, association of the parasite and the disease; they can only stand to each other in the relation of cause and consequence. The way in which the cause operates is made sufficiently apparent by the anatomy of the diseased structures, and arguing from what has been observed of the habits of other penetrating filariae, I have concluded that the essential feature of elephantoid disease—obstruction of the lymphatic circulation—is produced by the mechanical interference of the parent parasite with that circulation, higher up the lymphatic system than the seat of the elephantoid disease.

It may be asked, "If the filaria sanguinis hominis is the cause of elephantoid disease, why are embryos not invariably found in the blood; and why when embryos are found in the blood are they not invariably associated with elephantoid disease?"

The second question is easily answered. Disease in the host is not a necessary consequence of the existence of filaria in or near the lymphatics. The filaria immitis seldom inconveniences the dog in whose heart it lives and breeds—so the filaria sanguinis hominis may live and breed in or near a man's lymphatics without inducing disease. The disease, so to speak, is only an accident, though a very frequent one, in the history of the parasite.

But the accident or disease having happened we argue that the cause of it is or has been present; how can we account then for the absence of the other evidence of the parasite's presence, its embryos in the blood? Why were they found in one only out of ten cases of elephantiasis of the leg, in four only out of 15 cases of elephantiasis scroti, and be so frequently absent in the lymph scrotum and varicose groin glands? I do not know enough about the habits of the parent worm to give an exhaustive and quite satisfactory answer to this question, but I can account, in part at least, for this apparent anomaly. As I have already mentioned, embryos are often temporarily absent. This very often happens in cases where, from the small number of embryos found even at the time they are most abundant, we may infer that parent parasites are but few in number. . . .

It is evident from this that as most of the cases of elephantiasis, especially of elephantiasis of the leg, were examined once only, embryos may have been temporarily absent at the time of examination and present at other times. Case 28 was examined four times before embryos were discovered in the blood. Had this case been an ordinary one of elephantiasis of the leg, and not one of great interest, with chyluria and lymph

scrotum, the search for embryos would probably have been abandoned after the third or fourth failure, or more probably the patient would never again have returned to the hospital. This accounts for the absence of embryos in a certain number of cases; but there are undoubtedly others in which embryos are permanently absent. I proved this by examining frequently, often daily, the blood of patients recovering from the operation for elephantiasis scroti during the whole of their residence in hospital, perhaps many weeks. In such cases the absence of embryos may be accounted for in some of the following ways.

(1) The parent worm or worms, after permanently damaging the channels by which the lymph passes into the circulation, may have died. Filaria tumours and cicatrices are often found in the esophagus and aorta of the dog, the worm or worms which caused them having died or escaped. The same may happen in man.

(2) If still alive, they may be encysted in some situation where there is no opportunity of discharging embryos into the blood or lymph, and yet near enough the lymphatic vessels to occlude them. The accidents to which the filaria is constantly exposed are so numerous, that very few ever attain maturity. Very few embryos get further than the first step in development; probably very few of those that make a second advance, in the way I shall hereafter describe, reach the third step in man; and probably many of those that do enter man, and start fairly on their final journey, lose themselves among the tissues and fail to find their proper home and breeding place. Such wanderers may do infinite damage to man, though they never succeed in fulfilling their functions as regards their own species. Instances of wandering filariae that have lost their way I have met in the dog, and such I am sure do much more mischief than those who reach and breed in their proper habitat. Filaria sanguinolenta, whose home is undoubtedly the esophagus, sometimes penetrates the pleura, sometimes the walls of the aorta, becomes encysted and pregnant in these situations and discharges eggs uselessly into aorta or pleural cavity. A similar miscarriage may happen to Filaria sanguinis hominis. The eye worm of the horse is also a wanderer that has lost its way.

(3) The filaria may be present in the usual situation but only one sex may be represented; or if both sexes are present they may not have come

together. I have found unimpregnated female filaria immitis in the heart of the dog, no male being present, and vice versa. In such cases there could be no discharge of embryos.

In one or all of these ways the absence of embryos may be accounted for in elephantoid disease, and as they are most frequently absent in elephantiasis of the leg, the form of the disease that is usually longest in existence before coming under observation, it is probable that the most frequent cause of the absence of embryos is the death of the parent filariae.

Hydrocele is another disease frequently associated with haematozoa. It is not difficult to understand why this should be, and how a very slight obstruction in the lymphatic vessels connected with the tunica vaginalis would derange the delicate balance of secretion and absorption in that sac. The prevalence of hydrocele in warm countries may be thus accounted for. . . .

The Development of Filaria Sanguinis Hominis

Development cannot progress far in the host containing the parent—Fortunately, it is an almost universal law in the history of the more dangerous kinds of entozoa, that the egg or embryo must escape from the host inhabited by the parent before much progress can be made in development. Were it possible for animals so prolific as the Filaria immitis of the dog, or Filaria sanguinis of man, to be born and matured, and to reproduce their kind again in an individual host, the latter would certainly be overwhelmed by the first swarm of embryos escaping into the blood, as soon as they had made any progress in growth. If, for example, the blood of embryo filariae at any one time free in the blood of a dog moderately well charged with them were to begin growing, before they had each attained a hundredth part of the size of the mature filaria their aggregate volume would occupy a bulk many times greater than the dog itself. I have calculated that in the blood of certain dogs and men there exist at any given moment more than two millions of embryos. Now the individuals of such a swarm could never attain anything approaching the size of the mature worm without certainly involving the death of the host. The death of the host would imply the death of the parasite before a second generation of filariae could be born, and this of course entails the extermination of the species; for in such an arrangement reproduction would be equivalent to death of both parent and offspring, an anomaly impossible in nature.

The embryo must escape from the original host—It follows therefore that the embryo in order to continue its development and keep its species from extermination must escape from its first host in some way. After accomplishing this it either lives an independent existence for a time, during which it is provided with organs for growth not possessed by it hitherto; or it is swallowed by another animal, which treats it as a nursling for such time as is necessary to furnish it with an alimentary system. The former arrangement obtains in the filariae inhabiting the intestinal canal, the lumbricus and thread worm; the latter is followed by the several species of tape worm, and also by other kinds of entozoa.

I find that in cases where embryo filariae are not in great abundance in the blood, that is where we may infer that there are only one or two parent worms—they often disappear completely for a time, to reappear after the lapse of a few days or weeks. From this circumstance I infer, first, that reproduction is of an intermitting and not of a continuous character; and, second, that the embryos after a certain time either are disintegrated in the blood or are voided in the excretions. The latter does occur, I know from personal investigation, in the urine; and we have Dr. Lewis's testimony that he has found the animals in the tears. In this way then they may have an opportunity of continuing development either free, as in the case of the lumbricus, in the media into which the excretions are voided; or in the body of another animal, which has intentionally or accidentally fed on these, as in the case of the tapeworms. Man, in his turn, may then swallow this hypothetic animal or other thing containing the embryo suitably perfected, and so complete the circle. This is the history of many entozoa; but I have evidence to adduce that, if it be one way in which Filaria sanguinis hominis is nursed, it is not the only way, and therefore probably not the way at all.

The mosquito found to be the nurse—It occurred to me that as the first step in the history of the haematozoon was in the blood, the next might happen in an animal who fed on that fluid. To test this idea I procured mosquitoes that had fed on the patient Hinlo's . . . blood, and examining the expressed contents of their abdomens from day to day with the microscope, I found that my idea was correct, and that the haematozoon which entered the mosquito a simple structureless animal, left it, after passing through a series of highly interesting metamorphoses, much increased in size, possessing an alimentary canal, and being otherwise suited for an independent existence.

History of the mosquito after feeding on human blood—I may mention that my observations have been made exclusively on the female of one species of mosquito. I have never in many hundreds of specimens met with a male insect charged with blood.[1] There are two species found during the summer here; one quite a large insect about half an inch long with a black thorax and black and white banded abdomen; the other about half that size and of a dingy brown colour. The former is rare comparatively, the latter is very common and is the insect my remarks apply to.

After a mosquito has filled itself with blood (which it can do, if not disturbed, in about two minutes), it is evidently much embarrassed by the weight of its distended abdomen, so that it no longer can wheel about in the air. It accordingly attaches itself to some surface, if possible near stagnant water, where it remains in a comparatively torpid condition, digesting the blood, excreting yellow gamboge looking faeces, and maturing its ova. In the course of from three to five days these processes are completed, and the insect now betakes itself to the water, where the eggs are deposited, and on the surface of which they float in a dark brown mass looking like a flake of soot. The eggs do not take long to hatch (they are beautifully shaped objects, like an Etruscan vase) and the embryo emerges by forcing open a sort of lid placed at the broad end of the shell. The larvae now escape into the water where they swim about and feed, and become the "jumpers" we are familiar with, found in every stagnant pool.

If the contents of the abdomen are examined before the mosquito has fed or after the food has been absorbed, the following parts can easily be distinguished; two ovisacs containing from 60 to 100 ova; two large glandular masses; intestine and esophagus; and a very delicate transparent fibrous bag, the stomach. If the blood contained in the dilated stomach is examined soon after ingestion, the blood corpuscles are seen quite distinct in outline and behaving very much as when drawn in the ordinary way; but changes rapidly occur. First the corpuscles lose their distinctness of outline, then crystals of haematin appear; corpuscles and crystals give place to large oil globules, and the mass is deprived of its fluidity, and before the eggs are deposited, all colouring matter disappears; the white material is absorbed or expelled, and by the time the eggs are deposited the stomach is quite empty but for the embryo filariae it may contain.

How to procure mosquitos containing embryo filariae—It may be useful to those who wish to repeat and test my observations to know the plan I found most successful in procuring filaria-bearing mosquitos, and how their bodies were afterwards treated for microscopic observation. Such details may appear frivolous and unimportant, but by following them the observer will be spared disappointment and will economise his time and patience.

I persuaded a Chinaman, in whose blood I had already ascertained that filariae abounded, to sleep in what is known as a mosquito house in a room where mosquitos were plentiful. After he had gone to bed, a light was placed beside him and the door of the mosquito house was kept open for half an hour. In this way many mosquitos entered the house, the light was then put out and the door closed. Next morning the walls were covered with an abundant supply of insects with abdomens thoroughly distended. They were then caught below a wineglass, paralysed by means of a whiff of tobacco smoke, and transferred to small phials into some of which a little water had been poured. A cover providing for ventilation was then placed over the mouth of each phial. The effect of the tobacco smoke, if it has not been applied too long, is very evanescent, and seems to have no prejudicial influence on the future of the mosquito. From the phials they may be removed from time to time as required, by again paralysing with tobacco, and seizing them by the thorax with a fine forceps. The abdomen is then torn off, placed on a glass slide, and a small cylinder such as a thin penholder rolled over it from the anus towards the severed thoracic attachment. In this way the contents are safely and efficiently expressed, and observation is not interfered with by the almost opaque integument. If the contents are white and dry a little water should be added and mixed carefully with the mass so as to allow of the easy separation of the two large ovisacs. These can be removed in this way by the needle and transferred to another slide for separate examination. A thin covering glass should be placed over the residue, which will be found to contain the filariae either within the walls of the stomach, or, if these have been ruptured by too rough manipulation, floating in the surrounding water.

Large proportion of filariae ingested by the mosquito—The blood in the stomach of a mosquito that has fed on a filaria-infested man, usually contains a much larger proportion of filariae, than does an equal quantity of blood obtained from the same man in the usual way by pricking the finger. Thus six small slides, equivalent to about one drop of blood, from the man on whom most of my observations were made, would contain from ten to 30 haematozoa; whereas the blood drawn by a single mosquito, about as much as would fill one slide only, contained from 20 to 30 as a rule and sometimes many more. One slide in which I had the curiosity to count them had upwards of 120 specimens. From this it would appear that the mosquito has the faculty of selecting the embryo filariae; and in this strange circumstance we have an additional reason for concluding that this insect is the natural nurse of the parasite. . . .

Future history of the filaria—There can be little doubt as to the subsequent history of the filaria; or that escaping into the water in which the mosquito died, it is through the medium of this fluid brought into contact with the tissues of man, and then either piercing the integuments, or, what is more probable, being swallowed, it works its way through the alimentary canal to its final resting place. Arrived there its development is perfected, fecundation is effected, and finally the embryo filariae we meet with in the blood are discharged in successive swarms and in countless numbers. In this way the genetic cycle is completed.

The bearing of these observations on the explanation and prevention of elephantoid disease—The statistics I have given above are amply sufficient to prove the association of Filaria sanguinis hominis and Elephantoid disease as cause and effect; and now that I have

shown that the mosquito is a necessary element for the perfection of the parasite, the limitation of the distribution of elephantoid diseases to certain districts and zones of the earth's surface receives an explanation. Such disease is endemic only where the mosquito flourishes, *i.e.* in tropical and subtropical climates. Elephantiasis is more common in certain districts than in others; and I venture to predict that in those districts where it prevails the mosquito will be found to abound, and that in those localities where the disease is absent or uncommon, the mosquito will be found to be rare, or to be represented by a species incapable of nursing the infant filariae. The habits of the people, with regard to the use of water and mosquito nets, will also undoubtedly have an influence in determining the amount and spread of filaria disease. This is a point deserving investigation, for from the fact of the disease depending on so tangible a link as the mosquito, it is quite possible to prevent its spread, if not to secure its extermination. . . .

---

[1]This is explained by the arrangement of the appendages and proboscis of the male mosquito, which prevents it from penetrating the skin. As the male is provided with a complete alimentary apparatus it is presumed that he feeds on the juices and exudations of plants and fruits.

DISCOVERY OF THE ADULT REPRESENTATIVE OF MICROSCOPIC FILARIAE

Lancet, 2: 70–71, 1877.

Joseph Bancroft
(1836–1894)

A native of Stretford, near Manchester, his medical studies began at Manchester Royal School of Medicine and Surgery. In 1859 he graduated with the M.D. from St. Andrew's University. He practiced in Nottingham briefly but he went to Queensland in 1864 because of ill health. His interest in botany was almost equal to that in medicine and he made many unique observations on Australian plants. In 1877, after his discovery of filaria, he spent a year in England and left his son Thomas Lane Bancroft in medical school in Edinburgh. Returning to Australia, he continued to practice surgery and to continue his studies in such diverse fields as grape hybridization and banana production and even invented a new means of preservation of beef known as "pemmican." He was a public-servant and honored by his community.

T. Spencer Cobbold communicated Bancroft's original findings of the adult female Wuchereria bancrofti *in the following article. The plate accompanying this article illustrated Cobbold's paper, ''On Filaria Bancrofti,'' which appeared in* Lancet, 2: 495–496, 1877.

To the Editor of *The Lancet*

Sir:

Permit me to announce an interesting addition to our knowledge of parasites, seeing that it is calculated to throw light upon the question of the origin of one or more obscure diseases.

The brilliant discoveries of Lewis, followed up as they were by Sonsino in Egypt, and by Welch and others in this country, have at length been verified and extended by the observations of Dr. Bancroft, in Australia, who has become acquainted with the sexually mature form of at least one of the various kinds of minute nematoid hematozoa.

As has already been stated in the pages of one of your contemporaries, I received, in the spring of 1876, some capillary tubes from Australia, charged with blood taken from a chylurous patient. The donation came through Dr. Roberts of Manchester, who, prior to my investigation, had himself examined the contents of similar tubes, and had personally verified Dr. Bancroft's discovery of the microscopic hematozoa in question (Plate 58). In the notice which I published at the time, and which was reprinted in the *Veterinarian* (July, 1876) I mentioned that I had detected a nematoid ovum in the Australian blood—a fact which rendered it almost certain that the adult worm must be sought for in the human bearer. I sent Dr. Bancroft a copy of the article, and what was therein stated induced him to continue his investigations. These further researches have resulted in the record of novel facts which, in response to his courtesy, I now make public.

In a communication dated from Brisbane, Queensland, 20 April 1877, Dr. Bancroft writes as follows: ''I have labored very hard to find the parental form of the parasite, and am glad to tell you that I have now obtained five specimens of the worm, which are waiting to be forwarded by a trustworthy messenger.

''I have on record about 20 cases of this parasitic disease, and believe it to be the solution of chyluria, some form of hematuria, one form of spontaneous lymphatic abscess, a peculiar soft

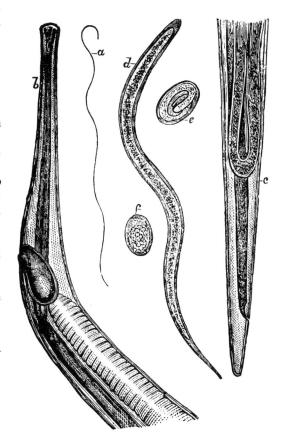

Plate 58. *Fig. a.* Filaria bancrofti, female, natural size. *Fig. b.* Head and neck, showing esophagus and vagina. *Fig. c.* Tail of same, showing fold of tuba, and termination of intestine. *Fig. d.* Free embryo. *Fig. e.* Intrachorional embryo. *Fig. f.* Egg.

varix of the groin, a hydrocele containing fibrinous fluid, another containing chylous fluid, together with some forms of varicocele and orchitis. These I have verified.

''In the colony there are no cases that I can find of elephantine leg, scrotal elephantiasis, or lymph scrotum; but, from the description of these diseases in the volume on Skin and Other Diseases of India by Fox, Farquhar, and Carter, and from Dr. Roberts's article on the latter in his volume on Urinary Diseases, I am of opinion that the parasitic nature of the same will be established.

''The worm is about the thickness of a human hair, and is from three to four inches long. By two loops from the center of its body it emits the filariae described by Carter in immense numbers.

"My first specimen I got on 21 December 1876, in a lymphatic abscess of the arm. This was dead. Four others I obtained alive from a hydrocele of the spermatic cord, having caught them in the eye of a peculiar trocar I use for tapping. These I kept alive for a day, and separated them from each with great difficulty. The worm, when immersed in pure water, stretches itself out and lies quite passive. In this condition it could be easily washed out of hydroceles through a large-sized trocar from patients known to suffer from filariae.

"I will forward you full particulars of my cases (and the worms) at an early date."

Such, Sir, is Dr. Bancroft's account of his "finds," and from the brief description furnished I propose to call the adult nematode *Filaria Bancrofti*.

If I refrain from lengthened comment on the significance of the facts it is because I know how ill you can afford the space necessary to do full justice to the subject. The literature of the hematozoa has already become intricate and of great extent.

I will only add that I share with Drs. Bancroft, Lewis, Sonsino, Fayrer, and others the opinion that a considerable group of morbid conditions, hitherto obscure as to their modes of origination, arise from the injurious action of microscopic filariae.

I am, Sir, your obedient servant,
T. Spencer Cobbold, M.D.

ADDITIONAL NOTES ON *FILARIA SANGUINIS HOMINIS* AND FILARIA DISEASE

Medical Reports, China Imperial Maritime Customs, Shanghai (or China: Inspectorate General of Customs, Medical Reports, according to Union Serials list), No. 18, pp. 36–39, April-Sept. 1879 (published in 1880).

Patrick Manson
(1844–1922)

Manson's biography will be found in the chapter on Malaria.
   Manson records the periodicity of Filaria sanguinis hominis (W. bancrofti) *in this paper.*

   . . . The Periodicity observed by the Embryo of Filaria Bancrofti in the Blood—Two years ago, writing on the habits of filaria sanguinis hominis (filaria Bancrofti), I remarked that in filarious patients the embryos were frequently temporarily absent from the blood. I was not aware at that time of any law governing this. My examinations were usually made in the early morning or late in the evening, and of the two assistants I employed one worked during the day, the other after 6 o'clock in the evening. I remarked that the former made very few finds in comparison to the latter, but attributed this to accident. Several months ago I gave directions for a filarious patient's blood to be examined daily, and a register to be kept of the examinations. On some days there appeared to be great abundance of filariae, on other days none, or very few. I noticed that when they were abundant the examination was made on busy days, when there was much work to be done in the hospital, and extra work of this sort had to be got through in the evening; and that when they were absent, the examination was made during the day. Recollecting the different results obtained by my assistants according as they worked during the day or after dark, and suspecting now that this was not altogether an accident, I made a series of systematic examinations every four hours in this patient and in others, with the view of ascertaining if this periodicity was maintained in every case. I examined a number of patients in this way, with the result of finding that unless there is some disturbance, as fever, interfering with the regular physiological rhythm of the body, filaria embryos invariably begin to appear in the circulation at sunset, their numbers gradually increase till about midnight, during the early morning they become fewer by degrees, and by 9 or 10 o'clock in the forenoon it is a very rare thing to find one in the blood. Till sunset they appear to have completely deserted the circulation, but with the evening they come back again, to disappear in the morning, and so on with the utmost regularity every day and from day to day. The circle is completed every 24 hours, and there are no longer spells of absence, as I at one time supposed, than from morning to evening.

   Subjoined is a register of some of the examinations from which I have drawn these conclusions. I have to apologise for the incompleteness of the series of observations in some of the cases, but I often found it very difficult to get a Chinaman to submit during a number of days to the necessary manipulations, and consequently the evidence in such cases is fragmentary. But the numbers, taking them together, are quite sufficient to justify my deductions. . . .

Register of Filaria Embryos Found in One Drop of Blood From the Finger, Obtained at the Hours Indicated

NAME AND DISEASE:

Oah. Case 53. Elephantiasis scroti and lymph scrotum

A.M.

DATE	4	5	6	7	8	9	10	11	12
1879									
June 16	.	.	.	.	.	.	.	.	.
" 17	6				2				1
" 18	23				1				0
" 19	18				0				0
" 20	15				0				0
" 21	2				1				0
" 22	2				0				0
" 23	5				0				0
" 24	23				0				0
" 25	7				0				0
" 26	14				0				0
" 27	11				0				
" 28	5				0				
" 29	17				0				
" 30	14				0				0
July 1	33				1				

P.M.

DATE	1	2	3	4	5	6	7	8	9	10	11	12
1879												
June 16	.	.	.	.	.	.	.	43				.
" 17				0				24				57
" 18				0				105				21
" 19				0		1	10	29	37			
" 20				0				29				89
" 21				1				53				41
" 22				0				17				34
" 23				0				24				43
" 24				0				14				
" 25				0				10				13
" 26				0				19				
" 27				0				10				
" 28				0				12				
" 29				0				13				
" 30				0				12				35
July 1	.	.	.	.	.	.	.	.	.	.	.	.

. . . These figures are abundantly sufficient to establish the diurnal periodicity of the embryo's appearance in the blood. For the meaning of it I think we have not far to look. The nocturnal habits of filaria sanguinis hominis are adapted to the nocturnal habits of the mosquito, its intermediary host, and is only another of the many wonderful instances of adaptation so constantly met with in nature. On establishing this fact these questions occurred to me: first, is the disappearance of the embryos brought about by their death, and have we therefore a fresh swarm every 24 hours? second, if they do not die, where do they conceal themselves during the day? third, has this periodicity any pathological significance? With regard to the last of these questions I cannot as yet give any answer. One could speculate very ingeniously with this for a starting point, but as yet I have no fact of any great importance to offer. My conviction is that the pathological significance of filaria sanguinis hominis in tropical disease is as yet by no means fully understood, nor the importance of the parasite completely apprehended. . . .

A NOTE ON FILARIA SANGUINIS HOMINIS (WITH A DESCRIPTION OF A MALE SPECIMEN)

British Medical Journal, 1: 1050–1051, 1888.

Alfred Gibbs Bourne (1859–1940)

A native of Lowestoft, Bourne entered University College in London to study the biological sciences, but simultaneously attended the Royal School of Mines. It was perhaps this dual interest in science and technology that enabled him to become one of the earliest makers of microdissection instruments.

In 1886 he assumed the chair of biology at the Presidency College in Madras, after having received the D.Sc. from the University of London and after having spent two brief periods working at the Zoological Station in Naples.

Although his major scientific work dealt with the anatomy of the Hirudinea, his interests began to turn in the direction of administration. He became the principal of the Presidency College in Madras, then director of public instruction in the same city, and finally director of the Indian Institute of Science at Bangalore. Upon his retirement from the last of these posts, he returned to England, settling in Dartmouth.

Male specimens of Filaria bancrofti *are exceedingly rare even today. Bourne records the first male specimen found.*

Our knowledge of the adult form of this worm is still incomplete. It was discovered by Dr. Ban-

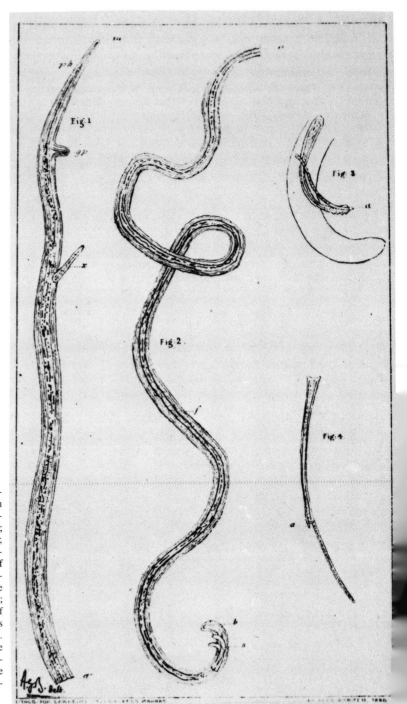

croft, in Brisbane, in 1876. It has also been found by Dr. Timothy Richards Lewis, in Calcutta; Dr. Patrick Manson, in Amoy; Dr. Silva Araujo and Dr. F. dos Santos, in Brazil. Dr. Bancroft's specimens were described by Dr. Spencer Cobbold. Drs. Lewis and Manson have both given descriptions of their specimens. All these specimens were imperfect, and they are stated by Cobbold to have been all females. This authority states in his book (*Parasites: A Treatise on the Entozoa of Men and Animals,* 1879) that the male parasite is unknown. This was not, however, strictly correct, as Lewis in the paper referred to by Cobbold, states that he found portions of two specimens: the one was about one inch and a half long, and belonged to a female from which the caudal extremity had been severed, while the other was a fragment of a male worm. Of this latter he says: "It measured half an inch in length, and 1/180 of an inch transversely; it was thinner than the female, but of considerably firmer texture—so firm, indeed, that while endeavoring to make out its anatomy a considerable portion of it was lost by one of the needles used for dissecting snapping, and carrying a portion of the worm along with it. On tearing the helminth across, the severed surface does not present a ragged edge, but an even outline. The male manifested also a great tendency to coil, and it was only with difficulty that it could be separated from the specimen of the female parasite, around a portion of which it had twisted itself. It is unfortunate that its caudal end, especially, could not be found, as the definite decision of the genus to which it should be referred depends in great measure on the characters which the posterior end of the male worm presents."

Brigade-Surgeon Sibthorpe has had several cases of filarial disease in the General Hospital at Madras, and has always made a search for the adult worm; this has hitherto proved fruitless. Recently, however, after an amputation of a lymphoid scrotum, he found two worms which he had mounted and identified as adult filariae. He had found embryo filariae swarming in the patient's blood on the previous evening. He very kindly sent these specimens to me for examination, and I found that one was a female, while the other was a male. The female specimen agrees very closely with Cobbold's figure, but the vagina is everted or protruded. Dr. Smyth, resident surgeon to the hospital, who mounted the specimens, tells me that the eversion took place during mounting; it is probably a normal act during life. The caudal portion is wanting. The male specimen is about an inch and a quarter long; the anterior extremity is wanting, but the caudal extremity is intact, and presents two spicules. The structure of these spicules will doubtless form a valuable specific character. Unfortunately, only one of these spicules remains in situ; the other has dropped out in the mounting and lies nearly isolated on the slide. The spicule is broad at its proximal extremity, and gradually tapers until it becomes capillary in character. About halfway down there is a lateral prominence, and when in situ the spicule is folded on itself so that this prominence forms the actual free extremity of the spicule, while the broad end and the capillary end lie near to one another.

A description and figures (Plate 59) of this specimen, which, with the exception of Lewis's fragment, is, I believe, the first recorded specimen of the adult male filaria sanguinis hominis, will be published in an ensuing number of the *Transactions* of the South Indian Branch of the British Medical Association. [The plate appeared in the *Transactions* 2 (6): 396-398, 1888, illustrating Bourne's article, "Note on Two Specimens of Adult *Filaria sanguinis hominis*" — Eds.]

It is interesting to note that in this case, as in Lewis's case, the male and female were found in close contiguity.

A SUPPOSED NEW SPECIES OF *FILARIA SANGUINIS HOMINIS* FOUND IN THE INTER-IOR OF BRITISH GUIANA

British Guiana Medical Annual, 9: 24–27, 1897.

Albert Tronson Ozzard
(?–1929)

Ozzard served British Guiana for 40 years (1887–1927) in various capacities as district medical officer and resident surgeon in Georgetown. His studies on hookworm led the Rockefeller Commission to begin its first hookworm control campaign in British Guiana. He contracted malaria in 1926 which forced his retirement.

Mansonella ozzardi, so named by Patrick Manson, is first described in this article and our knowledge of this parasite remains almost as obscure as the publication in which it first appeared.

The filaria sanguinis hominis (nocturna) has long been known to be very prevalent in British Guiana. Its presence, I believe, was first recognized by Dr. Hillis some 20 years ago. Its accompanying lesions, such as elephantiasis, chyluria, lymph-scrotum, &c., are also well known and are recognized as being dependent on the existence of the filaria sanguinis hominis.

Recently also the parent forms, filaria bancrofti, have been found by Dr. Daniels, and were described by him in the last volume of this Annual.

Out of 100 patients undergoing treatment for various diseases in the Public Hospital, Berbice, I found the filaria nocturna in no less than 28. These patients included Negroes, coloured Creoles, Coolies and Portuguese, and were taken haphazard without any reference whatever to the particular disease from which they were suffering.

Beyond the filaria nocturna and its parental forms, however, I am not aware that any other variety has been recognized as existing in British Guiana.

In December of last year it was my fortune to be sent on special duty some 130 miles up the Demerara River, and whilst there I collected 14 slides of blood taken at night from the Aboriginal Indians. These slides I sent home to Dr. Patrick Manson, who kindly examined them and found the following somewhat surprising result. No less than six of these contained filariae, not filaria nocturna however, but apparently two other var-

ieties, one a blunt-tailed animal resembling filaria perstans, and the other a sharp-tailed animal about the size of filaria demarquaii and somewhat resembling it in shape, but not possessing a sheath. In none of the slides were they numerous. In two slides both sharp-tailed and blunt-tailed filariae were present.

For some time after this I was unable to come across any more Aboriginal Indians. During the last few months, however, being in New Amsterdam, every now and again I have been able to examine the blood of several Indians from the Berbice River who were sent to me by Mr. Gordon, of the Crown Lands Department. In all I have thus been able to examine 57 Indians and 1 coloured Creole who has lived the greater part of his life up the Berbice River.

Out of these 58 cases, filariae blunt-tailed or sharp-tailed or both, occurred in no less than 39. Adding the previous 14 cases we have a total of 72 cases, filariae occurring in 45.

It is thus seen that considerably more than half of our Aboriginal Indians harbour these parasites in their blood. But that it is not confined to the Indians is proved by a case of mine beforementioned, in which a coloured Creole who had lived many years up the Berbice River had a plentiful supply of them in his blood, tending to show that their presence is dependent on locality and is not confined to any one particular race.

The question now to be settled, of course is as to their identity. Are they two distinct species? or are they one and the same animal? and have they ever been described before?

At first Dr. Manson was inclined to look upon the sharp-tailed animal as filaria demarquaii, and the blunt-tailed ones as none other than the filaria perstans. His opinion now is that the former is an entirely new specimen and the latter filaria perstans. My own observations lead me to consider the blunt-tail and the sharp-tail as one and the same animal, the blunt-tail being simply the very fine sharp-pointed tail retracted, and I look upon it as a new species.

If a slide containing filaria nocturna be de-haemoglobinised and stained with logwood, the latter being washed off after about ten minutes, most of the filariae will be found to show two spots under a high power of the microscope—one about a third back from the head, known as the "v" spot, and one near the extremity of the tail—the "caudal" spot. Also the whole length of the animal shows a central granular appearance. Now these appearances, together with the presence or absence of a sheath, afford an easy method of distinguishing the different species of filariae. Filaria nocturna and filaria demarquaii both possesses a sheath and show the "v" and "caudal" spots and the granular appearance. Filaria perstans, on the other hand, possesses no sheath and shows neither spots or granular appearance; but simply seems to be perfectly homogeneous throughout.

If now slides of blood containing the parasites under question be similarly prepared, both the blunt-tailed and sharp-tailed animals will show equally well the two spots alluded to and the granular appearance. And it is for this very important reason, therefore, that I think we have a new species and not filaria perstans.

Further if the different animals be carefully examined, they will not all appear as possessing either a very sharp-pointed or a perfectly blunt tail; but some will be seen to end in a small little knob, so that one cannot describe the tail either as being very sharp-pointed or on the other hand as abruptly blunt. These seem rather to be intermediate between the two forms. I consider these, therefore, to be the sharp-tailed animal with the tail partially retracted, and am inclined to think that the blunt-tailed animals are simply the sharp-tailed ones with a good deal more retraction of the tail.

If further a living specimen be carefully watched under the microscope it will at times be seen to assume the sharp-tailed form, at others the blunt-tailed form. I am bound, however, to admit that I have not as yet examined a sufficiently large number of living specimens to be absolutely sure of this and so rapid and energetic are their movements that one might easily be deceived.

Again in a recent letter from Dr. Manson he states that filaria perstans is always blunt-tailed and filaria demarquaii always sharp-tailed and filaria diurna always has a sheath. Out of 30 slides of filaria perstans which he recently examined there were 39 filaria in number and all were blunt-tailed; also of 123 filaria demarquaii all were sharp-tailed.

Now this is very different with the filariae so commonly found amongst the Aboriginal Indians. In the majority of slides which I have examined the two kinds—blunt and sharp-tailed—could be generally found together, and I am very strongly of the opinion that if sufficient search be made it will always be possible to find the sharp-tail along with the blunt, because as I think they are one and the same animal.

In making some permanent cover-glass preparations I have noticed that, of the blood obtained from one individual, one slide will sometimes contain all sharp-tails, another all blunt-tails, while a third will perhaps contain both varieties.

Another important point against the blunt-tail being filaria perstans is the fact that occasionally a sheath can be made out in these animals. I have permanent preparations which show a very distinct sheath in some of the blunt-tailed animals. Now filaria perstans is said never to possess a sheath and this is one of its distinguishing characteristics. Similarly also a sheath can be made out in the sharp-tailed animals.

It is a noteworthy fact, therefore, that the anatomical appearances of the blunt and sharp-tails, as seen under a high power of the microscope, agree in every detail. They both show the "v" and "caudal" spots—the central granular aggregation—almost the same measurements—and whereas at times neither seems to possess a sheath, at others a sheath can be made out in both.

Like the filaria perstans and filaria demarquaii, these parasites can be found in the blood at all hours of the day or night.

With regard to the measurements of these filaria I am as yet unable to speak with any certainty. I have not yet obtained a living specimen sufficiently moribund to be amenable to measurement and it is utterly impossible to measure them during their many and varied evolutions in life.

The dead dried specimens which I have measured give roughly speaking from 1/140 to 1/100 of an inch in length, and from 1/6000 to 1/9000 of an inch in breadth: the blunt-tailed animal being as a rule shorter and broader than the sharp-tailed one, which fact tends to support my view that the former are simply the latter with their sharp-pointed tails retracted. The length from the "caudal spot" to the tip of the tail in the sharp-pointed animals is about 1/600 of an inch: in the blunt-pointed animal about 1/1000 inch.

ON FILARIAL PERIODICITY

British Medical Journal, 2: 644–646, 1899.

Patrick Manson
(1844–1922)

Manson's biography will be found in the chapter on Malaria.

Manson had described the nocturnal periodicity of Wuchereria bancrofti *in Imperial Maritime Custom Reports of China No. 18, pp. 36–39, 1879 (published in 1880). In report No. 20, pp. 13–15, 1880, he found microfilaria and adult filaria in the lymphatics of scrotal elephantiasis. In this report he reviews the localization of adult* W. bancrofti *and describes the localization of the microfilaria in the capillaries of the lungs.*

Filaria bancrofti discharges its young (Filaria nocturna, the *Filaria sanguinis hominis* of Lewis) into the lymph stream. In the lymph stream the embryo parasites are carried to the general circulation, where they exhibit the peculiar phenomenon known as "filarial periodicity"—that is, they appear in countless swarms in the cutaneous circulation during the night, and disappear from it during the day.

This singular phenomenon suggests certain questions:

I. What is the object of it?

II. Is it constant?

III. What becomes of the young filariae during the day? (*a*) Do they die after a brief life of a few hours, and is there, therefore, a fresh swarm launched into the circulation every evening? or (*b*) do they live for many days, retiring every morning to some organ or organs, and remaining there during their daily absences from the peripheral circulation?

IV. If the latter be the case, how is it brought about?

I.

The answer to the first question, What is the object of filarial periodicity? has already been supplied. The mosquito has been shown to be an efficient intermediate host for the filaria. Bancroft in Australia has recently confirmed the original observations made in China on this point. The particular species of mosquito concerned are nocturnal in their habits. It is therefore reasonable to conclude that the nocturnal appearance of the filaria at the surface of the body is an adaptation of the habits of the parasite to those of the mosquito, its intermediate host.

II.

Is filarial periodicity constant? Yes; unless during fever, and unless the usual habits as regard the times of being awake and of sleep be inverted. In the former case periodicity is disturbed; in the latter, as shown by Stephen Mackenzie and confirmed by myself, it is correspondingly inverted.

III.

What becomes of the filaria during the day? This question a recent experience enables me to answer.

I had already ascertained by examinations of the fluids escaping in various forms of filarial lymphorrhagia that the embryo parasite is more or less constantly being passed into the lymph stream in which the parent worm lies, and that therefore filarial periodicity is not caused by a quotidian periodicity in the act of parturition. I had also ascertained, by examining blood collected from spouting arteries severed during surgical operations performed on filariated subjects at a time when the parasite is normally absent from the cutaneous circulation, that it was present, though in inconsiderable numbers, in the smaller arteries at such time; but until recently I had no opportunity of acquiring any fairly complete conception of its exact distribution in other organs during its daily temporary absence from the surface of the body.

On February 19, 1897, a man in whose blood Filaria nocturna abounded committed suicide by swallowing prussic acid. The case is recorded by Mr. Young in the *British Medical Journal*. As proved by numerous observations made at intervals during the previous nine months, this man's filariae invariably had observed the usual quotidian periodicity, appearing in the cutaneous circulation about 5 or 6 P.M. and disappearing from it about 8 A.M. The dose of poison swallowed was apparently large. Death took place almost instantaneously about 8:30 A.M., that is just about the time when it may assumed that the filariae had retired from the peripheral circulation for the day. The man's body was removed to Charing Cross Hospital and a *post-mortem* examination made the same afternoon.

Seventeen adult *Filariae bancrofti*—16 females and 1 male—were found in an enormous lymphatic varix which occupied a great part of the pelvis and abdomen; probably many more parental worms were present, but, owing to the small size of this parasite and the difficulties of the dissection, were overlooked. At the time of the examination a hurried microscopical scrutiny of the blood from various organs gave the following result:

A pulmonary vein contained very many embryo filariae.

A pulmonary artery contained very many filariae.

The margin of a lung contained prodigious numbers.

A small clot in left ventricle of heart contained a large number of filariae.

A small clot from aorta contained a large number of filariae.

A coronary artery and vein contained a very few filariae.

The right ventricle of the heart contained a few filariae.

The femoral vessels (a doubtful observation) no filariae.

The bone marrow contained no filariae.

The basilar artery of the brain contained two filariae.

The middle cerebral vein contained a few filariae.

The spleen contained no filariae.

The liver contained no filariae.

At the same time drops or smears of blood from the following organs were spread on microscope slips. The films were subsequently fixed with alcohol and stained with methylene blue or logwood. The filariae on the films were then counted with the following result:

Organ	No. of Slides	Aggregate No. of Filariae	Average per Slide
Liver	3	2	2/3
Spleen	3	3	1
Brachial venae comites	4	111	28
Bone marrow	1	0	0
Muscle of heart	3	365	122
Carotid artery	1	612	612
Lung	10	6,751	675

The number of filariae in the blood expressed from the lung was prodigious, as many as 30 or 40 being visible in some fields of one-sixth of an inch objective. In proportion to the amount of blood examined they were even more numerous in the thin film obtained from the carotid artery. In the lung blood they appeared to occur in groups. In the newly expressed blood most of the parasites were dead; only a few exhibited languid movements. They had the usual anatomical characters of *Filaria nocturna*; when stained the sheath could readily be made out.

Through the kindness of Dr. Mott, F.R.S., pathologist to the London County Council's asylums, sections were cut from the following organs, and the filariae, or rather fragments of filariae (for most of the parasites were necessarily cut across in making the sections), which they contained carefully counted. The sections were all of the same thickness and, approximately, of the same size. From three to ten sections of each organ were made, each section being from a different part of the organ. The following is the result of the count:

Organs	No. of Sections	Aggregate No. of Filariae	Average per Section
Liver	10	3	0.3
Spleen	4	0	0.0
Kidney	8	13	1.6
Brain	4	4	1.0
Muscle (voluntary)	3	2	0.33
Heart muscle	4	68	17.0
Lung	6	301	50.16
Lobe of Ear	4	1	0.25
Scrotum	4	0	0.0

From these facts and figures it may be concluded that *Filaria nocturna* during its temporary absence from the cutaneous circulation is present in the larger blood vessels, particularly the arteries; that a few are to be found in the capillaries of the muscles and brain, a few in the vessels of the kidneys, a considerable number in the muscle of the heart; but that the majority are lodged in the blood vessels of the lungs. In the last-mentioned situation the sections showed that the filariae are somewhat irregularly distributed, occurring in clusters in the larger vessels, or singly and more or less coiled up in the capillaries.

IV.

What is the mechanism determining this distribution of the filariae, and what causes their absence from the cutaneous circulation during the day and presence there during the night?

This question I am unable to answer. It has been suggested that the capillaries of the skin are relaxed during sleep and so permit at that time the entrance of the filariae. I would point out, however, that the parasites begin to come into the cutaneous circulation about 5 or 6 in the evening, and are present there in vast numbers by 9 P.M.— that is to say, long before the usual time for sleep; and that they begin gradually to diminish in number about midnight or 1 A.M.—that is, when sleep is usually profound. Therefore, although the appearance of the filariae at the surface of the body concurs to a certain extent with the hours of sleeping, their presence there is not caused by sleep. Rather, it seems to me, their presence in the cutaneous circulation is dependent on something that tends to accumulate in the body, or in certain parts of the body, in consequence of the activities of waking life, and which tends to disappear during sleep. Manifestly, the cause is not meteorological; for, as already mentioned, the inversion of the times of waking and sleeping suffices to bring about an inversion of the periodicity.

The question suggests itself: By what means do the filariae maintain their position in the organs they elect to occupy? How, for example, do they stem the current of blood in the aorta, or in the carotid artery, where they are in vastly greater numbers than in the slower flowing blood of the veins, as the observations I have enumerated indicate? For example, in the case of the carotid artery, the quantity of blood which I examined was insignificant—a mere trace— and yet it contained over 600 parasites; whereas large drops from the veins contained only about 25 filariae each. In the brain and voluntary muscles a few of the filariae occupied the larger vessels, but the majority were in the capillaries, in which they lay lengthwise, filling the little vessels. In the lungs some were in the arterioles and outstretched, usually in company with others; many were coiled up in the capillaries and smaller vessels, the disposition of their bodies suggesting that they had assumed this particular attitude so as to jam or fix themselves in the vessel. In the kidneys they occupied principally the vessels of the Malpighian bodies; in one instance I saw three filariae in one Malpighian tuft.

It is difficult to account for their complete absence from those highly vascular organs—the spleen, the liver, and the bone marrow.

It might be suggested that the absence of the filariae during the day from the vessels of the skin was owing to a contracted condition of these vessels at this time. Against this supposition is the fact that there is another blood worm, *Filaria diurna*, which also observes an equally regular periodicity, but appears in the peripheral circulation during the day, and disappears from it during the night, an arrangement exactly opposite to that which obtains in the case of *Filaria nocturna*. Then there are at least two other blood worms of

man—*Filaria perstans* and *Filaria demarquaii*—which are constantly present in the peripheral circulation both by day and by night. The two latter parasites are very much smaller than *Filaria nocturna*; it is therefore conceivable that they might enter vessels through which the latter could not pass.

Filaria diurna, however, is practically identical in size, shape, and structure with *Filaria nocturna*, so that what in respect to size of vessels applies to the one should equally apply to the other.

The facts seem to point to the existence of some physiological product, the outcome of the activities of waking life, which either drives *Filaria nocturna* from the surface of the body during the day, or attracts it to certain internal organs, particularly to the lungs and large arteries, during the night. What this substance may be it is for physiologists to say.

The Periodicity of the Malarial Parasite

In conclusion, I would point to another blood parasite of man which at one period of its life is in abundant evidence in the peripheral circulation, and which at another period elects to lie up in the vessels of certain of the deeper organs. This parasite also exhibits a periodicity almost as regular as that of *Filaria nocturna*. I refer to the malaria parasite. In certain varieties of this parasite, whilst the young forms are readily obtainable in finger blood, the mature forms are almost entirely confined to the capillaries of the deeper viscera. Strange to say, the principal of these viscera are just those which are shunned by the filaria, namely, the spleen, the liver, the bone marrow, and the brain.

It is a singular and suggestive circumstance, and one which, to my way of thinking, points to some important underlying biological law, that the two blood parasites of man subserved by the mosquito exhibit during what I might term their anthropal phase a well-marked diurnal periodicity, and, at the same time, a well-marked predilection for special but different organs during their periods of temporary absence from the peripheral circulation.

A RECENT OBSERVATION ON *FILARIA NOCTURNA* IN CULEX: PROBABLE MODE OF INFECTION OF MAN

British Medical Journal, 1: 1456–1457, 1900.

George Carmichael Low
(1872–1952)

A Scotsman by birth, Carmichael Low was educated at St. Andrew's and Edinburgh, where he received his M.B. and C.M. degrees in 1897. He studied under Manson at the London School of Tropical Medicine. With L. W. Sambon and Signor Terzi he attracted world-wide attention in 1900 by escaping infection with malaria by residing in a screened habitation in a highly malarious area of Italy.

He was active in the London School of Tropical Medicine, eventually becoming director of clinical tropical medicine. An effective and entertaining teacher, he retired in 1937 and died in London in 1952.

At Manson's insistence Low went to Vienna and Heidelberg to learn the colloidin embedding technique. At this time Manson had received many infected mosquitos from Thomas Lane Bancroft (son of Joseph Bancroft) of Australia accompanied by his notes that filaria were probably injected into man at feeding. Low proceeded to use this embedding technique to document the presence of filaria in the proboscis. He specifically noted that this was not conclusive evidence of infection by inoculation. Grassi and Noe demonstrated mosquito inoculation of Filaria immitis *in the dog later in 1900.*

The method by which Culex transmits Filaria bancrofti *is outlined in this paper.*

While working during the last three months in the London School of Tropical Medicine under Dr. Manson on a series of filariated mosquitos (*Culex ciliaris*) forwarded to the latter by Dr. Bancroft of Australia, I have been able to add some facts to our knowledge of the life-history of *Filaria nocturna*, facts which have special reference to the probable mode in which the human subject is infected by this parasite. They give also, if only indirectly, strong support to the inoculation theory of malaria, and add an additional argument, if such be required, for pushing forward the schemes now on foot for the protection of the human body from mosquito bite.

As is now well known, the filaria embryo, after being swallowed by certain species of mosquito, undergoes a metamorphosis in the thoracic muscles of these insects. In the stomach (Plate 60, Fig. 1) it casts its sheath. It then quits the stomach and enters the thoracic muscles (Fig. 2), in which it passes through various changes (Figs. 3 and 4). These result in the acquisition of vastly increased size, a mouth and alimentary canal, and a peculiar trilobed caudal appendage (Fig. 7). Until Bancroft's recent observations it was sup-

posed that the filaria on the death of the mosquito—an event which was generally believed to occur in the water on which the insect had laid her eggs for the first and last time—quitted the body of its defunct intermediary host, entered the water, and through this medium obtained access to the alimentary canal, and ultimately the lymphatic system of man. The principal reasons for this supposition were:

(*a*) That mosquitos confined in vessels after they had fed on human blood deposited their eggs about the end of a week and almost immediately thereafter died, and

(*b*) That the developed filaria on the completion of its evolution in the mosquito exhibited remarkable activity when placed in water, and a capacity for living in this medium for, at all events, several hours—an activity and capacity suggesting that water is its natural habitat at this stage of its life.

Ross, and subsequently Bancroft and others, have now shown that the female mosquito if fed can go on living and laying for many weeks after the meal on human blood and after depositing her first batch of eggs, provided she is supplied with nutriment, whether in the form of animal or of vegetable juices. It is manifest, therefore, that any filariae she may contain must find some other means for quitting the body of their intermediary insect host, and of getting access to the tissues of the definitive human host. Bancroft made two suggestions—(*a*) that the filaria might be swallowed by man while still in the mosquito—a somewhat improbable as well as unnatural event; (*b*) that it might be stimulated to re-enter the esophagus of a mosquito when the latter came to feed again on a human subject, and so creep along the proboscis by the natural channel and thus into human tissues. How near suggestion *b* is to the truth the following observations show:

To study the anatomy of the mosquito in reference to any possible migrations of the worms, sections of filariated mosquitos were cut after embedding in celloidin and stained. In serial sections of infected insects, killed at various times both before and after the final stage of the metamorphosis, it was found that the young filariae, after reaching their highest stage of development in the insect, instead of lying passively in the thoracic muscles, leave that tissue, and, in the vast majority of instances, travel forward in the direction of the head of the mosquito, and pass into the loose cellular tissue which

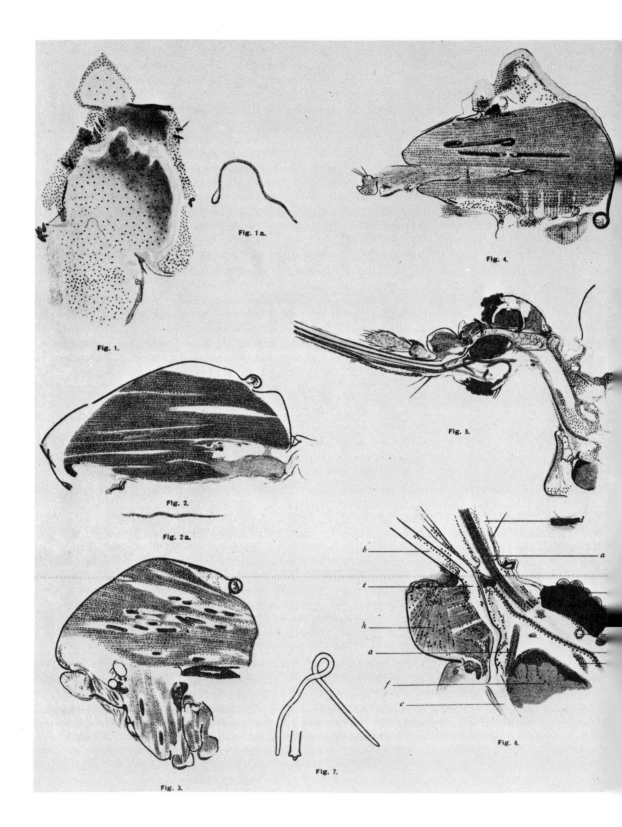

Fig. 1.

Fig. 1 a.

Fig. 2.

Fig. 2 a.

Fig. 3.

Fig. 4.

Fig. 5.

Fig. 6.

Fig. 7.

b

e

h

a

f

c

a

abounds in the prothorax in the neighbourhood of the salivary glands. Although the large majority of the filariae take up this position very constantly, an occasional straggler is seen in the tissues between the thorax and abdomen, or in the abdomen itself even as far back as the Malpighian tubes, or in the neighbourhood of the ovisacs. The situations last named are distinctly unusual. If we disregard these exceptional stragglers it will be found that the worms, after a short stay in the prothorax, pass along the neck, enter the lower part of the head, and coil themselves up in the loose connective tissue immediately below the cephalic ganglion and the salivary duct (Fig. 5). Rarely are they found above the cephalic ganglion. From the head they can be traced, in fortunate sections, passing into the proboscis; not along the salivary duct as is the case with the malarial parasite, for this channel is manifestly too minute to accommodate a body relatively so gigantic as the filaria; not along the esophagus or pharynx, as Bancroft suggested; but by making an independent passage through the base of the labium, and pushing forward along the proboscis between labium and hypopharynx amongst the stilets. Here I have frequently found them stretching along almost the entire length of the proboscis, the head being invariably in advance (Fig. 5 and 6). Strange to say two worms nearly always lie together in the proboscis, their heads being, so to speak, *téte-à-téte*.

It is difficult to avoid the deduction that the parasites so situated are there normally, awaiting an opportunity to enter the human tissues when the mosquito next feeds on man. The sections when made on filariated insects at any period after the third week in every instance contained parasites either in the head, or in the proboscis, or in both.

It is interesting in connection with this fact to remember that these insects after their meal on human blood had subsequently frequently fed on fruit juices. To keep them alive for the necessary time to permit of the evolution of the filariae this mode of feeding had to be resorted to. From this we may infer that the parasite has the power of discriminating between vegetable and animal juices. For did it not possess this faculty of discrimination our mosquitos would have shown no filariae, as the parasites might have been expected to have passed out into the bananas on which they had been feeding long before the date at which they were killed.

Without actual and somewhat dangerous experiment it would be rash positively to assert that the filaria is inoculated directly into man by mosquito bite. Nor may we absolutely ignore the possibility of its gaining access to the human tissue through the medium of water or of vegetable into which it might have escaped by way of the proboscis, the cloaca, or along with the insects' eggs. But the evidence of design implied by the position taken up by the parasite in the proboscis, and its declining to quit this position when the mosquito feeds on vegetable juices, are suggestive, and almost prove that the mosquito bite is the natural and, probably, the constant and only opportunity for the filaria to enter upon its next and final stage of development in the definitive host.

It is interesting to note that although degenerative changes appear to be produced in the muscles of the mosquito, especially by the more advanced forms of the filaria, nothing of the nature of inflammatory change or of encystment, as in the case of trichina infection of vertebrate muscle, is ever observed. And, further, that the rate of development is not uniform; sometimes advanced forms are found as early as the eleventh day, or immature forms so late as the third week from the presumed time of infection.

Bancroft is enclined to doubt Manson's statement that the filaria casts its sheath before quitting the stomach of the mosquito; in several of my sections the empty sheath is plainly visible in the blood contained in the stomach, thus proving that ecdysis is not an artificial phenomenon.

Plate 60. Fig. 1. Filaria nocturna in the blood in the stomach of newly fed mosquito. *Fig. 1a,* the same, isolated. (Australia.) *Fig. 2. F. nocturna* lying in thoracic muscle of mosquito after quitting stomach; first day after feeding, *Fig. 2a.* the same, isolated. (China.) *Fig. 3. F. nocturna* in thoracic muscle of mosquito 9 days after feeding. Great increase in size; commencing differentiation of alimentary canal. (Madras.) *Fig. 4. F. nocturna* in thoracic muscles 11¾ days after feeding; development nearly complete. (Australia.) *Fig. 5. F. nocturna* in head and proboscis of mosquito 20 days after feeding. Shows parasites coiled up below cephalic ganglion and extending along proboscis between labium and hypopharynx; part of another filaria can be seen passing along the neck from the prothorax to the head. (Australia.) *Fig. 6.* High power view of another section showing exact route by which the filaria enters the proboscis. The salivary duct is seen entering base of hypopharynx. (*a*) Fragments of filaria; (*b*) labrum; (*c*) base of hypopharynx; (*d*) labium; (*e*) pharynx; (*f*) cephalic ganglion; (*g*) eye; (*h*) muscle; (*j*) salivary duct opening into base of hypopharynx. (Australia.) *Fig. 7.* Filaria dissected out of mosquito 50 days after feeding. The tail with its appendages shown more highly magnified. (Australia.)

CHAPTER 21

Loaiasis

ON A WORM FOUND UNDER THE CONJUNCTIVA, AT MARIBAROU, SANTO DOMINGO

Sur un ver trouvé sous la conjunctive, à Maribarou, isle Saint-Domingue. Journal de Médicine, Chirurgie, Pharmacie, etc., Paris, 32: 338–339, 1770. Translated from the French.

Mongin

M. Mongin was a French surgeon who obviously worked in Maribarou, Santo Domingo. We have been unable to obtain biographical information.

This is the first description of the Loa loa. *Another early description is attributed to Guyot (1778) in Africa.*

The Earl of Cokburn called me to examine a Negro girl of his household. She was complaining of a severe stabbing pain in the eye of some 24 hours' duration; there were no signs of inflammation.

At first glance, I saw a worm which seemed to crawl superficially on the eye, but when I tried to catch it with forceps, I realized that it was between the conjunctiva and the cornea. When it approached the transparent cornea, the pains became more severe. In order to remove it, I opened the conjunctiva and extracted the worm through that incision.

It was one and a half inches long, the width of a violin string, and dark-colored. One end was bigger than the other, although both ends were very pointed. Nothing else was remarkable.

I believed it to be a worm from the blood; it did not seem possible to me that it could have grown in this area without causing pain and inflammation. But how could it have penetrated the body without causing the same disorders?

CASE OF *FILARIA LOA* IN WHICH THE PARASITE WAS REMOVED FROM UNDER THE CONJUNCTIVA

Transactions of the Ophthalmological Society of the United Kingdom, 15: 137–167, 1895. Selections from pp. 137–141, 162–167.

Douglas Moray Cooper Lamb Argyll-Robertson (1837–1909)

After preliminary medical training at the University of Edinburgh, Argyll-Robertson received his M.D. from St. Andrew's in 1857 and immediately thereafter was appointed to the Royal Infirmary. He went to Berlin to study under von Graefe, and upon his return developed a distinguished practice in ophthalmology. Despite the demands of this busy practice, he taught the first laboratory course in physiology ever offered by the University of Edinburgh.

*Although Argyll-Robertson is best known for the pupillary sign indicative of syphilis of the central nervous system that bears his name, he made many other important contributions to medicine. For example, his early studies on the Calabar bean (*Physostigma venenosum*) began a significant chain of chemical discoveries of great importance in neurology. Interestingly, and appropriately for a graduate of St. Andrew's, he was an avid and expert golfer and attributed his good health to this sport.*

This is the first detailed description of Loa loa.

On the 29th of June last I was consulted by Miss J. H— on account of what she termed the presence of a worm in her eye.

She is a slightly anaemic, prematurely grey-haired, but otherwise healthy-looking lady, 32 years of age. She has resided at Old Calabar on the West Coast of Africa at intervals, for nearly eight years altogether. She twice had to return home on account of debility following severe intermittent fever. During her last visit to Old Calabar, which extended to about 18 months, she suffered almost the whole time from chronic dysentery followed by severe remittent fever, which necessitated her return to this country last January in a very weak state of health.

She stated that the worm was first observed by her in February of this year, immediately after her return home. It frequented both eyes, but showed a preference for the left one, sometimes coursing over the surface of the eye under the conjunctiva, sometimes wriggling under the skin of the eyelids—causing a tickling, irritating sensation, but not real pain. It had latterly restricted its visits entirely to the left eye. On account of the remittent fever from which she was still suffering, her bedroom, when she first came home, was kept well heated, and until she recovered from the fever she noticed that the worm was particularly lively, occasionally causing the eye to become bloodshot, and the eyelids to swell and blacken slightly. As long as she was confined to warm rooms the worm was almost constantly moving about in the neighbourhood of the eye, causing such irritation as to prevent reading or work of any kind. This irritation with accompanying injection always passed off in the course of the day, and never resulted in severe inflammation.

She thus found that the worm was sensitive to cold, coming to the surface when the temperature was high, and disappearing to deeper parts when she was exposed to cold. As soon as she had recovered strength so far as to be able to go out of doors and visits of the worm to the eye became fewer, perhaps a week or longer occurring between them. It usually put in an appearance when she was near a cosy fire or in bed. Its last disappearance was for two months, during July and August, and as she at that time passed a worm *per rectum* she thought she had thus got rid of it. During these two months she was mostly in the open air, but as soon as, in September, the rooms began to be heated, it again came to the surface.

When I first saw Miss H—, in June, I very thoroughly examined the eye, but failed to observe any trace of the parasite, unless perhaps the appearance of a minute bluish vesicle at the extreme outer angle of the conjunctival cul-de-sac corresponded to one of the extremities of the worm, but the vesicle, though watched for a time, did not alter in position or appearance. I gave her strict injunctions to return at any time whenever she felt the worm on the move.

I saw her twice at the eye wards of the Royal Infirmary about the beginning of July, but on these occasions careful inspection was again negative in its results.

On the 12th of September, however, she again came to the Infirmary, stating that she had felt the worm moving about in the left eye that forenoon, and to prevent it leaving the surface she had kept the eye well covered with a warm cloth till she made her way to the Infirmary. On this occasion, after examining the eye for a minute or two, I observed the worm moving in a tortuous, wriggling manner under the conjunctiva, the surface of which became slightly elevated as it moved along.

It passed with a pretty quick movement over the surface of the sclerotic at the distance of about 5 mm from the outer margin of the cornea. It glided from the upper outer towards the lower outer part of the globe. There was increased lachrymation and slightly increased injection of the conjunctiva,—just such an appearance as would result from a particle of dust in the eye.

I at once placed my finger on the surface of the globe in such a manner as to prevent the parasite passing backwards until the conjunctiva was pretty well anaesthetised by the application of cocaine. I then got my friend Dr. Maddox, who was present, to apply his finger while the necessary preparations were hastily made for an operation.

She was placed on a couch and the speculum applied, when the pressure of the finger having been removed the wriggling movements of the worm were resumed, as briskly as before the application of the cocaine. I now grasped with a pair of toothed fixing forceps a good fold of conjunctiva over the centre of the wriggling worm, taking care to include in the fold all structures superficial to the sclerotic. I next made with a pair of scissors an incision through the conjunctiva a little nearer the cornea, in such a manner as to lift up a small flap of conjunctiva, and after a little careful separation of the tissues found one extremity of the worm, which I seized with a pair

of iris forceps. On now relaxing the fixing forceps the parasite came away readily. No irritation
or inflammation followed the operation.

The worm presented the appearance of a piece
of fishing-gut, being round, firm, transparent,
and colourless. It wriggled slightly for a few
minutes after removal while held in the forceps,
but on being placed in a solution of boracic acid,
so as to prevent it becoming dry, it seemed completely to lose its vitality. It measured 25 mm in
length and barely half a millimetre in breadth. It
terminated rather abruptly at one extremity,
scarcely tapering at all, but at the other it gradually tapered to a pretty sharply curved fine point.
Twisted round the worm, and apparently attached
to it near its centre was a much finer, less firm,
transparent filamentous body, which I at first
thought might possibly prove to be a second
young filaria, or even the male filaria, but which
on further careful microscopical examination appears to be the alimentary canal of the worm protruded through an opening in its musculo-
cutaneous wall, caused by the forcible grasping
of the parasite with the forceps.

The worm after removal was, on the suggestion of Dr. Muir, Pathologist to the Infirmary,
placed in a mixture of equal parts of glycerine
and methylated spirits, but the cork of the bottle
in which the mixture was put had retained some
of the blue colouring matter (methyl violet) of a
solution previously in the bottle, and thus the
preservative mixture became faintly blue-tinted.
The parasite absorbed the colouring matter
slightly, but the filamentous body projecting
from it absorbed it more freely, becoming markedly blue-tinted. After remaining in the solution
between three and four weeks the parasite was
carefully mounted as a microscopic preparation
in glycerine jelly by Mr. Simpson, assistant
keeper of the University Anatomical Museum.

It is not my intention to attempt an account of
the natural history of the parasite, as I propose to
submit the specimen to some special authority in
that department.

I have had some sketches of it made by a com-
petent artist, and these, as well as the preparation
itself under the microscope, I have pleasure in
exhibiting to you (Plate 61).

It appears to me not improbable that this
specimen may be found to supply what has
hitherto been a missing link, namely, the male
animal.

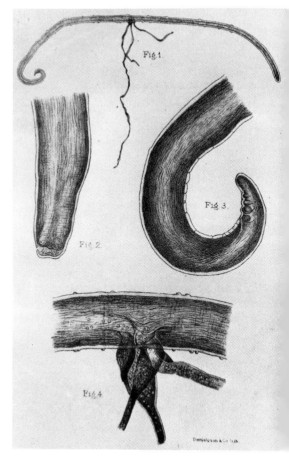

Plate 61. Male Filaria Loa. *Fig. 1*. The whole worm. Portions
the testicles and alimentary canal protruding through a rupture
the wall of the parasite. *Fig. 2*. The head of the worm. *Fig. 3*. T
curved tail of the worm with its papillae. *Fig. 4*. The ruptured p
of the worm with protruding alimentary canal and testes.

Since writing this I have had the opportunity of
submitting the specimen to Dr. Manson, who at
once recognised it as the male worm, and has
undertaken to make a careful microscopical
examination and description of it. . . .

Further Note of Case of *Filaria loa*

At a meeting of this Society on the 18th of
October last I narrated the case of a patient, Miss
H—, affected with *Filaria loa,* and I exhibited a
male worm which I had removed from under the
conjunctiva of her left eye. I purpose now to give
a short account of the further history of that pa-

tient, and a description of a female *Filaria loa* which I succeeded in removing from her right upper eyelid (Plate 62).

After the removal of the filaria from under the conjunctiva, Miss H— was not troubled with the sensations she associates with the presence of a worm for a period of about six weeks, when again she experienced a burrowing sensation at the back of her left eye. It affected her at intervals, and especially when she was occupying a hot room.

On the 3rd of February she distinctly felt a worm moving about in her left upper eyelid, and came at once to me, but before she arrived this feeling had gone, and I failed to discover any signs of the parasite. She returned on the 6th of February with the statement that not only had she felt the worm moving about in the left lower lid, but that it had also been distinctly seen wriggling under the skin. I saw her three different times that day, but failed to observe anything that might indicate with certainty the presence of a parasite, although she sat in front of a hot fire and had a succession of hot poultices applied, so as to tempt the worm to the surface. On the third visit, as she felt the wriggling of the worm, and as there seemed to be a little fulness at one point in the left lower lid, I decided to cut down at that point and search for the parasite. This I did with Dr. Mackay's assistance, having first of all applied clamp-forceps so as to prevent the worm escaping if it were there. I failed to find any parasite, although I made a careful search, and the patient showed great nerve and steadiness under operation, but I noticed a distinct narrow channel or burrow parallel to the edge of the lid, and crossing about the middle of it, which gave me the impression of being a burrow by which the worm had moved across the lid.

Two days later Miss H— came complaining of a swelling in the right temporal region. This swelling seemed pretty deeply situated, and firm palpation failed to reveal any corded feeling such as might indicate the presence of a worm.

On the 13th of February she felt the worm wriggling across the right upper eyelid, and then it appeared to her to remain coiled up under the skin. She bound the eye carefully up and came at once to the infirmary. I examined the lid and noticed a fulness at the upper inner part, which might be a coiled-up worm. By pressure of the fingers I attempted to force the swelling towards the edge of the lid, but I could neither see nor feel any movement such as might be expected from the presence of a worm. As, however, the patient's sensations were very distinct, I determined to make an exploratory incision. I applied the clamp-forceps and made a free incision over the region of the swelling, but found the chief cause of the fullness to be a small deposit of fat, which I cut away, and then proceeded to explore the neighbourhood carefully. After some dissection I found a very fine transparent filamentous body. On drawing upon it with forceps it came away with a snap. It was much smaller in calibre and shorter than the usual *Filaria loa,* and I concluded that it was only a portion of a filaria—the main part being caught between the blades of the clamp-forceps. The forceps being removed, further exploration was made, in which I was assisted by Dr. Mackay, and after some dissection a well-marked *Filaria loa* was discovered deeply embedded in the muscular tissue and removed with forceps. The edges of the incision were brought together by a couple of fine sutures, and healing occurred by first intention.

The worm thus removed measured about 30 mm in length and nearly 1 mm in thickness. It was firm and transparent like a small piece of fishing-gut. It tapered at either extremity to a blunt point, the tail being rather sharper-pointed than the head. At the distance of about 9 mm from the caudal end an opening existed in the wall of the parasite, through which protruded a filamentous coil, which subsequent microscopic examination revealed to be the uterine tubes filled with ova in all stages of development up to embryo filariae. Notwithstanding the amount protruded, the interior of the parasite was yet to a great extent occupied by oviduct, the alimentary canal being apparently comparatively small in size. The wall seemed to be chiefly composed of muscular fibre, the transverse striae of which were readily visible at all parts. The semicircular projecting tubercules, which Dr. Manson is inclined to view as serving to facilitate the gliding movements of the parasite by enabling it to get a purchase on surrounding parts, were very numerous towards the caudal end, fewer in number at the centre, and very sparsely distributed at the head extremity. Near the oral end of the worm a small general projection of the wall existed on one side, probably due to a partial rupture produced by injury.

The small piece of the worm I first removed in the course of the operation proved on microscopic examination to be part of the oviduct containing embryo filariae.

I will submit my specimen for more careful and thorough examination and report to Dr. Manson, who is entitled to speak with such authority on this subject.

During the last six months I have at intervals examined blood drawn from Miss H— at various periods of day and night, but have never been able to discover the presence of any filariae.

My patient has several times directed my attention to ill-defined swellings under the skin of the forearms a little above the wrists, over the dorsal surface of the radius, more marked generally in the right arm. The surface of the swellings was not quite uniform, but did not give one the idea of being produced by a coiled-up worm. The swellings measured about half an inch in diameter. They were not painful, but occasioned a feeling of stiffness when the arms were used. The swellings occurred at irregular intervals, and were generally most marked in the mornings. Cold had no influence in dispelling them; on the contrary, the application of cold water on one or two occasions seemed to bring the swellings forward.

My patient informs me that natives of Calabar, and others resident for a time there, are subject to such swellings in the forearms and wrists, to which the natives apply the term ''Ndi töt,'' or swelling. These swellings she has only suffered from since her return home.

I have further a correction to make in the history of my patient I previously submitted. It would appear that while she was most careful with regard to the purification of her drinking-water by boiling and filtering, she was for ten days prior to leaving Old Calabar so completely prostrated as to be unable to attend to any household matters, and the person who undertook her duties was unacquainted with the procedure employed for purifying the water. It might thus readily happen that she at that time partook of impure water containing embryo filariae. As she had no symptoms of filaria till after her return home, this *might* explain their entrance into her system.

It is easy to understand how the embryo filariae may enter the system, although their presence in impure water has not yet been demonstrated. And it is easy to conceive that, having entered the system from the alimentary canal, they may breed and bring forth a large crop of embryo parasites. But the chief difficulty consists in determining how these embryo filariae escape from the bodies of those affected with the disease, and get deposited in the impure water and thus propagate the disease.

In the case of the *Filaria sanguinis* this is accomplished by the mosquito which constitutes the

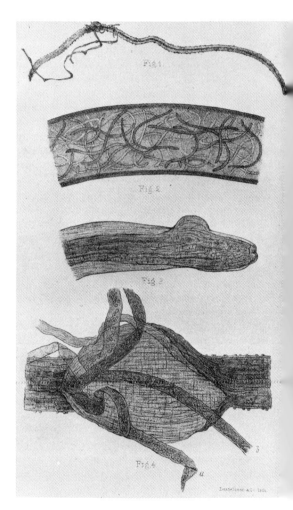

Plate 62. Female Filaria Loa. *Fig. 1*. The whole worm. Port of alimentary canal and uterine tube protruding through an oper in the wall of the parasite. *Fig. 2*. A portion of uterine tube, hig magnified, showing embryo filariae in interior. *Fig. 3*. Hea worm, with rounded projection of wall of worm at one point, du injury. *Fig. 4*. Part of worm where rupture of wall occurred. alimentary canal; (b) uterine tube with embryo filariae.

intermediate host; but as in the case of my patient, as well as in the case reported by Dr. Logan of Liverpool, careful examination of the blood failed to reveal the presence of embryo filariae, some other system of propagation than that by blood-sucking insects must be looked for. Possibly the embryo parasites may be discharged along with some of the excreta from the body, and from faulty sanitary arrangements find their way into drinking-water. Whether this be so or not, future investigation will probably show.

Report on the structure of the female parasite (by Dr. Manson)—Female *Filaria loa*: length, 3.25 cm; breadth, 0.5 mm; ova at morula stage, 0.03 by 0.02 mm; length of outstretched embryos in uterus, 0.25 mm.

As regards her general appearance, the female *Filaria loa* resembles the male parasite, only she is considerably larger and her tail is straight, tapers to a diameter of about 0.1 mm, and is then abruptly truncated. The mouth, the head, the stout muscular ring posterior to the mouth, the stout longitudinal muscular bands, and the bosses on the integument resemble exactly those of the male worm. In consequence of the mutilation of the specimen it is impossible to say where the vagina opens, or where the anus is placed. The uterine tubes are stuffed with embryos at all stages of development. The more mature embryos resemble in size and shape those of *F. nocturna* and *F. diurna,* but in consequence of the method of mounting it is impossible to say if they are possessed of a sheath or not. If they are possessed of a sheath, I should say that they are practically indistinguishable from the parasites mentioned.

(March 14th, 1895.)

NOTE ON THE FURTHER HISTORY OF THE CASE OF *FILARIA LOA* PREVIOUSLY REPORTED TO THE SOCIETY

Transactions of the Ophthalmological Society of the United Kingdom, 17: 227–232, 1897. Selections from pp. 227–228.

Douglas Moray Cooper Lamb Argyll-Robertson
(1837–1909)

My patient, Miss H—, affected with filaria loa, whose case was brought under the notice of this Society at the meetings in October, 1894, and March, 1895, having improved greatly in general health, returned to Old Calabar about a month after my last report.

Before leaving this country she had remained free from the sensations due to movements of the parasite, but scarcely had she returned to the tropics when her symptoms recurred. In a letter written in January, 1896, she mentions that she had frequently experienced itching behind her eyes, but that no worm had made its appearance in front. The swellings in the arms had recurred at intervals, and a medical man in attendance thought that they indicated beri-beri. She further stated that she had had a conversation with Miss Kingsley, the lady explorer, who informed her that nearly every one on the Ogowe River near Gaboon suffered from these worms. My patient also, as requested, sent specimens of mosquitoes and sand-flies, which were subjected to microscopic examination by Dr. Manson and myself. We failed to detect in their interior anything that could be viewed as embryo filariae.

I did not hear again from her till July last year, when she wrote informing me that one night on going to bed she felt a little nip in the side like a mosquito bite, but upon looking found a worm wriggling about under the skin. Fortunately one of the missionaries, who had received a little medical training, was at hand, and managed with knife and forceps to extract it. She put the worm into preservative solution in a bottle, and sent it to me for examination. She also mentioned that she had for some weeks previously been troubled with a worm occasionally appearing under the conjunctiva. Since then she had on two occasions had incisions made on the knuckles for a worm that seemed to wander down her arm and suddenly appear at the wrist or back of the hand. She stated that insects do not bite her often, that mosquitoes are few where she was staying, and that she did not think she had suffered from a sand-fly bite since she came out.

Miss H— did not stand the climate of Calabar well, and became again affected with severe colitis and dysentery, so that she had to be sent home about the middle of January, arriving in this country in the beginning of March in a very feeble, exsanguine state. She is residing in the neighbourhood of Edinburgh, and I have seen her twice since her return, the last time being on the 3rd of June, when I found her much improved in her general health, the dysentery having almost entirely ceased. She explained to me that the worm removed from her at Calabar had been extracted from the abdominal wall in the left lumbar region. She also stated that she always has nausea and headache at the times the worms are troubling her, and that occasional swellings in the arms such as she has are not uncommon among natives of or residents in Old Calabar, and that all of those thus affected whom she questioned were troubled with worms.

She has recently had visits of the worm to the lids of both eyes, to the side of the nose, the crown of the head, the left shoulder, and under the skin of both hands, especially over the knuckle of the middle finger of the left hand, but the worm's visits were of very short duration.

On the 15th of last month the parasite reappeared in the abdominal wall, on this occasion close to the umbilicus. Attempts were made by the doctor in her immediate neighbourhood to secure the worm, but they failed, the parasite disappearing before suitable forceps could be got to seize it.

REPORT OF THE HELMINTHOLOGIST FOR THE HALF YEAR ENDING 30 APRIL 1913

Tropical Diseases Research Fund: Report of the Advisory Committee for the Tropical Diseases Research Fund for the Year 1913, p. 86, 1914.

Robert Thomson Leiper
(1881–1969)

Leiper's biographical sketch appears in the chapter on Schistosomiasis where his work is more extensively reported.

Chrysops had been implicated in the transmission of Dracunculus *by Fedchenko in 1870. This is the first report of the transmission of* Loa loa. *Many aspects remain unsolved today.*

The whole of my time for the past six months has been occupied by a visit to West Africa for the purpose of ascertaining the carrier of *Filaria loa*: the causal agent of Calabar Swelling. The results of the investigation are as follows:

No evidence of infection was obtained from series of mosquitoes of various species fed upon a patient in whose blood very many filaria embryos were present. With the same patient *Stomoxys calcitrans, Stomoxys nigra, Glossina palpalis, Cimex rotundatus, Pulex irritans, Tabanus par, T. socialis, T. fasciatus, T. secedens,* also gave negative results. In *Haematopota cordigera* and *Hippocentrum trimaculatum* I obtained a slight degree of infection but development was unequal and slow.

In *Chrysops dimidiata* and *Chrysops silacea* I obtained a rapid and uniform development of filaria diurna embryos taken up from a patient upon whom the flies had been induced to feed. No experiments were made with *Chrysops longicornis*. This species was only obtained once at Forcados, and none of the four flies which were captured could be induced to bite.

Chrysops appears to have a marked seasonal incidence and the experiments were brought to an abrupt close early in January owing to the lack of material.

Being advised that these flies would not become common again in Calabar until June, I proceeded to Lagos to investigate meanwhile the nature of the organisms reported as ancylostome embryoes which had been found in the wells of Lagos and Ebute Metta. These proved to be harmless free living nematodes, sexually mature, and showing but slight resemblance to the young of parasitic worms. . . .

CHAPTER 22

Dracunculiasis

EXTRACTION OF GUINEA WORMS [Plates only]

Exercitatio de Vena Medinensi, ad Mentem Ebnsinae sive de Dracunculis Veterum. Specimen Exhibens Novae Versionis ex Arabico, cum Commentario Uberiori, cui Accedit Altera de Vermiculus Capillaribus Infantium. Augusta Vindelicorum. Imprensis Theophili Goebelli, 1674. 456 pp. (Plates only.) Legends for Plates 63–66 translated from the Latin.

Georg Hieronymus Welsch
(1624–1677)

A native of Augsburg, Welsch trained in medicine in Tübingen, Strassburg, and Padua. Though he practiced as an internist in Augsburg, he was a sickly, melancholic person and devoted most of his time to writing.

In 1674 he published a 456-page monograph in Latin. It is considered to be the first lengthy discussion on a single helminth. His understanding of the parasite and his confusion reflected the knowledge of the times. Cobbold wrote, "We are amused, if not edified, by the numerous plates representing the old Persian surgeons extracting Dracunculus.*"*

ON THE STRUCTURE AND NATURE OF THE *DRACUNCULUS* OR GUINEA WORM

Transactions of the Linnean Society, 24: 101–134, 1863. Selections from pp. 101–102, 106–117, 119, 129–130.

Henry Charlton Bastian
(1837–1915)

Although Bastian devoted most of his professional life to neurology and achieved his greatest fame in that field, his unusually early election to the Royal Society when he was only 31 years old came in recognition of his work in the field of parasitology. Educated at Falmouth and the University of London, he received his first appointment after taking the degree of medicine at St. Mary's Hospital. Soon, however, he resigned to become professor of pathology and assistant physician at University College Hospital, and ultimately he succeeded to the chair of medicine at that institution. Strangely for a man of his training and era, he persisted in believing in the theory of spontaneous generation of life (he claimed to have produced microorganisms from liquid in 1872), contending that his contemporaries had not given sufficient consideration to the possibilities of error in the experimentation that supported the opposing and almost universally accepted view. He published two volumes entitled The Beginning of Life; Being Some Account of the Nature, Modes of Origin, and Formations of Lower Organisms.

Bastian gives us the first detailed description of the anatomy of Dracunculus.

Among the numerous parasites which infest the human frame, the Guineaworm (*Filaria medinensis*) is one of those which have been known from the most ancient times, the first undoubted reference to it being made by Agatharchidas, the philosopher and historian of Cnidus, who lived about 140 B.C., in the time of Ptolemy Alexander. Küchenmeister, however, discusses the question whether Moses was not the first writer who mentioned the worm, and whether the "fiery serpents" referred to in the Book of Numbers were not in reality *Dracunculi*.

Owing to the tedious and very painful nature of the consequences entailed by the presence of this worm in the human body, more perhaps has been written concerning this parasite than upon any other single Entozoon. The statements regarding its nature have, however, been most conflicting, as may be seen by reference to the works of Küchenmeister, Bremser, and Moquin-Tandon. Up to within comparatively recent times its very animality has been denied, and that too by the distinguished French surgeon Larrey, who might

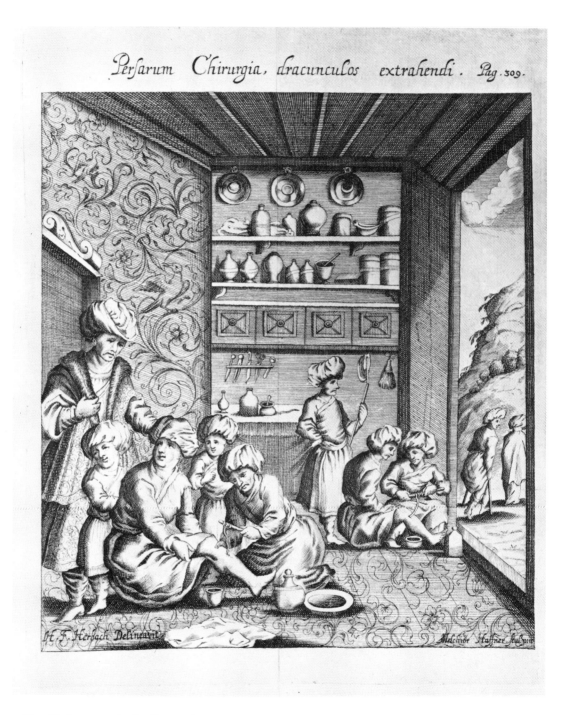

Plate 63. Surgeons extracting *Dracunculus*.

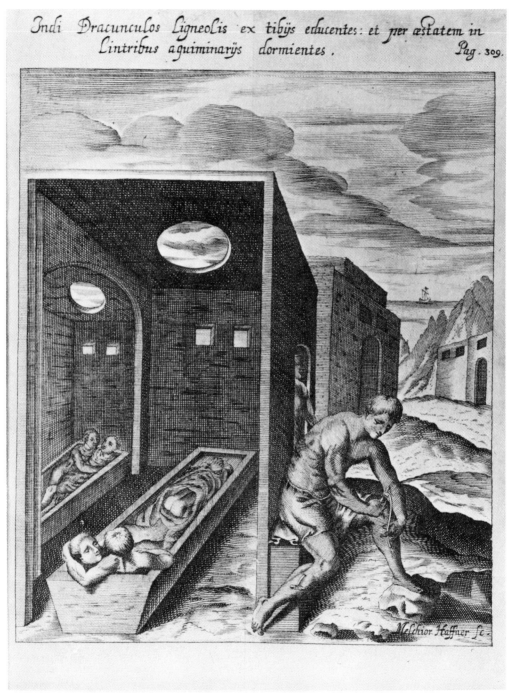

Indi Dracunculos Ligneolis ex tibijs educentes: et per æstatem in Lintribus aquiminarijs dormientes. Pag. 309.

Melchior Haffner fc.

Plate 64. The illustration shows a Hindu drawing out "little snakes" (dracunculos—meaning the Guinea worms) by means of a stick while others sleep through the summer in troughs.

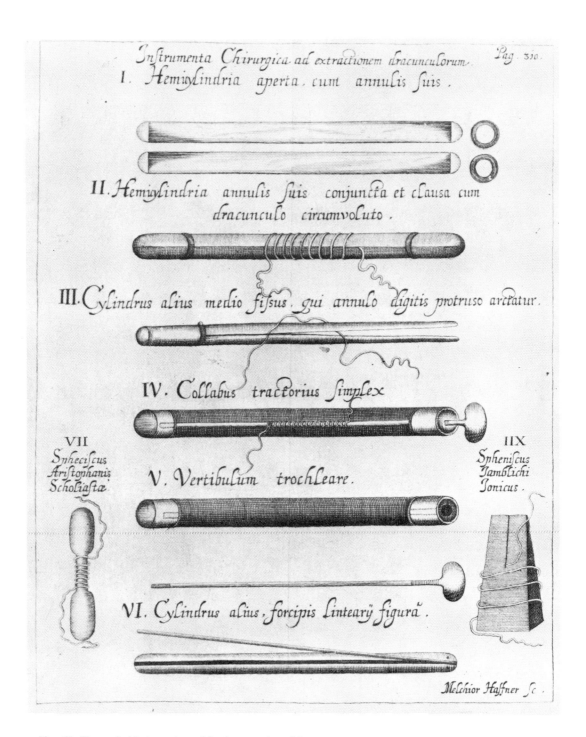

Plate 65. The surgical instruments used for the extraction of the worms.

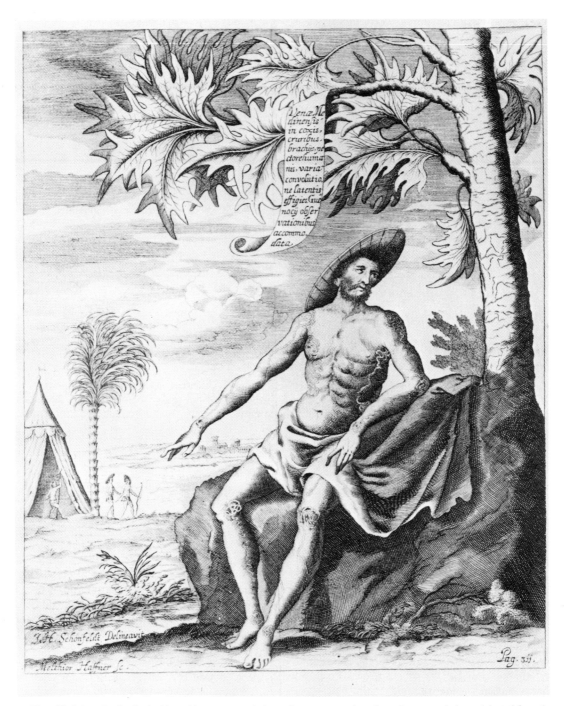

Plate 66. Infected veins in the hips, shins, arms, and chest of a man, spread out in various convolutions. Adapted from the observations of Guenocius.

well have acquired a more exact knowledge of its real nature during his residence in Egypt. He held that it was nothing more than a portion of "dead cellular tissue;" Richerand, that it was a "fibrinous concretion;" whilst Ambroise Paré declares that the effects produced by the presence of the worm are due only to a kind of tumour or abscess proceeding from "acidity of the blood." For other views equally novel, as well as for a history of the effects produced by the worm whilst lodged in the subcutaneous tissue of the body, and the medical treatment of the disease, also called *Dracunculus*, I would refer especially to the works before mentioned, as well as to other papers, to which reference will be made, in the Indian journals, as in the present communication I shall confine myself to the natural-history aspects of the question.

Gmelin was the first to assign the Guineaworm its place amongst the true Helminthes, in the order Nematoidea; but a more thorough investigation of its anatomy will, I think, lead us to doubt the propriety of considering it a species of the genus *Filaria*.

It is endemic in the tropical parts of Asia and Africa, in the island of Grenada, with the small neighbouring Grenadine group, and doubtfully so in the island of Curaçao; but it has not been met with anywhere in the tropical regions of the continent of America. It is not, however, universally distributed over the countries in which it is endemic, but is confined to certain limited areas, and is much more abundant at some times than at others—both which facts will be seen further on to have their special significance.

In the regions where it is prevalent, this parasite is met with principally in the subcutaneous tissue of persons who have exposed themselves to certain conditions known to be favourable to the production of the disease. In about four-fifths or more of the whole number of recorded cases, these worms have been situated in the lower extremities, below the knees; and taking into consideration the fact that the people so affected mostly go about with bare legs and feet, and other evidence of a similar nature which will subsequently be alluded to, it is generally admitted at the present day that the worms are contained in some imperfectly known condition in the waters and damp places of these regions, and that they also in some unascertained manner make their

way through the integuments of the body, and then acquire extraordinary dimensions in the subcutaneous or intermuscular cellular tissue.

Having once located itself within the body, the worm grows rapidly, without producing any signs of irritation, or attracting much notice, for a period varying from eight to 12 or 14 months. This has been aptly termed by Mr. Busk the "latent period" of its existence. After a time, however, the head begins to make its way to the surface, and then commences the long category of troubles peculiar to the disease, till the parasite has been completely extracted.

The worms are usually stated to vary in length from six inches to ten or 12 feet, and to be about two-thirds of a line in thickness. When fresh, they are of a milk-white colour, and nearly cylindrical. All that have hitherto been examined have been found to be undoubtedly female and viviparous, with the exception of three specimens, to which allusion will again be made further on. . . .

I have examined six specimens of *Filaria medinensis,* all of which were taken from the lower extremities of a well-known surgeon of Bombay, by whom they were given to Dr. Harley. The specimens were all of the same age, though of different sizes—four being about 30 inches long, one only 18 inches, and the other three feet long. All were female and viviparous, and perfect specimens, with the exception of one, in which the head was wanting; and their good preservation was probably owing to the method of their extraction by a native of Bombay, who, after making a minute aperture in the integuments, as nearly as possible opposite the middle of the worm, passed under its exposed body a small hook, and then by gentle traction, at the same time that the skin around was kneaded, each worm was extracted at a single sitting of perhaps an hour or less, instead of by the tedious process of rolling it daily round a small piece of wood.

As the manner in which this gentleman became affected with these parasites is pretty definite, both as to their mode of entrance and their age, I shall quote his account from a Report read to the Pathological Society of London by Dr. Harley.

After stating that he had been many years in Bombay, and never affected with Guineaworm, though accustomed often to be out shooting and drink freely of the water of wells, without being very particular as to quality, he says:—"At last, however, I one day discovered that I had what at first appeared to me to be varicose veins, but which in a day or two I found to be Guineaworms in my legs. At first I was at a loss to account for the presence of a Guineaworm in my body, till I remembered that one day, whilst out shooting, one of my boots burst, and being too impatient to wait till another pair was brought, I took off both boots and stockings and went on shooting barefooted over a piece of swampy stubble; and I believe that the worms entered my feet on this occasion; for after an interval of six or eight months the first worm appeared, and that is about the time generally allowed for the worms to come to maturity in the human body."

I will now proceed to give the results of my own observations.

External Characters: Worms varying in length (Plate 67, Fig. 1) from 18 inches to three feet, and from 1/10th to 1/15th of an inch in diameter, of a milk-white colour (or light straw when kept in spirits), mostly quite smooth, but sometimes slightly annulated by rugose contractions; cylindrical, or more or less flattened laterally, and tapering gradually towards both extremities. About 1/20th of an inch from the posterior extremity the body becomes more abruptly narrowed, and terminates usually in a sharply curved tail or point. In some cases, however, the tail is straight, and in others, as pointed out by Carter, it is more acutely bent upon itself, and seems connected to the adjacent portion of the body by a delicate membrane (Plate 67, Figs. 4–7). On opposite sides of the body are seen, extending along its whole length, two opaque bands, corresponding with the dorsal and ventral muscles, and two more translucent intermuscular spaces. For a short distance from the anterior extremity, two narrow, white lines may also be seen running along the body, each being midway between the lateral spaces. No vulva discoverable; anal aperture doubtful—if present, situated in the concavity of the tail.

The integuments are so elastic, that the worm may be stretched to nearly twice its natural length.

Examined with a low power of the microscope, the head presents the following characters:— Mouth punctiform, about 1/2000th of an inch in diameter, situated in the centre of a somewhat flattened terminal disk, and surrounded by a circular eminence or lip (Plate 67, Fig. 2) 1/270th of an inch in diameter. Around the mouth are four papillae, two of which (much larger than the others, and also nearer the oral aperture) are continuous with the narrow white lines before mentioned, and are therefore situated vertically; whilst the two lateral, more remote from the mouth, not prominent, and scarcely more than opaque spots are situated at the commencement of the gradually widening, lateral, intermuscular spaces. The upper and lower papillae are prominent, and well seen in outline (Plate 67, Fig. 3), being about 1/1000th of an inch in height, 1/500th of an inch in breadth at the base, and 1/200th of an inch apart, whilst the small lateral papillae are 1/125th of an inch apart. The mouth and papillae are situated in the midst of an opaque, whitish, quadrangular space, about 1/100th of an inch from side to side, the papillae being situated towards the angles, from which also proceed the two opaque-white, gradually widening, lateral spaces and two narrow dorsal and ventral lines, which are only about 1/2000th of an inch wide. Between the white lines surrounding the head may be seen longitudinal muscular fibres—the origins of the four longitudinal muscles.

Integuments.—The integuments of the worm are composed of a transparent, almost structureless, chitinous substance, arranged in a number of concentric lamellae, presenting peculiar linear markings. Altogether it forms a very tough and highly elastic cylindrical investment.

Analogy would point also to a deep cellular layer of integument; and though I have not been able to discover any trace of it, this may be due to the fact that the worms examined were not recent specimens, but had been preserved in spirits of wine.

The integuments of the Nematoid worms have been described by Von Siebold, Dujardin, Owen, and other writers, as composed of a structureless epidermis, and a corium made up of layers of longitudinal and oblique decussating fibres; but, after a most careful examination, I have been unable to discover that any such distinction can be drawn between the different portions of the integument of the Guineaworm—the whole thickness being almost identical in structure, and apparently composed of successive excreted

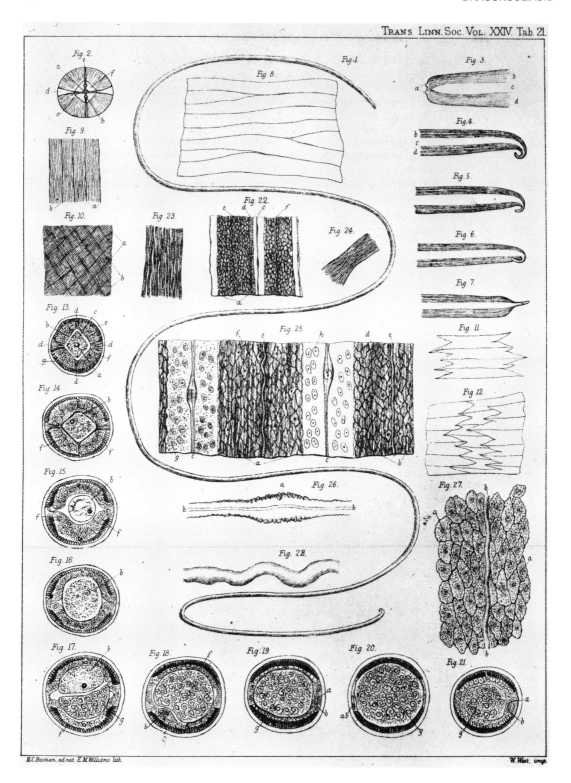

TRANS. LINN. SOC. VOL. XXIV. Tab. 21.

H.C.Bastian. ad nat. E.M.Williams lith.   W. West, imp.

epidermic layers. I think it will be possible to show also that what appear to be layers of decussating fibres, in the Guineaworm and some other Nematoids that I have examined, are not such in reality. A true corium or enderon, as before stated, I have failed to recognise.

The average thickness of the integuments is 1/400th of an inch, though it is considerably thinner towards either extremity of the body. It may be divided into two principal parts—an external portion with transverse markings, constituting about one-half of the whole thickness, not divisible into lamellae; and an internal portion, made up of about thirty very delicate lamellae, having longitudinal or oblique markings.

The *external* portion of the integument is composed of a thick, chitinous layer, tough, elastic, transparent, and perfectly structureless, save that it presents transverse markings at intervals. These lines (Plate 67, Fig. 8) have an average distance of 1/1400th of an inch from one another, though near either extremity of the worm they are as little as 1/6000 of an inch apart, the distance between the lines gradually diminishing up to this point. They are about 1/7000th of an inch in breadth, and easily recognisable when most of the lamellae covering them internally have been stripped off. They vary slightly in their distance from one another, are wavy, but do not preserve any parallelism between themselves; and moreover they frequently join one another or bifurcate, so that they by no means form perfect circles round the body.

The external surface of the integument seems perfectly smooth, there being no appreciable depressions corresponding to the annulose markings

Plate 67. Fig. 1. An average-sized Bombay Guinea worm measures 30 inches in length by 1/15 of an inch in breadth. *Fig. 2.* Head of Guinea worm, magnified: (a) orbicular mouth surrounded by a slight prominent lip; (b) one of large papillae; (c) one small lateral papilla; (d) lateral intermuscular space; (e) dorsal intermuscular space; (f) quadrangular or nearly circular opaque space corresponding to sheath of esophagus. *Fig. 3.* Anterior extremity seen in profile: (a) upper and lower papillae; (b) one of dorsal muscles; (c) lateral intermuscular space; (d) one of ventral muscles. *Figs. 4, 5, 6, 7.* Different forms of caudal extremity: letters as in Fig. 3. *Fig. 8.* Irregular transverse markings of the external portion of integument. *Fig. 9.* Set of superimposed lamellae with longitudinal markings: (a) the lines of superficial lamellae; (b) lines of lamellae, seen beneath. *Fig. 10.* Two sets of superimposed lamellae with lines in opposite directions: letters as before. *Fig. 11.* A portion of a single glass-like lamella, with its linear markings and jagged torn edges. *Fig. 12.* Three portions of lamella of unequal length, showing that the markings of the under layers correspond with some portion of the intervals between the lines of the layer above. *Fig. 13.* Transverse section of the worm just behind the head; (a) section of small thick-walled esophagus; (b) quadrangular esophageal sheath; (c) granular matter within sheath, with esophagus; (d, d, d, d) four strong mesenteric processes; (e) thin origin of one of the four longitudinal muscles; (f) one of the glandular processes; (g) integument.

Figs. 14, 15, 16, 17, 18. Transverse sections at gradually increasing distances from head up to 1½ inch, showing the speedy disappearance of mesenteric processes, the disposition of the four longitudinal muscles and their fasciculi, the varying dimensions of the peritoneal sheath of the esophagus, the diminution in thickness of the glandular layer, and, in Figs. 17 and 18, the sudden encroachment of the blunt end of the dilated oviduct or uterus distended with young upon the peritoneal cavity. *Fig. 19.* Section about two inches from the head, showing the great thickness of the longitudinal muscles, of which the two dorsal and two ventral have come so closely in contact as apparently to form a single muscle only in each situation; (g) dilated uterus, occupying nearly the whole of the cavity of the body, and compressing the intestine (a) enclosed in its sheath (b). *Fig. 20.* Appearance of transverse sections through nearly the whole extent of the body of a mature worm, showing great distention of the uterus, whose walls have become adherent to the parietes of the body; the glandular layer lining the body has been obliterated and absorbed by the pressure, and the muscles diminished in thickness: (a, b) intestine enclosed within its sheath, compressed into a flat band along the thin edge of one of the longitudinal muscles.

Fig. 21. Transverse section through the worm, about one inch from the tail; showing the uterus, near its termination, not so much distended, and the reappearance of the glandular layer lining the peritoneal cavity. *Fig. 22.* Integument slit open through the right lateral intermuscular space, showing, (a) two ventral muscles; (c) ganglionated nervous cord in centre of lateral space; (d) intestinal canal lying parallel and in contact with the edge of one of the longitudinal muscles; (e) median ventral vessel; (f) median dorsal vessel. *Fig. 23.* Communications of the muscular fasciculi with one another. *Fig. 24.* Portion of one of the muscular fasciculi made up of exceedingly slender fibrillae.

Fig. 25. Portion of the parietes slit open through the left longitudinal dorsal muscle: (a) two ventral muscles; (b) two dorsal muscles; (c) ganglionated nervous cord; (e, e) median, dorsal, and ventral vessels; (f) tessellated arrangement of glands on surface of muscles, each including a nucleated gland-cell; (g) one of similar gland-cells situated in a pulpy stratum over lateral space; (h) appearance of gland-cells when much altered from some cause, as noticed in some specimens. *Fig. 26.* A nerve-ganglion and adjacent portion of nervous cord, highly magnified, with appearance of the lateral vessel as seen through it: (a) irregular crenated margin of the ganglion; (b) lateral vessel. *Fig. 27.* Mosaic-like collection of glands with longitudinal vessel, scraped from the surface of the two dorsal muscles: (a, a) included spherical, light, granular, nucleated gland-cells; (b) median vessel. *Fig. 28.* Portion of median dorsal vessel, showing its sinuous course and irregular calibre.

such as may be seen to a slight extent in *Ascaris lumbricoides* and *A. mystax*; but there is some considerable alteration in the refractive power of the membrane in these situations, as when seen a little beyond the proper focal distance these markings become most distinct, appearing as bright white lines.

The *internal* portion is composed of three different sets of very delicate lamellae, each being very transparent, glass-like, and structureless with the exception of certain faint rectilinear markings at regular intervals, which correspond in breadth to those between the transverse lines of the outer portion of the integument, viz. about 1/1400th of an inch. These lines also seem due to some variation in structure producing an alteration in the refractive power of the lamellae.

Each set appears to be composed of about ten superimposed lamellae, the markings of the external being longitudinal, whilst those of the inner two sets are oblique, in opposite directions. When seen superimposed, the markings of the middle set of lamellae are found to intersect those of the internal set at an angle of about 85°, or nearly at a right angle, leaving diamond-shaped spaces between the points of intersection, and constituting a system of spirals in opposite directions around the body of the worm (Plate 67, Fig. 10).

These linear markings preserve a nearly uniform distance from one another, and pursue a straight course, without dividing or communicating in any way, similar to those of the external portion. And there is this in common with the three sets, that the lines, whether longitudinal or oblique, of the several superimposed lamellae do not correspond in position; so that when those of the most superficial lamellae are in focus, there may be seen generally about nine fainter lines of deeper lamellae shining through, and closely filling, what would otherwise be each clear interlinear space (Plate 67, Fig 9).

This appearance is very deceptive, and gives *each set of lamellae* the aspect of a *single striated or fibrous membrane,* as I, for some time, believed them to be, until on examining one of these supposed membranes with a high power, I discovered that a portion of a very delicate lamella had been torn off from those subjacent, leaving a toothed edge. The linear markings of this superficial lamella could be traced distinctly

up to the torn edge; and in this situation also the lines of the uncovered portion of the subjacent layer were plainly visible, corresponding with a portion of the interval between the lines of the lamella above (Plate 67, Figs. 11, 12). This I have frequently seen since; and the observation evidently affords the key to the arrangement of these markings generally: and the fact is most important, as showing that this anomalous appearance of fibrous membranes in the integuments of these worms is a mere optical delusion, and that the membranes have no real existence, but that instead there exists a series of delicate and successively excreted chitinous lamellae, having linear markings in definite directions—an arrangement fully in harmony with what we know of other analogous structures.

The two internal sets of lamellae may be readily isolated by tearing a small piece of integument to pieces with needles; but the external set with the longitudinal markings is very difficult to separate from the outer portion of the integument, to which it is intimately adherent. These longitudinal lines are not so rectilinear as the oblique, and they are all rather difficult of detection, requiring a high power to distinguish those of the superficial lamellae plainly from those of the lamellae beneath. In this respect they are very different from the transverse markings of the outer half of the integument,—the greater distinctness of these being apparently due to the fact that the alteration in texture, on which the markings depend, extends through the whole thickness of this outer portion, whereas the lines which have a similar direction in each of the three sets of lamellae do not correspond in position, and, being produced by an alteration in the texture of one delicate lamella only, are necessarily very faint.

There seems to be some slight difference, too, between the texture of this thick outer portion and the internal lamellae, since its torn edge is generally even, whilst that of the lamellae is always sharply jagged and toothed. . . .

Muscular System: This is composed of four powerful longitudinal muscles firmly attached to the inner integumental layer, two of which occupy the dorsal and two the ventral region. They are made up of non-striated muscular tissue. As the longitudinal fibres run along the convexity and the concavity of the tail respectively, and the intestinal tube will afterwards be seen to terminate in the midst of the fibres occupying the concavity, as first pointed out by Mr. Carter, we must look upon these as ventral, and those along the convexity as dorsal, whilst the curve of the tail is thus ascertained to be in the median longitudinal vertical plane of the body, having a direction from above downwards.

Only two longitudinal muscles have been described by other observers; but I think a more careful examination, particularly of the anterior extremity of the worm, will show that there are in reality four of these muscles, as in many other of the Nematoidea, two being dorsal and two ventral. The origins of the four muscles completely surround the head with a thin layer of fibres, the boundaries of each being marked off by the four crucial lines (Plate 67, Fig. 13). The two dorsal, running close together for two or three inches, one on each side of the middle line, then become fused as it were into one great muscle—though a trace of the original division continues apparent throughout the whole length of the worm, and becomes again rather plainer towards the tail. The two ventral muscles are arranged in just the same manner; so that a broad, lateral, intermuscular interval is left on each side between the dorsal and ventral group, equal in breadth to one-sixth of the circumference of the body. The four muscles are all of nearly the same size, each being of just the same breadth as one of the lateral spaces (Plate 67, Fig. 19). Each is composed of fasciculi of very fine fibres, about 1/40000th of an inch in diameter, whilst the breadth of the fasciculi themselves is about 1/500th of an inch (Plate 67, Fig. 24). Frequent interchange of fibres takes place between contiguous fasciculi (Plate 67, Fig 23).

The arrangement of the muscles and their fasciculi may be well seen in the series of transverse sections shown in Plate 67, Figs. 13–21.

The four muscles, after leaving the head, soon acquire a perceptible thickness; and it may be seen that the adjacent borders of the two dorsal and two ventral muscles respectively are very thin, whilst each gradually increases in thickness towards its free border bounding the lateral spaces. The irregularity of the inner surface of the muscular bands, owing to the arrangement of the fibres into prominent fasciculi, is very evident for about the first two inches from the head. Further on the fasciculi are less prominent, and, the muscles acquiring a more uniform thickness, each pair becomes fused, apparently, into one great muscle, occupying the dorsal and ventral regions respectively. Where much compressed by the distended ovisac, the muscles seem to undergo partial absorption (Plate 67, Fig. 20).

Nervous System: The only traces of a nervous system I have been able to discover are two delicate ganglionated cords, extending the whole length of the worm, one occupying the centre of each lateral intermuscular space. They are situated, with a minute vessel to be afterwards described, in the midst of a pulpy substance, between the peritoneum and inner layer of integument, on which they lie. Some slight change, too, is produced in the texture of the integuments at this place, by which its refractive power is increased; for when quite bared on the inner side, and seen a little beyond the proper focal distance, a bright line is observed, of the same position and breadth as the nervous cord which had lain over it.

I have traced these cords close up to both extremities of the worm, but have not been able to discover any connecting central ganglion anteriorly, or distinct termination posteriorly. The two cords pursue a slightly wavy course, and seem to give off no branches in any part of their length. Each is about 1/1400th of an inch in diameter, and marked with distinct, elongated swellings, or ganglia, at intervals of about 1/13th of an inch (Plate 67, Figs. 22, 25, *c, c,* 26). The average breadth of the ganglia, at the widest part, is 1/400th of an inch, each having an irregularly crenated margin. The intervals between the swellings are not perfectly equal, neither do the ganglia on opposite sides of the body correspond in longitudinal position.

Much doubt and uncertainty prevails amongst anatomists concerning the nervous system of the Nematoid worms; so that little or nothing definite can be said with regard to its arrangement in the order generally. . . .

Organs of Circulation: The representatives of this system met with in the Guineaworm belong, doubtless, as in its allies the Taeniadae and the Trematoda, rather to the "water-vascular system" and the function of respiration than to the propulsion of true blood; yet still, in the present imperfect state of our knowledge, I have thought it better to describe them under the above head.

Four equidistant longitudinal vessels extend through the whole length of the body, situated, like the nervous cords, in the midst of a pulpy substance beneath the peritoneal membrane. The two which occupy the median line of the dorsal and ventral regions respectively are much larger than the two lateral vessels. All four extend from one extremity of the body to the other; but how they terminate in either direction I have been unable to determine, neither have I succeeded in finding any external aperture with which they communicate, such as is generally met with in connexion with the water-vascular system of the Annuloidea.

The dorsal and ventral vessels are in all respects similar, occupying the median intermuscular interval in each situation (Plate 67, Fig. 22, *e, f*). They have an opake-white colour when seen with a powerful lens; but when examined under the microscope by transmitted light, they are found to be very delicate thin-walled tubes (Plate 67, Fig. 28). They pursue a very undulating course and are by no means of one uniform calibre, being frequently bulged at intervals. Throughout the greater part of their extent they are about 1/666th of an inch in diameter, but anteriorly and posteriorly are reduced to 1/1000th of an inch.

The lateral vessels are very much smaller, being only about 1/6000th of an inch in diameter, and near the extremities of the body not more than 1/10000th of an inch. They are situated outside the nervous cords, and may be seen through their substance pursuing a gently undulating course and having a uniform double contour (Plate 67, Fig. 26). These vessels may sometimes be seen lying on the integuments after the nerve has been stripped off, and on one occasion I saw the broken extremity of a vessel distinctly projecting alone from the membrane on which it was lying. . . .

Filaria medinensis would seem to present us with a higher type of development, in which lacunar channels in the axis of peculiar "fat-canals" are replaced by distinct walled vessels.

Glandular System: Lining the whole interior of the body is a bed of pulpy granular matter, containing numerous interspersed gland-cells. This system is most highly developed dorsally and ventrally, especially in the anterior part of the body, where it is situated on the corresponding muscles, and forms distinct circumscribed projections; but in the lateral regions, where it lies on the inner layer of integument, no regular projections can be seen. In both situations its inner boundary, or investing membrane, seems formed by the peritoneum lining the general cavity of the body. . . .

Organs of Digestion: The alimentary canal consists of a very narrow oesophagus and a wider intestine presenting no distinct stomachal dilatation, and throughout its whole extent enclosed in a loose peritoneal sheath, on which distinctly flattened epithelial cells can be recognized. The oesophageal portion is also lined with a distinct layer of muscular tissue. In its course through the body the intestine is for the most part unattached to the parietes, and winds several times round the genital tube before terminating, about 1/60th of an inch from the posterior extremity, in the concavity of the tail. . . .

Organs of Generation: The genital apparatus consists of a large, highly organized sac or uterus, distended with young *Filariae* and a little fine granular matter. It occupied the whole of the peritoneal cavity in the specimens examined, except from one to two and a half inches from the anterior extremity and about a quarter of an inch or less from the tail. Both anteriorly and posteriorly, this sac terminates abruptly in a small tube twisted several times round the intestine, or forming a knotted glandular-looking mass. Each tube is about one inch in length, and the two are in every way alike. In common with other observers, I have been unable to discover any vulva or vagina; but the symmetrical formation of the two extremities of the genital tube leads me to believe that the genital aperture, if it does exist, must be situated a short distance behind the middle of the body—regarding the two terminal tubes as ovaries, and the large sac as a double oviduct or uterus, which by its enormous development appears to form one great tube, and which has obliterated the vagina. This point could only be satisfactorily cleared up by the examination of very young specimens, before the genital apparatus had assumed such an unusual development. . . .

Young Filariae: The whole uterus is distended with a dense mass of young of pretty nearly the same size, whilst intermingled with them in every part are crowds of germs, or "pseudova", and all intermediate grades between these and the most perfect form of the young worm met with within the body of the parent. Mixed up with these young, in the various stages of their development, are the remnants of the membranes which at first enveloped them, and some fine granular matter. . . .

General Observations on the Nature and History of the Guineaworm

As before stated, all the specimens of Guineaworm hitherto carefully examined have been found to be female and viviparous; and the only writers who mention male worms (so far as I have been able to discover) are Professor Owen, M. Leblond, and Dr. M'Clelland; but in each case the observations are, as will be seen, incomplete, and scarcely definite enough to turn the overwhelming balance of evidence on the other side. . . .

I think, then, we are fairly entitled to consider that no satisfactory evidence has yet been brought forward of the detection of a male parasitic Guineaworm; and such being the case, the reason why females only are met with is a very interesting question.

This may be explained, it appears to me, in one of two ways: either both male and female representatives of the species, of which the Guineaworm is an after-development, make their way through the integuments of persons exposing themselves to the conditions favourable for their penetration, but that the males in their new situation never attain any great size, and consequently, producing no inconvenience, do not attract attention, whilst the females, by the enormous development of their genital organs and contents, under the stimulus of high temperature and abundance of nutriment, soon attain such a size as to be palpable in superficial situations. It seems very probable that the male, if it penetrated, would never attain any considerable magnitude; and that it might remain in its new habitat without producing irritation is rendered very likely, seeing that during the whole period of the growth of the female, till the maturity of its young, it does not cause any inconvenience, and but rarely attracts attention; and this has in consequence been termed by Mr. Busk the "latent period" of its existence.

Or it may be that females only penetrate the integuments, impelled, as is frequently the case

with the females of other animals, by a sort of instinct to seek a new habitat for the production of their young. But if, as we have supposed, the young worms penetrate before the genital organs are completely formed, this latter explanation would be rather improbable, as the sexual instincts could not then be reasonably supposed to come into operation.

But however this may be, whether both males and females penetrate, or females only, I think there can be little doubt that this occurrence (at all events as far as warm-blooded animals are concerned) must be regarded as an exceptional rather than an invariable event in the history and development of these microscopic worms, when we consider the vast number in which these creatures, low in the scale of organization, are found in situations favourable to their existence. So that these worms may be considered to have an *ordinary* existence in the waters and damp places which they naturally frequent, having then their sexual organs fully developed and capable of producing true ova in the usual manner, as well as an exceptional or *extraordinary* existence as parasites of certain warm-blooded creatures, in which condition females only have been met with, that seem to have the outlets of their sexual organs undeveloped, and to contain young which have been formed from internal buds or pseudova by a process of zooid development.

Whether or not the young so produced are capable of existing externally, in their natural medium, there does not seem at present sufficient evidence to enable us to decide. But there are no real grounds for the belief, on the other hand, that the disease is contagious, as it has been sometimes stated to be. There is, indeed, no evidence to show that the young can or do continue their existence beneath the integuments, where they have been reared, although they are frequently liberated in this situation by the rupture of the parent worm. In these cases the young die and are discharged with the pus and other inflammatory products which are the invariable sequence of such an accident. . . .

CONCERNING THE STRUCTURE AND REPRODUCTION OF THE GUINEA WORM (*FILARIA MEDINENSIS* L.)

Izvestiia Imperatorskago Obshchestva Liubitelei Estestvoz-naniia Antropologii i Ethnografii—Moskva, 8: columns 71–81, 1870. Translated from the Russian.

Aleksej Pavlovich Fedchenko (1844–1873)

Fedchenko was born in Irkutz, near Lake Baikal, on 7 February 1844. After his father's death his mother sold the estate and moved to Moscow to continue her family's education. During his studies as a physics major at Moscow University he joined his brother, a professor in the Moscow Technical Institute, in studying the flora of the salt lakes of South Russia.

He taught at Moscow University after graduation and in 1866 became assistant dean of the student body. After his marriage to a student, O. A. Armfeld, he traveled to Finland and Stockholm, where he completed work on the anthropometry of Finnish skulls and added to his insect collections.

Accompanied by his wife, he spent the following three years (1868–1871) in the relatively unexplored areas of Turkestan, Samarkand, and Tashkent compiling an exhaustive study of this region. His original observations on Dracunculus medinensis *were made during this time.*

In the summer of 1873, Fedchenko visited T. S. Cobbold in London and reported his findings to him.

His fascination with the glaciers of Switzerland prompted a visit to compare them with those of Turkestan. In the company of two French guides, he met his death in a storm on Col du Geant at Mont Blanc in September of 1873 and was buried in the English cemetery at Samöens.

Fedchenko was the first explorer of central Asia. His encyclopedic works on geography, flora, and fauna of that region were published posthumously, from 1873 to 1876, in the Bulletin *of the Society of Natural Sciences of Moscow which he had helped to organize.*

He was well acquainted with most of the important zoological laboratories in Europe and probably obtained his solid background in helminthology under F. R. Leuckart (1822–1898). Leuckart was responsible for his observation on Guinea worm. Leuckart had shown (1858) that embryos of Cucullanus, *a nematode parasite of freshwater fish, were swallowed by* Cyclops *and underwent development in them. He predicted a similar life history for* Dracunculus *and is said to have instructed Fedchenko to search for it. Fedchenko's residence, and his extensive travels in Turkestan, brought him in contact with numerous cases of dracunculiasis and led to the research reported in his classic article.*

Fedchenko was a founding member of the Imperial Society of Friends of Natural Sciences, Anthropology,

and Ethnography, before which the paper was presented on 21 January 1870, being published in the Proceedings *of the Society later that year. The structure of* Dracunculus medinensis *and its development in* Cyclops *are lucidly described in this beautifully written paper. These observations led Fedchenko to an accurate conclusion on how man becomes infected with this parasite.*

The inhabitants of certain areas of Central Asia suffer severely from a sickness that is caused by a parasitic worm lodged under the skin and known by the natives as "guinea worm." In April or May there appears under the skin a foreign cylindrical body that lengthens gradually, about 1 inch a week; it lies either stretched out or rolled up in a ball. Often several of them lie together, forming a ball about 1¾ inches in diameter. Subsequently, on the spot of skin underneath which lies the head of the parasite, an abscess appears. In the wound thus formed one can see the head of the worm. Depending upon the area of the body in which the parasite develops, the pain of the attack differs. Since most often the parasite appears in the lower extremities, the diseased person usually lies on his back while the abscess is acute, trying to avoid pain by not moving his legs. An abundance of malodorous pus flows from the wound. In Samarkand during the summer, one can see such afflicted persons lying in the market square, in the mosques, and in the caravansaries. If the whole parasite is extracted successfully from under the skin, the wound heals quickly. However, if the parasite is torn and part of it remains in the wound, inflammation occurs and develops into an abscess. In such instances, recovery is not infrequently retarded, the sickness lasts many months and is accompanied by great exhaustion. It is said to cause death in rare instances.

The parasite that provokes such agonizing attacks is not found exclusively in Central Asia. The same guinea worm (*Filaria medinensis*) is found in many localities in India and in Egypt, and among inhabitants of many other parts of Africa, as well as among Negroes who brought it with them to some islands of America.

The worm, once removed from a human being, presents a long, thin, cylindrical body of milk-white color. If torn apart or cut, from it flows a milk-like fluid containing an extraordinarily great number of small, fast-swimming worms. Thus, the worm is viviparous. That is why the first observers regarded it as a sack full of small worms—the embryos. With time, this idea changed; but, in general, knowledge of its anatomy was extremely limited, and only 6 years ago the English scholar, Bastian, published his first complete work concerning this worm.

My microscopic findings pertaining to the anatomy of this worm, begun in Samarkand and now continued here in specimens in alcohol, supplement considerably the known data and in some respects completely alter them (Plate 68).

Like every round worm, the filaria is made up of the following parts: a cutaneous integument, with inner muscles grown to this integument, makes up the walls of the body; within this lie the narrow intestinal canal and the wider uterus distended with embryos.

A cutaneous integument, which on the average is 0.07 mm thick, consists of six layers. The innermost granular layer forms the hypodermis (it is useless for Bastian to reject its presence, for from this layer the cutaneous integument is formed). The layers adjoining it and actually forming the cuticle of the worm are transparent; if one looks at them from above, one can see (through them) the deep-lying layers that present a system of crisscrossed lines meeting at a 90° angle. On the surface of the topmost layer are noticeable circular grooves, which give the worm annulation.

The muscles adjoining the inner side of the cuticle go along the dorsal and ventral side of the worm like two wide ribbons. These muscles are separated in the midline by outgrowths of the hypodermis. These excrescences are very narrow but noticeable, for to them are attached, pinnately, little muscles. These "ribbons" consist of long, flat, muscular fibers that, as in many other round worms, are made up of two highly distinct parts: a fibrous part and a blebby (bullous) part. The fibrous one is dense and has the shape of a plate. One side of the plate grows into the hypodermis; the opposite side usually has a groove, so that the plate appears pentagonal. The bulging ends of the plate are transformed into a membrane that covers the bullous part. Here, one discovers granular contents and nuclei, which often reach considerable size. The bullous part of the muscles is greatly developed at the anterior and posterior extremities of the body. However, in the main part of the body, which contains the highly developed uterus overloaded with embryos, the bullous part atrophies, and the walls of

the uterus press closely the fibers of the muscles. This fact, in the past, led to the belief that the guinea worm was simply a sack filled with embryos, the bullous part of the muscles being a glandular layer that is developed in some parts of the worm.

Contrary to the conviction of Bastian, I have discovered in the filaria a strongly developed system of little transverse fibers. From the bullous or bladder-like structure arise appendices that have the appearance of thin fibers. However, they differ from similar appendices in *Ascaris,* in that often interlacements are formed from which extend, still further, several branches leading into the middle lines. Furthermore, this net of transverse little fibers lies on the inner surface of the bullous structure but does not go through its mass as in the instance of *Ascaris*; this is why one cannot notice it in cross-sections.

The lateral lines, as opposed to the central ones, are distinguished by unusual width, but there are no traces of any protuberances such as are seen in *Ascaris*. On the hypodermis, between the dorsal and the ventral muscles, there lies a thick layer of fine, granular substance in which nuclei are scattered. Along the center of the lateral lines there is a wide duct belonging to the system of so-called "excretory vessels" so prevalent in many worms. It has a membrane in which nuclei can be seen at regular intervals. I could not find any transverse branch which, in other round worms, connects the ducts of two opposite sides and opens to the outside by a special aperture. If such apertures do exist in the guinea worm, they exist separately for the duct of each side and lie near the mouth.

At the anterior end of the body lies the orifice of the mouth. Until recently there existed only very unclear and scanty information concerning the mouth or the so-called "head." In working with cross and longitudinal sections, I succeeded in concluding that this part of the worm has a rather complicated structure.

On the anterior extremity is a disk, shining through the cover of the skin, and consisting of a granular substance. In the middle of this disk, in the cuticle, there is an oval depression of rather considerable size, which is surrounded by a roller-like thickening. From the top and the bottom, following along where the middle lines begin, there stand large tactile protuberances with depressions. Along the sides of the mouth orifice

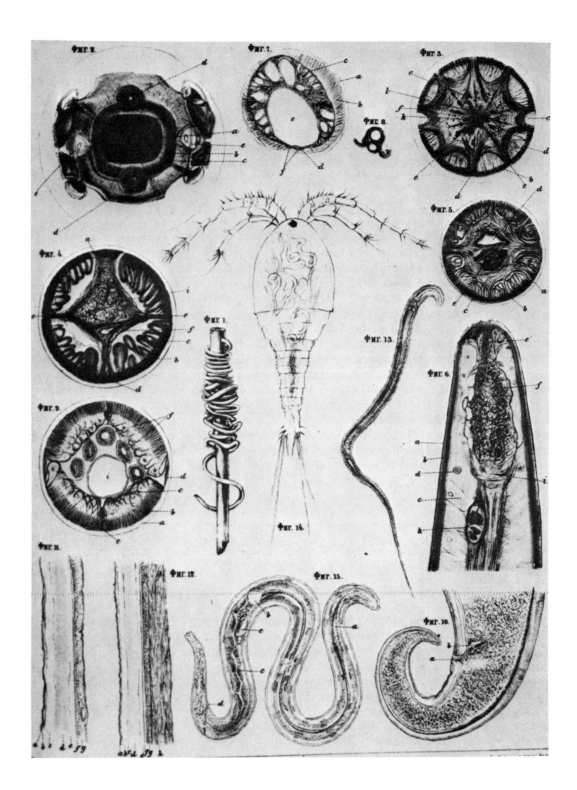

are found six whitish spots; in the middle of one of these spots a pair of these protuberances can be seen. Since the excretory organ passes in the lateral lines, could its opening possibly be here? On the sides of the disk are found four small plates of granular substance.

The mouth presents a flat, oval depression in the center of which can be seen the beginning of the esophagus, which is rounded in form. Further down in the section, eight muscle fibers can be seen leading out like rays from the cavity of the esophagus and adhering to the walls of the body; thus, at its beginning, the esophagus will have, in the section, an octagonal shape. The cavity of the esophagus presents, in that part of the section, a triangular form. Besides a significant number of ray-like muscular fibers, the esophagus has many longitudinal fibers; on the whole, it presents here a rather strong, muscular, sucking apparatus. A certain number of granules lie between the fibers, but this granular substance predominates in the following three sections of the intestinal canal.

The first section is square-shaped and, by means of fibers, adheres to the lateral and medium lines. In this section, the cavity does not lie in the center but is closer to the ventral side and has on this side very fine membranous walls. On the dorsal side, the walls are very thick and are formed of fibers among which granules are scattered.

The second section is surrounded on the outside by a ring composed of rather small fibers leading from lines and muscles in cross, longitudinal, and oblique directions. By analogy with other round worms, the central nervous system must be found in this fibrous ring; however, I have not yet quite succeeded in fully observing its structure.

On the ventral side in this same fibrous ring there lies a peculiar and highly interesting formation, probably having glandular properties: an oval body divided by partitions and containing as many as four nuclei; toward the back of it are found two excretory canals. On cross-sections one is convinced that this gland is not paired; it is found on one side only, but it is doubled: inside a common membrane one can see two accumulations of nuclei, which are covered by their indi-

Plate 68. Photograph of the plate that illustrates Fedchenko's article, courtesy of the Harvard Museum of Comparative Zoology. Legend edited by Dr. Robert Briggs Watson, former editor of the Am. Jnl. Trop. Med. & Hy.

Fig. 1. Guinea worm (*Filaria medinensis* L.) in its natural size, rolled up, after its removal, from the body, on a stick. This is the method used by Russian physicians; the Tuzem tribesmen pull it straight out, with their fingers or pincers, at one pull. *Fig. 2.* The superior surface of the head: (a) the mouth, located in an oval depression, (b) surrounded by a circular thickening. (c) Large papillae attached to the base of the dorsal and ventral longitudinal lines, (dd) with a depression at their center. At the base of the lateral longitudinal lines there are light colored papillae (ee) on which are noted two apertures (?). (The question mark is that of Fedchenko—Editor.) *Fig. 3.* Cross section immediately posterior to the previous figure, somewhat schematized. (a) The cuticle, (b) muscle, (c) lateral longitudinal lines, (d) ventral longitudinal lines, (ee) the lower paramedian lines, (f) connective tissue supporting the digestive system, (i) muscle cells surrounding (k) the esophagus, (l) longitudinal muscle fibers in cross section.

Fig. 4. (a) Cuticle, (b) muscles, (c) the muscle cell, (dd) ventral longitudinal lines, (ee) lateral longitudinal lines, (f) the esophagus, (i) upper wall, consisting of elastic tissues. *Fig. 5.* (a) Cuticle, (b) muscles, (c) connective tissue, extending from the lateral lines and surrounding the stomach, (d) midgut cavity, (e) vas deferens (?). (Translation of e may not be precise—Editor.) *Fig. 6.* Longitudinal section through the anterior parts of the intestinal canal; it is made in such a way that the cavity of the intestinal canal does not enter the section. The preparation is stained with osmic acid. (a) Cuticle, (b) muscles, (c) muscle cells, (d) muscle nuclei, (e) muscular portion of the esophagus, see Fig. 3, (f) elastic portion of the esophagus (esophageal gland—Editor), see Fig. 4 (i) fibrous ring (nerve ring—Editor), see Fig. 5, (k) longitudinal section of vas deferens, in Fig. 5. *Fig. 7.* Cross section of the intestinal tract, lying freely in the body cavity. The preparation was made from a specimen with atrophic midgut muscles. (a) Cuticle, (b) muscles, (c) walls of the intestine, (d) lateral longitudinal lines, (e) its cavity, (f) two tubules of the vas deferens (cervical papillae?—Editor).

Fig. 8. The same canal at posterior level, under the same magnification. *Fig. 9.* Cross section of the anterior ovary, forming coils. (a) Cuticle, (b) muscles, (c) central muscle cells (d) the lateral longitudinal line, (e) the ventral longitudinal line, (f) ovary, (i) cavity of the intestinal canal. *Fig. 10.* The tail of the guinea worm with remaining traces of the excretory pore. (a) Excretory pore, (b) translucent remains of the intestine. *Fig. 11.* Longitudinal section of the walls of the body on the lateral lines. (a-g) External layers (i) nuclei in lateral lines. (No i is found on the plate—Editor.) *Fig. 12.* Longitudinal section of the wall of the body on the muscle. Identical letters signifying corresponding layers in both sections: (a–f) layers of cuticle, (g) subcuticular layer, (h) muscular layer.

Fig. 13. Larva from the uterus. *Fig. 14. Cyclops sp.* with seven larvae in the body cavity. The length of the *Cyclops* is 0.8 mm, its width 0.3 mm. *Fig. 15.* The filaria larva after moulting and a one-month sojourn in the *Cyclops*. (a) Esophagus, (b) cavity at the beginning of the stomach, (c) stomach with large hepatic cells, (d) excretory pore, (e) rudimentary genital organs.

vidual membranes. There are also two excretory canals; these extend for a long distance along the walls and then disappear.

Where it is surrounded by the fibrous ring, the excretory canal has a unique structure: it is eccentric and lies closer to that side where the abovementioned glandule is found. On this side its walls are fairly thin, but on the opposite side they are thick and are made up of transverse fibers with granules suspended among them. The cavity of the intestinal canal here is of considerable size and is full of granular material, apparently ingested food.

The intestinal canal has such a structure also in the third division, only there it lies absolutely free in the body's cavity; its walls on the dorsal side become progressively thinner and the inner cavity widens considerably. At a certain distance from the mouth, the intestinal canal suddenly becomes extremely narrow, and its walls thicken; in such form it continues along the whole length of the body, ending blindly at the tail. I had been convinced that in a fully matured guinea worm there is no anus, but in one specimen which, judging by its size, evidently had been extracted when young, I found traces of an anus in the form of a half-healed slit. It was discovered on the side of the body into which the tail coils. I must note that that parasite probably died prematurely in the human being because, instead of the usual contents (embryos), it contained an incalculable number of live vibrios. As it nears the tail, the intestinal canal, previously lying loosely, now attaches itself to muscular appendages. In other round worms (in *Ascaris* for example), adhesion occurs not to the muscles but, on the contrary, directly to the intermuscular cavities.

Now I take up the last system, the reproductive. As is known, these organs are made up of a very elongated uterus full of embryos and two appendages, each up to 1 inch in length, on its extremities. I am convinced that these appendages are ovaries. I base my conclusion not on their position, but on the nature of their structure, which is the same in each appendage; namely, their walls present an evident trace of cells. At the time of the worm's exit, egg formation probably had ceased; at least I did not find any eggs in the process of development, and only once did I see, in an ovary, two embryos, which were identical to those found in the uterus. It is impossible to agree with Bastian (he accepts parthenogenesis

for the guinea worm) that the eggs or the pseudova are formed in the uterus. The histolic structure of the uterus strongly contradicts this: it consists of an external membrane, a layer of longitudinal fibers, a layer of ring-like fibers, and a nonstructural membrane. There is no outer sexual opening, and it is difficult to say where it occurs in early stages. In any instance, it is not on the head near the mouth, as Schneider quite recently assumed. I did not find anything that indicated the separation point of the two uteri. Once I discovered an invagination of the uterus, but I cannot maintain that this resulted from the coming together of the two uteri elongating in opposite directions. There, in general outline, is the structure of this parasite.

Let us now take up another question concerning which I have made a new and very substantial observation: How does the guinea worm, or its embryos, get under the skin of man?

At the present time it is impossible to concur with the conclusion of Professor Eversman, the first scientific observer of the guinea worm in Bukhara, who insists convincingly that it occurs under the skin of man as a result of an arbitrary infection. This theory concerning parasites is now fully rejected. In order for the parasite to appear, it is necessary that either it or its embryo enter a human being. An elucidation of the ways in which the parasite can enter is the most practical method of deliverance from it; only by becoming informed can one successfully counteract a permanent and, by the way, a very strong infection by any kind of parasite in certain given areas, i.e., the guinea worm in Bukhara.

In India, where the population of many areas suffers severely from this parasite English physicians have tried to find an explanation for the manner of infection. Carter, doing research in natural history in Bombay, concluded that the embryos of *Filaria* develop in a small worm, *Urolabes palustris* Cart., which lives freely in stagnant, half-salty waters, and, during bathing and on other occasions, enters the skin of man probably through the pores.

The most important arguments offered by Carter in support of his theory are as follow: *Filaria* is strongly developed in those areas where there is an abundance of small worms (Urolabidae) living freely in the water and where the natives are exposed to conditions that would permit the worms to enter their bodies. On the other hand, this parasite is very rare in those areas where thorough investigation did not reveal the presence of microscopic *Filaria* in the waters. Finally, Carter calls to witness the strong resemblance in anatomical structure between *Filaria* and its embryos and the free-living Urolabidae.

Carter's theory concerning the free-living embryos of filaria was met with great doubt. Truly, the above-mentioned conclusions are indecisive. In water, in silt, and in similar circumstances, live very many free worms close to *Filaria*. Recently, the investigations of Eberth, Bastian, and Schneider have revealed hundreds of worms, all resembling one another to a certain extent by their internal structure, although they also present indisputable differences. The question has thus far remained unanswered.

In June, upon returning from a trip across the plain, I learned that the native doctor, a specialist in extracting guinea worms, already had had the occasion of removing several parasites from persons arriving in Samarkand from Bukhara. According to my instructions, these specimens had been placed in water and were delivered to me. Since they had remained with the doctor for several days, the water had spoiled and now gave forth a most disgusting odor. However, microscopic investigation revealed the presence in this water of a great number of living embryos. Thus I received my first material for experimentation. However, carelessness deprived me of it and slowed down the work. Wishing to get rid of the water's disgusting odor which was permeating all the rooms of our apartment, I added some fresh water and all the embryos died. The water used for this purpose was well water, rather cold (near 13°C) and very rich in lime salts. Obviously, embryos cannot survive in such water. In all my later experiments with embryos, I used pond water.

Once again, it was necessary to obtain living embryos; by the end of June, I had them at my disposal. This time I placed them in my small aquarium in which lived different water animals that had been found in the stagnant waters of Samarkand. I made this arrangement in the hope that the guinea worm, like so many parasites, would live at first in some animal and later pass on to man. However, an incident helped me in my research.

In the month of July, guinea worm infection became very common in Samarkand. Every morning the doctor would bring me an ordinary guinea worm that had been extracted the previous day. On the 5th of July, in the small bottle in which he had brought a guinea worm, I noticed a pair of small water crawfish—the *Cyclops*. Placing them under the microscope, I saw in each one several familiar looking embryos of the guinea worm.

To convince myself that the embryo of the guinea worm really enters the *Cyclops* and in it continues its development, I conducted the following experiment. By puncturing a guinea worm, I released its embryos into a small watch glass. As I mentioned before, there is no opening for discharge in the sexual organs of filaria; however, the embryos come out easily through a small puncture in the cuticle. In addition to the muscular walls of the uterus, the muscles adhering to the cuticle help with the ejection. The worm retains its round shape only so long as it is distended by the embryos. When an artifical outlet is created for the embryos, the semicircular dorsal and ventral muscles push on the ovary, squeeze out the embryos, and straighten out, and the worm becomes flat.

After a puncture, a thick, mucilaginous liquid, in which wriggle masses of embryos, flows out of the worm. This liquid was poured into vessels containing *Cyclops;* after several hours a significant number of embryos appeared in most of them, especially in males and particularly in young specimens. By this process I obtained a considerable amount of material for continued observation of further development during the month. To exclude every possibility of error, since the embryos of many round worms are very much alike, I conducted the infection experiment on a small scale in a watch glass. In addition, both the water and the *Cyclops* had been examined previously under the microscope, and both had appeared free of any embryos.

I did not succeed in observing how the embryos enter the little crawfish, whether through the opening of the mouth or directly through the cuticle, namely, the spot where the segments join. The latter manner, judging by an observation of the embryos of *Mermis,* seems to me more probable. Besides, I have observed embryos that were found dead in the intestinal canal of *Asplanchna* after being digested and ejected through the anus. In the *Cyclops,* the embryos are lodged in the cavity over the intestinal canal.

Their number varies; usually there are five or six, but occasionally I have observed a whole dozen.

Before following the changes that the embryo of the guinea worm undergoes in the *Cyclops,* it is necessary to become acquainted with the structure of the embryo as found in the uterus of the guinea worm.

The size of these embryos is almost uniform, 0.65 mm. The body is very narrow, not thicker than 0.02 mm; the anterior extremity is somewhat narrowed and rounded. In the center is found a small opening, the mouth, at the side of which arises a conical prominence; the latter probably plays a role during entry into the *Cyclops* and may serve in the penetration of the tissue. Posteriorly, the embryo's body narrows and becomes a fine, straight tail, which constitutes almost one-third of the embryo. On the outside the cuticle of the embryo presents rather distinct, rounded grooves and rollers. These disappear where the body starts to narrow. The small aperture of the mouth leads into a narrow intestinal canal, which is as yet hardly differentiated, and is not connected with the anus which is found at the beginning of the tail. In the intestinal canal one can distinguish the esophagus and the stomach. The rest of the embryo's contents consist of a granular mass.

During the first days after the embryo's entry into the *Cyclops,* its changes are limited to internal development, namely the setting apart of the intestinal canal. The esophagus and the stomach become more clearly differentiated. The esophagus is a narrow tube; the stomach, however, occupies a greater part of the body cavity. The anus becomes more distinct, and one can see, leading obliquely from it, the rectum. One cannot, as yet, see a clear connection between anterior and posterior sections of the intestinal canal; the rings on the cuticle are still distinct.

After 2 weeks the embryo changes greatly in form; it fades, and its body length is shortened, because, as it throws off its cuticle, it deprives itself of a tail. Evidently, its tail had served as a motile organ in the water; now, being inside the *Cyclops,* this tail is superfluous. In addition, the character of the embryo's movements change. Previously, it had moved almost exclusively by means of the tail; now it crawls snake-like, wiggling its body. The size of the embryo is now 0.45 mm, instead of 0.65 mm. Its body, in this second stage, does not have even a trace of any rings; its cuticle is completely smooth. The posterior extremity ends with two small tooth-like projections, of which the ventral is slightly larger. The mouth does not undergo any changes, but the conic protuberance disappears. Internally, the most important changes involve the intestinal canal: the esophagus stands out more clearly, its walls thickening and elongating, until it occupies one-half of the body; the stomach stands out sharply; with its dark yellow color, which derives from a great number of granules. The features of the rectum and anus also become sharper. The granular content of the anterior half disappears almost completely; the walls of the intestinal canal almost reach the cuticle. In the posterior third the contents are still strongly noticeable as a mass of small granules; this envelops the rectum and fills out a part of the anus lying in the rear. I once succeeded in seeing inside its canal, as if it were opening to the outside, between the two small, tooth-like terminal projections. Could it not be that same outgoing canal of a specific gland that has been observed in certain embryos of round worms and that characterizes the whole family of Urolabidae? Once, I saw what looked like a third little tooth-like projection between the two terminal ones, but I could not be sure that it was not the discharge of a small tail gland which had hardened on its way out. After 3 weeks, the differentiation of the internal organs becomes still more pronounced; the structure of the stomach becomes especially clear. Its cavity starts with a widening, which results from the walls of the esophagus leading into it, becoming sharply thinner and forming a conic cavity. After this, the cavity of the intestinal canal again decreases; its walls thicken considerably and are lined with large, brightly demarcated cells with a yellow, granular content, between which remains a narrow, zigzag-like canal. These cells probably play a hepatic role. By this time, food intake occurs by way of the mouth because one notices, in the esophagus, granular contents that flow from one side to the other as the animal moves.

At the same time, rudiments of the genital organs appear as, on the dorsal side, at the beginning of the stomach, one notices a little, dark, oval body that contains a small nucleus. If one observes the embryo from the dorsal side, one can notice small sprouts leading backward and forward from this body. At this stage, my observations on the development of the embryos terminate.

What, then, happens to the embryo at a later stage? It seems to me that, taking into consideration the known facts concerning the development of other round worms, one can state the following: *Cyclops,* with the embryo, enter the stomach of man through drinking water; here, under new conditions, further development occurs pertaining primarily to the genitals. The differentiation of males and females occurs, and copulation takes place. Thereafter, the males die; however, the females, to develop their offspring, take off by unknown means, or by way of the blood vessels, or by burrowing through the tissues of the body toward the skin where they place themselves subcutaneously.

Many facts are explained by my assumptions:

(1) All guinea worm specimens that were studied by the various observers had been viviparous females. The error of Owen and MacClelland, who had stated that they had seen males, has been proved already by Bastian. The males do not penetrate to the subcutaneous point but, like the trichinae, are disgorged from the intestinal canal and go directly out to the exterior.

(2) Regarding its position, the guinea worm always lies with its head toward the outside. There are instances when the parasite lies not subcutaneously but between the muscles; however, even then, the head is pointed toward the skin.

(3) Occasionally, the guinea worm has been discovered, during autopsy, in the internal organs and cavities of the body (i.e., in Egypt, when Pruner-Bey found it in the membrane of the liver).

(4) In Central Asia the natives become infected with this parasite only in those areas where they are compelled to use stagnant water. I am informed, for certain, about three such areas: Dzhizak, Bukhara, and Karshi. These three areas have one thing in common in that they are located at the terminal point of rivers: Dzhizak, Djelan-Uti; Bukhara, Zaravshan; and Karshi, Kashgar-Darya. During the summer, at the end of their flow, these rivers have very little water. The natives then are compelled to use pond water. The ponds, called locally *haouzi,* are small rectangular holes that are lined with trees. Water is gathered into these through a gutter. When the pond is cleaned, another small gutter serves as a drain. Next to every mosque, rural or urban, such a *haouz* is indispensable. Besides serving as cooling places, they have still another function: the muddy water, flowing through the ditches and rivers of the area, settles when it reaches the *haouzi.* In freeing itself from the minerals, the water in these ponds becomes bad from another source for another reason: in it appear innumerable quantities of different kinds of tiny water animals. Among these, in the majority, appear those *Cyclops* in which I have observed the development of the embryos of *Filaria.* The natives are not squeamish about such water, and once I, too, had to use such water from a *haouz* to quench my thirst. On that occasion, the main inhabitants of the pond were the reddish Daphniae, easily seen by the naked eye. The natives drank the water unconcernedly. Besides, it is possible to drink, unnoticingly, the very tiny whitish *Cyclops,* which one can hardly recognize in the water.

(5) Carter's theory about mode of infection—bathing and going bare-footed—is inapplicable to Central Asia. Here, the population rarely bathes and does not go barefoot. Everyone, whether or not he goes barefoot at home, upon going outside, puts on shoes or galoshes.

The ablutions, which the law of Mohammed prescribes must be performed five times daily, do not serve to the advantage of Carter's theory, for the main argument of this theory is the prevalence of the guinea worm in the feet. During the ablutions, however, the face, feet, and hands are wet and all by means of the hands; therefore, the hands, coming in contact with the water most frequently, should house the guinea worm most often, but this does not occur.

The ablutions may play another role in infection, in that they may make it possible for embryos adhering to the body of a sick man to get into the water, for these ablutions take place most frequently in those very ponds from which water is taken for drinking. There are many other ways for the embryos to get into this pond water; for example, the ditches that bring water to the ponds are open, and all kinds of impurities get into them. Finally, the number of embryos in every guinea worm is tremendous—several million—

and a few of these will always find a way of getting to the water.

Assuming that infection takes place through the *Cyclops,* one can make use of this observation: if water in which the *Cyclops* are swimming is drawn into a medicine dropper, no matter how fast the water is sucked up, virtually not one *Cyclops* will remain inside the medicine dropper. Finding themselves in the current of water, they quickly get away from it. This information is useful when one wants to separate the *Cyclops* from the *Daphnia,* for the latter always gets into the tube. It seems to me that, to a large extent, it would be very simple to ward off the danger of infection by the guinea worm if the inhabitants would take the water not directly from the ponds but from the little streams that flow out of them. Then, I suppose, the *Cyclops* would all remain in the ponds. The embryos do not develop in other animals, e.g., *Daphnia.*

In conclusion, I should like to sum up the results of my research on the guinea worm: so far as anatomical considerations are concerned, the most important and completely new factor pertains to the structure of the esophagus. In addition, it seems that the guinea worm has a strongly developed ingesting organ and takes food, as is shown by its contents, until the very end of its sojourn in man.

A vital observation has been made that puts the question of method of infection on a completely different level: the embryo enters the *Cyclops* and in it continues developing. Now, experimentation is needed—similar to the feeding experiments conducted in studying other tapeworms or parasitic worms— to prove whether the *Cyclops,* with the embryo of *Filaria,* swallowed by a human being, is the cause of guinea-worm disease.

I repeat that, although my observations are purely scientific, at the same time they may have practical meaning in that they can contribute to the destruction or at least to a considerable weakening of this agonizing parasite. In this respect, one must heed the above-mentioned observation regarding the reaction of the *Cyclops* to running water. I shall also note that the final resolution of the question of infection by the guinea worm is necessary for still another reason: with the taking over of Turkistan by the Russians, the national life there obviously became more active; communication between different areas through

the pacification of this region increased 10-fold, as did the chances of spreading this disease. It can easily become endemic in various areas of our Central Asian possessions. There are many places in Central Asia poor in water and where the use of pond water is rather widespread. It is not necessary to cite ancient legends about devastating epidemics caused by this worm; the transportation of the guinea worm to the New World—on the islands of America—occurred recently, causing a deadly epidemic. [Probably the epidemic of *Dracunculus* cited by Bastian in the island of Grenada. H.C. Bastian, On the structure and nature of the Dracunculus or guinea worm. Trans. Linnean Soc. London, 24: 101–134, 1863—Eds.]

THE ETIOLOGY AND PROPHYLAXIS OF DRACONTIASIS

British Medical Journal, 1: 129–132, 1907.

Robert Thomson Leiper

Leiper's biographical sketch appears in the chapter on Schistomiasis where his work is more extensively reported.
    Leiper showed that the larvae of Dracunculus medinensis *would survive exposure to gastric juice.*

Dracontiasis is very common and widely disseminated throughout the native races of our West African possessions. During the last five years it has twice assumed epidemic proportions among the black troops stationed there, and on the more recent occasion severely hampered military operations in Nigeria. These outbreaks indicate how, by aggravating the difficulty of maintaining the necessary supplies of labour, the disease may materially retard the commercial development of these colonies in the future. The authorities are at present deterred from initiating any active prophylactic measures by the varied and conflicting nature of the theories now in vogue as to the life-history of the parasite, and the manner in which it gains access to the human body.

In order to investigate these points in more detail, and, if possible, to determine the means by which the disease might be mitigated or controlled, I was sent to West Africa in August,

1905, by the Committee of the London School of Tropical Medicine.

The aim of the present paper, is first, to record the results of experiments undertaken to test the truth of previous theories; secondly, to define the conditions essential to the complete development of the parasite; and, thirdly, to base upon the facts ascertained some suggestions for the prevention of the spread of the disease.

The hypotheses of infection that have been advocated from time to time may be classified as follows:

I. Those in which the development of the embryo is supposed to occur without the intervention of any intermediate host, human infection being caused by:

    a. The embryo, as discharged from the parent worm; or

    b. The mature larva, evolved from the embryo in water or marshy soil; or

    c. The young adult, the product of the continued growth of the larva in water.

II. Those in which an intermediate host is considered essential for the development of the larva in order that it may become fitted to reinfect man:

    d. The only, and in itself sufficient, host being cyclops.

    e. A second, and at present unknown, intermediate host being necessary to continue and complete the changes begun in cyclops.

Further, there remains to be considered under each heading a still more controversial and important question: By what route does the parasite enter the human body? Does it do so passively with the ingestion of fluid or actively by penetrating the skin? . . .

It has frequently been shown that the embryos discharged from the parent can only live in water for quite a short time, and that they undergo no metamorphosis. In my observations, on the vitality of these embryos in water the vast majority died on the third day, though some survived until the sixth. In mud they lived a day or two longer, probably because in this they move more slowly, and are consequently less quickly exhausted. Although provided with a mouth and digestive tract they are still unable to obtain food for themselves.

This inability on the part of the embryo to infect man by the skin or by the mouth, to undergo any further development, or even to remain alive in water, points to an intermediate host as an *essential* factor in its life-cycle.

This conclusion brings us to the consideration of the theories in Section II. The conditions under which the embryo becomes a larva were discovered by Fedschenko about 1870. He observed that the embryo made its way into the body cavity of a small crustacean of the genus Cyclops, and there, after a period of 12 days, underwent metamorphosis. Having followed the growth of the larva until the fourth week, he then endeavored to complete the life-cycle of the parasite by feeding cats and dogs upon the infected cyclops. These experiments were unsuccessful. Nevertheless, Fedschenko concluded that cyclops was undoubtedly the efficient intermediate host of the Guinea worm, and that probably the larvae were taken into the alimentary canal of man while still within this host, and there set free. His view was that in the intestine they then attained sexual maturity, and the females when fertilized made their way into the connective tissues, whilst the males died and were discharged in the faeces.

The failure of Fedschenko's efforts to produce infection artificially led many to doubt the accuracy of his conclusions. It has been argued that "possibly cyclops is not the real host of the *Filaria medinensis,* notwithstanding that the nematode might attain a certain stage of development in its body" (Sambon). Others maintain, upon the analogy of the behaviour of the ankylostome larva, that the larvae by becoming free-living later, may infect man through the skin. They are thus able to offer an explanation for the remarkable fact that the parasite occurs in the lower limbs in 90 per cent of all the cases of dracontiasis. While my own experience does not confirm Fedschenko's observations and conclusions in their entirety it brings no support to these later views.

I obtained the materials for experimental purposes most satisfactorily by the following means. Cases of dracontiasis were selected in which the vesicle caused by the worm was still whole or had only recently burst, and a damp compress was bound over the sore. When this was taken off, a few hours later, there would be found upon it an almost solid mass of embryos. With the material obtained in this way one had complete control over the degree of infection of water containing the cyclops. The worm discharged its young by a prolapse of the uterus, as described by Manson, though this extrusion never occurred through the mouth but by an opening just outside the circumoral ring of papillae.

Cases in which there was considerable suppuration or abscess formation were useless for our purpose, the accessible part of the worm being filled by white cells, which had destroyed the embryos. To secure a supply of cyclops, likely pools were swept with a fine silk net (60 meshes to the linear inch) into the apex of which had been fitted a wide-mouthed bottle of about 10 oz. capacity. When this bottle was filled with creatures of various sorts it was emptied into large jars, which were then corked and transferred to the temporary laboratory. After a time, possibly because the oxygen became exhausted, the cyclops collected near the surface. The upper layer was then decanted into a large Petri capsule and gently "swirled" round until the solid contents gathered in a vortex in the centre. By means of a large syringe with a fine nozzle all the dirt and the innumerable small creatures could now be got rid of—except the cyclops, which always darted away from the current into the clean water at the sides. In this way it was easy to get a large and fairly pure supply from the most miscellaneous catch.

Although most of the animals that prey upon cyclops were excluded by this method, there was some difficulty still owing to the evaporation and concentration of the water, and the growth in it of paramecia which destroyed large numbers. The bulk of the water had consequently to be drawn off and replaced by fresh every third day. Moreover, the cyclops themselves are carnivorous, and in absence of their usual food supply consume their fellows, so that it became necessary to add some organism that was suitable as food and yet harmless. The best results followed the use of rain water, which contained numerous nauplii and cladocera, to refill the tanks.

Of all the other organisms found in the ponds none was capable of infection with Guinea worm embryos. In a few instances these were swallowed, especially by mosquito larvae, but they were invariably digested and their cuticles evacuated. Cyclops on the other hand, was very susceptible, no resistance being met with even in adult forms carrying brood capsules. This fact provides a strong argument against the suggestion

of Graham that the greater incidence of the disease in May and June is due to the prevalence in these months of young forms of cyclops, which he supposes are much more liable to infection. . . .

There are, however, two episodes in the embryo's life that are of sufficient practical interest to be dealt with here, and regarding which I find myself at variance with previous observers, namely, the mode of its entry into cyclops, and the time required for the completion of metamorphosis. The teaching of the present day is that the embryo bores its way through the integument at the intervals between the "ventral plates," and so directly reaches the body cavity. I was never able, in spite of repeated endeavours, to observe this process, and there are several considerations which make it somewhat improbable. The cuticle of cyclops is continuous and almost uniform. There are no distinct "ventral" plates or intervals between them. In fact, as may be seen after the soft parts of a dead cyclops have been completely cleared away by paramecia, the cuticle is a rigid and uninterrupted exoskeleton. The Guinea worm embryo possesses no boring apparatus with which to pierce this resistant layer. Its movements, moreover, intermit regularly, and are insufficiently powerful to maintain its own weight against gravity. For it, the presence of a cyclops in its neighbourhood is a matter of indifference—a strong contrast to the swarming of the miracidia of trematodes around their special hosts. If by chance an embryo does come in contact with one of the cyclops's appendages it loops round it in the form of a Greek α, but it has no means of firmly affixing itself and quickly relaxes again. The coiling appears to me to be essentially spasmodic. It may be produced by salt solution and other chemical irritants. This peculiar flexion followed by sudden straightening, while useless for penetrating a resisting object from without, seems very well calculated to help the embryo to explode one or other of its extremities through the walls of a soft containing tube like the cyclops's intestine. Further, where more than half a dozen embryos gained access to the body cavity, the infection generally resulted in the death of the host. In these cases it could be seen that the intestinal wall at one part was severely lacerated. Lastly, we have the analogy of *Cucullanus elegans,* the similarity of the embryos of which to those of the Guinea worm suggested to Leuckart the possibility that the cyclops was an efficient host for both. Although the *Cucullanus* embryo is provided with a special "perforating tooth" (Blanchard), it is an accepted fact that it infects the cyclops through the intestine. The question can only be settled finally by serial sections of recently-infected specimens, and these I have hitherto had no opportunity of making. Meanwhile it is, I venture to submit, at least an open one.

As regards the time necessary for the completion of metamorphosis, Fedschenko, who continued his observations into the fourth week after infection, states that it occurs on the twelfth day. Manson, working in London with English cyclops, found that ecdysis was postponed until the sixth week, owing, doubtless, to the cold. In Africa I found that the striated cuticle of the embryo was cast generally on the eighth day. The larva which emerged lost, two days later, a very delicate enveloping pellicle, and from that time onwards underwent *no* further ecdysis. The subsequent changes were confined to the differentiation of internal structures, the larva apparently becoming mature in the fifth week.

The next point to be considered is the way in which the mature larvae quit the cyclops. If infection of man is to occur by the skin, it is clear that they must leave the cyclops and become free-swimming. If, on the other hand, infection occurs by the mouth, there is no necessity for them to do so till they arrive in the human stomach. Now, in the six weeks during which I was able to observe them developing, the larvae showed no inclination to leave the cyclops. On the contrary, as time went on they became more quiescent, and even when, as happened only too often in the later stages of the experiments, the cyclops died, they did not escape, but were found dead in its interior.

The manner in which they can be set free I have already described in a previous communication. When an infected cyclops was transferred to a 0.2 per cent solution of hydrochloric acid it was immediately killed, but the larvae, far from being destroyed, were awakened to great activity, and eventually escaped into the fluid, in which they swam about freely. This experiment pointed clearly to the probable way in which the larvae are released in nature, for if such a cyclops were swallowed the action of the gastric juice would give the same result.

In order to clinch the argument, I fed a monkey on bananas containing cyclops which had been infected for five weeks and which had in them larvae which appeared mature. Six months later a careful *post-mortem* examination was made for me by Dr. Daniels, and in the connective tissues five filariae were found which, as I have stated elsewhere, possessed the anatomical characteristics of *Filaria medinensis*. There were three unimpregnated and obviously immature females about 30 cm long, and two remarkable small males (22 mm), which were obtained one from the psoas muscle and the other from the connective tissue behind the oesophagus.

These results point strongly to the truth of the theory that infection of man takes place from the drinking of water containing infected cyclops.

The suggestion that a secondary intermediary host is necessary for the complete development of the Guinea worm larva is disposed of by the fact that this is actually attained in cyclops.

The finding of both male and immature female forms in the connective tissues relieves us of the more improbable alternatives previously open to us, namely, that either the filaria was hermaphrodite or that the larvae became sexually mature in the intestines, and the fertilized females only migrated into the body. The view that the larvae at once make their way through the gut wall and become sexually differentiated later in the tissues of their host, brings the after-development of the parasite much more into line with that of other filariae.

We have already referred to the extraordinary frequency of the parasite in the lower limbs in human cases, and discussed the possibility of the larva directly reaching its final position in the connective tissue by piercing the overlying skin. Those who reject this explanation suppose that the pregnant worm is attracted to these parts by a maternal "instinct" which bids her seek to discharge her young into water. In the case of our monkey, however, the three female worms, although immature and unfertilized, had already made their way into the limbs, being found *post mortem* in the forearm, the axilla, and the popliteal space. I venture to suggest that in these wanderings of the Guinea worm we have an example of one of those "-tropisms" that, as Loeb has recently shown, dominate the movements of many lowly-organized creatures. Geotropism seems to me to afford a rational explanation of the remarkable distribution of the parasite in man.

Two further statements must be briefly dealt with before we can proceed to summarize the circumstances controlling the complete development of the parasite. It has been repeatedly affirmed that the embryos as they come from the patient are able to withstand desiccation, and thus be spread widecast by the wind, or in the dry season await a favourable rain to carry them to a cyclops-infested pool. Were this true it would present an almost insuperable difficulty to the prevention of the spread of dracontiasis. The embryos are, however, immediately killed if dried by natural evaporation, and they cannot be revived by the readdition of water.

The presence of numerous large lagoons along the Guinea coast has been thought to explain the great prevalence of the disease in that part of Africa. At Accra there are two lagoons, but neither contains cyclops. The water was distinctly saltish. This excludes them as a source of infection, for on the one hand the species of Cyclopidae are, with one or two rare exceptions, fresh-water forms, and, on the other, water taken from these sources was found to kill the Guinea-worm embryos in half an hour. Sea water had the same effect.

We are now in a position to define with some accuracy the conditions essential for the completion of the life cycle of the parasite.

The young must be discharged directly into fresh water soon after the parent worm has succeeded in creating a break in the overlying skin and before the wound has become markedly septic. The embryos must find a cyclops within a few days. They must, moreover, succeed in entering its body cavity. Five weeks later they will have developed into mature larvae. These must, thereafter, be taken into the human stomach, and having been set free from its host by the gastric juice, reach the connective tissues by penetrating the gut wall.

The life-cycle of the parasite will necessarily be broken: (1) By the death of the embryos, either from sepsis while still within the parent worm, or after their discharge, by saltish water or drying. (2) If cyclops are not present in the water, or if the infected cyclops die or are not taken into the human stomach. (3) If the larvae, ingested by the final host, are immature or fail to escape from the chitinous sheath of the cyclops. Though they do gain their final habitat, the cycle will still be incomplete if (4) there are not both males and females among the matured adults, and if in their wanderings the females are not impregnated.

It will at once be seen from the above summary that the isolation of infective man from healthy cyclops and of infected cyclops from man must be the object of any organized effort to stamp out dracontiasis. . . .

From the nature of the disease it is evident that dracontiasis will disappear from the Coast towns when the provision of a properly-controlled water supply, obtained either from artesian wells or through pipes from some rapidly-flowing stream, permits the filling-in of the surface collections of rain water and the shallow wells upon which the natives now depend for their supplies. Care would have to be taken that any artificial reservoirs constructed were efficiently protected by their isolated situation from the possibilities of infection.

We have to adapt our prophylactic measures in the meanwhile, however, to the conditions as they now are in the towns, and as they will probably always remain in the inland villages. The simpler and less costly these are the likelier they are to be put into practice.

The native, more concerned with quantity than purity, takes his drinking water wherever it is most accessible—from rivers or rain tanks, from shallow wells, or the large ponds usually found at each village.

The question of the infectivity of these sources depends primarily on the presence of cyclops. It is said that cyclops does not occur in swiftly running waters, and this I found true of the Volta and the Sekum, the only rivers I had an opportunity of examining owing to the drought. It is noteworthy that in the village Oblogo, which depends solely on the latter stream for supplies, I could get no information of the occurrence of dracontiasis among the inhabitants. If, therefore, the scheme for providing Accra with its water becomes a reality it is expected that dracontiasis will disappear from the town. An examination of the rain tanks and the wells in and around Accra, Christiansborg, and Labadie was likewise negative. The reverse was the case with the village pools. Those at Akuse and Christiansborg were found to contain vast numbers of cyclops and other forms of crustacean life. In the latter village the evidence seemed irrefutable that the disease is endemic, and a small pond situated centrally, which supplied a proportion of the small population at least during the dry season, appeared the likely centre of infection. In cyclops obtained there I frequently found a nematode larva differing only from that of the Guinea worm in its greater size and the sharp chitinous tips of its triradiate tail. Probably it belongs to the genus Cucullanus, but it deserves mention as a possible source of error in the examination of suspected water.

At Akuse, numerous cyclops were found where the natives drew their drinking water, and where at another spot they could be seen washing.

In most of the villages of the plains I was able, while passing through, to procure cases of dracontiasis, and the histories were suggestive that the infection had been locally acquired. Unfortunately the ponds at most of these places had become dry, and consequently the presence of cyclops could not be determined.

The village pond seems to me undoubtedly the most likely source of the vast majority of the infections. Attention must, therefore, be mainly directed, on the Gold Coast at least, to their protection. My negative results seem to show that the wells are relatively less important. The wells should be surrounded by a stone parapet of about 2 ft. in height and the village pools stoutly fenced around in order to prevent the natives from bathing there or from wading into the water when filling their storage vessels. Each pool would have to be provided with a sufficient number of ''drawing'' wells dug at a short distance from the pool and connected with it by underground pipes in such a way as to ensure a constant supply of water. The openings of these would be protected by a stone or cement wall. In this way by preventing water in contact with the legs of the drawers returning into the pool the chances of infection would be reduced nearly 90 per cent. The ''drawing'' wells would most likely be used freely by the natives, as less labour is involved in obtaining water by draw-bucket or pump than by collecting it with a calabash. Nor would the prevention of the use of the pools for washing prove as great a difficulty as might be supposed, for at several places the natives have already learnt to do this at a place apart from where the drinking water is

drawn. At Accra, the filling of the large reservoir by a thunderstorm a few days before I left gave me the opportunity of observing that there those using the water for washing purposes carried it over the embankment to the lower ground. These precautions were, however, rendered unavailing, as far as dracontiasis was concerned, for those drawing the water for home use frequently entered it for some distance in order to secure a more copious supply than that obtainable at the margin.

If by these or other and more practical methods the infection of the open ponds in the villages could be prevented there is little doubt that a considerable diminution in the disease would soon result.

There still remain for careful investigation in relation to the prophylaxis of dracontiasis many details regarding the life of the intermediate host. We have still to determine more accurately the conditions under which it lives and multiplies in these tropical countries, what are its natural enemies, and upon what other forms of life it depends for its food supply; whether it can survive the drought of the summer, buried beneath the sun-caked mud, or if, when once a pool has dried, it must be restocked from another source; lastly, if, by the addition of chemicals, we can destroy the cyclops in suspected waters without rendering these useless or dangerous to man.

No account of my investigations on the Gold Coast would be complete were I to leave unacknowledged the kindly interest with which Sir John P. Rodger and Major Bryan encouraged my work, the generous way in which the Principal Medical Officer and his deputy aided me with every facility the medical department could have provided, and the daily help and forbearance of Dr. Buée, who had charge of the Government hospital, and Dr. C. H. D. Ralph, the Medical Officer of Health for Accra.

REPORT OF THE BOMBAY
BACTERIOLOGICAL LABORATORY FOR THE
YEAR 1913

Report presented by Major W. Glen Liston. Bombay: Government Central Press, 1914, pp. 14–16.

Dnyaneshvar Atmaran Turkhud
(1868–1926)

Although he was born in India and spent almost his entire career working in that country, Turkhud received his medical education at the University of Edinburgh. From 1908 to 1915 he held appointment as temporary doctor on plague duty, Satara District, Bombay Bacteriological Laboratory, at Matunga Leper Asylum, and as professor of bacteriology, Grant Medical College. In 1916, Turkhud became officiating director of the Bombay Bacteriological Laboratory and carried on the duties of that post in addition to the activities involved in the other positions he held concurrently. In 1926, the year of both his retirement and his death, he became acting director of the King Institute of Preventive Medicine, Guindy, Madras.

Turkhud experimentally demonstrated the complete life cycle of Dracunculus medinensis.

The Distribution of Guinea Worm Disease in India

It is impossible to define accurately the distribution of Guinea Worm disease over India because of the want of data concerning the prevalence of this disease. The only official figures available dealing with this disease are those recorded in the Annual Reports of the Sanitary Commissioner with the Government of India which pertain to native troops and prisoners; even in these reports the figures for the troops have been discontinued since 1908. From a study of these statistics Dr. Turkhud has come to some interesting conclusions regarding the distribution of this disease which is very widely disseminated throughout India.

Geographical Areas

For the purpose of collecting medical statistics, and also for the tabulation of meteorological data for the medical department, the whole of India has been divided into 11 geographical groups which are so arranged as to "represent areas which are fairly homogenous so far as the chief prevailing diseases and climatic conditions are concerned". These groups are:—

    I.—Burma Coast and Bay Islands.
    II.—Burma Inland

    III.—Assam.
    IV.—Bengal and Orissa.
    V.—Gangetic Plain and Chutia Nagpur.
    VI.—Upper Sub-Himalaya.
    VII.—North-West Frontier, Indus Valley and North-Western Rájputána.
    VIII.—South-Eastern Rájputána, Central India and Gujarát.
    IX.—Deccan.
    X.—Western Coast.
    XI.—Southern India.

The Distribution of the Disease among Indian Troops Stationed in Certain Geographical Areas

The division in which dracontiasis is most prevalent among native troops in south-eastern Rájputána, Central India and Gujarát. Here the disease prevails to the extent of 18 cases per mille of the average strength per annum. A ratio of 13.4 per mille is found in Gujarát. The other divisions where the disease prevails are:—

Deccan Proper,	ratio 7.1	per mille of average strength.
Western Coast,	ratio 5.72	do.
Gangetic Plain,	ratio 5.5	do.
Upper Sub-Himalaya,	ratio 5.22	do.
Sind,	ratio 5.12	do.

While in these divisions the disease is common, all the hill stations appear to be free from it except those situated in the North-West Frontier Province. Inland Burma also appears to be free from the disease.

The Distribution of the Disease among Prisoners

The incidence among prisoners in jails probably more accurately represents the prevalence of the disease in the various parts of India, for the majority of prisoners live under normal Indian conditions in the same districts in which the jails are situated in which they are confined. Judged by the incidence of the disease among prisoners, the western part of the Madras Presidency is the most afflicted area (39.64 of average annual strength per mille). The division which in intensity of infection follows the western portion of the Madras Presidency is the Deccan with the very high ratio of 28.10 per mille of average annual strength. The other localities where dracontiasis is common are:—

The Northern Circars,	ratio 12.09 per mille.
Madras and Carnátic,	ratio 11.86 do.

Gujarát and Káthiáwár,   ratio 10.66   do.
The Western Coast,   ratio 10.53   do.
The Indus Valley and North-Western
    Rájputána   ratio 10.11   do.

The Hill Stations, Burma (Inland and Coast) and the Andamans are all free from the disease.

The Distribution of the Disease among Prisoners, a More Reliable Guide to the Extent and Distribution of the Disease among the General Population than that Known to Exist among Indian Troops

The high ratio among the sepoys stationed in a locality showing a low ratio among the prisoners may perhaps be explained on the ground that the sepoys contracted infection in their native villages while on leave or before their transfer to the stations in which they were reported to be sick with the disease. Again a low ratio among the troops in the localities where the disease is prevalent among the prisoners, may be attributed to the superior sanitary surroundings in which the sepoys dwell.

The Extent of the Guinea Worm Disease in Sarsola Village with an Account of how the Disease is Spread in that Village

Some interesting observations were made in the village of Sarsola near Thána on the incidence of Guinea worm disease by Major Glen Liston, I.M.S., and Dr. Turkhud, M.B., C.M. (Edin.). With the assistance of Mr. Bhave, a graduate in science, and an influential Indian gentleman residing near the village, a census of the inhabitants was taken. It was found that 10.78 per cent of the villagers had suffered during the current year from the disease and that approximately 39 per cent of the villagers had at one time or another suffered from the disease. Of the whole population the males were affected in the proportion of 43 per cent, while 26 per cent of females suffered. The source of the disease was traced to an old well belonging to the villagers. The well contained numerous cyclops, of which 38.6 per cent harboured young Guinea worms, as ascertained at the first examination. Although instruction was given to the villagers regarding the precautions which ought to be taken to avoid the disease, and attempts were made by Mr. Bhave to assist them in securing pure drinking water supply, owing to the suspicion and indifference of the population

no attempt to adopt remedial measures had been taken several months later when their village was re-visited.

The Presence of the Disease in Other Villages and the Cause of its Existence in Them

In addition to the visits paid to Sarsola, excursions were made to Kadav and Takve in Kolába district, Yeola and adjoining villages in Násik district and Shetbunder (Elephanta). In these villages Guinea worm disease is very common and our observations made at these places confirmed our views that ignorance, indifference and prejudice on the part of the people are the chief causes which favour the spread of the disease. The parapets of wells are allowed to remain in a state of disrepair so that surface water, after being fouled by bathing and washing operations which are promiscuously carried on near village wells, easily finds its way back into the wells. It is a common sight to see the village wells, the water of which should be scrupulously guarded against contamination, being utilised as swimming ponds, and where a well is provided with steps, to see people washing themselves in the well water. It seems likely, that although this disease is one of the most easily prevented of all diseases we know, little progress will be made in eradicating it from the country till the people of themselves demand a higher standard in the purity of their drinking water; so long as they are content to drink water which has been used for bathing purposes the disease is likely to prevail.

Experiments to Determine the Method of Infection by Guinea Worm. Monkeys Apparently Not Susceptible to Infection

Experiments made on monkeys in the Laboratory to ascertain the mode of transmission of the disease gave the following result. Two series of experiments were carried out. In the first series various methods were employed for bringing about infection. Thirteen monkeys were used, some of them were fed by the mouth on infected cyclops and some with living Guinea worm embryos, while others were injected subcutaneously with the blister fluid containing living embryos, or with embryos suspended in normal saline. *Post mortem* examinations on these monkeys were carried out after intervals varying from one month to one and a half years from the date of experiment. The examinations were conducted very carefully but the results in all instances were negative. The monkeys injected subcutaneously showed no *local lesions,* and in none of them were any Guinea worms found.

In the month of April 1913, a sample of water obtained from the well at Sarsola showed the presence of a large number of cyclops harbouring Guinea worm embryos. About 38.6 per cent of the cyclops were found infected with Guinea worm embryos. Advantage was taken of this, and a second series of experiments was instituted on 12 monkeys which were fed on this naturally infected well water, each monkey being given about 100 cc of the water through a stomach tube. More than 100 cyclops were present in 100 cc of water, so that each monkey swallowed about 38 infected cyclops.

Nine of these monkeys were examined at periods varying from one to ten and a half months after the date of feeding. Careful *post mortem* examinations were made but the results were negative in all the animals examined. The remaining three monkeys out of the series are still alive and well. The monkeys used were all *Macacus sinicus.*

Successful Experimental Infection of Man by Guinea Worm: The Disease Produced by Swallowing Infected Cyclops

Owing to our failure to infect monkeys and the observed absence of the disease among the animals living in infected villages, we thought that the worm might only develop in man; volunteers were therefore called upon to drink water containing infected cyclops. As stated in our last report, five persons came forward. Each volunteer was given five infected cyclops to swallow in a small quantity of sterile water. The experiment was inaugurated on the 5th of April, and the cyclops used had been infected on the 24th of March 1913. On the 18th March 1914, *i.e.,* 348 days after drinking the infected water, one of the volunteers a Laboratory assistant, developed a very small blister on the dorsum of his right foot. The appearance of the blister was accompanied with fever, vomiting and diarrhoea. On the 30th, the blister had assumed the size of a marble and it was then found to contain Guinea worm embryos. From this date large number of embryos were daily collected from the worm until the 14th

April. The worm then broke; some local swelling and suppuration supervened, but this eventually subsided. In this case the volunteer, with the exception of two or three little ulcerations about the body in the rainy season, showed absolutely no symptoms until the appearance of the blister, nearly a year after he swallowed the infected cyclops.

The other volunteers showed no signs and symptoms of the disease with the exception of a little occasional urticaria. In the case of one of the volunteers the blood examination showed an eosinophilia to the extent of 34 per cent in the month of October 1913, but he did not develop a Guinea worm.

These experiments go to prove that the cyclops is the actual intermediary host for the Guinea worm, that the monkey *Macacus sinicus* is probably naturally immune to the disease, and that man is to some extent resistant to infection, for only one person of five who swallowed cyclops containing six to eight Guinea worm embryos developed the disease.

Number of Young Produced by a Single Guinea Worm

An attempt was made to ascertain the number of embryos contained in an adult worm. This was done by dissecting out the uterus from a worm and counting the embryos in a measured volume of the fluid found in the uterus and thus estimating the total number contained in the uterus. The result showed that a mature Guinea worm contains about three million embryos.

Experiments with Potassium Permanganate to Test its Action on Cyclops, the Intermediary Host of the Guinea Worm

The following experiments were conducted to ascertain the efficacy of potassium permanganate for destroying cyclops:

(1) To a large bottle of well water from Sarsola containing many cyclops a quantity of permanganate of potassium in solution was added until the water assumed a pink colour. Two and a half hours afterwards all the cyclops were dead. The bottle was put aside in the laboratory: nine days later some living cyclops were again seen in the water.

(2) A standard solution of potassium permanganate containing 3.95 grammes to the litre was

first prepared and some of this solution in quantities varying from 1 cc–100 cc was added to a litre of water. Six cyclops were transferred to the water containing different strengths of potassium permanganate. The experiment showed that when 100 cc of the standard solution was added to a litre of water, all the six cyclops were killed in an hour. When 75 cc of the standard solution was added all but two cyclops were killed in one hour and six cyclops were dead in one and a half hours. When 25 cc and 50 cc of the solution was added, all cyclops were dead in one and a half hours, but with 20 cc, 15 cc, 10 cc, 8 cc and 6 cc, to the litre of water some cyclops were still alive after three hours. With 4 cc and lesser quantities of the standard solution some of the cyclops survived even after three hours exposure but all were dead in 24 hours.

Potassium Permanganate Destroys Adult Cyclops but Not Their Eggs so that after a Time Cyclops Reappear in the Water and These Cyclops in Favourable Circumstances Soon Become Infected with Young Guinea Worms

(3) Lastly, the well at Sarsola itself was disinfected on 16th March 1914 with nearly three lbs. of potassium permanganate so that a distinct pink tint was imparted to the water. On the 23rd March the water showed no cyclops. On the 30th of that month, however, it was found to contain a large number of daphnia and also a few cyclops. On the 8th April, the number of cyclops had increased, and in addition to daphnia, a few larvae of Anopheles rossi were found. On this date 5.9 per cent of the cyclops were found infected. By the 20th of that month the number of cyclops had considerably increased and the percentage of infection among them had risen to 14 per cent. Daphnia and Anopheles larvae were still present.

Summary

Our researches on Guinea worm disease have shown that:

(1) The disease is widely prevalent in India; in some parts of the country, as for example the western portion of the Madras Presidency, 39 persons per mille of the population annually suffer from the disease if prisoners admitted to jails represent the extent to which the disease exists among the general population. Even in the Deccan 28 persons per mile harbour the worm and in some villages as many as ten per cent of the inhabitants may be affected in a single year.

(2) Males appear to suffer from the disease more frequently than females. It does not occur among domestic animals living in infected villages nor can the disease be conveyed in the laboratory to monkeys (*Macacus Sinicus*). Even man is to some extent resistant to infection for only one of five persons who swallowed in water from six to eight Guinea worm embryos contained within cyclops developed the worm.

(3) The worm appears under the skin nearly a year after drinking infected water; during this long period the infected person shows no symptoms of the disease.

(4) The worm is very prolific, each female produces about three million young worms.

(5) No other intermediary host for the young Guinea worm than cyclops was found; the usual mode of infection is by drinking water containing infected cyclops.

(6) Cyclops were readily killed in weak solution of potassium permanganate but they reappear in the water after a time having probably developed from eggs which resist the action of this drug. After disinfection with potassium permanganate, wells may become infected again within a month if proper care is not taken to prevent reinfection. Cyclops can be easily removed from water by merely passing it through a piece of fine cloth.

(7) The existence of this easily prevented disease in India is due largely to the indifference, ignorance and prejudices of the people who are careless about the condition of their wells and do not mind drinking water which as been soiled by people bathing in it.

CHAPTER **23**

Onchocerciasis

ON THE PRESENCE OF A FILARIA IN "CRAW-CRAW"

Lancet, 1: 265–266, 1875.

John O'Neill
(1848–1913)

Two years after receiving his M.D. and M.Ch. from Queens University (now National University of Ireland) in 1870, he entered the British Royal Navy. His naval career was short-lived, and he joined the Indian Medical Service in 1875, where he rose to the rank of surgeon lieutenant colonel. He returned to Great Britain in 1896, and later retired in London.

The first recognizable description of Onchocerca volvulus *microfilaria is found in this article.*

Among the natives of the West Coast of Africa there is of frequent occurrence a peculiar skin disease called the craw-craw. Its intractability, contagiousness, and irritating nature so aroused my attention that I was induced to bestow much time on its microscopic examination, and succeeded at length in discovering a filaria which I believe to be the immediate cause of the complaint. I shall make some remarks on the nature, appearance, etc., of the craw-craw, and then proceed to the mode of procuring, and the description of, the filaria.

At first sight a well-marked case suggests the presence of extensive scabies in all its stages of development—the papule, the vesicle, and the pustule; showing itself first in the clefts of the fingers, front of the wrists, and back of the elbows, seldom being found on the face, and always accompanied with intense itching. It should be stated that all the cases examined, about six in number, were in the persons of Negroes, where the native hue of their complexion obscures the blush which, in the case of a "white man," would surround every eruption accompanied with irritation. The papules arise singly and at irregular intervals, increase to the size of a pin's head, feel firm to the touch, and, on account of the reason above stated, appear of the same colour as the surrounding integument. In some cases the papules arrange themselves in a crescentic form, like ringworm; still it appears this is accidental, and that the separate and scattered distribution is the more common. In about two days' time the papule becomes converted into the vesicle, with very little increase in size, and in the course of a couple of days the pustule is developed, rapidly enlarging, and uniting with those in its immediate neighbourhood. In the height of his suffering the patient tears the pustules, and their liberated and desiccated contents produce large and unsightly crusts. Night or day produces little alteration in the amount of itching, the cool of night tending, if anything, to lessen the irritation. The contagiousness of this diseases is so well known that those affected are most studiously avoided. Three days' time is said to be the period at which the complaint shows itself after productive contact, and it is popularly believed that, though a person affected should, in search of its riddance, proceed to the Cape of Good Hope, or some other cool latitude, the disease, which thus merely becomes latent, will burst out with all its former vigour when the unfortunate patient returns to the warmth of the tropics. Sulphur, so beneficial in scabies, is here of doubtful efficacy, and the nostrums of the native "medical man" have frequently failed in bringing relief after six months' application.

Having placed the contents of a pustule beneath the microscope, nothing could be seen except pure pus corpuscles; the vesicle gave no further information, and it was the papule which was at length successfully examined. After many trials I find the readiest way to procure the filaria is to take between the finger and thumb a fold of the skin, so that the papule will be the highest point, then with a very sharp scalpel slice off the epidermis, which may be discarded; now take another slice, which will remove the base of the papule and the cutis vera. This film, moistened with a drop of water, and magnified about 100 diameters, will very likely contain at least one filaria, easily detected in the field by its violent contortions. Thread-like in form, at one time undulating, and now twisted as if into an inexplicable knot, then, having rapidly untwined itself, it curls and coils into many loops. After some minutes beneath the microscope the motions of the little worm become less energetic, and it spends the last moments of its existence in gradually extending itself to near its full length. Measuring it now we find its length about 1/100 inch, and its breadth about 1/2000 inch, and with the exception of the abruptly pointed tail the filaria is of nearly equal breadth throughout its entire length. At the head, or blunted extremity, two small dots are noticed, but their nature could not be determined.

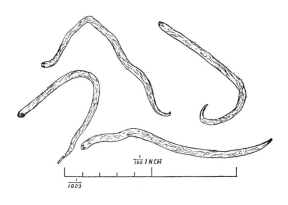

Plate 69. Filariae in "Craw-craw."

If the scalpel used be not sufficiently sharp to completely remove the slice to be examined, it should be detached by means of scissors, and not with forceps; and if the section be taken at a sufficient depth, five or six filariae may be seen in the field together, though the pain thus caused

the Negro has prevented me from obtaining many such specimens.

The accompanying drawing (Plate 69) is taken by means of the camera lucida.

I have to return my best thanks to Dr. Thomson, Glover Expedition, Addah Fort Hospital, for having placed at my disposal those cases of craw-craw which were under his care.

FILARIA VOLVULXUS

Filaria Volvulxus. *In* Andrew Hope Davidson's Hygiene and Diseases of Warm Climates. London: Young J. Pentland, 1893. 1016 pp. Selection from p. 963.

Friedrich Rudolf Leuckart (1822–1898)

Orphaned at an early age, Leuckart came under the influence of his uncle who was professor of zoology at Freiburg. Since, at the time, a medical degree was a prerequisite for zoological studies, he enrolled at Göttingen University which granted him the M.D. in 1845. He remained there as a privat-docent until 1850 when he became professor extraordinary of zoology at Giessen.

The Institute of Zoology and the Zoological Museum at Leipzig were his home from 1870 until his death. He attracted pupils (including Looss, Janicki, Kerbert, Fedchenko, and Lutz) from all over the world, and he wrote on almost every class of the animal kingdom. Many of his original observations are found in his textbook, Die menschlichen Parasiten und die von ihnen herrührenden Krankheiten.

Although this article is reprinted under Leuckart's name, it was written by Manson. He properly assigned credit to Leuckart on the basis of the latter's description which established a new species of parasitic nematode, Onchocerca volvulus. *Happy it is to see such cooperation between two giants of medical parasitology.*

Professor Leuckart informed me some time ago (1890) that he had received from a German medical missionary, practising on the Gold Coast, West Africa, two tumours, each about the size of a pigeon's egg, which had been removed from Negroes,—from the scalp and chest respectively. Both tumours contained several mature filariae—3 to 4 females, 1 to 2 males. These parasites were of considerable length—the female specimens from 60 to 70 cm., the males about half this. They were coiled up together in the form of a ball, about the size of a hazel-nut, and were difficult to unravel. Apparently in the first instance the individual parasites had occupied separate tunnels, but the partitions between them having broken down, these tunnels had become merged into a common cavity. This cavity, in addition to the mature filariae, contained a fluid laden with free embryos.

Professor Leuckart very kindly sent me a slide containing a fragment of the uterus of one of these parasites. It was stuffed with outstretched embryos, resembling in shape and dimensions *F. diurna* and *F. nocturna*. Possibly, compared to these parasites, the embryo *F. volvulxus* was somewhat shorter, and also somewhat broader proportionately, and more abruptly truncated at the cephalic end. Little value, however, can be attached to this observation, as in glycerine or spirit preparations, shape and dimensions are apt to alter considerably. One important feature of *F. diurna* and *F. nocturna* I did not see represented in the embryo *F. volvulxus*, viz., the sheath. Professor Leuckart makes the same remark. It is probable, therefore, judging from the absence of this structure, that *F. volvulxus* is not the mature form of *F. diurna,* and it is certainly not the mature form of *F. nocturna*. Judging also from the absence of sheath, it may be that the life history of this parasite is somewhat different in character from that of *F. diurna* and *F. nocturna*.

Doubtless, in certain districts of Africa this helminthiasis is not uncommon; but, beyond the facts just stated, we possess very little information on the subject. Observations on this and allied matters are very much wanted. From the numerous discoveries, notwithstanding very limited opportunities, made in recent years in African pathology and helminthology, it is evident that many novelties await the investigator of disease in that country.

A NEW DISEASE IN GUATEMALA

Enfermedad nueva en Guatemala. La Juventud Medica, 17: 97–115, 1917. Translated from the Spanish.

Rodolfo Robles
(1878–1939)

Born in Quezaltenango, Guatemala, Robles studied briefly in California, then returned to complete high school in Guatemala. His parents sent him to Rouen, France, where he prepared to enter medicine. In 1904
he received his medical degree in Paris and showed much interest in tropical diseases while under the influence of Emil Brumpt.

He returned to the private practice of medicine in his home town. In 1911 he moved to Guatemala City, where, in addition to his private practice, he held numerous positions in the Faculty of Medicine.

Few important scientific discoveries first appear in a newspaper, but the discovery of Onchocerca volvulus *in Guatemala was published in a fine article in* La Republica *on 29 December 1916. Details of the discovery were reported on 4 March 1917 before* La Sociedad de la Juventud Medica *and published in its journal a few months later. Most of the copies of the issue of* La Juventud Medica *in which the article appeared were destroyed by earthquakes of 1916 and 1917.*

In Latin America onchocerciasis is known as Enfermedad de Robles in honor of its discoverer.

I have the honor to present to you a study that I have been conducting for two years pertaining to the causes and treatment of the illness commonly known by the name of ''Erysipelas of the Coast.''

About two years ago a woman consulted me complaining of recurrent erysipelas of the face which was associated with a high fever, a burning sensation, and pruritis of the affected area; she also complained of losing her sight. A careful examination of the sick woman revealed that this was not erysipelas produced by the *Streptococcus,* but an illness hitherto unknown to me.

Later on, I examined a boy who lived in a place some distance from where my first patient came; however, his symptoms were exactly the same. The ocular symptoms consisted of redness of the conjunctivae and iritis; the usually brilliant and transparent corneas were now dull and without glossiness; there were scattered small leucomas as if the patient had suffered from an ulcerative keratitis; there were periorbital pains, constant severe headaches with periodic exacerbation, and very notable diminution of visual acuity. The boy complained of cloudy vision. Photophobia was so intense that the little boy always walked with the brim of the hat pulled down to shade his eyes from the light; at midday he experienced burning and pruritis in the eyes which felt as though they were full of sand. Occasionally, he would say he was in darkness, but this never lasted more than a quarter of an hour; usually for two or three minutes. There was edema of the eyelids, the forehead, and the superior lip. The cheeks were puffed up with shiny, dry, scaly lesions that resembled chronic eczema; also there was a greenish coloration of both cheeks as you would see in ecchymosis of several days' duration. When touched, the edema was hard, leaving no digital impression. The ears were much increased in size with the external ear pushed forward; the lobe was edematous, scaly, dry, and whitish.

On his forehead the boy had a tumor the size of a cherry which, according to his mother, had been there for several years. When the tumor was extirpated and opened, I found that it enclosed a fine worm, white and ball-shaped, with the characteristics of a filaria. I understood then that the "erysipelas" lesions surely were due to the presence of this parasite. The child's appearance the following day was completely different; the edema as well as the redness of the conjunctiva had disappeared. The child, endowed with rare intelligence, explained to me very clearly that the headaches and periorbital pain had ceased completely. The clouding of his vision had disappeared so that now he could see perfectly; the light did not bother him any longer; the pruritis and gritty sensation were no longer present, and he added, "It is curious that today I know I have a wound on my forehead but I do not feel the severe headache that I always had." The boy also explained to me that on the farm where he lived there were other children with the same illness.

The dissection of the parasite was extremely difficult because it seemed to be sewn into the tumor itself. Extremely fragile, it broke at the slightest pull. However, after a laborious effort, I extracted a whole piece that measured almost 30 cm [sic]. I showed the parasite to my esteemed companion and friend, Doctor Maximo Santa Cruz, who confirmed that it was a "Filaridia." The thick cuticle and the very obvious transverse striations made me suspect that it was of the genus *Onchocerca*; however, not having the head, the tail, or a male, I was unable to identify the parasite fully. It was not until later, having extracted other cysts and digesting them in a dog's stomach for five hours, that I obtained the samples which today I have the honor to present before this society.

Although complete identification has not been possible, it looks very much like the *Onchocerca*

volvulus described by Leuckart in 1893; however, the characteristics described in Brumpt and Castellani do not coincide exactly with my observations. The size of the adult female is always between 28 to 40 cm in length, 300 μ in width. In the examples of males that we have, there is also a variation in sizes: length from 24 mm to 42 mm, and width 200 μ. The papillas of the tail which Brumpt regards as characteristic are not constant in number or size. The details of the spicula are also slightly different. The eggs also have different details, as you may observe in the preparation that is under the microscope; they are elliptical, more round than the elongated form described by Brumpt. Only one longitudinal lengthening seems different, the other is rudimentary; this lengthening is formed by the overlapping of the cuticle. The embryo is 250 μ long by 8 to 10 μ wide; it is clearly marked with a V form. We were able to observe other spots, similar to those in nocturnal filaria. The female, now on display, was placed, live, under the microscope. We could follow the release of the eggs by the vulva; these came out in great abundance, one after the other, but almost immediately they opened at the cuticle. The microfilaria were initially sluggish; but after a few seconds, the movements became very rapid, especially at the posterior two-thirds. These movements consisted of moving the tail from right to left, curling and uncurling it very rapidly, and whipping forcefully the cells in the preparation. The anterior one-third has a slower undulation as is ordinarily seen in serpents. The female, pale yellow-white in color, has a blunt anterior extremity; in contrast, the tapering of the tail is uniform and progressive, unlike other authors have stated. It is found uncurled in the cysts, but, if it is touched with any instrument or if the animal is killed, it curls up instantly. The very small, circular, unarmed mouth is followed by a strong esophagus, but the cuticle is thick and folded at the lips. The body is striated. These thick striations, very conspicuous on the body, fade toward the posterior extremity. Because of these striations, the body is extremely elastic; however, if you pull it too much the external cuticle will break, leaving the internal organs intact, and since they are more resistant they give the appearance of a tail.

The cysts vary in size from that of a pinhead to that of a chicken egg, but the most common size is that of an almond. They are generally situated in the subcutaneous tissues, but we have found them on the dermis, in the aponeurosis of the muscle, and the cranial periosteum. When they touch the bone, either because of the continuous movement or because the animal secretes a toxin, a rarifying osteitis is produced which causes perforation of the cranium, leaving an orifice similar to Doyen's trephine [Eugene Louis Doyen (1859–1916), a French surgeon who described an operation for pericardial paracentesis requiring perforation of the sternum with a trephine— Eds.]. In four cases of 500 I operated upon, a complete perforation was found. In one of these four cases, the cyst rested directly on the meninges.

The cyst is formed by a hard, fibrous tissue, almost cartilaginous in some cases, and like recently formed avascular fibrous tissue. The thickness of the wall is ordinarily from three to five millimeters in the larger cysts and two millimeters in the smaller ones; the common shape is like a lentil, but they can be oval or round. They are located mainly on the head, where they tend to be localized in the temporo-parietal region. The order of frequency is as follows: the occipital region, then the frontal; commonly three to four fingers distant from the hairline; they may be present over the mastoid region and in the skin of the forehead, but here they are rare. On the hip they usually are found three fingers below the superior border of the iliac crest and a short distance from the anterior superior iliac spine. In addition, they can be found in the insertion of the muscles, of the thorax, of the abdomen, and of the extremities of the body; however, they are very rare in these regions, contrary to what other authors affirm.

Many times the occipital and cervical lymph nodes contained parasites. In other cases, lymph node enlargement did not exist in proximity to the cysts.

Those on the cranium may be motile, but more commonly they are fixed, simulating to expert hands a true exostosis. We call attention to this point since on many occasions what I thought was an osseous exostosis was in reality a subaponeurotic cyst. Those cysts that had perforated were found by accident as an incision was made. It is impossible to recognize them any other way, even by the most expert palpation of the scalp. In the other regions of the body they are mobile, and if there is slight resistance they are easily palpated; otherwise, they are difficult to palpate.

The cyst is hard; only on rare occasions, when the parasite is dead, is it soft. I have observed this in the cysts injected with a solution of mercuric iodide. When the parasite dies or for other reasons unknown to me the cyst turns soft, it diminishes in size and disappears. This phenomenon I saw in a boy kept in my house under observation for several months. Some patients also reported this occurrence to us. In general, the cyst does not disappear but persists up to ten years, according to trustworthy testimony from two of our patients; in these, the extracted parasites were found to be alive.

When carefully examined, these cysts were always found to have fibrous extensions. These are of variable length; in many cases there are two, one at each end of the tumor. This permits the hypothesis that the cyst is always open and in communication with the tissues that surround it and that the parasites pass through these openings to nourish themselves, leaving paths marked by these fibrous extensions. The exit of the embryos could not be explained otherwise; after all, the parasites could not live wrapped in an avascular fibrous layer and without nourishment for long years. A patient who lived far from the endemic area had a cyst for seven years in a very thick fibrous avascular layer, but with live parasites inside. In several cysts extirpated with part of the tissue that surrounded them we could see, after submersion in water, a parasite appear through a minute orifice.

When a cyst is opened with much care so as not to hurt the parasite, and the cyst squeezed vigorously, there appears at the openings a series of loops which are produced by the coiling of the filarias. These are attached to the mucofibrous tissue that forms the interior of the cyst and yet seem to have few connections with the internal wall of the cyst. With care the cyst can be everted like the finger of a glove. This mucofibrous tissue is impregnated with a yellow substance which is the same color as the liquid squeezed from it and in which thousands of eggs and embryos swim. In many cases upon opening the lymph node and finding this yellow coloration, we have been able to affirm immediately that it is parasitized.

It is impossible by dissection—unless done in

water, carefully, and requiring many long hours—to extract the parasite intact. To obtain our specimens, we digested the cyst for five hours in a dog's stomach; artificial digestion can be used also, but this takes a long time and is incomplete.

The disease is found in a wide strip of land that extends from the periphery of the Volcano of "Fuego" up to the Atitlan, heights that vary from 2,000 to 4,000 feet above sea level. In several places the division is abrupt. Of two farms, one at 2,000 feet and the other at 2,200, one could observe cases in the second and none in the first. We were able to make very interesting studies at the "El Baúl" farm where two ranches were located, one situated at 2,300 feet and the other at 2,000. Of the same farm, both ranches were in constant communication. In the higher ranch, all inhabitants have this disease. In the lower one none of those who never left there was afflicted. Only those workers who during the day picked coffee at heights varying between 2,300 and 2,500 feet were infected, although they had never slept at the higher ranch or stayed there after sundown. Consequently, we can say logically that these individuals acquired the illness during the day and at the higher ranch. Many of them have married women who have never been at the high ranch and, although they live with their husbands, they have never been infected. Similarly, men living at the lower ranch who are not infected are sometimes married to women from the higher level who are infected. Inhabitants of both ranches drink exactly the same water and have exactly the same customs and the same jobs; the infected farms are on the summit of a mountain or in a ravine, some near a river, others very far from water; consequently, the presence of water seems not to have any influence, contrary to what Brumpt says. These are plantations of sugar cane or coffee, and these cultivations do not have any influence.

The descending rivers start in regions where this illness does not exist, pass to the endemic zone, and continue their course through many other plantations which are situated below 2,000 feet and are free of the disease. On many farms where this parasite exists, water comes from a fountain which passes through iron pipes to the house; the farms below drink the same water, and they do not have the disease. In consequence, we can say, logically, that according to all probabilities, the illness is not transmitted by water. The Pantaleon farm uses unfiltered water from the river which drains all the infected farms; none the less, no cases are found there. The same is true with the Xata Farm. We can also add that there probably is no contamination by excrement in the water. The same insects and other blood-sucking parasites exist above and below the infected zone. We can even say, as you all well know, that in the farms of 2,000 feet, the number of these blood-sucking insects is considerable. From a careful investigation, we deduce that only two mosquitoes [sic] of the genus *Simulium*: the *S. sanboni* and the *S. dinelli,* exist between 2,000 and 4,000 feet above sea level. In the places where these insects were most numerous, the largest number of ill patients was found. . . . Mr. Howards, chief of the entomology office in Washington, tells me they differ a little. These mosquitoes that I am going to pass on to you are known by the name of "mosco rodadores" (vagrant mosquito). Black and red, they bite for five minutes, sucking blood to the point where you can see the abdomen fill progressively, giving them a red coloration. When they are completely full, they become so heavy they can hardly fly, and many times they fall to earth. In one of the farms, probably the most cruelly attacked, I undressed the torsos of 10 children and exposed them, at ten o'clock in the morning, to the bite of these mosquitoes, begging them not to make any move to brush the insects away. The majority of these insects rested on the ears, cheeks, and neck; an occasional one over the forehead or thorax. Among these children there was one with the disease in an acute stage; his face was red and swollen. For every mosquito that rested on the other chronically ill children, the child in the acute stage was bitten by five, as if the red color attracted the mosquitoes. On these farms where uncinariasis and malaria cause so much damage, the resulting anemia still leaves the ears with some color; it is precisely on the ear and around it that the mosquito chooses to bite. These insects do not bite on the anterior part of the face because the individual sees them and frightens them away. The hands and the legs are in continuous movement because of their work and are not bitten. The women who have long hair down their back, having their ears and neck covered, seldom suffer from this illness. For these reasons, I believe I can hypothesize that these are the intermediate hosts. At any rate, it is necessary to demonstrate this, and it has not been done. Hour by hour the blood has been examined in numerous preparations, during the day and during the night, and we have never been able to find the microfilarias except once, pricking a region near a tumor. The lymphangitis in the acute stage culminates in cracking of the skin where an abundant serous liquid flows and, here, we believe, the germ exists. The work we plan to undertake will be based on this point.

The symptoms of the acute and chronic stages differ. In the acute stage, when the cysts are in the head, which is common, a swelling appears all over the face. The skin becomes tight, red, painful, absolutely simulating facial erysipelas produced by the *Streptococcus*. The temperature is very high, 39° or 40° centigrade. The children become debilitated; convulsions and delirium occur; the conjunctivae are red and extremely injected; the ears are considerably enlarged. Their eyelids are swollen, preventing the patient's opening his eyes; the lips (usually the upper one) are swollen; the neck, too, shows slight swelling. The patient complains of generalized pruritis, of formication, a subjective sensation that animals are walking all over the face. If they scratch, they experience a burning sensation and severe pain. The symptoms in the eyes are very marked. Periorbital pains with terrible exacerbations, conjunctivae and cornea very injected, sensation of foreign bodies inside the eyelids and in some cases an iritis complicate with symptomatic courtship this dangerous clinical picture. The cornea has the characteristics of a punctate keratitis. The examination of the fundus by Dr. Pacheco has not revealed anything abnormal.

Other times there are terrible neuralgias in all of the trigeminal region. The patient hears humming and sounds of a hammer and develops intermittent or continuous deafness. Examination of the tympanum was normal. We have not observed anything that deserves pointing out regarding the tongue or the olfactory senses.

If the lesion is on one of the extremities, this swells considerably; the skin is smooth, shiny, red, tense, and warm simulating erysipelas. Dermography is very noticeable in the individuals of white skin, and pruritic eczema is found in children. After three to four days the fever falls slowly, and the patient enters a chronic stage. The swellings persist much longer, for days, up to months in the same stage; but usually at the end of 20 days they diminish notably. The periodic pain persists as much in the acute stage as in the chronic. We have never observed lesions on the thorax, the abdomen, or on the testicles, but we do not deny the possibility.

Chronic stage: The face: The cheeks are always indurated, the skin eczematous, pigmented and lustrous, with an absolutely typical greenish livid color; elephantiasis of the ears, which are doubled in size, bent forward with skin wrinkled and scaly; the ear lobe extremely thick, double the normal width. On the limbs of the body there is a uniform swelling with induration as seen in elephantiasis of the Arabs. However, the typical greenish color suggests the diagnosis instantaneously.

The eyes: The eyelids have very little edema, the conjunctivae always red with frequent pterygia and punctate keratitis. In the iris there is always a color change. It is dull, no longer shiny, the pupils are commonly deformed in very advanced cases. With time it becomes reduced to pinpoint size and completely closes; in many cases downward deviation occurs. If the cases are very old, sight diminishes progressively from seeing objects in a slight haze to complete blindness. Many of the patients with normal pupils are completely blind; this blindness can develop either abruptly or progressively. In all cases photophobia exists with greater or lesser intensity. There are some patients who complain of seeing very little during the night; the majority do not see well during the day, but can move around during the night.

When the tumors exist on extremities, there is always a slight numbness associated with them. One of our operated patients lived for five years outside of the infected zone, and extirpation of a solitary tumor on the hip brought a notable improvement in the ocular symptoms the following day. From this example, we can only conclude that the toxin of the parasite is the cause of the vision disturbances.

Treatment: We have used injections of "914" intravenously in high doses, without any results. The injections of mercuric iodide into the interior of the cyst kills the parasite, but there is an aggravation of the symptoms with considerable edema, diminution of vision, and so on, that does not cease until many days afterward. The best treatment that we have found until now is the complete ablation of the cysts with all the fibrous extensions. The technique we employ is extremely simple: with a cocaine solution, 2:1,000 and five drops of adrenalin, we make intradermal injections and infiltrate subcutaneously two cm around the cysts. We then outline between two incisions a strip of skin one and a half cm to two cm wide; with the skin removed we explore with the finger to detect the fibrous extensions, then dissect these and the cyst. We then suture very carefully, without concerning ourselves about hemorrhage which many times may be abundant, but which yields immediately to the strong compression bandage which we loosen after 12 hours. With this simple technique we have been able to perform more than 1,000 operations without a complication.

Using this very weak solution we have been able to remove up to 17 cysts in a single individual, not using more than nine centigrams of cocaine and five drops of adrenalin of the solution.

THE INSECT TRANSMISSION OF *ONCHOCERCA VOLVULUS* (Leuckart, 1893) The Cause of Worm Nodules in Man in Africa

British Medical Journal, 1: 129–133, 1927. Selection from pp. 129–132.

Donald Breadalbane Blacklock (1879–1955)

After receiving his medical education at Edinburgh University, Blacklock joined the staff of the Liverpool School of Tropical Medicine in 1911 as research assistant in its laboratory at Runcorn, thus forming a connection that was unbroken until his retirement in 1945. He was successively director of the Runcorn Research Laboratory; lecturer in parasitology; professor of tropical diseases in Africa; first director of the Sir Alfred Lewis Jones Research Laboratory at Freetown, Sierra Leone; professor of parasitology; and professor of tropical hygiene. During World War II, when over 60 years of age, Blacklock undertook a government malaria mission to Sierra Leone with the rank of surgeon captain in the Royal Naval Reserve. In addition to writing many papers, he collaborated with Dr. Thomas Southwell in publishing the Guide to Human Parasitology *which remains a standard work on the subject.*

The Simulium fly was proved to be the vector of Onchocerciasis as described in this original report.

Among the families of parasitic nematodes which infest man none surpasses in diversity of interest the family Filariidae. This is due both to the pathogenic effects produced by some species, and also to the strange biological adaptations in the human host and in those insect vectors so far known. Complex problems are presented by the larval habits of different species, some living in the blood stream, others having their chief habitat in the skin; some showing the remarkable phenomenon of periodicity, the causes of which are still obscure. No less important are its historical associations; since it was with the species *Filaria bancrofti* of this family that Manson worked when, in 1878, he made the discovery—destined to revolutionize the tropics—of the part played by insects in the transmission of human disease. From this observation dates all that research into the association of insects with disease which has already produced such significant results and which is daily achieving fresh discoveries in the ever-widening domain of human and animal parasitology.

The Genus *Onchocerca*

Included in the family Filariidae is the genus Onchocerca (Diesing, 1841), which has one species, *O. volvulus,* parasitic in man in Africa, another species, *O. caccutiens*—so closely allied with *O. volvulus* that some authorities consider it identical—parasitic in man in Central America, and several species parasitic in domestic and other animals in various parts of the Old and the New World. Naturally the two species which are parasites of man are of great direct importance. They have a restricted geographical distribution, the ill effects produced by them being confined to the limited regions in which they occur. Of a different order, and affecting man much more widely, are the indirect ill effects produced by those species which infest domestic animals, especially cattle.

Onchocerca volvulus (Leuckart, 1893) infests man in tropical Africa with an intensity which varies in different localities. In West Africa there are large areas in which a very high percentage of the total population is infested. Prout (1901) in Sierra Leone was one of the first to describe it. The worms live in nodules in the subcutaneous and deeper tissues, and give rise to larvae which find their way into the skin; an infested area of skin may contain vast numbers of larvae, so much so that not even the smallest portion can be removed without numerous larvae being found. Different observers have attributed to the worm an etiological significance in the production of very diverse pathological effects, which depend on the distribution of the worm itself in the body and of the larvae in the skin. Several forms of skin disease, itch, ulcers, as well as glandular enlargements, hydrocele, and elephantiasis, are some of the conditions with the production of which this worm is credited.

Mode of Transmission of Onchocerca

The transmitting agents of several of the Filariidae are already known, if we accept invasion of the proboscis as evidence of the insects being capable of transmitting; up to the present time, however, no one has succeeded in demonstrating by what means any species of the genus Onchocerca is transmitted from man to man or from animal to animal. As a result of investigations carried out at intervals during the past four years I believe that I am now in a position to state that the conditions essential to transmission of *O. volvulus* are fulfilled by a biting insect, a species of the genus Simulium, named very appropriately *Simulium damnosum*. These investigations were undertaken in the Konno district of the Sierra Leone Protectorate, where the worm is common. More detailed accounts are being communicated to the *Annals of Tropical Medicine and Parasitology,* in which the first experiments were published in February, 1926.

The Konno District

The Konno district of the Protectorate of Sierra Leone lies to the north of the railway line which traverses the Protectorate from west to east. It is a hilly region drained by several large rivers and a multiplicity of small streams; the hills are in most cases clothed with dense bush right to the summit. Each village has in its immediate vicinity several streams; swampy areas produced by silting up and overflow of the streams are numerous

and biting insects are plentiful. The population is largely agricultural, and both sexes spend much time working on farm lands situated in the dense bush; the streams are used for latrine purposes as well as for washing and drinking. The result is a goitrous population and one heavily infected with urinary schistosomiasis; intestinal diseases, helminthic, protozoal, and bacterial, are rife. The following facts concerning the disease caused by *O. volvulus* demonstrate its prevalence and illustrate the kinds of observation made in order to ascertain its pathogenic effects on the population.

The Subcutaneous Nodules

The character of the subcutaneous nodules produced by *O. volvulus* varies from a smooth, soft, just palpable nodule to a large, irregularly nodular, hard mass of the size of a large walnut. The first type is usually found in the region of the great trochanter, on the ribs, and on the scalp; the second is generally closely associated with joints, more especially the elbow and knee joints; neither type is usually adherent to the skin, but in some cases, especially over the region of the great trochanter, the skin over the nodule is thickened, partly adherent, and polished on the surface from pressure.

Distribution of the Larvae

The larvae of this species were seldom found by me in the blood, only a rare larva being present occasionally in the blood film, and that probably derived from the infected skin. The larvae are present in the skin, and may often be found there in large numbers, even when no nodules can be discovered. They are not, however, evenly distributed over the body; thus, while of 93 persons whom I examined by making four sections of the skin of each—that is, from the scapular, loin, thigh, and ankle region—over 45 per cent proved to be infected with *O. volvulus*. The larvae occurred in these sites in the following order of frequency from the highest to the lowest: loin, thigh, scapular region, and ankle.

Diagnosis of Infection

The presence of the worm in the body may be detected either by puncture of the nodules and the discovery of the larvae in the aspirated fluid, or by cutting off with a razor small pieces of the skin, which are then teased with strong needles in a drop of water, so as to liberate the active larvae; apparently the first discovery of microfilariae in the skin of man by this latter method was made by O'Neill in 1875 on the Gold Coast. The larvae, although they do not live in the blood, have nevertheless to be distinguished from those of *F. bancrofti, L. loa, A. perstans,* and also from *Ag. streptocerca,* the last named being a skin microfilaria described by Macfie and Corson (1922). It was found in the Konno district that only 40 per cent of those who had *O. volvulus* larvae in the skin had also subcutaneous nodules, while of those in whose skin larvae could not be found 16 per cent had nodules. The examination of skin gave, therefore, a higher percentage of positive findings, and it has the advantage of being easier to carry out in natives than puncture of the nodules.

Pathogenic Effects of the Worm

In view of the fact that many observers have recorded severe lesions of the skin, glands, and, in the case of the American human Onchocerca, of the eyes, it was advisable to ascertain whether similar effects would be found in Sierra Leone.

The Eyes—Sixty-one cases in whom the eyes were examined and the skin was searched for larvae yielded 29 instances of *O. volvulus* infection. Only six of the 61 had any abnormal conditions of the eyes and only four of these six belonged to the infected group. The eye conditions pterygium, blepharitis, and defect of vision were not associated with the presence of nodules in the head, and the last named appeared to be rather associated with advancing years than with the infection with *O. volvulus*. The examination revealed the fact that in the Konno population the eyes did not suffer notably from either toxic or other effects produced by the worm.

The Skin—In an examination of 60 people 17 were found whose skin displayed no trace of the disease visible to the unaided eye. This absence of obvious skin disease did not, however, prove to mean that none of these 17 cases was infected; for in point of fact no fewer than eight of them were proved to be infected with *O. volvulus* by the discovery of its larvae in the skin. It was thought that the age of the person might have some bearing on the question, on the assumption that skin disease as a result of infestation might be a tran-

sitory condition on the one hand or a late developing one on the other. Against this, however, was the fact that the youngest case showing larvae in a good skin was 24 years of age, while the oldest was 51. The conclusion reached was that infection with *O. volvulus* does not necessarily connote obvious disease of the skin, although it may often coexist with it.

The Glands—In 68 cases the glands were examined, and it was found that of those having *O. volvulus* larvae in the skin only 27 per cent had enlarged glands, while of those not having larvae in the skin 32 per cent had enlarged glands. Admitting that such skin examination as described must inevitably fail to reveal more than a fair percentage of cases, it may be said that on the whole this investigation did not yield definite evidence of pathogenic effects on the glands.

Thus neither in the case of the eyes, the skin, nor the glands did this Konno population show pathological effects definitely and solely attributable to *O. volvulus* infection. It is nevertheless probable that in localities where hyper-infection with the worm occurs a different clinical picture may be produced; very suggestive of this is the work of Ouzilleau (1913), who ascribes to the agency of *O. volvulus* lymphatic gland enlargement, hydrocele, and elephantiasis, occurring in a region in the Congo where *F. bancrofti* could not be found while *O. volvulus* was common. Dyce Sharp (1926), who has made a study of onchocerciasis in Nigeria, observes that the larvae of *O. volvulus* occur with great frequency in hydrocele fluid, and that, while possibly innocuous, they may well stand in some causal relationship to this condition as well as to elephantiasis.

Experiments to Discover the Transmitting Agent

The investigation of the problem of transmission was begun in 1923–24 and continued in 1925 and 1926. The question was approached from the view that, as the larvae occur not in the blood but in the skin, any blood-sucking arthropod to be capable of transmitting it would have to damage the skin and dislodge the larvae in its efforts to reach blood. The Congo floor maggot *Auchmeromyia lutcola,* common in Konno houses, seemed a possible agent in so far as producing damage to the skin is concerned, and specimens of this were first dissected, but no larvae were found. At several villages in December, 1923, and January, 1924, it was observed that *Simulium damnosum* Theob. was biting viciously and in great numbers beside the streams; it was noticed that although this species attacked the skin readily it was slow in reaching the blood and appeared to have difficulty in getting through the skin; this delay led to the belief that, in biting, this insect inflicted considerable damage on the skin, a belief which was strengthened by an examination of the biting apparatus of the fly. One hundred specimens captured were examined for larvae in the gut, but nothing was found, and owing to pressure of other work the search was abandoned temporarily.

Discovery of *O. volvulus* Larvae in the Gut of *Simulium damnosum*

In 1925 at another village the search was resumed, and this time with success; infection of the gut with larvae morphologically identical with those of *O. volvulus* was discovered in 20 out of 780 flies—that is, in 2.6 per cent— captured on unselected boys. Two men known to be infected with larvae of *O. volvulus* in the skin and in whom no other microfilariae could be detected were then submitted to the bites of the flies; as a result the percentage of gut infection in the fly rose at once to 17. The most heavily infected person was then submitted alone to the flies, the following regions being exposed to them in successive experiments: the loins and upwards gave 28 per cent of gut infections; the waist and hips only gave 59 per cent of gut infections; finally the person was exposed so that the flies could bite only on a four-inch-wide band of skin round the body, having the nodules, which were present near each trochanter, in the centre of the band; this experiment gave a positive gut infection in the flies of 80 per cent.

Development in the Thorax of *Simulium damnosum*

During the dissection of the thorax of 1,320 wild Simulium caught on unselected boys 15, or 1.1 per cent, were found to have developmental forms of some nematode larva present in the muscles of the thorax. Extensive examinations of samples of the population and of animals and a study of the biting habits of the fly led to the exclusion of other members of Filariidae and to

the conclusion that the thoracic forms found were in all probability derived from *O. volvulus*. Flies fed on selected cases as described above were kept alive as long as possible and the thorax dissected; the effect was seen in a progressive rise of the percentage of thorax infection, first to 10 per cent, then to 32 per cent, and finally, in flies fed on the four-inch band in the heavily infected case, to the high figure of 82 per cent. No development actually into the head was observed in the course of these experiments, although one form was found partly embedded in the posterior part of the head. It was therefore impossible to make any definite statement at this time beyond recording the fact that the larvae of *O. volvulus* are readily ingested by *S. damnosum,* and that development up to a certain stage occurs in the gut and thorax of this blood-sucking insect.

Development of *O. volvulus* in the Head of *Simulium damnosum*

In 1926 a further series of experiments was carried out and evidence was obtained that the development in the thorax continues with progressive increase in size and morphological modification till the larvae, having invaded the head region of Simulium, finally reach the proboscis. They enter the labium of the fly, where they remain coiled up and ready to emerge, which they do at once when provided with favourable conditions. The experiments are too numerous and long to give in detail here, but they may be summarized briefly as follows.

In six experiments 502 flies were allowed to feed freely on the heavily infected case referred to above; of this total 201 were dissected at a period later than the third day, and in the thorax of 127 of them (63 per cent) developmental forms were discovered; in the head developmental forms were found in 34 (16 per cent). The earliest infection of the posterior part of the head was five days, and of the anterior part of the head seven days, after the infecting feed. The development of *O. volvulus* in the fly from the time it is taken up from the skin until it reaches the labium and is mature and presumably capable of infecting a human being occupies about ten days. During this time the larva has undergone great changes in form; not only so, it has also increased in size from about 250μ long by 7μ broad to over 760μ long by 20μ broad.

Summary of Development in the Fly

The skin forms taken into the gut of Simulium accumulate at the margin of the blood coagulum lying between this and the gut wall. They are very active and the majority pass out of the gut within 24 hours and may be found in the posterior part of the thoracic muscles in 48 hours. They have altered completely in shape, having increased in width and acquired a characteristic caudal spine-like appendage which may be either straight or much curved; they have also lost a great deal of their mobility. Several moults appear to occur before the form is reached which is capable of invading the head. The advanced thoracic forms show progressive stages of development of the alimentary canal, which is differentiated first into anterior and posterior portions, of different calibre and separated from each other; these unite later to form the uniform gut of the proboscis form, which runs from the head to open in a slit-like anus in front of the tail (see Plate 70).

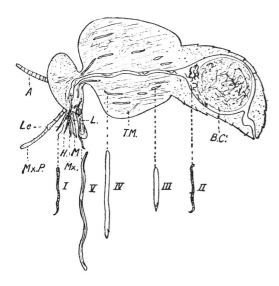

Plate 70. Diagram illustrating the development of *O. volvulus* larvae in the tissues of *Simulium damnosum*. (I) Larva from infected skin. (II) Larva in midgut. (III) Larva in thoracic muscles (early stage). (IV) Larva in thoracic muscles (late stage). (V) Larva in head and labium. (A) Antenna. (B–C) Blood coagulum. (T–M) Thoracic muscles. (L) Labium. (Le) Labrum-epipharynx. (H) Hypopharynx. (M) Mandible. (Mx) Maxilla. (Mx.P) Maxillary palp.

The Effect of Temperature on Development

Differences in the rate of development were noted at different temperatures. It became evident that, although almost identical percentages of flies had acquired infection at the higher and lower temperatures used, the lower temperature had a retarding influence on development to such an extent that the flies usually died before the head became infected. Thus of 78 flies which lived for six days or over and were dissected, the absolute maximum temperature being 88° F., the absolute minimum 49°, and the average minimum 58°, only five—that is, 6 per cent—became infected in the head. Better results as regards head infection were obtained with an absolute maximum temperatue of 87°, an absolute minimum of 63°, and an average minimum of 68°. In these circumstances, of 52 flies which lived six days or over and were dissected, 16—that is, 31 per cent—were found infected in the head.

Ovarian and Parasitic Development

In flies allowed to feed on severely infected skin and then kept in tubes a heavy mortality ensued. Part of this appears to be due to the large number of worms developing in the fly's tissues; part was attributable to the ill effects of retention of the ova owing to the experimental conditions not being suitable for oviposition. Low temperature retarded the development of the ovaries as well as of the parasites, and the two processes presented a definite correspondence in developmental rate. A correspondence of this kind is to be expected if the fly, after ovipositing, is to be capable of infecting at the next time of biting.

Emergence of Larvae from the Head of *Simulium damnosum*

When the larvae had taken up their final position in the labium and were fully developed they were observed to emerge spontaneously into a drop of monkey serum which had been warmed; this phenomenon evidently depends on a definite attraction exercised by such serum, because a drop of warmed normal saline solution did not produce the same stimulating effect on them. Apart from such spontaneous emergence the larvae were seen to emerge when very light pressure was applied to the head region with a needle.

Experimental Inoculations into Animals

Two monkeys were inoculated intra- and subcutaneously, the first in the flank and the second in the head, with advanced forms of larvae contained in the heads of flies. Neither of the monkeys showed any immediate reaction, the incisions healing by first intention, nor has any development so far become apparent. As, however, only two months have elapsed since the first animal was inoculated it is too early to express any opinion as to the ultimate result.

The Habits of *Simulium damnosum*

Simulium damnosum Theob. in the Konno district is a small stout fly about 3 mm long, almost black, and of inconspicuous appearance. It belongs to the same group of flies as those which are sometimes called Buffalo gnats, Turkey gnats, and black flies, and is common in many parts of equatorial Africa. It occurs in Uganda, where it is known as Mbwa, and in the Sudan, where it is called Kilteb; in the Konno it is called Mooli, and in Lokkoh, Poondee gootena = short mosquito. It is a notoriously vicious biter and is much dreaded in regions where it is numerous. The fly is to be found in the bush and grass in the vicinity of water; collectors always went to the waterside in order to find it easily. It dislikes strong sunlight and heavy rain; it likes shade and humidity; a great deal of its movement is by crawling and hopping, rather in the manner of a flea. In tubes it moves towards the light, a fact which can be made use of in changing flies from one tube to another. Only the female was found biting, and the biting habit is diurnal. It proved unwilling to come out far in strong sunlight to feed; it preferred to feed, if situated in fairly open country, during the hours when the sun was not strong, the early morning and late in the afternoon. It makes no sound and bites most frequently low down on the body, from the waist downwards, choosing especially shaded portions of the legs. The presence of overhead shade gives it an opportunity of biting higher up on the body. Palm-tree climbers state that it bites them in the dense palm bush even when they are far above the ground. The fly takes from one and a half to five minutes to engorge; when it has fed it looks remarkably distended, and is so heavy that it flies with difficulty. It was not found to follow man for any distance, and it is not a fly which attracts the attention by flying round the face. One may, in fact, walk along a path without seeing a single fly, although in the grass a yard or two away there may be dozens of them concealed. For this reason many Europeans who pass from rest house to rest house, and do not frequent the streams and marshy areas, may be entirely unaware of the presence of this noxious insect.

With this brief account of the habits of *Simulium damnosum* we may conclude the section dealing with *O. volvulus*. From the experiments recorded it appears extremely probable that this worm is transmitted from man to man by the bite of *Simulium damnosum*. At the same time it must be stated that the only unequivocal evidence will be that furnished by recovery of adult worms from animals or man infested by larvae which have developed in laboratory-bred flies as a result of feeding upon *O. volvulus* infested human beings. Such evidence I regret that I am not in a position to place before you, as up to the present time I have not been able to obtain laboratory-bred flies.

We may now pass on to consider very shortly two other species of the genus Onchocerca—namely, the American human parasite *Onchocerca caecutiens,* and a parasite of domestic cattle, *Onchocerca gibsoni*.

Onchocerca caecutiens

This species was erected by Brumpt not so much on morphological as on biological grounds; it is a parasite of man in certain parts of Central America, and produces in man worm nodules which occur almost exclusively on the head. Brumpt (1919) named this species *caecutiens* ("blinding") because of the very remarkable account given by Robles in Guatemala of the severe eye symptoms and lesions which are associated with its presence, and which disappear with dramatic suddenness after removal of the nodules from the head: Robles (1919) records several instances in which the nodules formed by this species had eroded right through the cranial vault and were lying directly upon the meninges. On epidemiological grounds Robles several years ago suggested that two species of Simulium locally called "coffee flies"—that is, *S. dinelli* and *S. samboni*—were possibly the transmitting agents of this worm.

This American species is considered by some

to be morphologically identical with the African one which has been discussed above. One of the points upon which Brumpt lays stress in the differential diagnosis of the two species is that the nodules caused by the American species are situated in the head in 99 per cent of cases, whereas the African species causes nodules which in only one per cent of cases are situated in the head. I may record here the fact that in one village in the Konno district I recently found that many of those who had nodules had them in the head. In a population of 66 examined, 33 (50 per cent) presented nodules in some region of the body. Of the 33 who had nodules, eight (24 per cent) had them on the head, the diagnosis being made by puncture. On searching for an explanation for this unusual incidence two points were noted which appeared suggestive. The first was that this little village of eleven houses occupied less space than any other village of the same

number of houses seen by me; the houses were arranged in a close ring practically touching each other. The second fact was that the village was shaded by large trees, as was also the path down to the river beside which the village was situated. In such a place as this it was possible for *Simulium damnosum* to attack the upper parts of the body without exposing itself to the sunlight. I concluded that it might be because of the local conditions as regards high shade that so many persons in this village presented nodules on the head. From inquiries which I have made from persons familiar with the conditions on the coffee plantation in Guatemala it appears that coffee in that country is most commonly grown under overhead shade. This fact might partly explain the incidence of the nodules of this species in the head, more especially if the lower parts of the body are covered by trousers and some kind of footwear. . . .

CHAPTER **24**

Trichinosis

DESCRIPTION OF A PECULIAR ANIMALCULE OBSERVED IN A HUMAN MUSCLE

Manuscript to the Editor of the London Medical Gazette, 10 February 1835.

James Paget
(1814–1899)

At age 16, Paget, the youngest of the nine survivors of 17 children, was apprenticed to a local surgeon in Yarmouth, his native town. At 20, he enrolled as a medical student in St. Bartholomew's Hospital in London.

As a result of financial reverses, Paget's father, a brewer and ship owner, could not pay the necessary dressing fee to the surgeon of St. Bartholomew's and, therefore, Paget became clinical clerk to a physician, who required no such fee. Nevertheless, at 22, he passed the examination for membership in the Royal College of Surgeons. He earned his living primarily by teaching and by acting as subeditor of the London Medical Gazette.

Although he is remembered chiefly for his original description of the diseases that bear his name, Paget made numerous contributions to medical education. So brilliant was he as a lecturer that he earned the praise of Prime Minister William Gladstone. He finally became president of the Royal College of Surgeons, surgeon extraordinary to Queen Victoria and sergeant surgeon to the Queen.

The chronology of the discovery of Trichina *larvae was recorded in a letter by Paget to* Lancet, *5 March 1866:*

On the Discovery of Trichina

. . . The man in whom the trichina was first observed died at the hospital on January 30th, 1835. Three days later the dissection of the body was commenced. The report soon ran through the dissecting-rooms that there was another body with spiculae of bone in the muscles. Examining some of these spiculae with a lens, I soon found that they were cysts, and almost directly afterwards ascertained that nearly every cyst con-

tained a small worm coiled up. I was anxious to observe them with a microscope, and, possessing none, I applied to the only man of science whom I at that time knew in London, Mr. Children, principal keeper of the Natural History collection at the British Museum. He, I think, had no microscope, and he therefore took me to Mr. Robert Brown; and I shall not soon forget the feeling approaching to awe when I went to one whom I had long looked upon as the first physiological botanist of his time. I remember that, when Mr. Children entered his room, he said, "Brown, do you know anything about intestinal worms?" and the answer was, "No, thank heaven—nothing whatever." Mr. Brown at once lent me his simple dissecting microscope, with which I soon observed structures in the worm which were before invisible. He himself dexterously pulled a worm from a cyst, and I believe I still possess my sketch of it. As soon as the discovery of the entozoon was made known in our dissecting-room, portions of muscles were distributed far and wide, and among those to whom they were first carried was Mr. Owen.

I was invited, as the discoverer of the entozoon, to communicate the facts respecting it to the Abernethian Society, and I did so on Feb. 6th, the chair being occupied by Dr. Arthur Farre, who had himself investigated the structures of the worm with great accuracy. An abstract of my communication is in the second volume of the Abernethian Society's Transactions. It contains a description of the entozoon—not indeed complete, but I believe not inaccurate, except in a blundering endeavour to assign its zoological relations. I proposed immediately afterwards, on the recommendation of Mr. Stanley, to send a description of it to the Medical Gazette, *but from this I was dissuaded; and the admirable memoir of Professor Owen, much more complete and exact in zoological detail than anything I could have written, was communicated to the Zoological Society on Feb. 24.*

> *I am, Sir, yours faithfully,*
> *James Paget*

We have chosen to publish Paget's hitherto unpublished report to the London Medical Gazette. *The material has been reproduced as faithfully as possible from Paget's handwritten notes which are difficult to decipher and erratically punctuated, and which bear many interlinear alterations.*

To the Editor of the London Medical Gazette.
Sir:

The following circumstances having excited considerable interest, I have at the suggestion of Mr. Stanley, drawn up the subjoined notes, which you will I hope deem worthy of insertion in your journal. I am Sir

Your obedient servant,
James Paget

St. Bartholomew's Hospital
10 February 1835—

The first case in which the existence of this peculiar animalcule was observed was in the body of an Italian, Paulo Bianchi aged 40 who had been admitted into St. Bartholomew's hospital two or three months previously under the care of Dr. Roupell, with slight cough with purulent expectoration, profuse diarrhea, edema of the lower extremities and great debility. At the time of his admission, the urine which he passed in very large quantities was albuminous, and it continued so in a slighter degree till his death which took place on the 30th of January. While he was in the Hospital the dropsy decreased and the cough and expectoration remained very slight but the diarrhea continued with great obstinacy and gradually exhausted him.

At the post mortem examination, both lungs were found to contain tubercules in various states, and in the right were three or four cavities of different sizes. The mucous membrane of the lower end of the ileum was ulcerated and the kidneys presented the peculiar appearance particularly described by Dr. Bright.

When the body was being dissected three days after death immediately on reflecting the integuments there were observed scattered over the muscles an increased number of minute whitish specks. On closer examination with the microscope these I found to be cysts containing small worms as represented in the accompanying drawing (Plate 71, Fig. 1). Each cyst is of an elliptical shape pointed at the extremities, about 1/40 of an inch in length, apparently closed at all points, and lying in the cellular tissue connecting the muscular fibres to which it is closely connected. Within

it, is contained another of an oval or vesicular form, the substance by which they are united being opaque and more dense at the extremities than at the sides. In this latter cell is the worm which is about 1/25 of an inch in length, and is coiled up in a spiral form. When removed from its cell in which it seems to float loosely in a clear fluid it is found to be thread-shaped, bluntly rounded at both ends, but tapering towards that which appears to be the head and which lies at the outside of the coil. Its organization appears to be of the most simple description—at the larger extremity is a linear opening in the communis cutis with a simple canal running along the whole length of the body—no appearance of fibres either longitudinal or circular can be detected though from the movements observed in the living animals, the former must necessarily exist. Its coats are perfectly transparent and through them may be seen two lines running along the axis of the body, marking probably the outlines of the intestinal canal, while towards the tail four or five lines are seen crossing the space between them transversely—in a fresh specimen.

When carefully taken out of its cell it may be seen to uncoil and uncoil [sic] itself with more or less rapidity, and when placed in a drop of water will continue for a considerable time to move the smaller extremity in different directions.

Nearly all the specimens examined presented the above characters—in some cases however two worms were enclosed in the same cell one lying at each end of the inner cavity and touching or overlapping each other in the middle—in a few others the worm instead of being coiled up spirally was in the form of a figure of 8 (Plate 71, Fig. 2). None were in a state of further development; very few cells were found empty and no worms were detected out of the cysts. There were found, too, occasionally small opaque bodies closely resembling cells but not containing any worms (Plate 71, Fig. 3).

They were abundantly distributed in all the muscles of the body, as well in the diaphragm, intercostals, and those most deeply seated as in the superficial ones, and not less numerously in the substance than on the surface of them all. Those in which they were most thickly set were the pectoralis major, latissimus dorsi, and sartorius, and some idea may be given of their number by stating that in a space one-quarter of

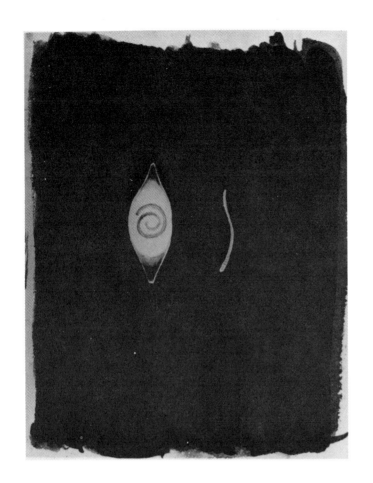

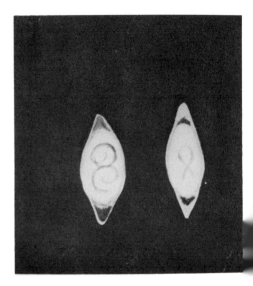

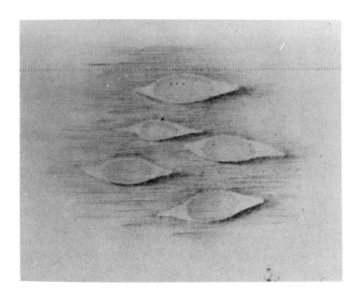

Plate 71. Fig. 1. "Whitish specks" found scattered over muscles. These were discovered, microscopically, to be cysts containing small worms. *Fig. 2.* Representation of cyst enclosing two worms and another containing a single worm in the form of a figure "8." *Fig. 3.* Small, opaque bodies closely resembling cells, but not containing any worms.

an inch square on the last named muscle, upward of 20 were counted.

They all lay with their longest diameters parallel to the direction of the muscular fibres, which seemed themselves perfectly healthy. None could be found in any of the other tissues of the body, nor did the blood which was carefully examined present any unusual appearance.

The genus to which this species (as far as its organization has been at present observed) approaches nearest in character is that described by Leder, under the name of Capsularia as "an acicular round worm, rather slenderer anteriorly, enveloped in a proper capsule, blunt at both ends, with a divided intestinal canal, and a fine blunt little hook." "The worms of this genus," he says, "live like Hermits each in its own peculiar cell. They lie coiled up on the liver to which they are attached by fine filaments. The membranes are with the worms flattened and compressed. The body is hard and very elastic, rounded at both ends. The tail is more blunt than the head and furnished with a short and blunt hook." He includes two species in it, one found in the Herring (*C. halecis*), the other in the salmon (*E. talaris*), and with the exception of the minute hook at the tail the drawings which he has given have a very great similarity to the present species.

There can be little doubt that the appearance of the muscles described by Mr. Hilton at the Med. Chir. Society, and published in the *Medical Gazette* for February 1833 was owing to the presence of cysts similar, or at least analogous to the above. (The organization of these worms, however, differs materially from that of the cysticerci to which that was ascribed.) This occurrence indeed appears by no means uncommon, having been observed many times in the dissecting rooms at St. Bartholomew's, but hitherto regarded as spicules of bone deposited among the muscular fibres.

Preparations exhibiting the appearances described have been deposited in the musuem of the Hospital.

February 12th—Mr. Brown showed me today some specimens to one end of which was attached a smaller membranous sac without any contained worm. Thus at the same time, with much more powerfully magnifying lens I drew the worm but could perceive no orifice at either extremity.

Mr. Farr has found some cells shrivelled and empty and with smaller cells affixed at one end, and again he has seen small cells separately with the interior filled with cellular tissue. The worms, for some time after being removed from the cell, are able to uncoil themselves moving especially the smaller end.

In a few, one or both of the extremities have been found not pointed. Dr. Wormald has found them abundantly in the tensor tympani, not in the levator nor in the iris.

The second instance in which they have been found was in the body of an Irish woman who had been admitted into St. Lawrence's Ward six weeks previously with a large sloughing ulcer just below the knee. She was very weak and emaciated, but by nutritious diet and the use of tonics and anodyne medicines with appropriate local application the slough separated from the surface of the sore, exposing a considerable portion of the upper part of the tibia. Her general health however was but little improved. She had frequent diarrhea and vomiting,—became gradually weaker and died, in an extreme state of emaciation, on the 20th of February, the body being taken to the dissecting room. The internal organs were not examined till six or eight days after death, but as far as was observed, there was no material organic alteration with the exception of a few crude tubercules in both lungs. . . .

The animalcules in this subject were in every respect similar to those found in the last, but having been obtained rather sooner after the death of the patient they were more generally alive, as to afford a better opportunity of observing their movements.

Portions of muscle were given to Mr. Owen who has since described this species at the Zoology Society by the name of *Trichina spiralis*.

Of either the causes or effects of this extraordinary affection little can be said. In the three instances in which it has been observed and whose history is known, the only circumstance common to them all, was that the subjects had died of disease in which they had been reduced by long, protracted suffering to a state of extreme debility and emaciation, (but without any further affection of the muscular power than might have been expected to have arisen from such a condition of the system generally). As far as can be remembered too, all the subjects in which they had previously been seen in the dissecting room and these have been upwards of 20, were in the same state. There seems, therefore, some ground to suspect that their development like their species of Entozoa is favored by a condition of body in which the vital powers have been reduced by the influence of some debilitating agents. It is not improbable that from their minuteness they may have very frequently been overlooked. They have occurred in abundance, as has been said, in the pectoral muscles, so that it will require in any post mortem examination whether in hospital or private practice, merely to dissect carefully a portion of either of those muscles, and examine it closely with a common magnifying glass, or should they exist in any number they will be visible clearly to the naked eye. But having already been observed in three cases in above about 100 which have been carefully examined, should this be a true average opportunities of seeing them will not be uncommon.

At present no symptom has been observed which could in any way be attributable to their existence. There was not observed any further affection of the muscular power than might have been expected to have arisen from the disease under which the patient labored.

It is scarcely possible to imagine such myriads of beings, however insignificant their size, deriving their support from an individual, without producing such a material effect on his health as it is hoped further observation will enable us to trace to its real cause. . . .[Two brief case reports have been omitted—Eds.].

ENTOZOON IN THE SUPERFICIAL PART OF THE EXTENSOR MUSCLES OF THE THIGH OF THE HOG

Proceedings of the Academy of Natural Sciences, Philadelphia, 3: 107–108, 1846. Selection from p. 107.

Joseph Leidy
(1823–1891)

A physician who was also one of the greatest naturalists in the history of American science and the father of American parasitology, Leidy was born in Philadelphia. He studied medicine at the University of Pennsylvania where he later became professor of anatomy and then professor of zoology; he also held high academic posts at Swarthmore College and at the Wagner Institute of Science.

The observation that pigs could become infected with Trichinella *was an important link in the life cycle of* Trichinella spiralis.

Dr. Leidy stated that he had lately detected the existence of an Entozoon in the superficial part of the extensor muscles of the thigh of a hog. The Entozoon is a minute, coiled worm, contained in a cyst. The cysts are numerous, white, oval in shape, of a gritty nature, and between the 30th and 40th of an inch in length.

The Entozoon he supposes to be the *Trichina spiralis,* heretofore considered as peculiar to the human species. He could perceive no distinction between it and the specimens of *T. spiralis* which he had met with in several human subjects in the dissecting rooms, where it had also been observed by others, since the attention of the scientific public had been directed to it by Mr. Hilton and Prof. Owen. . . .

OBSERVATIONS ON *TRICHINA SPIRALIS*

Beobachtungen über *Trichina spiralis*. Nachrichten von der Georg-August Universitat. Königliche Gesellschaft der Wissenschaften: 260–264, 1851. Translated from the German.

Ernst Friedrich Gustav Herbst
(1803–1893)

Herbst was born in Göttingen, Germany, and educated in the university of that city, where he won an academic prize with study in the field of hematology. He spent most of his academic and professional life in Göttingen.

Herbst's original and long unrecognized experiment of transmission of Trichina [Trichinella] spiralis *from animal to animal antedated the work of Küchenmeister and Leuckart, and is recorded here.*

On 25 November, Professor Herbst presented the Royal Society of Sciences with the following observations on *Trichina spiralis* and the transmission of intestinal worms:

Intestinal worms are so prevalent among men and animals that it is very difficult to determine the time of their first appearance; it is even more difficult to determine, with certainty, the manner of their origin in the respective host. The observations which I have the honor to present to the Royal Society, therefore, might merit some attention because they provide a way of clarifying this obscure subject by means of direct experiment and experiences.

My observations concern the *T. spiralis,* an internal worm, which, although it does not yet seem to be recognized by all helminthologists, because of its very rare occurrence and the ease with which its presence can be demonstrated, seems excellently suited for such experiments.

To date, I have observed three kinds of them. The first, which corresponds exactly to those found by Hilton, Owen, and Bischoff in human cadavers, I encountered in August of 1845 in countless numbers in all voluntary muscles of a large, old, male cat.

A second kind was found shortly thereafter in the mesentery of *Strix passerina* which had been submitted to me; unfortunately, I was unable to learn whether such entozoas had also been found in the muscle. The mesentery, however, was permeated abundantly with pinhead-size, yellow nodules in which the curled worm could be recognized by means of a magnifying glass.

These trichinae differed not only in circumference, which was twice as large, but also by the different structure of their ends. Their thicker head end terminated in a short, conical point covered with cilia. The thinner tail end seemed to be provided at its very tip with two papillary protuberances, as though with a funnel-like opening.

The third kind I first found in the summer of 1848 in the muscles of the extremities of a grown dog. At that time, however, I was busy with the examination of another subject and contented myself with examining some of the cysts and their contents; I neglected to investigate whether the trichinae were spread throughout all voluntary muscles. The cysts were very small and, not being visible to the naked eye, could only be discovered by means of the microscope. The worms therein were also smaller, but otherwise very similar to the first kind mentioned. Only the fact that the more recently observed trichinae which I shall mention below showed the same structure made me believe that the variation in size represented an incontrovertible difference between the third and the first kinds.

In November of the previous year an almost two-year-old female badger had died; I had fed her for a year and a half, partly with vegetable fare and partly with the remainders of many animals used in my work. Microscopic examination showed the presence of countless trichinae in all voluntary muscles in which, by the way, nothing abnormal was discovered. The longitudinal

diameter of the cysts was 0.1166''' [1/00''' = 1 line or 1/12''—Eds.], the transverse diameter 0.1''', the width of the worms 0.01'''. This time I considered it important not to lose the opportunity for investigating further the origin of these worms.

In 1845 I had experimented with the transmission of trichinae by inserting 30 cysts containing live worms between the skin and back muscles of a young cat. The results were negative in that after four weeks the cysts had become attached to the connective tissue beneath the skin and to the surface of the muscles. The worms therein, whose middle part seemed to consist entirely of granules, had become thinner and were dead.

As a result of this experience I devised a new experiment. The flesh of the badger was given to three six-week-old Pomeranians who ate it within a few days. One of the dogs was sent to the country where it was set free and under completely changed environmental conditions. The examination of the two others on 10 and 18 February of that year showed that all voluntary muscles were permeated with trichinae equally abundantly, as in the badger eaten three and a half months previously. The length of the cysts was 0.133''', the width 0.075''', the width of the worms 0.01166'''. It only remained to determine the condition of the the muscles of the third dog, which was sent back to me at the beginning of November after an interval of nine months. The dog was now fully grown, strong, and apparently healthy. On 11 November its sternomastoid muscle was exposed. With the naked eye nothing unusual was seen in this muscle, but under the microscope one could easily recognize the trichinae which were so numerous that from a two- or three-gram piece of muscle ten specimens could be dissected out. The length of the cysts was 0.133''', with a width of 0.0833'''; the length of the worms was 0.33''', the width 0.01166'''.

Since the trichinae are, in general, a very infrequent phenomenon, there can be no doubt that their growth in the aforementioned three dogs had resulted from the intake of the badger meat. This growth had been favored by the ability of these worms to survive and by the fact that they do not seem to be harmed by either heat or cold. However, the greatest difficulty lies in explaining the process by which the very small and very elastic, but solidly formed particles representing worm eggs have been able to enter the blood vessels from the intestinal cavity since the ample, simultaneous, and equal distribution of the trichinae through all voluntary muscles justifies the assumption that their eggs have been carried to their respective places of settlement by means of the blood circulation. My previous experiences provide no information on this point and, therefore, I do not believe it practical to attempt a more specific discussion, as this would necessitate a thorough consideration of the state of all substances reaching the blood during digestion. As, at this time, I still possess one of the animals infected with trichinae, and as several other less frequently occurring internal worms might be useful for similar experiments, I consider it possible to obtain, in the future, some further useful results on this subject.

ON TRICHINOSIS IN MAN

Ueber die trichinen-krankheit des menschen. Archiv für Pathologische Anatomie und Physiologie und fur Klinische Medicin, von Rudolf Virchow, 18: 561–572, 1860. Translated from the German.

Friedrich Albert Zenker
(1825–1898)

A native of Dresden, Zenker studied medicine both in Leipzig and in Heidelberg and then accepted an appointment in pathologic anatomy at the University of Leipzig. Eventually, he returned to Dresden, where he was finally appointed professor of general pathology and pathologic anatomy in that city's medical-surgical academy In 1862 he became ordinary professor of pathology at Erlangen, where he remained until his retirement in 1895. Zenker contributed significantly to the understanding of the pathology of many diseases besides trichinosis.

Henry Wood (1835) described clinical disease associated with Trichinella spiralis *in muscle. However, this article by Zenker is the first definitive study of the pathology of trichinosis.*

The *Trichina spiralis* [*Trichinella spiralis*], following its first description by Owen, has been seen for more than 20 years by a series of observers, but the cases were so sporadic that the parasite was generally considered to be very rare. It can probably be assumed that the number of cases described in the literature during this time indicates rather completely the total of cases actually seen. Lately, this has changed considerably since it has become increasingly apparent that the small number of cases observed has been due merely to a lack of sufficient attention to the subject. As proof of this, reference to Virchow's statements in the preceding issue of this archive and the fact that lately I have been apprised repeatedly by other private sources of unpublished cases of trichinosis will suffice. As far as I am concerned, I have convinced myself over a number of years of the relative frequency of this parasite. Thus, in 1855, I observed within eight months, among 136 autopsies, four cases with trichina. During the same time span cysticercus and echinococcus were each found only once. *Pentastomum denticulatum,* [Larval stage of *Pentastomum taenioides,* H. W. Stunkard, and C. P. Gandal, *Zoologica,* 53: 54, 1968—Eds.] on the other hand, was found 22 times. According to these figures, one trichina infection occurred for every 34 dead persons, certainly a very considerable rate. Yet, it is very probable that I have overlooked other cases, especially since I, like Virchow, have seen several cases in which the trichinae were so sparsely distributed that only a particularly fortuitous circumstance could bring them to our attention. I have certainly seen a dozen such cases.

Although this parasite caught the interest of individual observers and contributed greatly to the general theory of parasites and their migrations, the interest in it remained mainly zoological; pathologically, almost no importance was attached to it. It was thought that the worm caused no symptoms at all, which probably was going much too far. It was known only that no striking symptoms referable to the muscle system were present prior to death in the observed cases (perhaps with one exception). Whether infiltration by the parasite caused symptoms was not known because the finding was always accidental and it was not possible (nor seriously attempted) subsequently to gather adequate data about the history and physical examination. The trichina seemed to be one of those many unproductive toys with which impractical anatomists and microscopists waste their time and which practical men pass with a condescending smile. But, only too often, the toy gradually aquires flesh and blood, or suddenly inflates, like Faust's poodle, into an elephant. The latter picture might fit our case. The small hypocrites are unmasked.

I have always been of the opinion that the infiltration by so many worms could hardly occur without considerable symptoms. Because most of the symptoms are temporary, they are considered not worth mentioning and, therefore, do not come to the attention of the doctor. However, this was only a hypothesis until now. But on the basis of a case observed in the last few weeks and investigated in all aspects with the greatest care, I am now able to prove that the trichina, after penetration (probably in all cases where this is massive), is able to cause considerable, even dangerous symptoms. In fact, accompanied by the most severe symptoms, it can kill a strong, healthy person within a few weeks. Therefore, of all the animal parasites of man (not even excluding the echinococcus, which at least grows slowly and frequently is susceptible to therapeutic intervention), the trichina is the most dangerous and the most to be feared.

Disturbing as this fact is, it is gratifying that this one case gave such surprisingly clear and striking results in every respect. By means of the investigations and experiments directly connected with it, the whole theory of the trichina has been almost completely explained, zoologically and pathologically. No actual mystery is left in this heretofore so mysterious matter, and it only remains to complete the investigation of several less important points for which the way is now clearly outlined. These results are even more unassailable considering that, as far as the zoological part is concerned, they agree completely with the results of trichinae feedings made by Virchow last year and with those made by Leuckart which were simultaneous with my observations.

In view of the practical importance and novelty of the matter, I consider it necessary to report in detail the entire case and the related investigations. However, I wish to complete several aspects of my observations and hence will limit myself to a short resume of the essentials, reserving further details until later.

The case was as follows: a 20-year-old servant girl, previously healthy, was admitted on 12 January 1860 to the medical department of Dr. Walther in the local city hospital. She had become sickly around Christmas and had gone to bed around New Year's Day where she remained, first at her place of employment and then at her parents' home, until she was sent to the hospital.

The illness had started with great fatigue, insomnia, loss of appetite, constipation, fever, and thirst. The same symptoms were observed early in her hospitalization. The fever was very high, and the abdomen was painfully distended. Swelling of the spleen could not be demonstrated, and roseola was not present. The diagnosis, although made with some reservation because of the absence of an enlarged spleen, was typhoid. The total picture favored this assumption, and there was no support for the presence of any other known disease.

Suddenly a striking disturbance of the entire muscular system was added to the described symptoms. This consisted of extreme pain, especially in the extremities, so that the patient complained loudly day and night; due to the great discomfort upon contraction of the knee and elbow joints, any attempt at stretching was impossible. To this was added an edematous swelling, especially of the lower legs. Although this affection attracted our attention, we believed it to be only a complication, very rare in this form and severity, to be sure. For reasons that I will explain some other time, this assumption fascinated us.

Later on, pulmonary symptoms occurred which were in keeping with typhoid lung disease. After a marked apathy on 26 January, death ensued the morning of 27 January.

Prior to the actual autopsy, performed 28 January, I examined the muscles (those of the arms first). These showed a moderate development and an over-all pale red-gray. One can imagine my surprise when, in the first microscopic preparation, I saw at first glance, dozens of trichinae not yet encysted, but lying freely in the muscle parenchyma. They were rolled up or stretched out in all forms and gave clear indications of being alive. Further examination showed all muscles to be permeated massively with trichinae in a way that has never been observed before; with lower magnification one could sometimes see 20 worms in the field of vision. There could be no doubt that the animals were still in the process of migrating within the muscle tissue and that this was an instance of fresh infiltration. Moreover, the muscle fibers, as far as they were still preserved, showed generally extensive degeneration; this had been recognized, on cursory examination and on pulling apart, by their unusual brittleness. Microscopically, it was characterized by loss of transverse striation, by homogenization, and by countless fine transverse tears in the fibers.

Further autopsy showed absolutely nothing on which to base the assumption of typhoid; there was no swelling of the spleen and no involvement of the intestinal and mesenteric lymph nodes. Therefore, for the moment, I will skip some less important findings and mention only a rather extensive collapse, especially of the left lung, with interspersed small infiltrates; intensive bronchitis; and severe hyperemia of the mucosa of the ileum.

In view of all this, there can be no doubt that the trichinae infiltration caused the intense muscle symptoms and that the patient actually died from it. On the one hand, the autopsy did not indicate any other cause of death (the changes in the lung were undoubtedly of a secondary nature), and, on the other, such an intensive and extensive degeneration of the most widespread system of the body was incompatible with continuation of life.

Aside from numerous questions on detail, the task then was to study the case, pursuing a two-fold direction. First it was necessary to trace, if possible, the trichinae's route of infiltration; second, it was essential to investigate, by feeding experiments, the further development of the trichinae. For both objectives, this case seemed ideal.

Concerning the route of infiltration, in the muscles were found some bodies which evidently represented earlier stages in the development of the trichinae; they were similar in form to the latter, with one pointed and one more rounded end, but were much shorter, a little plumper, and without clear differentiation of internal organs. (Virchow confirmed this observation after examining the muscle which I sent him.) As was expected, the animals reach the muscles as embryos and there develop into trichinae. But is the infiltration of the muscle a purely active one, through the tissue, or is it at least partly passive, aided by the blood? Examination of almost all of the more important tissues showed no trichinae or earlier stages of their development. Also, there were no changes anywhere which would indicate that the tissues had been penetrated by such a massive number of worms. Nothing was found in the blood either. Since a positive starting point

was lacking, this negative finding, along with other things, seemed to speak strongly for an infiltration through the blood stream. Perhaps they come from the intestine first, into the chyle, and move along with it into the blood. This was suggested by observations of young trichinae in the mesenteric lymph nodes made by Virchow in his feeding experiments. I will examine the intestinal wall in this regard later.

I had, I must admit, little hope of finding anything in the intestinal mucus [sic]. According to the present state of things, two concepts seemed especially justified: either the trichinae came from one of the known intestinal helminths of man, according to Küchenmeister's concept from *Trichocephalus dispar,* but then they still would have been found at autopsy, which was not the case. Or the trichinae, like the cestodes, went through their various stages of development in different animals and, perhaps also, partly extrinsically. In order to migrate immediately from the intestine to the muscles, the eggs or embryos would have to have been swallowed by man with vegetables, water, or otherwise. In this case, however, the introduction of the embryos would surely have stopped with admittance to the hospital, and it could be assumed that the ones introduced earlier would have left the intestinal tract. In spite of my small hopes, I wanted, for the sake of thoroughness, to examine the intestinal contents, and I put it aside for this purpose. I returned to this examination only a couple of weeks later [sic]. To my most pleasant surprise, on microscopic examination, I found in the first drop of mucus (schleim) from the jejunum a mass of small worms; there was no doubt about their being sexually mature trichinae. Their form corresponded completely to that of the trichinae—pointed anterior end, more rounded posterior end—only they were much bigger and more slender. The females were 4 mm in length and the males 1-1/2 mm. They proved to be viviparous (a fact for which I had been prepared by a letter from Leuckart); the middle portion of all female bodies was filled completely with rolled up, fully developed embryos. The embryos already showed the form of a round worm. In many worms, a difference in thickness between the anterior and posterior ends was noticeable, although less prominent than it would be later on. I cannot confirm Leuckart's statement that the males are much less frequently encountered than the females. I found many of them and, taking into account the great difficulty in finding them because of their smallness and delicateness, would judge their number to be hardly less than that of the females. Likewise, I find, contrary to Leuckart, that in many of the males, the posterior end is slightly bent. Further details on this I am omitting for the present.

Thus, with this observation alone, the question pertaining to the further development of the muscle trichinae was solved. This was especially true since this finding completely confirmed the results of a feeding experiment made last year by Virchow, and since Leuckart, simultaneously with the observation of my case, had raised exactly the same sexually mature worms by feeding trichinous meat to dogs. Finally, feeding experiments which were made with muscles from my case led to the same result. I am, therefore, now adding what there is to be said about these experiments.

Jointly, with Dr. Küchenmeister, I fed four dogs with trichinous muscles. At the same time, I sent muscles to Professors Virchow, Leuckart, and Luschka, all of whom started feedings at once. We killed the first dog on the fifth day after feeding and found in the jejunum a number of the finest thread worms. They resembled exactly those raised by Virchow, but they were further advanced in their development, in that the egg cells had already developed into spirally coiled (but not completely mature) embryos. The worms were even smaller than those from our patient's intestine. There were no trichinae in the muscles. The second dog was killed in the fourth week, but no trichinae were found either in the intestine or in the muscles. The third dog died six weeks after feeding, after having lost his appetite and having become very emaciated. In this case, too, there were no trichinae either in the intestine or the muscles. The fourth dog is still alive, but under the circumstances offers little hope for success. Nevertheless, this changes nothing because of the complete proof offered by the rest of the observations and experiments.

Professor Virchow himself reported the very wonderful results of his feeding experiment. The raising of sexually mature trichinae in the intestine of a fed rabbit; the infiltration of the embryos into the muscles of the same animal and their growth into *Trichina spiralis*; the death caused by this infiltration—all formed the most surprising experimental duplication of my case in man, just reported.

According to correspondence with Professor Leuckart, he fed to a dog flesh which I sent him and found, while dissecting the intestine seven days later, few but sexually mature trichinae very similar to the ones found in earlier experiments. At the same time he wrote me that a piglet fed with sexually mature trichinae and their brood became seriously ill immediately after the feeding with symptoms which indicate involvement of the intestinal tract. After eight days symptoms of paralysis appeared, first affecting the posterior extremities and soon thereafter the front ones. This associated with incontinance of urine, and other symptoms. The animal recovered and even regained partial use of its extremities. It was killed four weeks after the feeding. At autopsy, in addition to clear traces of a subsiding peritonitis, countless trichinae were discovered in the muscles. These muscles, as I convinced myself with a piece which kindly had been sent to me, showed entirely the same picture of fresh trichinae infiltrations as the muscles of my case. Thus, we have here a highly interesting, experimentally caused example of trichinosis followed by recovery, for which I will immediately report an analogous one in humans.

One of the dogs fed by Professor Luschka died 14 days later, according to a letter just received; the autopsy revealed intensive intestinal catarrh, but no worm.

If we summarize the results of all these experiments and the earlier ones of Virchow and Leuckart, it becomes evident that the trichinae grow to sexual maturity in the intestine of the dog, but that the dog is not the most suitable experimental animal for these feedings, since all dogs examined 12 days after the feeding were uninfected. It seems, therefore, as Leuckart also assumed, that the trichina spends only a short time in the intestine of the dog, and the migration of the young into the muscles seems to occur less easily in the dog. Only the older experiments, by Herbst, indicate that the latter takes place in the dog at all. In further experiments, we shall probably have to use mainly rabbits and pigs with which they were so successful.

I now return to our patient: Finding the sexually mature trichinae in the intestine of the patient proved that the trichina goes through the whole developmental cycle in one and the same host. This refuted the previously held concept about the manner in which trichinae infiltrate humans. One must now assume that the parasites were swallowed in the form of muscle trichinae and that, therefore, the infection followed the consumption of trichinous meat. I now reminded myself: the patient had worked on a farm—she fell ill there immediately after Christmas—on farms, pigs are usually slaughtered at this time— trichinae have already been observed in the pig. What was more obvious than to assume a connection here; namely, that the patient had infected herself by eating raw pork during slaughtertime. It was worthwhile investigating this concept. I went, therefore, to the nearby village of Plauen and to the estate owner concerned. To my pleasure I found a very intelligent farmer who readily agreed to all my intentions and gave me all the desired information. He actually had slaughtered a pig on 21 December of last year (he had also slaughtered an ox at that time and another pig in November). The girl had become sick soon after the slaughter. Whether she had eaten any raw meat, he did not know; yet she had loved to pick at food. Some provisions from all three slaughtered animals were still around, and I received a piece of the ham and the corned beef for examination. The first preparation from the ham of 21 December, and every later preparation, showed numerous encysted trichinae in the familiar form. On the contrary, the other pig and the ox were clean. Later, I received some cervelat sausage and blood sausage from the first pig, and trichinae were immediately found in both. Accordingly, there no longer can be any doubt that the patient had been infected by the consumption of trichinous pork.

It was also of interest to know whether other people on the farm had been infected. I had already inquired about this during my visit. It was discovered that the housekeeper had become ill a few days after our patient and had been in bed for several weeks, ostensibly because of "nerve fever." At first she had had stomach cramps; then she became very fatigued and had had headaches, and so on. Now she felt well again. Although the symptoms offer little proof, they suggest that a trichinae infection, now cured, had

been present here also. The estate owner himself had become sick in January, but only for a short time, with a stomach catarrh; however, it is difficult to reach a conclusion in this case. The estate owner also added that, at that time, everyone on the farm had been fatigued. I was most interested in the butcher who had slaughtered the pig, since butchers, as is well known, like to eat the raw meat during slaughtering. Therefore, I went to his home and learned from his wife that he had been very sick in January; he had been in bed at least three weeks with the "gout." It was as though his whole body had been paralyzed; he could hardly lift his arms or legs, nor had he been able to move his neck; in addition, he had suffered from heavy sweats. She had believed that he would not recover. He was a strong, healthy young man and had never had anything like this before. He was now back at work but still had not regained his full strength. To my question, how he might have contracted this disease, she immediately replied that he had thought he must have caught a cold during the slaughter in question because the illness began immediately thereafter. It seems to me that these wholly spontaneous statements speak for themselves and I do not hesitate to call this disease, with conviction, a trichinous infection. Undoubtedly, someone one day will find the encysted trichinae in him. Thus, we have the first diagnosis of trichinosis during life.

With this, the theory regarding trichinosis is pretty well rounded out. Clearly, this theory is important for pathology dietetics and medical policing, as well as for agriculture. In the latter respect, I have reached an agreement with the estate owner to find out first of all whether this disease is prevalent in the stables there and, if so, to work on the elimination of this dangerous enemy. It will also be in order to investigate whether the trichinae occur more often in the pig, which is probable in view of the demonstrated frequency of the trichinae in man. It can hardly be doubted any longer that the infection of man results (as a rule or always) from trichinous meat and that he does not acquire his trichinae from the dog, as Leuckart assumed. However, there is the additional question whether the infection is caused only by fresh, raw meat or whether the various products of the same such as ham or sausages are also able to cause infection. The latter is not unlikely, particularly for those products like hams, which are not subjected to a high degree of heat, and cervelat sausage, the meat for which is only chopped and smoked. In this regard, I remember particularly the experiences (which I was able to confirm some time ago) regarding the revival of dried, round worms by moistening them. In the interest of the now-frightened devotees of these delicacies, it is very important to resolve this question experimentally. I have at least made a start on this. The worms in the ham are simply shrunken, without further change. On addition of water or of dilute acetic acid they assume the form and appearance of live worms, but even with addition of warm water they exhibit no signs of life. Furthermore, I fed a piece of ham to a rabbit which, when killed seven days later, showed no trichinae in the intestine. According to this, the ham at least seems to be harmless. Nevertheless, to arrive at a reliable conclusion, a larger number of experiments are necessary. I must add that the recognition of the trichinae in the ham is very difficult for the naked eye because they are, to a large extent, in the heavy fat layers and, in part, are completely covered by them.

Whether cases of trichinosis ending in death occur often or whether our case is a rare exception cannot yet be decided. It is surely possible that many cases remaining unexplained after the autopsy belong here. How often do the anatomists appease their not too sensitive consciences by assuming typhoid in the blood. What explanation would have been offered in our case without microscopic examination of the muscles? In the literature on trichinae I find a case which might possibly belong here. Reported by Henry Wood, it is one of a 22-year-old man who was admitted to the Bristol Infirmary because of a violent rheumatic fever which was complicated by heart trouble. When he died after eight days, inflammation of the lungs and the heart sac was found at autopsy; trichinae were present in the muscles. The data given in Schmidt's yearbooks, which is all that is available to me, are too sparse to permit a decision as to whether it was a case of articular rheumatism in which the trichinae were only an incidental finding.

If the foregoing has shown that the trichina is able to complete its whole cycle of development in one individual, the question remains whether this is always the case or whether the development sometimes is divided between two animals: the intestine of one and the muscles of the other. That the latter does occur, at least experimentally, was proven by Leuckart. He raised sexually mature trichinae in the intestine of a dog and, by feeding these to a pig, infected the muscles of the latter. Since pigs have a greater opportunity, it is really more probable for them to infect themselves by licking up sexually mature intestinal trichinae eliminated in the feces of the dogs than by swallowing muscle trichinae which must first develop in the intestine. In this way, too, the opportunity and danger of one pig infecting another, thus making the disease endemic on a farm, are obvious. Then, the infiltration can continue for a longer time and can occur very gradually. It is surely different in man, in whom swallowing of sexually mature trichinae cannot take place so easily. The infection is probably caused by the consumption of contaminated meat; thus it occurs quickly and at one time, thereby increasing the danger to him considerably.

These investigations have solved further the problem of whether life in muscle is a necessary transitory stage of the trichina or whether it should be considered an aberration. The latter conjecture seems improbable both a priori for teleological reasons and because of the very definite location of the parasite in transverse striated muscle. The embryos must bore into the muscles in order to nourish themselves. Complete development of the muscle trichina takes less than three to four weeks. If they do not get into the intestinal tract of another animal sooner than this they wait in the encysted condition with strange patience for another opportunity. On the other hand, if this transitional stage in the muscle is necessary, the successful feeding experiments made with the flesh of my case show that previous encystment and a long, quiescent stay in the muscle is not necessary for continued future development. The muscle trichina of man, if it does not fall into the hands of the feeding-happy anatomist, does not attain further development. This does not change the principal interpretation (whether aberration or necessary intermediate stage).

Another observation may be mentioned in this connection. I have not found in the trichinae in my case or in Leuckart's analogous case of the pig the frequently discussed small grainy organ in the front part of the genital structure. It seems that this develops only during the encystment and in some fashion is specific for the encysted condition.

So far as the spread of the trichinae in my case is concerned, it extended to all striated muscles. It must be emphasized, in contrast to previous observations, that even the heart was not free of them. While I was busy with the autopsy, Dr. Küchenmeister found a trichina in one preparation of the heart muscle and the assistant physician, Dr. Forster, and I found several of them in other preparations. Here, in contrast to the voluntary muscles, they were extremely sparse, so that even if complete immunity does not occur, there must be factors which do not favor infiltration of the heart. Perhaps this is due to the heart's constant contractions which, to be sure, cannot make the worms very comfortable.

One very remarkable circumstance which I noticed repeatedly in earlier cases and which appeared very pronounced in this case was that the trichinae were particularly crowded in the direction of the tendon insertion. One is reminded immediately of an animal herd or a crowd of people which, on pressing ahead, is suddenly checked by a barrier. Evidently the tendons are such a barrier for the trichinae. From this it was clear to me, even in earlier cases, that before their encystment the trichinae must travel through the muscles in the direction of the fibers. My present case offered the most complete information on details of the intramuscular life of our worm.

Virchow, in his article appearing in the previous issue, tried to point out, on the basis of his earlier observations, that the trichina was not situated between (as was generally assumed previously) but *in* the primitive fibers and that the cyst capsule was altered sarcolemma. During the first days I had not turned my attention to this point, mainly because I was occupied with other business and, at that time, I was not acquainted with his report. After receipt of my material, Professor Virchow had the kindness to call my attention to this point with the remark that he finds his previously developed opinion strikingly confirmed by my case. At once, I was able to confirm this completely. As soon as one studies it, there remains little doubt that all trichinae lie inside the primitive fibers. The worm stretches the

sarcolemma sheath into a spindle shape. Furthermore, the sheath is completely collapsed at some points, but can be followed plainly and isolated easily. The sarcolemma itself is noticeably thicker, doubly outlined, and shiny. In these fibers, cross-striations are missing completely. The sheath in the collapsed portion is, in part, completely empty and, in part, contains only a little of a fine granular mass or of small clumps (remains of the contractile substance and excrements?). It is evident that the worm crawls along in the fibers and eats up the contractile substance; this is also indicated by its frequently elongated shape. If it wants to encyst, it rolls itself spirally; inside the sarcolemmal sheath a fine granular mass is formed around it, especially in front and behind. In my case, this mass enclosed unusually large, vesicular nuclei with large nuclear corpuscles. Evidently it is from this granular substance that the later solid cyst is made, since it shows, in part, the characteristic form of the same. The thickened sarcolemma only form a cover which, perhaps later, like the rest of the collapsed part of the sheath, disappears or fuses with the cyst. Quite a few worms on the point of encystment were found; however, the majority were evidently still free, that is, still migrating within the muscles.

STUDIES ON TRICHINOSIS

Johns Hopkins Hospital Bulletin, 8: 79–81, 1897.

Thomas Richardson Brown
(1872–1950)

Born in Baltimore, Brown received his M.D. at The Johns Hopkins University in 1897 and was associated with that institution throughout his professional life. Brown was known primarily for his work in gastroenterology. In 1943 he received the Julius Friedenwald Medal of the American Gastroenterological Association, and the July 1950 issue of Gastroenterology *was dedicated to him. Until his retirement, he was physician-in-charge of the Division of Digestive Disease at The Johns Hopkins Hospital, and he was a trustee of the University. He also served as chief of the Medical Division of the League of Red Cross Societies in Geneva.*

When he was a medical student, Brown associated eosinophilia with the clinical diagnosis of trichinosis.

The clinical history of the case which forms the basis of these remarks resembles in some respects the classical picture, though the symptoms were unusually mild. The patient, a man 23 years of age, was admitted to the hospital on March 3, 1896, complaining of general muscular pains. He had been ill six weeks, and for the two weeks before entry the pain had been so severe that he had scarcely been able to move about. There were irregular fever and extreme muscular tenderness, particularly in the arms and legs. The diagnosis of a myositis, probably due to trichinosis, was made and confirmed by the finding of actively motile trichinae in pieces of muscle removed from the arm.

He remained in the hospital for over two months, being discharged well.

During his stay in the hospital the blood was examined daily. The number of leucocytes per cm was determined and a differential count was made of the various forms; frequent examinations of the urine were made with quantitative determinations of the uric acid, urea, and total nitrogen. The two small pieces of muscle which were removed were subsequently subjected to careful microscopical examination. The results of the studies may be summarized as follows:

(a) *The blood*. The study of the blood was carried on continually during the course of the disease, a determination of the leucocytes and a differential count of the various forms of leucocytes being made daily. The result of these observations showed: (a) A gradual rise of the proportion of eosinophiles reaching 68.2 per cent—35 per cent higher than any previous record—and from this point a gradual decline to 16.8 per cent on the patient's discharge; (b) a coincident depression of the polymorphonuclear neutrophiles, reaching at one time 6.6 per cent., while for two weeks these forms showed an absolute decrease in the blood, notwithstanding (c) the marked leucocytosis, reaching on some occasions above 30,000 per cubic millimetre.

In fact, the neutrophiles and eosinophiles showed at all times an inversely proportional relation, and the eosinophilic rise could be seen to be distinctly at the cost of the neutrophiles, the other forms showing relatively little fluctuation.

The presence of such quantities of eosinophiles suggests their possible diagnostic value in trichinosis, and perhaps, if it be found on further studies to be characeristic of this disease, may help to clear up the cases which are regarded *intra vitam* as rheumatic in nature and which, years afterward, the autopsy table shows to have been cases of trichinosis.

As an association has for a long time been noted between the eosinophiles and the Charcot-Leyden crystals, various experiments were made with the blood which contained such large quantities of eosinophiles, to see if the crystals could be derived directly from these cells. In all cases, however, the results were negative, seeming to show that the crystals are, at least, not direct crystallization products from the eosinophiles, but that something besides the presence of these cells is necessary for their formation.

(b) *The urine*. The quantitative determinations of the uric acid, urea and total nitrogen were carried on mainly in connection with the ideas of Horbaczewski, that the uric acid, derived from the destruction of nuclein-holding material, comes normally in large part from the leucocytes and is therefore increased in leucocytoses.

Although the uric acid per 24 hours was determined on 23 different days, and on four of these the urea and total nitrogen also, on no occasion did the total uric acid excretion, or the relation between the nitrogen of the uric acid to that of the urea or to the total nitrogen exceed the normal limits, showing that the views of Horbaczewski are not universally correct. In this case, however, the leucocytosis differed somewhat from the ordinary in that here the eosinophiles were the cells markedly increased; in his cases the ordinary polymorphonuclear neutrophiles.

(c) *The muscle*. The changes in the muscle were extensive. There was a great proliferation of the muscle nuclei throughout the section; about the fibres containing trichinae this proliferation was very marked, especially in the second specimen; not so extensive in the earlier specimen. In fact, in a few places where the parasite had but just wandered into the primitive bundle no change in the muscle substance nor any proliferation of nuclei was visible. Most of the fibres containing the worm showed a conversion of the muscle substance into a finely granular faintly-staining material containing many large swollen nuclei, *i.e.* the proliferated muscle nuclei; and about many of the proliferated nuclei, both in the more and in the less degenerated portions, distinct vacuoles could be made out.

Throughout the specimens the muscle showed various forms of disintegration, in some places a longitudinal splitting of the fibres into fibrillae, in other places the formation of what might be called muscle cells, the muscle nucleus taking about itself some of the muscle substance and separating itself from the fibre; while in still other places a peculiar transverse splitting up of the muscle into disks, the nuclei here proliferating transversely instead of in the usual longitudinal method, was noted.

Besides these changes there were seen in the first specimen many polymorphonuclear cells, some showing a finely granular protoplasm which did not stain to any extent with acid stains (the so-called neutrophiles), some distinct eosinophiles with large deeply-staining granules, and beside these, cells which somewhat suggest transitional forms, showing in the protoplasm of the cell body fine granules, but with a distinct affinity for the acid stain; and all these cells seemed to be acting as phagocytes in the disintegrating muscle, being often seen in little lakes or bays in the degenerating bits.

In the second specimen there were decidedly fewer neutrophiles and many more eosinophiles than in the first. That in both cases these were typical eosinophiles was shown by staining them in the different acid stains and in the Biondi-Heidenhein triple stain.

At the same time with this greatly increased proportion of eosinophiles in the extra-vascular leucocytes in the muscle, *the blood vessels in the interfascicular connective tissue showed the same proportion of neutrophiles and eosinophiles as was found in the blood count for that day.*

In another specimen of muscle from a case of acute trichinosis which was obtained from the pathological museum, great quantities of eosinophiles were also found.

The study of the blood, showing the steady increase of the eosinophiles at the expense of the neutrophiles, together with the identical character of the nuclei of the two forms, would tend to support the view held by some observers, that the former variety of cells is derived by some transitional change from the latter.

That such a change might take place in the muscle is suggested by the presence here of neutrophiles, eosinophiles, and what may be regarded as transitional forms, in large quantities. Particularly suggestive is the great disproportion between neutrophiles and eosinophiles seen in the second muscle specimen. Here the eosinophiles were much increased, the neutrophiles correspondingly decreased, while the blood vessels in the interfascicular connective tissue showed but the same proportion of these forms as was to be made out in the specimens of the peripheral blood for the same days. It is further noteworthy that the eosinophiles increased in number soon after the increase in severity of the muscle symptoms, and shortly after the decrease of those symptoms, diminished gradually, descending toward the normal point as the symptoms abated. Suggestive also is the presence of large numbers of eosinophiles in a specimen of muscle from another case of acute trichinosis.

Dr. Osler—This is the only case of trichinosis which has been in the hospital, or it is safer to say the only case recognized, since we know that not infrequently the disease escapes recognition or is mistaken for some other disorder. This is the second case which I have seen clinically, while in the post-mortem room I have found on eight or ten occasions the calcified cysts. Mr. Brown is to be congratulated on the very thorough way in which he has followed this case. [Dr. William S. Thayer included in his comments the following, "With regard to the actual blood condition—the increase of the eosinophiles—no similar case exists in the literature; the percentage of eosinophiles in this instance is more than twice as large as has been reported in any other case." This was supported by Dr. Lewellys F. Barker's comment, "The occurrence of such an enormous number of eosinophiles in the circulating blood is truly remarkable and makes the case unique in the bibliography"—Eds.]

CHAPTER 25

Schistosomiasis Mansoni—Haematobium

A CONTRIBUTION TO HUMAN HELMINTHOLOGY

Ein beitrag zur helminthographia humana. Zeitschrift für Wissenschaftliche Zoologie, 4:53–76, 1852. Selections from pp. 53–55, 59–62, 71–76. Translated from the German.

Theodore Bilharz
(1825–1862)

Bilharz was born in Sigmaringen, Germany, the son of a manager of royal estates, and studied medicine at the universities of Freiburg and Tübingen. In 1849 he accepted a post as prosector at the Freiburg Institute of Anatomy, but one year later left to become the assistant to his former Tübingen professor, Griesinger, who was personal physician to the Khedive of Egypt and director of medical services in that country. When Griesinger returned to Germany in 1852, Bilharz remained in what had become his second homeland and successively became head physician of the medical department and professor of the medical clinic of Kasr el Aini Hospital in Cairo and then professor of descriptive anatomy in that city's university. He died in Cairo of ''typhoid'' fever contracted while serving as the physician on a journey up the Nile headed by the Duke Ernst von-Coburg Gotha. This remarkable man, in a letter, described three human parasites for the first time: Heterophyes heterophyes, Hymenolepis nana, *and* Schistosoma.

Bilharz did not publish his observations directly but sent them to Professor C. T. von Siebold in Breslau, who was also editor of this journal. In these letters to von Siebold, Bilharz describes the ova and adults of Schistosoma. *He appreciated that two different types of eggs could be found. Cobbold and Meckel created the genus* Bilharzia, *but priority has since been ascribed to* Schistosoma. *The sections of the letter describing* H. nana *and* H. heterophyes *are included in their respective chapters.*

From the letters of Dr. Bilharz in Cairo to Professor C. T. von Siebold in Breslau, with comments by the latter

When Dr. Bilharz, whom I was permitted to count among my most industrious pupils in Freiburg, informed me that he would follow Professor Griesinger to Egypt for an extended stay in that strange country, he asked me which subject of natural science he should observe particularly; I recommended, among other things, the human helminths for his attention since that country seemed to me to be a particularly fruitful source for such investigations. My supposition was not inaccurate; after a rather short time I received from Dr. Bilharz, who had had the opportunity of performing many autopsies at a large hospital in Cairo, very comprehensive helminthologic notes. I am reporting them here in the hope that he will keep his promise to me and soon publish his special investigations on this subject. How frequently men are plagued by helminths in these eastern regions of Africa can be seen from the following portion of a letter which Dr. Bilharz sent from Cairo on 1 May 1851:

"So far as the helminths in general and those of man in particular are concerned, I believe that Egypt is one of the most suitable countries for their development and study. Nematodes in particular populate the intestines of the natives, often in unbelievable numbers. It is not at all rare to find, at the same time, in one cadaver, some 100 specimens of *Strongylus (Ancylostoma) duodenalis,* 20–40 specimens of *Ascaris lumbricoides,* 10–20 specimens of *Trichocephalus dispar,* and some 1,000 *Oxyuris vermicularis.* Three or four times in the 200 cadavers that I have dissected since last fall, I found *Taenia solium*; in one case I found five specimens. One of the cadavers was that of a Negro, the second that of a slave from Abyssinia. There, I am told, the tapeworm is so common that the Abyssinian considers it abnormal when no tapeworm segments pass from him. No slave is sold there who does not get a quantity of Cusso (Brayera anthelminthica) to take. This medicine, therefore, is obtainable from the slave dealers. (Some time ago, Professor Griesinger sent a large quantity to a dealer in Stuttgart.) The frequency of the tapeworm in Abyssinia is ascribed to the ingestion of raw meat; people who refrain therefrom—Schimper, our compatriot, for instance—supposedly have been spared. Is it possible that the tapeworm embryos choose animal tissue as a vehicle while the round worms are ingested chiefly through plant food? Insofar as I remember, in Europe, the *Ascaris lumbricoides* and pin worms are attributed to spoiled flour and bread; here in Egypt the population consumes many vegetables (especially raw leaves and roots) and is plagued in particular by round worms.

"I found *Echinococcus* three times in the liver, once several together of different sizes. On the inner surface of the cysts were small, loosely attached semolinalike corpuscles or vesicles with a number of tapeworm heads inside which behaved exactly like the *Taenia* from the snail [sic] that we had examined earlier. The only difference was that they were attached to the wall of the cyst with the small, tail-like end of the body. In the native *Taenia solium* I found a rostellum. Also the neck was wider than the European *Taenia,* as I remember it, and as Bremser and Goeze, whose books I have here, describe it. Because of the favorable opportunity for helminthologic investigations (there is no better site than in Egypt; we did two or three autopsies daily this winter, all of which I performed myself), I hope to find still much more that is interesting in this undisturbed land of helminthology. The *Filaria medinensis,* unfortunately, does not occur here; in the course of two or three years one case or so might be seen. On the other hand, it is very frequently encountered in the Sennaar and in Berber and Shendi in Nubia, and it is worth a trip there although the climate is supposed to be extremely dangerous; I feel that the dangers can be mitigated by caution and an appropriate way of life. By going there, as I would like to do, I hope to be able to send you the *Filaria medinensis* in various stages of development. Burckhardt says that the

Negroes in Shendi claim that the worm enters the body with the drinking water after the flooding of the Nile; its presence, therefore, must have had a certain relation to the seasons."

One of the helminths of man observed by Bilharz in Cairo is the *Distomum haematobium Bilh.* That the inhabitants of Egypt are plagued by a hematozoon will certainly interest physicians and zoologists alike. Dr. Bilharz first reported this surprising discovery to me in the following communication dated 1 May 1851:

"Soon after my attention had been directed to the liver and its associated structures, I found in the blood of the portal vein a number of long, white helminths which, with the naked eye, I considered to be nematodes, but soon recognized as something new. A look into the microscope revealed a splendid *Distomum* with a flat body and a spiral tail at least ten times as long as the body. However, the tail was not loosely inserted, as in the case of the cercariae, but was a continuation of the flat body of the worm itself, rolled sideways toward the stomach surface in a half canal; the forked, blind end of the intestinal canal extended into it very plainly. The intestinal canal contained numerous blood corpuscles throughout its whole length. The end of the tail was slightly indented; a small canal opened at this point, having been formed from two thinner canals which, without showing further ramification, could be pursued toward the front for some distance but were then lost. They did not appear to be filled with anything and, therefore, I am unable to state whether this organ corresponds to the calcium-secreting organs of the *Distoma* or belongs to the excretory system. In different places, close to the free edge of the half tube formed by the tail, I observed a rather large vessel but could not explain its relation to the above-mentioned duct. I found no mature sexual organs; the only evidence of their existence was one or more highly transparent bodies lying behind the ventral sucker. Although I could not determine their structure or content, I do consider them developing genital organs; however, the area could just as easily be a germinal center, similar to the one you [von Siebold—Eds.] described in *Gyrodactylus.* What, then, is this animal? In spite of its long tail it probably cannot be called a cercaria, which is completely different, histologically and morphologically."

On 28 August 1851, Dr. Bilharz communicated his subsequent investigations on this hematozoon:

"I have not yet reported to you the new stages of my portal vein worm. It did not, as I had expected, develop into an old wives' tale but into something more wonderful, a trematode with *divided sex*. The worm I described in my last letter was a male. When I searched the intestinal veins more carefully (and more expediently by holding the undamaged mesentery against the light), I soon found specimens of the worm which harbored a gray thread in the groove of their tail. You can imagine my surprise when I saw a trematode projecting from the frontal opening of the groove and moving back and forth (Plate 72, Fig. 11a); it was similar in shape in the first, only much finer and more delicate. Instead of the groove-shaped tail it had a ribbonlike posterior end which was completely enclosed in the groove-shaped half canal of the male posterior, similar to a sword in its scabbard. The female was easily pulled out of the male's groove and was recognized most clearly by its internal structure. The intestine in the female divides anterior to the ventral sucker and unites again posteriorly, to form a large gray-brown tube which winds down along the midline of the posterior segment of the body and ends in a blind pouch shortly before the tail (Plate 72, Fig. 11 b,c). Up to its forked division, this simple intestine is surrounded on both sides by ramifications of the vitellaria; at the division they combine to form an excretory duct. Here also lies the ovary from which an oviduct runs anteriorly between the bifurcating intestine. It contains complete eggs (provided with germinal cells and shells), and it ends at the posterior edge of the ventral sucker (Plate 72, Fig. 13c). The eggs are oval and are pointed at one end; this point is always oriented posteriorly, both in the uterus and the oviduct. The oviduct forms a long, thin-walled canal of uniform diameter (Plate 72, Fig. 13f). I recognized in the ovary the same delicate cells that I had seen earlier in the ovary of hermaphroditic trematodes. After this discovery, I had to reexamine the *Distoma* about which I first wrote to you. I did not hesitate to explain those mysterious organs between the body and tail as male genital organs, but not decisively, for I had not seen the spermatozoids. One notices, at the spot where both sides turn inward to form the groove,

five or six spherical or oval organs, the four or five rear ones which are packed with delicate cells (Plate 72, Fig. 12a), while the foremost one contains a transparent substance. The walls of this latter organ show, in addition, a double contour and turn frontward and down into a duct which ends free with a bulged lip toward the outside (Fig. 12d). The shape and the appearance of the posterior organs remind me of testicles; the large number of them does not confuse me since an increased number of testicles has also been observed in other trematodes."

In December of 1851, Dr. Bilharz supplemented the above description with the following:

"I am sending you *Distomum haematobium in natura* and in illustration. On the front end of the body, the male has a smooth, soft membrane; conversely, its tail is studded with many little knobs which are covered with short hairs. The two suckers and the lining of the gynecophoric canal are covered with innumerable tiny granules which give the surface of these areas a grainy, leatherlike appearance; however, the midline of the canal is free of the granules. The leathery appearance of the canal seems to be spiny, while in the suckers it is due to numerous flat granules."

These observations led Dr. Bilharz to introduce this worm into the helminthic system with the following nomenclature which he communicated to me in his last letter:

"*Distomum haematobium,* distinct sexes
"Male: soft, white, filiform body, anterior 'forebody' flattened, narrow, ventrally concave, dorsally convex, smooth surface remaining portion of the body = 'hind body' behind the acetabulum (sucker) the ventral surface is rolled in to form a 'gynecophoric canal,' the external surface is rough, and the surface of the canal is smooth. The oral acetabulum subapical, triangular. The ventral acetabulum arises at the end of forebody, the diameter is equal to the oral sucker. The surface outside the acetabula is finely granulated. The esophagus has no pharyngeal muscle and divides anterior to the ventral acetabulum and reunites in hind body. Genital pore originates between ventral acetabulum and gynecophoric canal.

"Female: different shape, more delicate, thin, taeniform body. The anterior sensory organs are attenuated with a smooth surface; the tail ends in a narrow point. Acetabula and esophagus are similar to the male. The genital pore is present at the margin of the ventral acetabulum.

"Length: 3–4 lines [1 line = 1/12 inch—Eds.] but the length of the female is greater.

"Country: Egypt. In human portal vein before bifurcation. Female within male gynecophoric canal always found in mesenteric veins, intestinal veins, hepatic veins [sic], and splenic vein."

I have just received more information from Dr. Bilharz in Cairo (letter dated 16 March 1852) which gives the following new data concerning the life of *Distomum haematobium*.

"Yesterday Griesinger and I performed an autopsy on a boy who died of meningitis. Upon opening the urinary bladder we found lentil-to-pea-size, soft, spongy excrescences (encountered frequently here but unknown in Europe). They were ecchymotic and often encrusted with urinary salts. In the older lesions, we observed dark gray, leatherlike areas of mucosa covered with salt crusts; in the earlier lesions we saw areas surrounded by varicose capillaries coated with mucus and blood. When I cut through the largest of the excrescences, a white thread adhered to the knife. Examining it more closely, I recognized our *Distomum haematobium*. I searched the depth of the incision and pulled out several more. Inside the excrescence were several large, communicating cavities filled with the above-mentioned worms. These smooth-walled cavities were continuous with blood vessels, so that I can only consider them as being very dilated capillaries. The worms were males, and almost all of

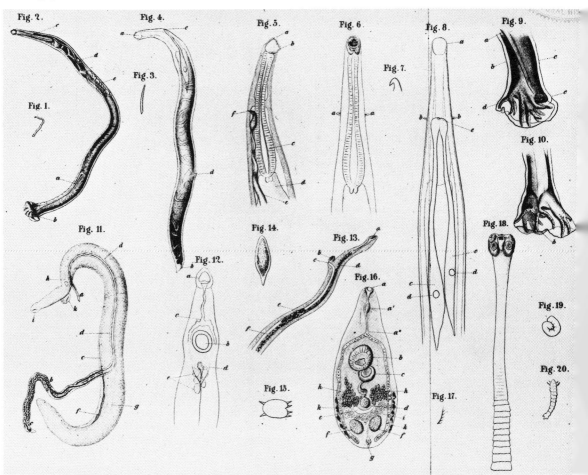

them enclosed females in their gynecophoric canal. The latter differed from the females found in the mesenteric veins by greater clarity of their internal structure, with respect to size and distinctness of the ovary and, even more so, with regard to the abundance of eggs noted in all stages of development. The areas of the bladder mucosa where the earliest stages of the tumors appeared were covered with viscous, clear mucus containing large numbers of *Distomum haematobium* eggs, singly or in clumps. Some of the eggs were enclosed in brittle, calcified capsules which broke into sharp pieces. The eggs had a thin, delicate membrane, a pointed appendage (Plate 72, Fig. 14) and, on the inside, a transparent mass with randomly scattered small granules in which no sharp details could be seen. In other areas were empty egg membranes in which no trace of the inhabitant could be discerned. I then turned my attention to the small blood clots on the surface of the mucosa. Some were in small blood vessels whose lumina ended on the surface of the mucosa. Often, these blood clots were attached to small white clumps which consisted of a number of the above-mentioned eggs.''

Another letter received later that month contained further observations on the *Distomum haematobium* living in the portal vein of man and its relation to certain pathologic formations.

''When I showed Dr. Lautner the *Distomum haematobium* found in the bladder of the boy's cadaver that I had dissected on 15 March, he remarked that he, too, had seen the eggs of *Distomum haematobium* while studying the pathologic changes of the bladder but had not been able to explain them. He and Dr. Griesinger encouraged me to examine the pathologic changes of the bladder which were so similar to those found in dysenteric degenerations of the intestine. On 22 March, I was fortunate enough to get a case for examination which presented the described excrescences of the bladder, as well as extensive dysenteric changes of the large intestine. The bladder excrescences contained no worms; however, embedded in the parenchyma were a number of eggs in spherical heaps. Many of these eggs contained mature, actively motile embryos; next to them lay broken, empty egg shells. The mucosa of the large intestine was loose and easily detached from the submucosa.

Plate 72. [Only Figures 11-15 pertain to schistosomiasis. We did not delete Figures 1-10 and 16-18 which were also drawn by Bilharz. Figures 19 and 20 are from Pruner's paper—Eds.]

Fig. 1. Ancylostoma duodenale, male. *Fig. 2.* The same, seen from the side. (a) The one long penis; (b) anal region; (c) region of the opening of the two secretion organs; (d) lower enlarged part of the one of the secretion organs with the nucleus; (e) the windings of the testicles. *Fig. 3. Ancylostoma duodenale,* female. *Fig. 4.* The same, side view. (a) oral opening; (b) anus; (c) opening of the two secretion organs; (d) vulva. *Fig. 5.* Front end of an *Ancylostoma duodenale,* side view. (a) lower edge of the oral cavity turned to the ventral side; (b) upper edge of the oral cavity turned to the rear side; (c) muscular esophagus; (d) intestine; (e) secretion organ of the left side; (f) opening of the secretion organ on the ventral side of the worm.

Fig. 6. Front end of an *Ancylostoma duodenale,* seen from the back. One can see the tooth apparatus through the oral cavity turned upward; (a, a) two lateral papillae. *Fig. 7.* One of the four teeth from the oral cavity of the same worm. *Fig. 8.* The same worm seen from the ventral side. (a) lower arch of the oral cavity; (b, b) the lateral papillae; (c, c) the two secretion organs, (d, d) the nuclei of the same; (e) opening of the same. *Fig. 9.* The lower end of a male *Ancylostoma duodenale,* side view. (a) right penis; (b) rear side; (c) the ventral side; (d) the middle unpaired radius of the eleven parenchyma radii supporting the split tail bladder; (e) anus region. *Fig. 10.* The same seen from the back. (a) the right lobe of the split tail bladder; (b) the middle unpaired parenchyma radius.

Fig. 11. A male *Distoma haematobium* holding a female enclosed in its gynecophoric canal. (a) front part of the female which projects out of the front end of the gynecophoric canal; (b, c) posterior of the same which hangs out of the back part of the canal; (b) place where both tubes of the split intestinal canal reunite; (c) place where the again simple intestine ends blind; (d, d) place where the body of the female enclosed in the gynecophoric canal shines through; (e) closed groove of the gynecophoric canal; (f) slightly opened groove of the same; (g) bottom of the gynecophoric canal; (h) location of the male sex organs; (i) mouth disc; and (k) stomach disc of the male. *Fig. 12.* Front part of a male *Distoma haematobium,* seen from the abdominal surface. (a) mouth disc; (b) abdominal disc; (c) forking of the intestinal canal; (d) cirrus pouch; (e) testicles.

Fig. 13. Anterior section of a female *Distoma haematobium,* seen from the side. (a) mouth disc; (b) abdominal disc; (c) mouth of the oviduct; (d) place of separation of the intestine; (e) eggs in the oviduct; (f) empty oviduct. *Fig. 14.* Egg from a calcified tubercle of the liver, corresponding in every respect with those of the *Distoma haematobium. Fig. 15.* A flat body provided with pointed appendages which was found encysted simultaneously with an egg (Fig. 14). *Fig. 16.* A *Distoma heterophyes.* (a) oral suction cups; (a') pharynx; (a'') place where intestine separates; (b) abdominal suction cup; (c) cirrus body; (d) germinal vesicle; (e) vesicula seminalis interior; (f, f) the two testes; (g) opening of the excretion organ; (h, h) pile of brown colored eggs; (i) pile of pale eggs (all of these eggs are in a multiple wound oviduct whose outlines have been omitted in the drawing); (k, k) traces of the lateral vitelline vesicles. *Fig. 17.* A prick from the cirrus sac provided with lateral branches. *Fig. 18. Taenia nana. Fig. 19.* A capsule from the liver which contains a *Pentastoma constrictum. Fig. 20.* This *Pentastoma* freed from its capsule.

From the middle of the transverse colon to the anus, the mucosa was somewhat swollen and delicate; it was markedly congested and covered with reddish mucus. In the region of the sigmoid colon and in the rectum were superficial erosions which were intensively and uniformly scarlet and were covered with thin layers of exudate. Between these hyperemic, inflamed areas were both more coarsely congested and almost or completely normal stretches of mucosa. Moreover, this was a very recent case of acute dysentery.

"While I was pulling the mucosa away from the hyperemic areas, I saw, on the submucosa, small white clumps—egg masses—which corresponded exactly with those found in the bladder. Thin cross-sections of the intestine showed large numbers of these clumps embedded in the submucosa; smaller clumps and single eggs were seen in the mucosa itself, between the Lieberkühn's glands and even in the capillaries which extend between these glands. In the uncongested, almost or completely normal areas of the intestine, I found no eggs. The egg masses from the submucosa contained partially opaque eggs filled with a vitelline mass; eggs in which the embryo was plainly visible through the vitelline mass which, for the most part, had been reabsorbed; and mature embryos with a few vitelline corpuscles. The latter moved briskly in all directions, now contracting spherically, now stretching out, and finally tearing the egg shell; in this process they stretch out to their full length and tear the shell with a strong sideward pull. In the cases I observed, the egg always slit lengthwise, with the edges turning outward; yet among the empty egg shells, transverse and oblique slits were also seen. The vitelline membrane would tear at the same time as the outer shell and the animal emerged, in the cases I observed, posterior end first. The ciliary covering of the posterior end would begin to vibrate slowly and the organism would endeavor to loosen itself from the egg by lively movements in all directions and occasionally took a long while. The organism that emerged had a long, cylindrical cone-shaped form which was thicker anteriorly and more rounded posteriorly, with a proboscislike protuberance anteriorly. It was completely covered with rather long cilia which enabled it to swim around in the added water with a lively rotating motion, contracting and stretching at the same

time. Through mucus, egg masses, and the like it crawled with a wormlike motion. The proboscis showed a cuplike indentation. Ventrally, two adjacent pear-shaped bodies were discernible from each one of which a thin stem extended to the proboscis. The posterior portion of the body contained numerous smaller, spherical bodies. It did not take any food. After it had swum around in the water for some time, blisterlike protuberances formed several places on its surface, so that the animal finally assumed a mulberrylike shape, lost its mobility, and gradually dissolved. I noticed these phenomena in the course of an hour in about a dozen specimens. They agree with the observations which you made on the *Monostomum mutabile*.

"I was not able to observe directly the further transformation of these infusorialike embryos. However, I was successful in discovering another fact which, if I am not mistaken, will throw some light on these conditions. Early in 1851, I had found in the calcified areas of the liver, along with eggs of *Distomum haematobium*, strange bodies (Plate 72, Fig. 15) provided with spines, approximately similar to those eggs in size. Last winter I discovered them again under the same conditions. They seemed to me to be long, yellow-brown bodies rounded on both ends. On one side, near the more rounded end, was a conical appendage, directed obliquely toward the pointed end. No content was recognizable in these strange bodies. Last summer I found one of these bodies in one of the first female specimens of *Distomum haematobium* that I studied. It was in the front part of the oviduct, the posterior of which contained the usual eggs. I made a drawing of the specimen at that time but, as the observation was not repeated, I did not attach any particular significance to it. However, I found the same bodies in the above-described dysenteric intestine; they were located singly in the submucosa; in the mucosa between the glands of Lieberkühn; in the blood vessels; and embedded in the bloody mucus covering the free surface of the mucosa. I found large numbers of these bodies in these locations, but always alone and not as frequently as ordinary eggs. I found only one in the lumen of a vessel. These bodies, compressed from all sides, are biconvex with a sharp edge from which the conical appendage protrudes. With respect to content, I found small, sparse granules massed against the edge opposite the spine. A few days ago, Professor Griesinger made an observation of greatest importance in the explanation of these bodies. He found, in a heavily pigmented large intestine (without a doubt the result of a previous dysentery) several bean-sized, deeply pigmented folds of mucosa projecting into the intestinal lumen and containing considerable numbers of the described bodies. These bodies contained living organisms which crawled out and swam around and which seemed to be similar to the specimens that I had observed. Whether or not they had cilia remains the question. Unfortunately, I did not observe any more of the living animals, only dead ones, as well as full and empty shells. The absorbed water caused changes similar to those in the embryos.

"Therefore, how should we regard these bodies? Are they a second type of egg or a kind of pupal covering assumed by the organism after leaving the egg? That these shells belong to the developmental stages of *Distomum haematobium* and not to another organism seems indubitable to me. I not only found them intermixed with eggs of *Distomum haematobium* in the calcified areas within the liver, in the submucosa, and in the mucosa of the large intestine in acute dysentery, but also, although only once, in the oviduct of a female worm which also contained ordinary eggs.

"The hypothesis that these bodies are true eggs is supported by the observation of such a shell in the oviduct and, also, by the emergence of an infusorialike animal similar to organisms from undoubted eggs. Against the two-egg hypothesis, however, is the rarity of such a phenomenon, which although described in some Turbellaria, to the best of my knowledge, has never been observed in trematodes and helminths; further, none of these bodies, neither the specimen in the oviduct nor those outside, showed any trace of the usual egg content, neither germinal vessels nor vitelline mass. Finally, is the fact that among the many dozens of female specimens which I examined during various seasons, such a capsule was found only once inside of the worm.

"In favor of the opinion that these capsules represent a further stage of development, perhaps a kind of pupal covering for the organism newly emerged from the egg, are, in addition to the above-mentioned negative reasons, their fre-

quency, their apparently exclusive presence in old dysenteric lesions, and their relative rarity in the tissues of the acute dysenteric intestine. In addition, this hypothesis is supported by their occurrence on the free surface of the mucosa where the ordinary eggs could not be found. The eggs themselves were found much more frequently in the tissues of the mucosa than within the capsules. Against this is the fact that the animals coming from these capsules seem to be very similar to the organisms originating from the true eggs and seem to be very simply organized. (By the way, a careful comparison of both organisms has not yet been made.)

"I must confess that, with the facts at hand, it is not possible to explain the capsules definitely at this time. However, the most likely supposition is that they represent a protective cover with which the delicate embryos coming from the true eggs of *Distomum haematobium* surround themselves in order to survive after leaving the human body. The specimen found in the oviduct could have undergone this metamorphosis abnormally early, while those found in the tissues of healed dysentery could have gone prematurely through a development which usually occurs outside the human body because cessation of the disease prevented their escaping to the outside.

"I limit myself to these conclusions since I hope to have an opportunity, soon, of deciding this question with certainty by observations. Further investigations in this country, which I shall continue zealously, as well as those being carried out in Europe, investigations to which I invite my colleagues, will have to decide whether *Distomum haematobium* stands in the same relation to dysentery as *Acarus scabiei* does to the itch."

FURTHER COMMUNICATIONS ON *DISTOMUM HAEMATOBIUM*

Fernere mittheilungen über *Distomum haematobium*. Zeitschrift für Wissenschaftliche Zoologie, 4: 454–456, 1853. Selections from pp. 454–455. Translated from the German.

Theodore Bilharz
(1825–1862)

Bilharz' biography will be found with the preceding article in this chapter.

The following are extracts from Bilharz' letters to Professor C. T. von Siebold.

In a letter to Professor von Siebold of 17 May 1852:

My ideas expressed previously concerning dysentery appear to me more and more probable since I have found eggs in a number of cases. In one case the intestine contained many empty egg shells at places where the ulcers were located; in other locations I found inflammation but no ulcerations, and intact eggs were present. I no longer have any doubt that the worms cause the changes in the bladder, ureter, and the seminal vesicles, and so on. I, therefore, believe that the worm is related to a large extent to the frequency of bladder ailments, calculi, and also certain renal diseases. I am enclosing the completed drawings of the eggs and embryos.

From a letter of 2 August 1852:

The eggs of *Distoma haematobium* have been found repeatedly in the dysenteric intestine. However, cadavers of dysenteric patients are somewhat rare at the present time. Some time ago I found an ulcer in the urinary bladder which had the identical appearance of a dysenteric ulcer of the intestine; at its base it contained a large number of fresh eggs just as I had described them in dysenteric intestinal ulcers. They were mainly clumped in small white balls—different areas of the bladder appeared hypervascular without ulcer formation. Other areas showed leathery crusts with calcified eggs. I believe that this case confirms my view concerning the unity or identical nature of the pathologic process in the intestines and the bladder. In the diseases of the bladder the worm is without a doubt the necessary condition, *sine qua non*; however, in dysentery, I have found two cases in which eggs could not be found. Is my ineptness to be blamed or is the worm attracted by the initiation of primary disease of the intestine or is the worm the direct and immediate cause of the disease—but not solely responsible? I have not been able to reach a decision about these important questions. Recently, I examined a patient who complained of heaviness and burning in the bladder for some time. I therefore concluded that he might be suffering from a bladder calculus. I examined him, but could not find a stone. During withdrawal, the catheter passed over a rough surface which I was able to press

between my finger and the catheter on rectal examination. It was immobile, and the bladder was thickened at this point. I am convinced that this was one of those leathery areas previously observed which resulted from the accumulation of chalky [sic] eggs. Unfortunately, I was not able to examine the urine of this patient. I believe I have already advised you that I found fresh eggs in the urine of a young man who had moderate hematuria of unknown etiology. I have also found eggs in the stool of a patient with acute dysentery.

From a letter dated 4 January 1853:

I do not have any new facts of importance to add. The eggs were found in all cases of the described pathology of the bladder and the ureters (they are doubtlessly the main cause of bladder stones which occur so frequently here). Last summer I had occasion to see the embryos from the capsules as observed by Griesinger. They were present in a small intestine from a case of dysentery in which the disease, although not new, had not yet entered the chronic stage. In the tissue of the mucosa, the capsules were found in large numbers; however, the true eggs were not seen. The capsules were not pressed together laterally, as previously noted, but were round (in transverse section). The embryos were alive and were so similar in form, size, and behavior to those which emerged from the true eggs that I could not differentiate between them. They were covered with abundant cilia, and they swam around and disintegrated like the others. Furthermore, the inside of the thin shell was lined with a membrane (yolk) which tore during emergence. The capsules seemed to me to be empty specimens which, like the empty shells of the true eggs, remained in the tissue [See Plate 73, Fig. J—Eds.] and then became filled with calcified deposits. This process can be seen in calcified areas of the liver and, more extensively, in the mucosa of the bladder and the ureters. Here, the described leathery-gray or yellow-stained patches (which creak a little under the scalpel) do not consist of urinary salt deposits, as I had previously believed, but of billions of empty egg shells filled with a chalky mass. On the intestinal mucosa a much more complete ejection of eggs takes place.

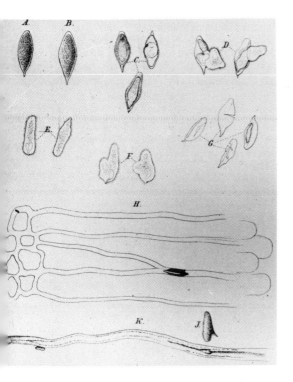

Plate 73. Figures A–K. Fig. 1. Calcified egg from the liver ¹/50′′′ wide, 1/18′′′ long. *Fig. B.* Egg from the open vessels of the bladder mucous membrane. *Fig. C.* Three eggs with living embryos. *Fig. D.* Two eggs with emerging embryos. *Fig. E.* Two free embryos. *Fig. F.* Embryos on the point of decomposition. *Fig. G.* Four empty egg covers (C–G from the bladder and dysenteric intestine). *Fig. H.* Capsule in an injected capillary vessel in the mucous membrane of a dysenteric large intestine. *Fig. J.* The capsule free in bloody mucus from a dysenteric large intestine 1/18′′′ long, ¹/46′′′ wide, and 1/32′′′ wide. *Fig. K.* Front part of a dead female specimen of *Distoma haematobium,* with capsule in the ovarian tube.

CLINICAL AND ANATOMICAL OBSERVATIONS ON THE DISEASES OF EGYPT

Klinische und anatomische beobachtungen über die krankheiten von Egypten. Archiv für Physiologie Heilkunde, 13: 528–575, 1854. Selections from pp. 561–575. Translated from the German.

Wilhelm Griesinger
(1817–1868)

Griesinger's biography will be found in the chapter on Hookworm—Ancylostoma duodenale.

It was Griesinger who invited Bilharz to go to Cairo as his personal prosector. Griesinger's observations on the pathology of schistosomiasis haematobium were the first to be published.

Distomiasis

Distoma haematobium was found by Dr. Bilharz in our autopsies shortly after the *Ancylostoma.* It is three to four lines long [1 line = 1/12 inch—Eds.] and lives in the blood of the portal and mesenteric veins and in the vessels of the bladder; it is probably very abundant in the vessels of the ureter and may at times reach the kidney pelvis. Dr. Bilharz found that the vessels of the bladder wall sometimes contain masses of its eggs; that these eggs very frequently are found in the mucus on the inner lining of the bladder; and that certain pathologic changes in the bladder and ureters, occurring so very frequently in Cairo, stem from deposits of these eggs (Plate 74).

I noted these changes 117 times in 363 autopsies. In some instances, however, especially at the beginning, the mildest cases may have been overlooked. The changes which had occurred in at least one-third of all the cadavers coming to us for autopsy were the following kind:

The simplest, mildest, and most recent change of the bladder mucosa consisted of foci of severe hyperemia, sometimes sharply outlined, sometimes somewhat blurred at the edges, containing many fine extravasations of blood. The mucosa was somewhat swollen or protruded and often, but not always, was covered either with viscous mucus or with a soft, grayish-yellow, hemorrhagic exudate. In these secretions the eggs of the *Distoma* were found, en masse. In some cases, almost the entire mucosa of the bladder was severely congested and showed ecchymoses; in the great majority of cases, the process was confined to small, lentil-up-to-20-cent-piece-size areas, particularly on the posterior bladder wall. In some cases, the urine within the bladder was thick, but generally it was light and clear.

In many cases, we found—a later stage of the disease—polypoid patches of the mucosa which were grayish-yellow, yellowish, discolored, and mixed with many pigmented spots. This protruded mucosa occasionally looked very smooth and leatherlike, as if it had been preserved in alcohol for a long time. Often, however, it showed a brittle crust which, on the surface, was very easily detached in fine crumbs, but which, in its deeper layers, was tightly adherent to the mucosa. In many cases this crust was permeated with urinary salts and a fine sand consisting of masses of eggs or egg shells. It was not possible to detach these crusts completely without also removing the upper layer of the mucosa. These crusts were, at times, as much as one line thick, very soft and friable, partly mixed with blood, and, as noted, very often encrusted with sand. In some cases nothing could be found but dirty red,

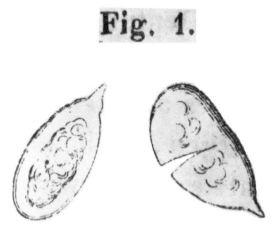

Fig. 1.

Plate 74. Fig. 1. Eggs of *Distoma haematobium,* one with an embryo, and one torn and empty. In distomiasis, these are most numerous in the vessels of the large intestine and the bladder, and in deposits under and on the mucous membrane of these parts and the ureter.

gray, or black raised pigmented areas in the otherwise unchanged mucosa or lying next to fresh areas of hyperemia and hemorrhage. In one case we discovered the mucosa covered with many fresh 20-cent-coin-sized ecchymoses, deep defects of the mucosa, that is, ulcerations, under a thick layer of heavily encrusted urinary salts.

All of these changes could be attributed to extravasation and an inflammatory process resulting from invasion of small vessels by *Distoma* (in some cases they could be removed directly from the vessels), deposition of eggs, and penetration of the eggs through the torn vessels.

However, in many cases the process may look entirely different. In some instances solitary or clusters of pea-to-bean-size, yellowish or ecchymotic papillomata or vegetations one to three lines high were found on the mucosa. They were wartlike or fungiform, divided superiorly into individual lobules, and thus similar to a coxcomb

or raspberry-shaped condyloma; they were often narrowed at the base or pedunculated. As a rule, the external mucosa appeared undamaged, only it was somewhat thicker and perhaps was more tightly adherent to the underlying layer. It often appeared to be heavily congested, and the body of the papilloma was formed by edematous submucosa; this was sometimes soft, yellow-gray, brittle, friable, marrowlike, sometimes solid, tissuelike, infiltrated or, at other times, permeated with clotted blood or pigment. Occasionally, the yellowish-gray "exudate" could be recognized between the mucosa lamina propria so that some cases resembled the cross-section of a fresh typhoid Peyer's patch. In some solid old papillomata, cross-sections at the base showed cellular pedicles which extended and spread into the surrounding uninvolved submucous tissue. Most of the time nothing of this kind was seen; usually, only a soft, yellowish-gray mass mixed with small ecchymoses or pigment was present. Frequently, the whole papilloma was so soft and friable that small pieces could be detached with the greatest of ease; in such cases the mucosa over the protuberance was found to be merely softened in some places or even completely absent. If the mucosa was absent, the core of the papilloma—the submucous tissue—could be easily fragmented.

Among the above-mentioned type of diffuse patches, which are elevated only slightly if at all, there are countless transitional and intermediate stages of the pedunculated papillomata and fungiform lesions. They often occurred in the same bladder, so it was quite clear that the latter constituted more advanced degrees of the same process involving the submucous tissue. The muscle coat of the bladder showing these changes is seldom altered, even in severe cases of this disease; however, it may be slightly hypertrophied. A very odd finding was once made: the serosa of the bladder and the parietal layer of the peritoneum in the vicinity of the bladder showed exactly the same strongly pigmented papillomata similar to a coxcomb.

Dr. Bilharz was successful in extricating the *Distoma* which causes the papillomata from the submucous tissue and from the smooth-walled cavities which, communicating with the vessels, were vessels themselves. From this and the fact that he found a number of *Distoma* eggs in the mucus on the surface of the papillomas as well as in the yellowish-gray exudates of the diffuse patches, it is clear that all these changes are related to the parasite's presence in the bladder wall. It is highly probable that their infiltration and lodging in the bladder wall is connected with egg deposition.

In many cases, these same changes were seen not only in the bladder, but in mucosa of the ureters as well (at times, only the latter and not the bladder). In very rare, exceptional cases they were found even in the renal pelvis. In the ureters, the lesions usually consisted of irregular, isolated, yellowish-gray, slightly raised patches which were formed by a soft, brittle but tightly adherent crust which was sandy to the touch and, as a rule, contained much dark urinary gravel as well as a number of *Distoma* eggs. The consequences of these pathologic processes were much more serious here than in the bladder. Deposits on the mucosa and frequent thickenings of the submucosa caused stricture of the ureter; in addition, there may be spindle-shaped or saclike dilation of the lumen, muscular hypertrophy, and/or urinary retention with its complications. Even in more recent and less severe lesions of the ureters, the kidneys were frequently somewhat swollen and hyperemic and the mucosa of the pelvis was congested. In cases where these changes had been present a longer time, fatty degeneration, pyelitis, hydronephrosis, and complete atrophy of the kidney parenchyma were found. The abundant gravel deposits, in which uric acid crystals could be demonstrated, had as a nucleus a mass of *Distoma* eggs. In addition, large urinary stones often formed in the kidneys, ureters, and bladder with serious consequences. Thus, as Prosper Alpinus [*de Medicina Egyptiorum,* 1829] suspected, the endemic lithiasis of Egypt is based on processes initiated by the *Distoma* and nothing else.

Following are some examples of the late stages of this disease with involvement of the ureters as they appeared to us in 15 cases:

(1) 4 February 1851. A powerfully built man died one hour after admission to the hospital. Autopsy findings included: fresh, reddish-gray hepatization of the right middle lobe of the lung; moderate hypertrophy and dilation of the left ventricle with thickening of the valves; extensive, streaky hemorrhagic erosions of the stomach mucosa; areas of fresh, very intense "diphtheric" dysenteric process with countless follicular abscesses from the distal part of the ileum to the

rectum, along with some older, fibrotic ulcers in the lower large intestine; the calyces and pelvises of both kidneys were markedly dilated, the kidney parenchyma in many places was completely destroyed except for the renal capsule. The mucosa of the pelvis was congested and contained a cloudy somewhat hemorrhagic liquid. Both ureters showed a number of constrictions throughout their entire course which allowed only partial passage of a fine probe; in the area of the constrictions, the muscle layers of the ureter stood out on the inner surface as a markedly restiform, plexiform, and trabecular tissue (very similar to the hypertrophied muscle layer of the bladder). The ureters also had dilations which, proximally, were about the caliber of the small intestine of a cat. The most severe constrictions were found bilaterally, at the entrance of the ureters into the bladder. The mucosa of the ureters was covered, especially in its lower half, by a number of irregular, yellowish-gray, somewhat sandy exudates which were fused with the mucosa and intermixed with ecchymoses and congested areas. The urinary bladder was distended, the muscularis considerably hypertrophied, and the whole mucosa which showed intense hyperemia and hemorrhage was covered with blood and a thin, soft, yellow-gray, sandy exudate; it also had many wartlike, soft, and friable papillomata which could be easily broken off peripherally at the top but remained attached at the base by a solid pedicle. Only microscopic investigation permitted us to recognize that these abnormalities in the urinary apparatus were the result of *distomiasis.*

(2) In a similar case (15 July 1851) with dysentery of about four weeks' duration, the right kidney was again atrophic with marked dilatation of the pelvis and the calyces; the ureter was distended throughout its length to the size of a swan's quill, and deposits of sand were found firmly attached to its inner surface. One inch above the entrance of one of the ureters into the bladder there was a stricture in the form of a diverticulum, more than a few lines wide, its opening facing upward, similar to the valve of a vein, and filled with fine sand; the tissue around it was deeply pigmented, and there was considerable hypertrophy of the muscularis. In the left ureter, which was also distended, there were many soft, yellowish-gray, thin patches of the kind previously described. On the right, the changes were so old and secondary that their origin can only be explained by analogy to the other cases.

In another very similar case (22 August 1851) with a valvelike stricture of the ureter, the mucosa of the bladder showed no changes. In still another similar case (8 November 1851), a valvelike stricture formed by a hypertrophied transverse muscle was found in the left ureter one-half inch above its entrance into the bladder. Posteriorly a diverticular herniation of the ureter was present; the mucosa of the bladder was entirely smooth as the serosa and yellowish-gray, though preserved in alcohol for a long time. There were also scattered spots of gray pigment (the original and obviously very intense process had terminated long ago and its evolution could be explained only by analogy with other cases). In several (five) such cases the mucosa of the ureter was found to be covered with numerous light-colored poppy-to-millet-seed-size cysts which, unfortunately, were not closely examined; one such cyst was the size of a mustard seed and had a milky content.

(3) 30 August 1851. A 20-year-old, emaciated individual died of bilious typhoid; the kidneys were pale and somewhat swollen, the left ureter was dilated and thickened in its wall distally. Proximally, scattered deposits of dark sand and a soft, yellow-gray substance were in the mucosa. Two inches above the bladder there was a hazelnut-thick, spindle-shaped swelling where all layers were found to be thickened; on the inner surface there were many raised (in part, more than line-high), whitish-yellow, soft, granular or wartlike protuberances covered with much sand. Cross-sections showed that the protuberances stemmed from a deposit under the mucosa. On the bladder mucosa, especially on the posterior wall, there were some older wartlike vegetations, along with some linewide, fresh, yellowish-gray, friable deposits as well as some very recent, markedly hemorrhagic areas; in many places, everything was covered with lightly adhering sand.

(4) In another case (1 February 1851), in addition to fresh processes, we found hemorrhage and precipitates of urine salts; on both ureters and the mucosa of the bladder there were many wartlike excrescences one of which, located on the posterior wall, reached the never-before-observed size of a hazelnut. It had the appearance of a cauliflowerlike chancre (villous carcinoma); in cross section it showed a hard, fibrous pedicle radiating into the small tumor, surrounded by a spongy, soft, hypercellular mass. Microscopic examination was lacking, but analogy points to the likelihood of this larger formation being a proliferation of the mucosa of the bladder and its submucous tissue initiated by the *Distoma*. A similar hazelnut-size excrescence was once found in the large intestine of a patient with dysentery.

(5) Finally (on 11 April 1851), at the autopsy of an emaciated soldier from the clinic, the secondary renal changes of calculous pyelitis, caused by the processes described, reached their greatest severity. The left kidney was transformed into a tumor twice head-size, with indication of shallow lobulation; in its over-all form it resembled the bean shape of the kidneys. It consisted in part of apple-to-fist-size communicating compartments, whose membranous walls were several lines thick and which contained at least 12 pints of thick, grass-green pus; there was no trace of kidney parenchyma. At the entrance of the ureter was a dark,

hazelnut-size urinary calculus which was partially fragmented (as if decayed); the walls of the ureter were markedly thickened. In its lower third the lumen was severely constricted; the mucosa was a deep slate-gray. The mucosa of the bladder presented gray or coal-black patches.

It must be deducted by analogy that the formation of stones in this diseased kidney was unusually intense as a result of the *Distoma* infection, traces of which were found in the pigmentation of the ureter and bladder.

These diseases—the various disturbances in the function and nutrition of the urinary tract—do not exist without being injurious to the whole organism. We know of a series of cases which resulted in a generalized chronic illness and eventual death. Most of these individuals die, after complete debilitation, of pneumonia, dysentery, anemia, and the like. It is natural to think of the direct depletion of the blood by the animals living in it and to ascribe to them, as well as to the *Ancylostoma*, an influence on the development of "chlorosis," but I have never seen a simultaneous occurrence of "chlorosis" with *Distoma* that was as striking as its occurrence with the nematodes of the small intestine. The general marasmus which accompanies far-advanced distomiasis seems to me to be more of the sort that can accompany every severe chronic illness, especially one involving the urinary tract; I, therefore, do not find it likely that the development of chlorosis is caused by the presence of the *Distoma* alone.

Distomiasis is closely allied with no other illness, as with dysentery. They are not necessarily always combined. The described changes in the urinary tract occur occasionally in a normal intestine. Frequently, in dysentery, changes are found in the large intestine which morphologically resemble distomiasis in the bladder (hemorrhage; sub- and supramucosal deposits; wartlike, fungiform excrescences, and the like). Microscopic examination in these cases reveals massive deposits of *Distoma* eggs in the vessels of the intestine, the mucosa, and the submucous layer in and under the diphtheritic exudates which at times covered the intestinal ulcerations; they were found even on the free surface of the mucosa which they reached, undoubtedly by penetrating the vessels.

In a black-pigmented large intestine showing scars of healed ulcerations and many warts and spines, I found (19 March 1852) an enormous number of *Distoma* shells (eggs?) [sic] provided with a lateral spine. I was fortunate enough to see massive hatching of the organisms (Plate 75). Following this, and more frequent finding of characteristic eggs of the organism on the intestinal walls of dysentery cadavers, the thought occurred to me that the *Distoma* might be related to the endemic acute and chronic diseases of the large intestine, "like Acarus to scabies" (that is, all endemic dysentery of Egypt could be ascribed to the *Distoma*.)

However, during my brief time in Egypt after this finding, I did not see, even with the most painstaking effort, egg deposits in the intestine or mucosa in several cases of dysentery (among them, a case of the gangrenous type). Apparently related to this fact is that an over-all consideration of the pathology of Egyptian dysentery leads to the conclusion that it is similar to the follicular disease, diphtheria, and croup varieties. The incontrovertible clinical fact that most cases of dysentery arise from originally slight, but neglected diarrheas, contradicts the distomiasis theory completely. I believe, therefore, that ordinary dysentery of all types arises from causes other than distomiasis; further, that distomiasis of the large intestine—egg-containing deposits on the mucosa, infiltration of the submucosal tissue with eggs, formation of the wart- and spinelike swellings of the mucosa, lodging of the *Distoma* eggs in rows in the blood vessels of the mucosa—is only one, but nevertheless a highly important complication of these diseases. But I do consider it possible that, in some cases, *Distoma* alone can effect changes in the large intestine which, at least to the naked eye, seem very similar to those of true dysentery.

My autopsy records show that of 117 reported cases of distomiasis of the urinary tract, 50 occurred along with acute and chronic dysentery and more than 20 cases were accompanied by changes associated with bilious typhoid. However, this does not necessarily indicate a direct connection between distomiasis and the ailments mentioned because the numbers given are directly proportional to the total number of cadavers which generally died of dysentery and bilious typhoid.

I cannot say whether distomiasis is related to the formation of liver abscesses. One will have to consider this possibility since, at times, the entire portal vein is filled with mature worms, and their eggs have been found in liver tissue. In the hot countries, where liver abscesses occur even more frequently than in Egypt, a thorough investigation of this subject will have to be made. The same holds true for liver atrophy which is also found frequently in Egypt.

I can add only little to the question of which symptoms are caused by the described processes during life and whether they can be diagnosed in the patient. Only shortly before my departure from Egypt was the subject clarified so that its application became feasible. The clinically treated patients in whom the autopsy showed distomiasis usually had suffered from other serious diseases which overshadowed some of the minor symptoms of distomiasis. The major signs of the disease are manifest in the urinary tract, primarily in the urine itself. Transient hematurias of unknown origin in more or less marasmic individuals have come to us several times in Egypt. We no longer doubt that this condition is caused by distomiasis. The eggs of the *Distoma* were found by Dr. Bilharz while microscopically examining the urine of a boy who developed hematuria during convalescence from typhoid fever. The diagnosis can be established with this finding alone.

The symptoms of pyelitis or simple bladder ailment must be present in many cases; acute exacerbations of obscure and undiagnosed bladder and kidney ailments have come to our attention several times. In Egypt, an undetermined chronic illness with occasional disturbances in urine formation must call to mind the disease under consideration here. In the most serious and less frequent cases (such as No. 5 above), the associated enlargement of the kidneys could be diagnosed during life. We also have had some cases which in themselves gave rise to the supposition that the *Distoma* disease can run its course as a serious, acute ailment, sometimes leading to death. Twice, in the cadavers of individuals who had died after very brief, unfortunately not more accurately diagnosed illnesses, we found abundant, fresh *Distoma* lesions (hemorrhages, exudates, and the like) in the bladder, fresh mucus in the kidney pelvis and an even, severe hyperemia of the kidney tissue in the absence of other changes. In three cases, after alleged typhoid disease of short duration, we found characteristic lesions in the bladder and ureters; once with a very limited hepatization of the lung, once with a wedge-shaped splenic in-

Fig. 2.

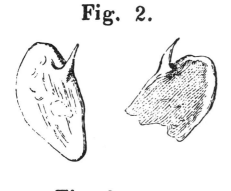

Fig. 3.

a

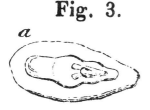

b

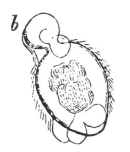

Fig. 4.

a

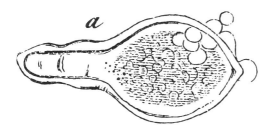

b

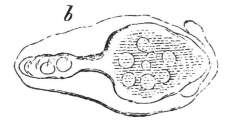

farct, and once with small meningeal hemorrhages. A number of possibilities present themselves here. First, one has to think of many causes of disturbances of urinary excretion by local processes and uremia; also, the possibility of a sepsis of the bloodstream due to the large number of worms living and dying in the portal vein; finally, the transportation of the worms or at least their eggs into the general circulation and to essential organs must be kept in mind. With respect to the latter, we have made (31 March 1852) an important and surprising discovery: the presence of some *Distoma* egg shells in the blood of the left heart. A report of the case follows:

The emaciated cadaver of a 20-year-old soldier showed edema of the legs; there was a serous-fibrinous effusion of moderate degree in both pleurae with compression of the lower lobes; there were disseminated pale, lobular, nongranulated, consolidated areas in the upper lobes which blended with the edematous surroundings. Other findings included: moderate ascites; a tough, solid, olive-brown liver reduced symmetrically to half its normal size, without granulation; moderately enlarged, waxy spleen; pale mucosa of stomach and small intestine. In the large intestine, up to the beginning of the descending colon, much thin bilelike exudate; from there, up to the rectum, there was only watery exudation. The entire intestine was edematous; the mucosa in the ascending colon pale, soft, and easily scraped off

Plate 75. Fig. 2. Seldom found saclike bodies provided with a lateral spike (eggs? pupal coverings?); in any case, belonging to the developmental cycle of the *Distoma haematobium*, since such a body was once found in the Fallopian tube of the organism. They were found on the completely black-pigmented walls of a large intestine which was covered with previously mentioned excrescences. *Fig. 3.* (a) One of the coverings from the aforementioned intestine (19 March 1852) with an embryo lying inside. The embryos moved for some time by contracting and stretching; suddenly the covering tore and the animal crawled out slowly. (b) Form of the animal 15 minutes after emerging. In the course of the next few hours, the neck of the animal became elongated and its form thus changed considerably, but it was lost in the mucus in which it lay. *Fig. 4.* Next to the external shell coverings in the same intestine, I found free animals. (a) One was living. Upon the addition of much water the movement of the animal ceased and (by lifting off or swelling of the outer covering as a result of imbibing water?) it took on form (b). It seemed to me as though the light balls which were noticed on and within the animals were drops of a liquid which were finally eliminated at the rounded end; however, I am not sure about this.

with the back of the scalpel; from the beginning of the descending colon to the rectum abundant pale, spotty, and striped hyperemias covered with thin, mucoid secretions; in some places in the colon dense hyperemic patches with superficial erosions of the mucosa; general softening of the mucosa; kidneys small, pale, and fatty; bladder full of clear urine; bladder mucosa pale.

I carefully examined the catarrhal intestine; neither *Distomas* nor their eggs were present, nor did I find any in the hepatized areas of the lung which were examined. However, I did find in the blood of the left heart a small group of six egg shells of *Distoma haematobium* lying together, very light and pale, containing no embryos. In the blood of the left and right heart and the splenic vein were bodies which resembled the dead embryos of *Distoma.* I do not dare to venture an explanation. Their size corresponded to that of the eggs, whose identical lifeless forms (at the time considered to be dead) I had found earlier (on 22 March) on the mucosa of an intestine from a case of dysentery.

One further point deserves mention. In Cairo, I noticed that, at certain times, *Distoma* infections are found almost daily in cadavers and then are absent for a considerable time. I suspected at that time a seasonal influence on the incidence of this disease; this cannot be proved completely by the autopsy reports currently available to me, though I do find a noticeable variation in the frequency of infection from month to month. For instance, among all the autopsies for the months of June and August, distomiasis was mentioned in half the cases; it occurred in only one-quarter of the cases in September, October, and January. I believe that this is not completely accidental. Future investigators will be able to get valuable information from observing and pursuing the differences in the life cycle and development of these entozoa, perhaps in their connection with the foods of certain seasons and with other pathological processes showing a seasonal cycle. The tedious investigation into the epidemic occurrence of distomiasis has to begin with the study of the influence of the seasons.

Had I remained longer in Egypt, I would have set myself two large practical tasks. First, I would wish to discover the ways in which these entozoa penetrate the body. This is relatively easy considering the simple food of the people (at least much simpler than in Europe). There are three main possibilities—either through consumption of (a) the unfiltered Nile water; or (b) bread and grain and/or dates; or (c) fish of which I am highly suspicious and which, served in a half-rotten condition under the name of *Physich,* is food and delicacy to the fellaheens. With patient investigation, fully mature organisms which appear in the intestine and in the blood such as *Ancylostoma* and *Distoma,* ought to be found in one of these organs—as eggs, at intermediate stages of their development, or as fully grown animals.

Second, on the basis of my experiences, I would have tried a new approach in the treatment of these widespread endemic illnesses. When I left the autopsy room after the autopsy on a case mentioned previously, I said to the Arabian assistant, "You must now try calomel for anemia." This hint hardly fell on fertile ground and yet it is obviously of the greatest interest to try all kinds of anthelminthics—partly against frequently occurring ailments of undetermined cause which, according to the newly acquired facts, can now be ascribed to distomiasis, and partly and in particular for the cure of "chlorosis." A priori, calomel and oil of turpentine might be especially advisable; future experience will have to show which of these is the most effective drug. Perhaps certain foods like onions and garlic exert a beneficial influence. The investigation of the ways in which the entozoa enter the body should result in large-scale hygienic measures for the entire country. I wish that these remarks would draw attention in Egypt, not only from the doctors, but also from those in authority who are entrusted with the health and care of an underdeveloped population and whose greatest interest should be to see that strong and vigorous people inhabit this beautiful country.

I shall not pursue further what consequences will result from this for the pathology of warm countries in general and of tropical regions in particular. The pathology of these countries should be subjected to new investigations from the standpoint of helminthology. Hematuria, lithiasis, dysentery, liver abscess, and tropical chlorosis are all still poorly understood. Perhaps even part of the tropical fever ought to be reinvestigated in the light of the latest helminthologic discoveries.

REPORT OF A CASE OF BILHARZIA FROM THE WEST INDIES

British Medical Journal, 2: 1894–1895, 1902.

Patrick Manson
(1844–1922)

Manson's biography will be found in the chapter on Malaria.

Manson's report of a laterally spined egg of Schistosoma *is recorded here; it is the first report of* Schistosoma *infection in the New World.*

With the exception of Mesopotamia, Cyprus, and Mauritius, bilharzia disease has hitherto been supposed to be peculiar to Africa. The following case shows that the parasite has a wider range. Personally, until I came across this case, I never encountered the disease in patients from the West Indies, but its occurrence in a white man from that part of the world practically proves that in some of these islands, if not in all, it must be by no means uncommon amongst the coloured population. Now that attention has been directed to the subject, we may expect to hear from time to time of similar cases. It is evident that the distribution of this and similar parasitic diseases depends on the presence or absence of the efficient intermediaries. Possibly our zoologists may be able to point to some mollusc or anthropod which the West Indies and Africa have in common, and thereby indicate the long-sought-for, but hitherto undiscovered, intermediate host of bilharzia haematobia. Another African disease, guinea-worm, was at one time said to be endemic in Curaçao and others of the West India Islands, and in a limited area in Brazil. I understand the disease has disappeared from Curaçao, and we hear no longer of its presence in the Brazils; it may be that bilharzia has obtained a similar precarious footing in the Western Hemisphere, and that subsequently it will disappear from that region; meanwhile we can assert its presence there as a fact.

I may mention that the patient, an Englishman and a professional man, came to me as a private case complaining of vague symptoms, lumbar pain, headache, etc. As I could not account for the symptoms, and as he looked anaemic, and knowing that he came from a place where Ankylostoma duodenale is very prevalent, the idea that he suffered from ankylostomiasis occurred to me. I made an examination of his faeces and discovered the ova of bilharzia. In this case, as so often happens in bilharzia ova from the alimentary canal, the spine is placed laterally.

I am indebted for the following notes to Major Ross and Dr. Daniels, of the London School of Tropical Medicine.

Previous History—The patient is an Englishman aged 38. Five years ago, in Antigua, after a heavy day's work he felt a dull pain in the lumbar region; it went off after rest, but would come on again after active exercise. During the last year this pain has increased in severity and duration; he was invalided home on account of it. Has resided in the West Indies chiefly for 15 years, and has had many attacks of malaria. Never passed blood in his urine; never noticed blood in his stools.

Present State—Temperature 97°; tongue slightly coated; is slightly anaemic; complains of right frontal headache; has some enlargement of liver and spleen.

Microscopic Examination—Faeces, bilharzia ova not numerous; generally distributed throughout the faecal mass; lateral spined. *Urine,* no ova.

Blood (By G. Duncan Whyte)—Haemoglobin, 84 per cent; red blood cells, 4,650,000; white blood corpuscles, 8,200; polymorphonuclear leucocytes, 49 per cent; lymphocytes, 21 per cent; mononuclear leucocytes, 17 per cent; eosinophiles, 12 per cent; intermediate, 1 per cent.

History of Patient's Residence in West Indies, by Himself—I went from England to Antigua in May, 1887. In the place I lived in there are a good number of swamps, but my house was a mile from the nearest; water was obtained from cisterns (iron) and ponds, was often stale, and contained visible living things; had two or three attacks of malarial fever, one severe.

I removed to Anguilla in 1889. It is a flat and dry island. The drinking water came from stone cisterns, the bath water from wells. My health here was fairly good.

Moved to St. Kitts in 1891. This is a mountainous island, no swamps within six miles of my residence; water from public service reservoir conveyed in pipes. My health was fair, but had two or three "run-downs" and one or two attacks of fever. Came to England in June, 1894, and returned to St. Kitts in January, 1895.

In September, 1896, I returned to Antigua— same district, but nearer to swamps; water from stone cistern; plenty of frogs in water, which was usually boiled; health very unsatisfactory; pain in back severe, but generally yielding to rest and treatment.

In June, 1898, I came to England and returned in January, 1899. In December, 1900, I returned to St. Kitts, but to a different neighbourhood; house 600 ft. above the level of the sea; nearest swamp three miles; drinking water from private mountain source; water for baths, etc., from open mountain source (very unsatisfactory at times), passing through a village, and used by everybody. On two or three occasions I got an "itch" in the bath, called locally "cow itch." My health at first good, soon failed, and for the whole of this year have had pain in the back, and headache in right side and right eye; also pains in the knee-joints, and always tired. Was invalided home in July.

I ought to have added that between 1891 and 1901 I have been to Nevis on short visits many times; water there is good. To Montserrat two or three times; water there also good. I spent five days in St. Thomas in 1894, and five weeks in Barbados in January, 1900. I have never been to Africa or anywhere else except the British Islands.

NOTE ON A NEW FORM OF LIVER CIRRHOSIS DUE TO THE PRESENCE OF THE OVA OF BILHARZIA HAEMATOBIA

Journal of Pathology and Bacteriology, 9: 237–239, 1904.

William St. Clair Symmers
(1863–1937)

Although he was born in South Carolina, Symmers went to Aberdeen, his father's native city, to study medicine, receiving his degree in 1887. After a short period in the general practice of medicine, he became assistant pathologist in the Royal Infirmary in Aberdeen and later pathologist to the Birmingham General Hospital and to the Lancashire County Asylum. Following a period of study at the Pasteur Institute in Paris, he became assistant bacteriologist in the British Institute of Preventive Medicine in London, now known as the Lister Institute.

In 1897, Symmers was appointed professor of pathology and bacteriology at the Government Medical School in Cairo and pathologist to the government hospital. Soon after his arrival in Egypt, he helped to terminate a serious outbreak of cattle plague.

He returned to the British Isles in 1904 as chairman of the Department of Pathology in Queens College, Belfast. He was elected secretary of the Pathological Section of the British Medical Association in 1907 and president in 1909. In addition to his medical interests (which included medical jurisprudence) he was an avid student of classical literature and philosophy.

The unique hepatic fibrosis of schistosomiasis was first documented by Symmers.

During the last five years I have observed, from time to time, in the post-mortem room of the Kass-el-Ainy Hospital, Cairo, a peculiar condition of the liver, in which there was an unusual distribution of cirrhotic tissue. The microscopic examination of several of these livers (six) has satisfied me that there is, in these cases, a constant concomitance of *Bilharzia* ova and periportal cirrhosis.

To the naked eye the liver is somewhat enlarged, often weighing 1800 grms. The surface shows a peculiar shagreened appearance, owing to a pronounced increase of the perivascular connective tissue, so that dull white markings appear through the capsule, forming a wide meshed network with irregular quadrate, pentate, or many-sided areas. There is also a variable number of flat, almost china white nodules, which project more or less from the capsule, particularly on the under surface of the organ toward the anterior margin.

These projections vary in size from a pin-head to a split pea, and occasionally are as large as the half of a white haricot bean. They are distinct growths of the capsule,—perihepatitic nodules,—and have no relation whatever, in appearance, structure, or origin with the hobnail projections of coarse cirrhosis. On section, the liver presents a remarkable appearance (Plate 76, Fig. 1), due to an enormous increase of the fibrous tissue (Glisson's capsule) which normally surrounds the portal canals. This periportal new tissue is white,—almost as much so as porcelain,—although it occasionally has a faint pink tinge.

When a portal canal is cut transversely, the mouths of the contained vessels and bile duct are seen embedded in the centre of a circular or slightly oval area of white connective tissue, the diameter of the mass being, on the average, from a sixth to a quarter of an inch; whereas, longitudinal sections of the canals (Plate 76, Fig. 2) reveals elongated masses of similar appearance and

490

thickness, so that the cut surface of the liver looks as if a number of white clay-pipe stems had been thrust at various angles through the organ. There is no naked-eye appearance comparable to the interlobular distribution of fibrous tissue that characterizes the usual forms of hepatic-cirrhosis. There is, therefore, no prominence of the liver lobules either singly or in groups, nor is there any of the retraction of the capsule, which, in the usual forms of cirrhosis, gives the granular or hobnail appearance to the organ. The parenchyma of the organ is homogeneous in appearance, and has a peculiar anaemic or drab colour which contrasts very markedly with the pinkish white of the new fibrous tissue.

Microscopic Examination

There is a great increase of the periportal connective tissue, especially of the sublobular and larger portal canals rather than those of interlobular distribution. This cirrhotic tissue is, for the most part, composed of well-formed bundles of nucleated fibrous tissue, but there are parts in which it is made up of young spindle cell tissue with occasional groups of nucleated round cells. The fibres are wavy and parallel, for the most part, but in certain places they are arranged concentrically, so that sometimes in a single field of the microscope, several such concentric masses may be seen.

Among this tissue are seen ova of the *Bilharzia haematobia,* often in considerable numbers. Very frequently an ovum is seen lying in the centre of the above-mentioned concentric masses of fibrous tissue. A small blood vessel may often be seen running up to, and widening into, such a mass of concentrically arranged young fibrous tissue, and lying in the centre of the newly formed mass, as if it had become impacted in the vessel, and had, by its presence produced the proliferation of tissue which resulted in the cirrhosis, an ovum. The tissue immediately surrounding such an impacted ovum is invariably composed of spindle cells arranged concentri-

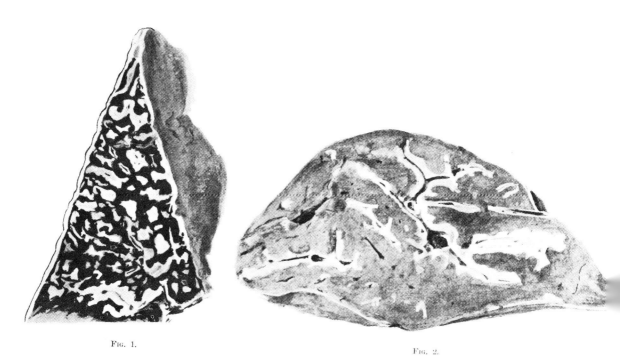

Fig. 1.   Fig. 2.

Plate 76. Fig. 1. Section of liver in which there is great increase of periportal fibrous tissue. *Fig. 2.* Longitudinal section of portal canals, which there is great increase in the amount of fibrous tissue around the vessels and bile ducts.

cally around the ovum, and at the periphery of the mass passes into the more fully formed fibrous tissue which makes up the general periportal cirrhosis.

These ova are usually empty, *i.e.* merely the shell or part of the shell remains, very frequently with a well-marked lateral spine; indeed, most of these ova are laterally spined. As a rule, the ova are broken and shrivelled, but are easily recognised by the peculiar translucent shining shell and spine. I have several times seen well-formed unbroken ova, which were filled with a mass of nucleated round cells which stained readily with logwood. Apparently these cells have wandered to the ova from without, and are probably phagocytic in action, being able to destroy the contents of the ova, but not to dissolve the shell.

I have only occasionally observed ova lying in the larger capillary blood vessels which permeate the new fibrous tissue, these eggs, as a rule, are found in the midst of the fully formed connective tissue, or else, as above stated, in the concentric masses of young fibrous tissue. No ova are seen lying among the hepatic cells. The cirrhotic tissue is well supplied with minute blood vessels; and the newly formed bile ducts are often seen.

The whitish nodules on the surface of the liver are composed of fibrous tissue containing ova. In the liver lobules, the capillaries running between the columns of liver cells are somewhat dilated, and in them are a great number of scattered cells which contain granules and amorphous masses of a sepia-brown pigment (melanin); these cells often appear round, and are almost full of a pigment which obscures the nucleus, but in most instances they are elongated, with tapering ends (*Stern Zellen* of Kupffer). There is also a small amount of pigment lying free in the cirrhotic tissue, particularly in the neighbourhood of the ova shells in the young fibrous tissue, but in the denser, old fibrous tissue the pigment is, as a rule, absent, though it is occasionally present within round cells which have apparently wandered into the tissue.

This cirrhosis is, I believe, due to the presence of the *Bilharzia* ova, a view which is strengthened by many observations of similar fibrous overgrowths in various other parts of the body, in which the new formation is accompanied by the presence of these ova.

NEW OR LITTLE KNOWN AFRICAN ENTOZOA

Journal of Tropical Medicine and Hygiene, 10: 117, 1907.

Louis Westenra Sambon
(1866–1931)

Sambon was born in England of Anglo-French parentage and was educated both at St. Bartholomew's Hospital in London and at the University of Naples, where he received his M.D. in 1891. His lifelong interest in cholera stemmed from his work during a terrible epidemic of the disease which occurred in Naples while he was still a student in 1884.

He started his professional career as a gynecologist in Rome, but the lure of England was too strong for him. When he went to London, he met Sir Patrick Manson and came under the influence of that great figure in tropical medicine. His early publications, which advocated the view that it was the parasites of the tropics, and not the climate, that killed human beings in those latitudes, were ridiculed almost to the point of ruining his career because his ideas were quite contrary to universally accepted opinion. Later, Sambon had the satisfaction of visiting Panama at the invitation of General William C. Gorgas, whose testimony vindicated Sambon's hypothesis, "My colleagues and I are pleased to have been able to prove that you were right."

He was a lecturer in epidemiology at the London School of Hygiene and Tropical Medicine. Sambon spent the last years of his life studying the epidemiology of cancer, leading him to develop the concept of "cancer houses" and "cancer streets."

Sambon proposed that the name "Schistosoma mansoni" designate the lateral-spined egg and that the terminal-spined egg be called "Schistosoma haematobium."

In a paper on Entozoa, read at the last meeting of the Zoological Society of London, 19 March 1907, Dr. L. W. Sambon, F. Z. S., described two new parasites of man for which he proposed the names of *Sparganum baxteri* and *Schistosomum mansoni*.

Schistosomum mansoni is very similar to *S. haematobium* in general appearance, and in both species the males present a tuberculated outer surface of the body, but the ova of the new species have a large, curved, lateral spine, which distinguishes them unmistakably from those of the old classic species with a short, straight spine at their posterior extremity. Like *S. japonicum*, *S. mansoni* does not affect the genito-urinary organs, its ova are eliminated solely by way of the intestine; they are never found in the urine. The patients harbouring this parasite suffer from a haemorrhagic enteritis, but they never present haematuria. *S. mansoni* has a wide distribution throughout Africa. In Egypt it is found, not infrequently, together with *S. haematobium,* but in the Congo Free State and in other parts of Africa it is the only species present. It is found also in the West Indies (Antigua, Porto Rico, and probably others), and very likely in other places within the Tropics.

The laterally-spined ova of *S. mansoni* have frequently been found in Egypt, but, as a rule, in cases of mixed infection, and hitherto they have been looked upon by the majority of observers as eggs with shell distorted during their passage through the intestinal wall. This explanation, soon dispelled by a comparative examination of the ova of the two species, is further contradicted by the fact that the laterally-spined ova have been observed within the uterus of the correlative female worms. Looss suggested that they might represent the product of unfertilised females, but morphological details as well as facts of geographical distribution and clinical examination place now beyond doubt the reality of the new species.

The Schistosomidae of man and cattle are all very much alike in general appearance and structure. The most striking and characteristic difference is that of their eggs, which differ markedly in each species. In *S. haematobium* they are ovoid and provided with a short, straight terminal spine; in *S. bovis* they are spindle-shaped and also provided with a short, terminal pear-shaped spine; in *S. mansoni* they are oval and provided with a large, thick lateral spine; in *S. japonicum* they are ovoid and have no spine. Moreover, each species has its own peculiar distribution and differs in its pathogeny.

Sir Patrick Manson having found laterally-spined ova in the faeces of a West Indian case, and no ova in the urine, suggested some years ago that the laterally-spined ova might represent a different species. In appreciation of this, one of his many genial intuitions, the new Trematode is dedicated to him.

CONTRIBUTION TO THE STUDY ON SCHISTOSOMIASIS IN BAHIA

Contribuição para o estudo da schistosomiase na Bahia, and Contribuição etc., Dezeseis observaçoes. Brazil-Medico, 22, No. 29: 281–283 and No. 45: 441–444, 1908. Selections from pp. 281–282 and 441–442. Translated from the Portuguese. (Continuation in No. 46, 451–454, not included).

Manoel Augusto Pirajá da Silva (1873–1961)

Pirajá da Silva was born in the town of Camamu, Bahia, Brazil, moved to Salvador for his early education, and studied medicine at the Faculty of Medicine of Bahia. After a period of practice in the interior, he returned to Salvador and, in 1902, was appointed to the first chair of clinical medicine in that city's university. After pursuing various investigations, one of which led to the microscopic confirmation of Treponema pallidum *as the causative agent of syphilis, Pirajá da Silva embarked on the studies which were to lead to the zoologic identification of* Schistosoma mansoni. *The resulting scientific controversy led him to travel widely through Europe for the sake of further study and consultation. Upon his return to Brazil, he was appointed head of the Department of Parasitology at the Medical School of Bahia, a post he held until his retirement in 1935. In addition to his work on schistosomiasis, Pirajá da Silva also pursued problems relating to leishmaniasis, Chagas' disease, skin-biting and burrowing flies, mycotic infections, and ainhum, and made notable contributions to historical and botanical researches dealing with his native land.*

Pirajá da Silva described in detail the adults and ova of Schistosoma mansoni, *the only medically important schistosome in the western hemisphere.*

On 20 April 1908, an 18-year-old, single Negro entered on the service of the first Department of Medical Clinics. He was an unskilled worker, born in this state and resident of Santo Antonio, in this city. Upon examining this patient's fresh blood [sic], we found crescent-shaped hematozoans and an egg which was very similar to that of *Schistosoma mansoni.* Because of this fact and other findings during his complete examination, we examined the patient's stools; the results of our studies will be given later. On physical examination we noted pallor of the skin and conjunctivae. The patient also was emaciated. Except for a slightly enlarged spleen, nothing else was remarkable.

Twenty-four hour urinalysis:
Quantity.................................1,000 cc
Specific gravity...........................1,012

Reaction ....acid
Sediment.....................................27.96
Urobilin ....small amount

We did not find abnormal elements in the urine. The urine was centrifuged, but nothing noteworthy was found in its sediment.

Hematologic examination:
Red blood cells 2,732,000
Leukocytes................................12,400
Hemoglobin..................................50%

Differential leukocyte count:
Neutrophils................................46.4%
Eosinophils.....................................9%
Transitional forms..........................10.4%
Mononuclears 8.8%
Lymphocytes, large........................18.2%
Lymphocytes, small 7%
Mast cells 0.2%

After entering the hospital the patient experienced slight fever which did not exceed 38° C, in spite of our having found many crescents in preparations made with freshly stained blood. Confusion and epistaxis were his chief complaints. It was not possible to examine the blood of the epistaxis, which might have had great importance in the disease with which we were dealing. The patient also stated that his stools had been somewhat bloody for quite a while; this led us to examine his stools more carefully for the presence of schistosome eggs (as we observed in the stool examination of a patient in the clinic about four years ago). In the stool we found laterally spined eggs, as well as ova of *Ascaris lumbricoides, Trichocephalus, Trichuris* [sic], *Uncinaria duodenalis,* and *Anguillula stercoralis.* Upon consulting textbooks on tropical disease we did not find, in the literature on schistosomiasis, any reference to the disease in Brazil nor is this country mentioned in the geographic distribution of the worm.

"Bilharzia" was the generic name used; the rules of nomenclature use the term "Schistosomum," and there are authors who use the word "Bilharzia" to identify the species of this genus. Until a short time ago, it was thought that human bilharziasis was caused by only two species of schistosomes: *Schistosoma haematobium* and *Schistosoma japonicum* (or *cattoi*). Now there are three known species of schistosome able to attack the human being:

Schistosoma haematobium, S. japonicum (or *cattoi*), and *S. mansoni.* The latter was so classified by Sambon to honor Patrick Manson, who was the first to describe this third species. . . .

Dimensions of the eggs of *Schistosoma mansoni* and its spine [based on 10 eggs—Eds.]:

Maximum dimensions: length 162μ; width 72μ; length of spine 27μ.

Minimum: length 126μ; width 49.50μ; length of spine 11.25μ.

Average: length 146μ; width 62μ; length of spine 18μ.

The eggs of *S. mansoni* have been found in the liver producing a particular cirrhosis. The eggs of *S. mansoni* are oval and provided with a lateral spicule; those of *S. haematobium* are more or less ovoid and have a straight terminal spicule; those of *S. japonicum* are ovoid and do not have a spicule. The workers do not agree about the way man becomes infected. It is generally accepted that the eggs expelled by humans find their way into the water and, in this medium, the miracidium is freed. The intermediate host and the migrations and transformation of this trematode are not presently known. . . .

After seeing the above-mentioned case of schistosomiasis, we had the opportunity of observing two other cases. One of these patients had died of another disease; we performed an autopsy. In the branches of the portal vein we found a worm which, when examined microscopically, seemed to us to be a female specimen of *S. mansoni.* It measured 13 mm in length, and 0.364μ in width more or less in its midportion. Plate 77 presents drawings of the eggs which were made from photographic slides by the distinguished fifth-year student Octavio Torres, intern of the Medical Clinic. . . .

Contribution to the Study of Schistosomiasis in Bahia, 16 Observations

About four years ago, while examining a patient's stools, we found, together with some ova of *Ancylostoma duodenale,* different eggs with lateral spines. This aroused our curiosity at the time, but we could not find a ready explanation. This year, we proceeded systematically to examine the stool of every patient who came into our clinic and, once again, we had the occasion to observe the ova with lateral spines. . . .

In the three autopsies which we have performed up to the present time, we found one schistosome in the portal vein of each of the first two cadavers and 24 of them in the third one. All of these worms were found in the portal vein and in its main branches. The 24 worms found in the last cadaver autopsied were classified as follows: 19 isolated males, one isolated female, and two males containing females in their gynecophoric canal. . . .

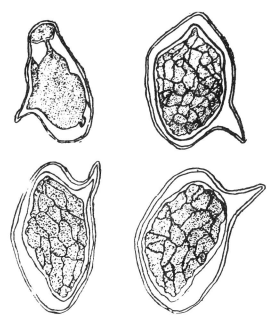

Plate 77. Eggs of *Schistosoma mansoni.*

With this material, we continued our studies already initiated with the ova; the first worm we microphotographed. For greater clarification of the anatomical structure and for identification of the above worm, we were able to microphotograph an ovum, a miracidium leaving the ovum, adult worms copulating, the sexual organs of the female, and the caudal and cephalic extremities of the male and female. . . . [Unfortunately, the quality of the microphotographs was too poor to permit their being included—Eds.].

It seemed to us that the cephalic extremity of the worm which we found differed somewhat from that of the *Schistosoma haematobium.* (We used for this comparative study a drawing by Looss of *S. haematobium* which is found in all textbooks of parasitology and tropical diseases.) The caudal extremity of the worm we saw becomes gradually thinner and then terminates.

Studying the male worm under the microscope on slides fixed by lactophenol which, besides fixing, has the property of clearing the preparation greatly, we saw that the digestive tract presented the same arrangement noted in *S. haematobium* and that the sexual organs were composed of six masses; the latter were composed of the genital glands, testes, and seminal vesicles.

The spinous papillae coating the external dorsal and posterior surface of the body did not seem to us to be as pronounced as those observed in *S. haematobium.*

EGYPTIAN BILHARZIOSIS

Researches on Egyptian Bilharziosis (A Report to the War Officers on the Results of the Bilharzia Mission in Egypt, 1915). London: John Bale, Sons & Danielsson, 1918. 140 pp. Selections from pp 3–4, 24–26, 36–44, 48, 93, 114–127, 131–132, 137–140. [Published originally in The Journal of the Royal Army Medical Corps, 1–48, 1915—Eds.].

Robert Thomson Leiper
(1881–1969)

A Scotsman, Leiper began his studies in zoology and medicine at the University of Birmingham and later transferred to the University of Glasgow, where he graduated in 1904. His interest in zoology, particularly helminthology, took him on extensive travels to Africa and the Far East. In 1914 he was sent to Egypt by the British Army to investigate the molluscan transmission of Egyptian schistosomiasis.

Shortly afterward, he was appointed to the chair of helminthology at the University of London and director of the Division of Medical Zoology In the London School of Hygiene and Tropical Medicine.

He was founder and editor of the Journal of Helminthology *for many years and was considered to be a sort of "international court of reference" by twentieth-century helminthologists because of his encyclopedic knowledge.*

Sonsino nearly succeeded in describing the life cycle of Schistosoma in 1885. The Japanese workers had demonstrated the snail's role in the life cycle of Schistosoma japonicum prior to Leiper's work. Leiper's travels to Japan and China with the first Wandsworth Expedition of the London School of Tropical Medicine provided an opportunity to become acquainted with the Japanese research. This report completes the life cycle of Schistosoma mansoni *and* Schistosoma haematobium.

Introductory

The lesions of bilharziosis are mainly due to the damage caused by the hard-shelled eggs of the parasite acting as foreign bodies in the tissues. Once the eggs are laid it is impossible to destroy them by treatment owing to the chitinous nature of the egg-shell. The effects continue with ever-increasing risk of complications and sequelae for a number of years; until, in fact, the eggs succeed in escaping from the organ, bladder or bowel, in which they are deposited.

The only mode of dealing successfully with bilharziosis is to prevent its spread to uninfected persons.

The great economic loss resulting from widespread bilharzial infection was commented upon by Lord Kitchener in his annual report on Egypt for 1913, and the view is therein expressed that "it is high time that serious steps should be taken to prevent the continuity of infection that has been going on so long in this country."

The intractable character of the disease and the corresponding financial burden can be graphically illustrated from the experience of the Army. During the Boer War 625 men were infected with bilharziosis in South Africa. In 1911, 359 of these were still on the list, exclusive of those meanwhile permanently pensioned. The cost to the State for "conditional" pensions for these 359 men was about £6,400 per annum. The "permanent pensions" already allotted amounted to an additional sum annually of £4,400.

In the Nile Delta, bilharziosis is much more widespread and more severe in its manifestations than in South Africa. With the concentration of troops in Egypt it became desirable that the preventive measures taken against this disease should be made with a clear appreciation of the factors and the conditions under which the disease is contracted and propagated. Unfortunately, although the parasitic nature of the disease had been established in 1851 nothing definite had yet been discovered of the life-cycle of the parasite or its manner of entering the human body. Early writers had supposed that the bilharzia worm, like other trematodes, required to undergo a metamorphosis in a molluscan intermediary before it became capable of infecting another person. In 1894, however, Looss formulated the hypothesis that the disease is communicable directly from man to man. In submission to his great authority in helminthological matters and his skill in dialectics, practically all research on the transmission of African bilharziosis undertaken during the last twenty years has been directed to the experimental verification of this hypothesis. During 1914 the author was in charge of the first Wandsworth Expedition of the London School of Tropical Medicine investigating the mode of spread of trematode infections of man in the Far East. Results which threw discredit upon the Looss hypothesis had just been acquired when the outbreak of war rendered field work impossible and necessitated an early return. The new facts were communicated to the War Office, and approval was given for the author to proceed to Egypt "to investigate bilharzia disease in that country and advise as to the preventive measures to be adopted in connection with the troops." Drs. R. P. Cockin and J. G. Thomson were associated with the author in the inquiry, and Private W. McDonald was transferred from the Sixth Essex (T.), as laboratory assistant.

The Committee of the London School of Tropical Medicine granted permission to all three members of their staff, while retaining their appointments, to accept temporary commissions for the period of the investigations. The requisite scientific apparatus was furnished by the School Committee. The Medical Research Committee (Insurance Act) allocated a special fund for all necessary field and other expenses incidental to the research. The Mission arrived in Egypt on February 8 and left again on July 15.

The Present Inquiry

As the province of Qaliubia had been shown to be heavily infected with bilharziosis it was decided to make Cairo the headquarters of the inquiry. . . . The province of Qaliub adjoins Cairo immediately to the north, lying between the eastern (Damietta) branch of the Nile on the west and the desert on the east, and is easily accessible by road and rail, being traversed by the highway and main line to Alexandria and their subsidiaries. At the request of Sir David Semple, Chief of the Public Health Department of Egypt, the vacant laboratories of the Professor of Parasitology in the School of Medicine in Cairo were kindly set apart for our use by the Director, and facilities for the keeping of experimental animals were provided at the Bacteriological Institute. The

C.M.S. Hospital at Old Cairo constantly supplied fresh material for observation from their clinical cases. The programme of work laid down and consistently followed was:—

(a) To collect and specifically determine all the fresh-water molluscs in the selected endemic area, i.e., within a half a day's journey from the laboratory in Cairo.

(b) To dissect large numbers of all species found for trematode larvae.

(c) To differentiate among the larvae found those showing the morphological characters peculiar to the bilharzia group.

(d) To ascertain which, if any, species of mollusc showed chemiotactic attraction for Bilharzia miracidia.

(e) To induce experimentally infection of animals brought from England with Bilharzia cercaria when found in the mollusc.

(f) To ascertain experimentally whether infection took place through the skin or by the mouth or in both ways.

(g) To ascertain experimentally the incubation period of the disease.

(h) To determine experimentally on infected animals the efficacy of medicines, reputed to be of value on clinical grounds, to destroy the bilharzia worms in the portal system.

(i) To observe the conditions favourable and inimical to the life of the free-swimming cercaria and the effect thereon of acid solutions and other medicinal substances.

(j) To study the bionomics of the special molluscan intermediary, if obtained, for facts upon which prophylactic measures could be formulated.

An examination of the banks of the Nile to the south of and around Gezireh, an island opposite Cairo, showed that, excluding bivalves, there were very few living forms in the main stream. Similar results followed from an examination of the Ismailia Canal at Mataria, north of Cairo, and of the Giza Canal, on the western bank of the Nile.

A study of a map of the environs of Cairo showed that there was a large number of collections of water in the Zoological and Botanical Gardens at Giza. With the permission of the Director, Major Flower, these ponds were exhaustively examined and were found to contain nearly all the described species of molluscs, with one or

two notable exceptions. With material from this source a type collection of molluscs was made so that specimens brought in later from infected areas could be rapidly compared and determined.

In the report of the ankylostomiasis campaign in Qaliubia it was noted that a small travelling hospital had been stationed at the village Qalama, 13 miles north of Cairo and near the main road to Alexandria. Of 95 inhabitants of this village, 43 had been found to harbour bilharzia. This small village seemed, therefore, at first sight, a suitable place in which to make an intensive study of the local molluscan fauna. It proved, however, more difficult of access than had been anticipated. There was, too, a very large pond or birket which could not be thoroughly examined. Finally, as will be noted from the map, the canal outskirting the village had passed through a number of other villages after it took off from the main stream. Infection acquired in Qalama might well have been due to infective larvae carried on from a higher part of the canal, and not actually derived from molluscs at Qalama itself. It was consequently decided to seek a more suitable village, if possible (a) of easy access, (b) without a birket, and (c) on a small canal coming almost directly off one of the main supply canals. . . .

Technique

The various molluscs, wherever and whenever collected, were separated into their different genera and, as far as possible, species, and examined for developmental stages: (a) by direct inspection, (b) by dissection. When an infected mollusc is kept in a glass vessel in clean water for a few days the cercarial forms are frequently discharged naturally by the mollusc, and may be easily seen swimming about in the water if the glass is held against the light and examined with a hand lens. By this method large numbers of the same species can be placed together in a vessel and tested without further technique. If, however, the larval development has not yet reached the stage for the discharge of the cercaria the results are apt to be misleading. Should a positive result be noted, the cercaria can be determined by microscopical examination and the infected mollusc isolated and kept alive for further observation. By dissection the earlier stages (sporocyst, redia, and immature cercaria) are obtained. The method has the disadvantage that the mollusc is necessarily killed in the course of the dissection and cannot be used for further work. The technique is simple though tedious when large numbers are involved. The shell, when hard and calcareous as in Cleopatra and Melania, is crushed with lion forceps, placed on a slide in a drop of water or weak formalin and the mass then torn apart with two dissecting needles. With the thin-shelled forms like Planorbis it suffices to fix the shell by piercing the central whorl with one needle and to cut outwards with the second. In our experience the spear-shaped steel points issued for use on gramophone records when fixed in needle-holders are far more satisfactory than ordinary dissecting needles for this work. With them a large window can be quickly cut in the hardest shells and the molluscan body rapidly dragged out complete. The liver, which occupies the upper or central whorls of the gastropod shell, is the usual site of election for the developmental stages of trematodes. But a detailed examination of the mollusc is practically never necessary for

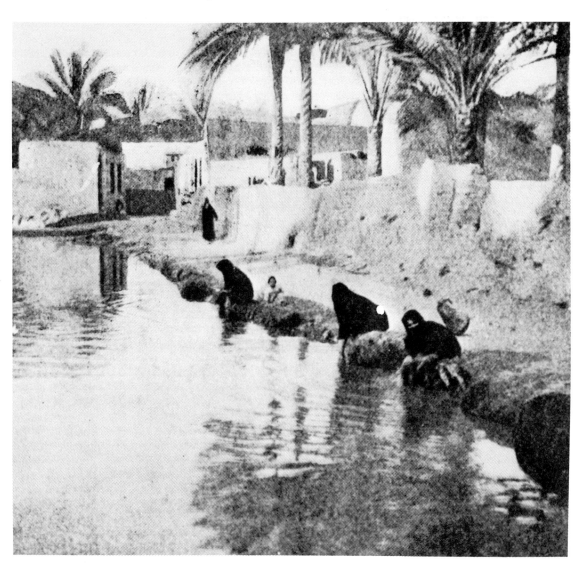

Plate 78. Women washing garments in the Marg canal.

the determination of an infection. With the first tear, as a rule, the characteristic bodies flood out in numbers into the surrounding plasma and water, while further search may be made under a low power by squashing the whole molluscan body slightly between two slides. In this way over 3,300 samples were minutely examined in the course of the inquiry. Seventeen species of Trematode larvae were identified during these dissections. A number of new species were found also.

Recognition of Bilharzia Cercaria

The adult bilharzia worm resembles the other distome trematodes in possessing well-developed oral and ventral suckers, but differs in two remarkable ways: the sexes are separate, and there is an absence of a definite muscular pharyngeal bulb at the commencement of the oesophagus. As in all parasitic worms the infective stage shows no sexual differentiation, consequently the absence of pharynx in the cercaria is the one reliable character upon which a bilharzia cercaria can be distinguished from the cercariae from other distomes, because the body of the cercaria without further metamorphosis grows to become the body of the adult worm. All cercaria have a motile tail at the posterior end. This appendage is a purely larval structure both morphologically and functionally. It serves the definite object of enabling the cercaria body to travel from the intermediate host to some favourable position where it can gain entrance to the final host. The tail is always shed before the actual arrival of the cercaria in the tissues of its host. Various cercaria exhibit different types of caudal appendage. In the four bilharzia cercaria that have come under the notice of the writer the tail was forked at its free end. This peculiarity, however, is shared with some other widely different forms among the distomes. It will be shown in the latter part of this report that four distinct sub-groups of bifid-tailed cercaria occur in the mollusca of Egypt.

Marg Molluscs Found Infected with Bilharzia

Large numbers of snails collected from the Marg Canal throughout its course, but more especially within the village (Plate 78), were infected with larval forms showing the morphological peculiarities of the bilharzia group. The infected shells were readily obtained at spots daily frequented, such as the praying ground at the embankment crossing, in front of the cafes, and at a bend in the canal specially used for washing.

The same species of mollusc was quite common at some distance from the village in the agricultural drains away from foot-paths, but was not infected. Nearer the village, however, and especially where crossed by public paths, these drains contained infected snails. So far the molluscan intermediary has not been found in birkets, but it occurs not uncommonly in large marshes such as that, lying to the south-west of Ismailia. . . .

Once a bifid-tailed cercaria has been placed in the bilharzia group on account of the absence of pharyngeal-bulb, further determination of its systematic position can only be effectively established in the first instance by experimental infection of a susceptible host and the subsequent examination of the adult worm resulting therefrom.

Attempts to Infect Animals Experimentally

Three cercariae of bilharzial type were found in four different species of molluscs. The first form met with differed considerably from the other two, more especially in possessing a pair of black pigment spots just anterior to the ventral sucker, and a delicate but well-defined cuticular expansion on each side of the two prongs of the bifid tail. This form was found exactly five weeks after the commencement of our search, and occurred in *Planorbis mareoticus* collected from the ponds in the Zoological Gardens at Giza. Apparently identical cercariae were found later at Giza and Suez in *Melania tuberculata,* and at Ismailia in *Planorbis boissyi.* The second bilharzia cercaria occurred in large numbers in *Planorbis boissyi* at El Marg, and was found later in similar canals between Inshas and Bilbeis in the Sharqia province. A very few cercariae, apparently identical with this, were recovered on one occasion only from a *Melania tuberculata* in the Zoological Gardens. A third cercaria, which on morphological grounds was only provisionally distinguished from that occurring in *Planorbis boissyi,* was also found at Marg in a certain number of specimens of *Bullinus.*

At Marg the *Planorbis boissyi* were so commonly infected with non-eyed *Bilharzia cercaria* that half-an-hour's collecting sufficed to ensure a large supply of active larvae. An extended series of experiments was instituted to determine the specific character of these forms.

Three species of *Bilharzia* worms are supposed to occur in Egypt: In man the *Schistosoma haematobium* (both varieties), in cattle the *S. bovis,* and in ducks the *Bilharziella polonica.* As bifid-tailed cercariae with eye spots have been found, though not identified, in snails both in Central Europe and in North America, and as this cercaria departed somewhat from the two other forms, it seemed a reasonable conjecture that this cercaria was the larval stage of an avian *Bilharzia,* and that the two remaining and similar cercariae probably attained their maturity in the two known mammalian hosts. Attempts were made to verify this conjecture experimentally. In order to exclude possible fallacies it was essential to infect ducklings immediately after hatching and before they had come in contact with other than filtered water. These were not obtainable in Cairo.

One was struck by the apparent entire absence of rats in the banks of the canals and in the fields. The authorities at the Giza Zoological Gardens stated that the common watervole does not occur in Egypt. A professional rat-catcher was commissioned to obtain rats and field-mice from around Marg. His search proved quite fruitless. It was possible that this extraordinary absence of rodents might be due to a susceptibility to Bilharzia disease.

The animals frequenting the canal at Marg were man, cattle, sheep, dogs (possibly rats), geese, ducks, chickens, and crows. Man and cattle were the most obvious sources of contamination of the canal water, and as each was a known host of species of *Bilharzia,* the probabilities were that cercaria normally developed in them.

Attempts to infect a calf and a lamb by allowing water heavily charged with the living cercaria to remain in the hollows of the groin for periods of ten to thirty minutes on several days gave entirely negative results at the post-mortems some weeks later. It was noted, however, in the case of the lamb, that the skin, where repeatedly exposed to infection, became markedly red.

A series of experiments was then made on mice, rats, geese, ducks, chickens, crows, and wagtails. The experiments on the birds proved entirely negative.

A positive result became apparent by July 13 in a young white rat, which had been infected on May 4. A black mouse which had been infected on May 2 died on June 24 with a number of Bilharzia worms in the liver and mesenteric veins.

In these early successful infections the mice and rats died from the occlusion of the portal system before the Bilharzia worms had reached sexual maturity. A comparative study of mature specimens of *Schistosoma bovis* and *S. haematobium* showed that these two species are so closely allied that, when experimentally reared in an abnormal host, a differential diagnosis could only be made with certainty upon the characters of the fully grown worms, and especially upon those of the egg shell. Further experiments were made. In those animals which survived for seven to eight weeks, female worms were found containing the characteristic eggs. This placed the diagnosis beyond question.

The animals used were variegated mice and white rats brought from London and fed solely on oats and filtered water. They had been kept in the laboratory under conditions entirely precluding the possibility of unobserved infection.

Animals Found Susceptible to Infection

In addition to tame white rats and variegated mice, the Egyptian desert rat, obtained from the neighbourhood of the Pyramids, was found to be susceptible to experimental infection, while guinea-pigs were peculiarly so. Mangaby monkeys died of acute bilharziosis within two months of infection. Experiments were not made on dogs owing to the quarantine difficulties that would have arisen on our return to England. At the conclusion of its field work the Mission brought back from Egypt four mice, 26 white rats, 16 desert rats, two guinea-pigs, and four mangaby monkeys, which had been submitted to infection shortly before departure. When examined shortly after their arrival in England all these animals had enormous numbers of bilharzia worms in the portal system.

Mode of Entry of Bilharzia into the Body

That something similar to this might occur in Bilharzia was suggested by a simple observation on the habits of the Bilharzia cercaria. These cercaria progress by swimming mainly through the activity of their tails or by creeping by means of their well-developed suckers. When actively swimming cercaria are poured from one dish into another it is very noticeable that they immediately fix themselves firmly by means of their ventral suckers to the surface of the vessel into which they are carried until the motion of the water has ceased, when swimming is again resumed. It seemed, therefore, quite possible that if heavily infected water was drunk, the cercaria, coming into momentary contact, might similarly adhere to the mucous membrane of the mouth, tongue and oesophagus and at once proceed to penetrate into the tissues. That this actually can take place is apparently borne out by the following experiment. Four sooty monkeys which had been taken out with the Mission in January and kept in separate cages in the laboratory until the experiment was completed, were subjected to infection with Bilharzia cercaria. In three cases the infected water was poured into the bottom of the cages and the monkeys were consequently exposed to infection through the skin of the hands, feet, buttocks and tail. The fourth monkey was fed for a day or two on dry food only, and then allowed to drink from a cup containing filtered water swarming with Bilharzia cercaria. Some effect, probably a prickly sensation, was produced almost immediately, for the monkey began to pull down the lower lip, to rub the mucous membrane of the mouth, and in other ways to indicate that the drink had not been pleasurable. After a second experience on the following day the monkey refused to accept water out of a cup although thirsty. The four monkeys eventually died and all showed a heavy infection with Bilharzia. The monkey infected from drinking water showed earlier and much more intense symptoms than the others. This experiment showed that in Bilharzia infection may be both oral and cutaneous. As in ankylostomiasis there is little doubt, however, that the infection enters through the skin in the bulk of cases.

As Brock has pointed out, the chances of infection are much greater in bathing than in drinking, because under the former circumstances a much larger quantity of water comes into contact with the body. . . .

Conclusions Based on the Results of the Present Inquiry

(1) Transient collections of water are quite safe after recent contamination.

(2) All permanent collections of water, such as the Nile, canals, marshes and birkets, are potentially dangerous, depending upon the presence of the essential intermediary host.

(3) The removal of infected persons from a given area would have no effect, at least for some months, in reducing the liability to infection, as the intermediate hosts discharge infective agents for a prolonged period.

(4) Infected troops cannot reinfect themselves or spread the disease directly to others. They could only convey the disease to those parts of the world where a local mollusc could efficiently act as carrier.

(5) Infection actually takes place both by the mouth and through the skin. Recently contaminated moist earth or water is not infective.

(6) Infection in towns is acquired from unfiltered water which is still supplied, even in Cairo, in addition to filtered water, and is delivered by a separate system of pipes.

(7) Eradication can be effected without the cooperation of infected individuals by destroying the molluscan intermediaries. . . .

Development of the Definitive Host

Once the cercaria has entered the definitive host it undergoes no further metamorphosis. There is gradual growth with differentiation of organs, and in Bilharzia with differentiation also of male and female individuals. The males are recognizable from the females by their greater breadth and the stouter formation of the ventral sucker. . . . The route taken by the cercarial body in its transit from the skin to the portal system is still under investigation. It is noteworthy here, however, that the cercariae do not all appear to arrive in the liver at the same time. Some of the smallest forms were obtained by teasing liver which contained also forms almost fully grown. This accords with Professor Looss's experience in ankylostome infection. A number of larvae probably become "lost" in the tissues. It may be, however, that a certain number enter the bloodstream direct, while others pass first through the lymphatic system. . . .

Adults and Ova

The morphology of the adult worms, and of the eggs recovered from cases of bilharziosis in Egypt, has been dealt with exhaustively by several previous writers, notably by Bilharz, Leuckart, Fritsch, Lortet and Vailleton, and particularly by Looss.

Variations

In parasites generally there are certain small variations within the limits of a species both in size, shape, etc., of adults and of eggs. In *Bilharzia haematobia* unusually striking and constantly recurring departures from the normal have been described. In Looss' monograph on the adult anatomy it is recognized that a number of these do actually occur, but others are, in his opinion, due to errors in interpretation by previous workers. These abnormalities, rather than the normal anatomy, are our more immediate concern. The differences that have been recorded in the shape of the eggs are of special interest. As early as 1851 Bilharz had noticed that certain of these, passed in the faeces, were distorted, the small terminal spine of the typical egg being apparently displaced laterally. These lateral-spined eggs he regarded as abnormalities.

Duality Theory

In 1864 Harley was so struck by the absence of these atypical forms in cases of bilharziosis seen in South Africa, that he named the South African parasite *Distoma capense,* to distinguish it from the Egyptian parasite which gave rise to both types of eggs. The subject remained one of merely academic interest until 1902, when Sir Patrick Manson saw in London a case of intestinal bilharziosis, contracted in the West Indies, in which lateral-spined eggs only were present. In the following year he put forward the suggestion that: "Possibly there are two species of Bilharzia, one with lateral-spined ova, depositing its eggs in the rectum only, the other haunting bladder or rectum indifferently." This view was revitalized by Sambon in a series of papers, commencing with one in 1907, in which he formally named the new species after Sir Patrick Manson, "in appreciation of this, one of his many genial intuitions." Sambon's new species met with an unsympathetic reception, more especially from Looss, who held, with many elaborate arguments, and with some apparent success, that vesical and intestinal lesions in bilharzial infections in Egypt were caused solely by the one species, *B. haematobia.* The whole controversy cannot be reviewed here, but the curious reader will find in the prolonged debate "a stimulating vitupera-

tiveness" which makes it highly entertaining, if somewhat cruel reading.

Sambon's Species

In his "Remarks on *Schistosomum mansoni,*" Sambon explained that his "determination is based principally on the characters of the eggs," but that, in addition, he had "taken into consideration their different geographical distribution, the different anatomical habitat, and the different pathogeny of the two species." He maintained that "the lateral-spined ova are not found occasionally only, within the distributional areas of *S. haematobium,* as would necessarily be the case if they were the product of this species, but have a peculiar and wide geographical distribution of their own, being absent in many places where endemic haematuria and its causative agent are prevalent (Cyprus, South Africa)."

Looss' Theory

The opposing theory put forward by Looss was, briefly, that "unfertilized females are not capable of producing other than abnormal eggs." These abnormal eggs were for the most part the lateral-spine variety, and where they contained a miracidium this was attributed to parthenogenesis. Looss' position, which met with clever criticism from Sambon, became somewhat changed later in the light of his own further observations, but his main tenets remained, and his final ground became, theoretically, unassailable without the aid of experimental evidence.

Looss' Arguments

In Looss' opinion "the strange and striking differences presented by the clinical and pathological pictures of bilharziosis as seen in various places" could be explained "on the presumptive life history of the parasite, in connexion with the habits of the host and the conditions of the country."

Commencing with his postulate that infection is direct and takes place at all times through the skin, he maintained that the miracidia proceed to the liver, where they developed into sporocysts, from which worms escape later into the portal veins. As at post-mortems it is not uncommon to find males, obviously of the same size and age, alone in the portal vein, he assumed that "they must have been generated at about the same time; this would become comprehensible on the assumption that they were generated in one sporo-cyst.'' The female worms which are less common likewise would originate from a sporocyst. Applying these postulates to the ordinary conditions found in the Delta, it appeared to Looss that ''several miracidia penetrate the body at short intervals and thus males and females will be present.'' ''In this case the females will not have long to wait for fertilization.'' While waiting they will have produced a few abnormal eggs but being almost immediately captured by the males are carried off to the pelvic organs, with the result that ''there is urinary bilharziosis characterized by the apparition of terminal-spined eggs in the urine; the same eggs may appear in the faeces, but the lateral-spined ones will be so scarce that they seem to be altogether absent.''

In countries where conditions are unfavourable for infection, i.e., where the population is scattered and the people do not bathe in crowds, or where water is scanty or swiftly running, and the chances of miracidia entering the skin are small, then the following train of events may be presumed: ''On a single occasion a few miracidia manage to enter the skin and one gets safely to the liver. It produces males. The worms grow to sexual maturity, but finding no females they wait for a certain time and then undertake the journey to the pelvic organs alone. The liver is again free from worms: the infection remains without consequences.'' This may recur as male producing miracidia are so common. Eventually a miracidium enters alone which gives rise to female worms. In due time these ''begin to lay lateral-spined eggs. The oviposition goes on, perhaps, for a long time. The number of lateral-spined eggs increases steadily; all are carried to the liver.'' Some of these worms may migrate successfully as far as the large bowel.

Eventually there will be a ''strong infection of the liver and some isolated patches in the wall of the intestine, but no terminal-spined ova will ever appear, nor will there be a regular infection of the bladder. After some time, the lateral-spined eggs of the liver begin to appear in the faeces, and they continue being voided in this way for several years.''

Looss details other circumstances under which a secondary infection with terminal-spined eggs may be contracted by a case showing originally Manson's intestinal bilharziosis if a sufficient interval has lapsed between the entry of the two miracidia. Lastly, infection by a large number of miracidia at a single exposure would result in a pure case of ''urinary bilharziosis.''

Looss concludes that, from his point of view, ''no sharp line of demarcation between the two types'' exists. ''They are simply the opposite ends of a continuous series of intermediary stages.''

Looss' Criticism of Sambon's Species

After detailed criticism of Sambon's arguments, Looss dismisses them with the conclusion that ''in all the evidence there is not the slightest detail which would really point to the existence of a distinct species in the West Indies and certain parts of Africa.'' He adds that one of the fundamental facts on which his views rest is that in 1852 Bilharz actually found in Egypt that ''the eggs of *S. haematobium* and *S. mansoni* may occur in one and the same individual.''

Sambon's Reply

Replying in 1909, Sambon pertinently points out that Bilharz's alleged observation has never been confirmed and that the interpretation that both lateral-spined and terminal-spined eggs were actually seen in the same individual worm does not necessarily follow from Bilharz's statement. In turn he attacks Looss' hypothesis, especially his assumption of the occurrence of parthenogenesis in the adults.

Looss' Readjustment

The effectiveness of this criticism is revealed by the readjustment of his position by Looss in 1911. He now recognized that ''the question of the formation of these eggs and the question of their fertilization are in reality independent.'' He is still of opinion that the uncopulated females are incapable of giving their eggs the normal shape. After fertilization the change to normal shape will not take place immediately; there will always be a transition period. There is thus no longer any necessity of admitting on the part of the egg cell a capability of developing by parthenogenesis.'' ''I have received the impression that when once the production of normal eggs begins, the others are, as a rule, quickly evacuated.'' ''That the females of *S. haematobium* can, and do, produce the two forms of eggs is beyond question even now.''

Via Media

American parasitologists attempted to settle the controversy by suggesting that possibly the eggs of *S. mansoni* were normal eggs similar to the abnormal forms, with distorted spine, produced by *S. haematobium*.

Bearings on Present Inquiry

Obviously the possibility that, in Egypt, man harboured two distinct species of bilharzia worm complicated the transmission problem, already rendered intricate by the presence there of bovine and avian infections.

It was realized, however, that the full solution was not an essential preliminary to the conduct of experiments which were more urgently needed to provide the necessary data on which to base prophylactic measures for the protection of the troops. The *Bilharzia cercariae* found in *Bullinus* and in *Planorbis,* as well as other cercariae, were found to react in a practically identical manner to changes in their environment; whether these were physical, such as exposure to heat, drying, etc., or chemical, such as exposure to dilute amounts of sodium bisulphate, etc. The *B. cercariae* showed the same limited capacity to survive in water and caused local irritation due to penetration of the skin in animals exposed to infection by immersion. Thus the earlier parts of this report were written with reference to "bilharzia," without touching (save inadvertently by the use of "B. haematobia" in the old inclusive sense) on the problem of the unity or duality of the parasite concerned in the causation of bilharziosis. Indeed, the success of these experiments led to a further delay. The lethal effect of very dilute solutions of coal tar derivatives on the cercariae raised the hope that if minute quantities of these substances could be got into the portal system unchanged, they might be found to destroy the bilharzia worms there. Thus, by cutting short the egg-laying period, the subsequent severity and duration of an infection might be considerably diminished.

Surgeon-General Ford was of opinion that a satisfactory method of treatment might prove of considerable service. Expert cooperation in the pharmacological aspects of the problem was obviously desirable. As soon, therefore, as it was evident that animals were being infected successfully, I decided to infect as many animals as were

then available and to return to England to carry on further work on these lines. Infections were accordingly made from *P. boissyi* and from *Bullinus*. It was hoped that these would provide material still needed for the zoological inquiries not yet completed. A return in the autumn was foreshadowed, if facilities were obtainable, in the event of the need arising for further investigations through failure of the material or the upcrop of new problems.

Experimental Treatment Negative

Most of the infected animals survived the homeward journey. Dr. H. H. Dale, F.R.S., kindly carried out a series of tests and the animals were afterwards dissected. It was agreed that none of the substances of known anthelmintic or cercariacidal value could be introduced into the portal system in doses lethal to adult parasites. This cleared the ground for a continuation of study of the specific nature of the cercariae found respectively in *Bullinus* and *Planorbis*.

The Cercariae in Planorbis and Bullinus

In addition to the cercaria provisionally identified as that of an avian bilharzia worm, three bilharzia cercariae were provisionally differentiated from material collected at El Marg. Of these, one infested *P. boissyi*; with it, later, but seen much less frequently, was a large form. This mollusc was not found in some other villages where bilharziosis was also prevalent. It was, therefore, apparent that even if eventually it was proved to be a carrier of infection to man, other species of mollusca must also be concerned. The search was therefore continued, and several weeks later, at the commencement of June, examples of the genus *Bullinus* were found to be likewise infested with *Bilharzia cercariae* of slightly different appearance. As cercariae, naturally discharged, became available from each source, animals were submitted to infection by immersion, and later by the mouth.

The animals first submitted to infection died from blockage of vessels by the growing worms before these had attained their full size. Such hyperinfection was at first courted to establish the fact that the animals in experimental use were actually susceptible. Later this had to be avoided to ensure that the infected animals would survive sufficiently long to show the effect of drug treatment on the worms in the portal system, and to give the growing worms sufficient time to attain sexual maturity and produce eggs whereby the specific character of the infection could be finally identified. This proved a much more difficult task. Too slight an immersion might result in a failure to infect or a failure to infect with enough to ensure the presence of females as well as males. Mishaps from all these causes befell in the animals taken to England, and as will be seen, necessitated a return to Egypt for further material.

Early Appearance of Lateral-Spined Eggs

Before leaving for London, two or three eggs only were seen. The first occurred in a female taken from the mesentery of a mouse that had survived until June 24. The others were seen a few days prior to sailing. These eggs were lateral-spined and the result of infection with cercariae from *P. boissyi*. According to Looss' theory these were the early abnormal products of young sexually mature females of *B. haematobia*; according to Sambon they should be regarded as characteristic ova of *B. mansoni,* the cause of intestinal bilharziosis; according to American parasitologists, they were merely early abnormal products of *B. haematobia,* simulating the true lateral-spined egg of *B. mansoni,* the cause of bilharziosis in the New World. Males were present as well as females, but this fact had now no significance, since Looss had himself abandoned the view that the females produced eggs parthenogenetically. The females found had only reached the egg-laying state. It was possible that they were just entering Looss' "transition period."

Sufficient time had not elapsed since the submission of animals to infection from *Bullinus* to warrant an examination of these prior to sailing.

After reaching London, in July, animals continued, as before, to die from hyperinfection with young adults. At the beginning of August, four monkeys which it had been hoped would survive several months, began to pass eggs and died within a fortnight of intense infection. These eggs were lateral-spined. The cercariae used had been obtained from *P. boissyi*. No other type of egg was found. It could not be said, however, that the worms had become mature sufficiently long to have passed through Looss' "transition period."

Later Results

Certain of the rats which had survived until September showed at post-mortem an extraordinary condition of the liver. This was enlarged and deeply pigmented with black amorphous granules. The surface was speckled with minute white spots. These were found to contain accumulations of lateral-spined eggs. The final peripheral veins were frequented by paired adult worms. The liver from these cases was macerated and the eggs released in enormous numbers. Every described variation in size and shape of lateral-spined egg was then found, but no terminal-spined eggs were seen. These animals had been infected from *P. boissyi*.

It had proved impossible to obtain material of the occasional large cercaria in *P. boissyi* for experimental purposes, but it was anticipated that in the very large series of infections made with cercariae from *P. boissyi* for the experiments with drugs this cercaria would give evidence of its presence. Neither in the eggs nor adults resulting, however, was any indication seen of another species. The nature of this large cercaria remained, therefore, a perplexing mystery.

Failure of First Bullinus Experiments

During September the animals submitted to very slight infection were still alive and were anxiously watched for evidence of successful infection. No eggs were passed, and as the length of time that had now elapsed since immersion was considered sufficient to allow of the worms attaining sexual maturity, those treated with cercariae from *Bullinus* were killed and examined. The results were disappointing. It was evident that in the attempt to infect so slightly as to ensure the survival of the animals for some months the number of cercariae that had actually entered had not been sufficient to ensure successful infection with paired adults. This experiment was repeated with certain of the animals slightly infected with cercariae from *P. boissyi*. No adult worms were found.

New Experiments in Egypt Successful

Reviewing the position early in October, I realized that the materials now available were insufficient to enable me to deal effectively with the question of the zoological relationship of the bilharzia worms that caused the symptoms of vesical and intestinal bilharziosis. Certain facts might justify a reopening of the Sambon-Looss controversy, which had reached a position of stalemate, but they would not render the final position taken by Looss untenable. With the *B. cercariae* available, it was clear that a complete solution was possible. The completion of this report was, therefore, postponed. I was granted permission to return to Egypt, and was enabled to do so by the Committee of the London School of Tropical Medicine, which allowed me to resume an unexpired portion of the Wandsworth Research Scholarship, which I had previously held.

Two series of experiments were seen to be required and were instigated immediately after I reached Egypt in November:—

(1) To lightly infect animals with *P. boissyi* cercariae so that they would survive several months and thus enable the female bilharzia worms to pass the "transition period."

(2) To heavily infect animals with *Bullinus* cercariae to ensure a successful diagnosis of the specific nature of this form. In view of the successful and heavy infections that had followed the administration of *P. boissyi* cercariae by the mouth, it was decided to make the crucial experiments by this method, which appeared to afford a more accurate means of control in the dosage. To ensure longevity monkeys were used. Additional experiments were made by immersing rats and mice in infective fluid, and other monkeys were subjected to skin infection.

These new experiments proved, after the necessary lapse of time, completely successful.

The smaller animals were killed week by week to watch the progress of the development. Worms were first recovered from a mouse, infected by immersion, on the seventeenth day. These were of course, very immature, but they showed differences in the development of the gut from those previously reared from *P. boissyi*. This difference persisted during the growth of the worms, as seen from later dissections, until the adult size was almost reached. The two lateral branches of the gut failed to unite early. In several of the experiments, males only were found. After five weeks, males and immature females were recovered from the mesenteric vessels of mice infected by immersion, but the numbers were small. A mouse, injected subcutaneously with cercariae obtained from *B. dybowski,* by dissection showed

eight adults, of which none were females, when killed 37 days later. In this series, worms were found after the sixth, seventh and eighth week, but the females had not yet begun to lay eggs. On the ninth week, however, the production of eggs had commenced.

Turning to the series of infections by the mouth, the following contrast is interesting: Two Indian monkeys, taken to Egypt from London for the purpose of these experiments, were given infective fluid to drink on the same day. The female monkey received fluid containing cercariae naturally discharged by *P. boissyi*; that administered to the male monkey contained cercariae naturally discharged by *Bullinus*. The female monkey began to pass lateral-spined eggs in the faeces on the forty-second day, and died from bilharzial dysentery on the sixtieth day. The male monkey showed no eggs in faeces or urine on the forty-second day and was killed. Many male and female worms were found in the liver and mesenteric vessels, but no eggs were found either free or in the females.

In the worms recovered from these older infections from *Bullinus,* the lateral branches of the gut had now united, and a short caecum was developing. The males showed a further point of difference from those found in infections by *P. boissyi,* viz., the testes were less numerous, numbering only four to five. As this number had been recorded for *S. haematobium,* and was found to occur normally in *B. bovis,* it was still impossible to say whether the *Bullinus* infection was due to the bovine or the human parasite, without the evidence provided by the eggs. A further monkey had meanwhile been infected from *Bullinus* by the mouth. This passed numerous eggs in the twelfth week, and died of intense intestinal bilharziosis five weeks later. No eggs were found in the urine nor were any found in scrapings of the bladder wall. The eggs were terminal-spined without exception and corresponded to those found in man, not those in cattle. Female worms found post mortem contained the eggs in numbers. This result confirmed the earlier find in mice which had been infected by immersion. Other animals gave confirmatory evidence. We had now established experimentally that the cercaria derived from *P. boissyi* gave rise to lateral-spined eggs, whilst those derived from *Bullinus* gave rise solely to terminal-spined eggs.

In both cases infection was restricted to the intestine, but this was probably due to differences in the venous connexions of the bladder. Undoubtedly the gut wall was the primitive habitat of all the bilharzia worms.

The young but sexually mature *B. haematobia,* derived from *Bullinus* infection, were well able to lay terminal-spined eggs. Although the very earliest efforts did not conform completely in full size and shape to the standard egg, no evidence of tendency to the formation of eggs with laterally-distorted spine was forthcoming.

To completely clinch the matter, a final experiment seemed desirable. Animals—monkeys and rats—were infected very lightly with *P. boissyi cercariae* and kept alive for nine months. The living female worms, found post mortem at the end of that period were still producing lateral-spined eggs; one or two only at a time. For these coupled worms, the "transition period" must surely have long since passed.

The terminal-spined and lateral-spined eggs found in bilharzial infections are, therefore, the normal and characteristic products of two distinct species, *B. haematobia* and *B. mansoni,* and are spread by different intermediary hosts. The young females in each species produce slightly atypical eggs, but these slight variations do *not* "form a continuous series of intermediary stages between the two types."

As transmitter of the parasite of urinary bilharziosis in Egypt, *Bullinus* fulfils all requirements as far as distribution is concerned. It is found in the larger canals, in the smaller irrigation channels and finally, in the village ponds or "birkets." *B. haematobia cercariae* have been found in the species *B. contortus, B. dybowski,* and once in a specimen which was recognized as *B. innesi.* These species would appear to correspond to the forms named *Physa alexandrina* by earlier workers.

The more restricted distribution of *Planorbis boissyi* would appear to correspond equally satisfactorily with the less universal occurrence of intestinal bilharziosis due to *B. mansoni* in Egypt. In the course of this inquiry, it was not found in the large canals or in the village "birkets." It appeared to frequent the smaller irrigation channels and drains where these were permanent. It was found also in marshes. Both carriers were found susceptible to drying, *Bullinus* extremely so. . . .

In his postulates Looss had argued in favour of sporocysts giving rise to adults of one sex only, to explain the frequent presence of males only in an infected person. This highly suggestive hypothesis may well prove true for the sporocysts and their resulting cercariae in the molluscan host.

Experience shows that if the cercariae discharged from one specimen only be used for experiment, the resulting worms may be of one sex only. Owing to the extreme fragility it was impossible to isolate a single "tube" of cercariae from an infected liver and so put the matter to experimental proof. Experimentally infected animals, like naturally infected persons, usually show a marked predominance of male over female worms. This would seem to be a happy provision of nature to ensure that no female that had successfully gained her way into the final host should lack opportunity of producing offspring.

Other Problems

There is one other matter relating to the bilharzia problem as presented by the village Marg which was for a long time puzzling, but for which a tentative explanation may be suggested. Urinary bilharziosis prevailed among the children in Marg to the extent of ninety per cent. The incidence of intestinal and particularly Manson's intestinal bilharziosis could not conveniently be ascertained. The presence there of infection with lateral-spined eggs was revealed by the find of specimens in the urine of one of the infected children. Now in the small canal within the confines of the village, *P. boissyi* was relatively more frequently infected with cercariae, i.e., with *B. mansoni* than was *Bullinus* with *B. haematobia.* After many visits the habits of the residents became fairly well known. The shelving banks of the canal served as a public latrine. The sides and uncovered bed of the channel were strewn with faecal deposits. The Egyptian squatting for the purpose of defaecation faces the bank to observe anyone approaching. Consequently, any urine discharged falls on to the dry surface at a higher level than that at which the stool is deposited. This urine sinks into the dry soil leaving bilharzia eggs on or near the surface where they are exposed to the destructive effect of sun and wind. The eggs passed in the faeces are not so readily killed. It is well known that bilharzia eggs will remain alive and unhatched, in a fairly consistent stool, for weeks under suitable conditions. At Marg the level of the water in the canal rises and falls with a varying periodicity owing to the control in the amount of flow by the irrigation department. The consequence is that the sides of the canal, and especially the flatter portions of the bed, are automatically and periodically washed. The bulk of the lateral-spined eggs will be set free and will rapidly hatch in the immediate vicinity of the proper intermediary *P. boissyi*. The terminal-spined eggs which hatch are only those that have been passed in the faeces, and to this limited extent the *Bullinus* snails will become infected. Within the village the stream is too shallow for bathing. In the summer the children proceed higher upstream and to the parent canal where *Bullinus* is unaccompanied by *P. boissyi*. It does not necessarily follow, therefore, that the incidence of bilharzial dysentery and haematuria due to *B. mansoni* and *B. haematobia* respectively should correspond to the incidence of infection in the respective intermediary hosts within the village. Unfiltered water for all uses is taken from this stream into every house in Marg, so that the chances of infection within the home seem very great, both from the use of the water for drinking and for washing. Practically nothing appears to be known of the prevalence of intestinal bilharziosis, especially among women.

Bilharz's "Fundamental" Observation: Suggested Explanation

Before leaving the Sambon-Looss controversy, I have necessarily to deal with Bilharz's original observation, as Looss regarded this find of lateral-spined and terminal-spined eggs in the same female as one of the fundamental facts on which his own view rested.

When first seen by Bilharz the lateral-spined egg was an enigmatical body. It was first thought to be possibly a kind of pupa; only later did Bilharz conclude that it was definitely egg. Bilharz's find of this peculiar body within the female is recorded, as translated by Looss, thus: "such a body was, though once only, but quite undoubtedly, found in the uterus of a female worm, the posterior part of which contained the normal ova."

Sambon contends that Bilharz did not here actually refer to a lateral-spined egg, but to a pigmented body and that "he only says that a peculiar brownish yellow body furnished with a lateral spine was found only once within the oviduct of a female worm, the posterior part of which contained the ordinary ova." There is no clear indication, according to Sambon, that the ordinary ova were terminal-spined ova or that the point of his remarks had reference to the position of the spine, rather than to the dark yellowish discoloration.

To this objection Looss replies later by quoting a further statement by Bilharz: "Strange to say, the eggs appear under two different forms. The two forms were found within the oviduct of the mother as well as in the tissues of various abdominal organs of man."

The latter quotation to my mind brings no support to the contention that Bilharz found the two types within the same individual worm. Here he apparently wishes to convey that the shape of the egg was already determined before the egg left the female and was not a result of distortion in passage through the tissues—a view that has been held later by others.

On the other hand, having read carefully the original text, I am fully convinced by its context that Bilharz really believed that he had seen the two types in the female, when he wrote the first statement, and that the shape of the egg, not its colour, was what he wished to bring under notice. Earlier in the same paper he describes the normal ova as terminal-spined.

An even more important paragraph in this paper has not been utilized by Dr. Sambon. Bilharz states that this body occurred in one of the first females that he examined. A drawing was made at the time, but no importance was then attached to the observation. A similar condition had not been met with again. Now it seems legitimate to infer that an observation made at the commencement of the research might not have the accuracy or detail of later results when more material was available. The eggs with lateral spine are very striking objects, even when seen through the body of the females, but the ordinary ova observed by Bilharz may have been only apparently terminal-spined. My own suggestion is that Bilharz met with one of those females seen occasionally in which egg-laying has only just commenced. I have figured a series of eggs from one such female in the *Journal of Tropical Medicine* for 1911. . . . The first-formed egg is lateral-spined, and lay just within the vulvar opening. The others . . . lay one behind the other towards the ootype, having just passed from the ootype. All the eggs were rolled to show the greatest amount of lateral displacement of the spine. The later samples, it will be noticed, were incomplete and did not contain an ovum. These were, in fact, casts of the ootype in egg-shell without normal content. If Bilharz met with a female similar to this one at the commencement of his investigations, he might well have concluded that the worm contained both types of egg.

. . . I thought [this] might give support to the view put forward by Ward that the terminal-spined type of worm produced at first abnormal eggs with a sort of lateral spine; not identical with the lateral-spined egg of the New World.

On this interpretation the female was actually in Looss' "transition period," but the formation of standard terminal-spined eggs had not been reached. I now believe that the female was one just commencing to lay; that ovulation had not fully set in; and that after producing one or two complete eggs a number of casts of the ootype in egg-shell were thrown off. I have since met with similar abnormal lateral-spined eggs in the material obtained by maceration of the liver of animals experimentally infected with *S. mansoni* in Egypt.

Other Modes of Infection

Among South African tribes there is a widespread belief that the cause of haematuria there, which we know to be bilharzia, enters the body through the orifice of the penis during bathing.

To prevent this certain races, such as Zulus, wear a basket-like protection. Pfister has shown that a similar belief and a like form of protection prevailed among the ancient Egyptians. Its mode of use is to this day figured on the walls of some of the ancient temples of Egypt.

The belief, so far as I am aware, is no longer current among the native populace in Egypt. It has however spread in South Africa among the white population although the protective measures do not seem to be in vogue with them. The matter is of interest here because, as I am told, troops proceeding to Egypt were instructed that they could avoid bilharzia infection while bathing in the canals there, if they took the precaution of wearing the European equivalent of this ancient speciality.

During the field work in Egypt certain observations seemed to afford a rational basis for this ancient belief. Often one found small and very agile leeches on the nets and collecting gear. These were indeed a great pest, for unless they were carefully excluded from the aquaria they rapidly destroyed the molluscs. Now I have heard of one or two cases where such a small leech entered the penis during bathing, and, lodging in the urethra, gave rise to profuse bleeding. This I believe is the probable origin of the association of a penile ingress with bilharzial haematuria and in so far as these penile sheaths have proved efficacious this is probably due to the exclusion of leeches.

In this report it has been shown that infection through the mouth is readily induced experimentally. As the acidity of the stomach destroys cercariae, it has since been argued that such experiments are of little practical significance, giving merely an extension of the area of skin infection. I am personally inclined to attach much more importance to this demonstration of mucous membrane invasion; more especially as it brings me into line with the conclusions of Day. This distinguished observer came to the conclusion from a close study of the conditions of infection in Egypt that the nasal and oral ablutions, carried out as a part of religious ceremony, played no small part in the repeated infections with bilharzia seen in the Egyptians, more especially of male sex. One of the most heavily infected sites in Marg was at the water's edge immediately in front of the local praying ground upstream of the village.

Extent of Risk to Troops

From the established facts regarding the mode of spread and of infection it is evident that troops deriving their water supply for all purposes from the large public waterworks run no risk of infection, even though the washing places become accidentally contaminated with urine containing bilharzia eggs. The risks were among those stationed in small parties on the various bridges, roads and canal crossings throughout the Delta and among the troops occupying new camps on the fresh water canal, in the Fayum and elsewhere. Although supplied with pure water for drinking purposes, this had often necessarily to be supplemented by local supplies for general purposes. At one such place it was pointed out to me that the daily ration of water could be supplemented with ease "from a wee bit burn" which seemed to be of clear good water. A brief examination showed however that there were many *Bullinus* in the stream, which was simply an irrigation channel derived from a main canal on which was a large native population a mile or two inland. . . .

As the chief monographs on the anatomy of the adult bilharzia worms were based on materials collected in Egypt, such material quite probably came from mixed infections. A comparison of the anatomy of adults of *B. mansoni* from uncomplicated cases in the New World with these published descriptions of *B. haematobia* was not likely to lead to acceptable conclusions.

It is evident then that a final settlement of the specific differences between the adult worms of *B. haematobia* and *B. mansoni* must be based upon a comparison of specimens taken from cases of unmixed infection and preferably from cases in South Africa and the West Indies respectively, where such infections occur.

The bilharzia worms that have been reared experimentally from *Bullinus* and *Planorbis,* unfortunately, do not attain in the laboratory animals the full growth met with in their natural hosts. Although sexually mature and actually producing eggs, the worms are still young and small. Differential characters based upon measurements are likely to be fallacious under these circumstances. Morphological differences, may, however, be relied on; especially where these can be verified by reference to full grown adults taken from the human body in unmixed cases of vesical and intestinal bilharziosis. Unfortunately, an opportunity of obtaining such material has not been forthcoming hitherto. The following account of the differential characters as seen in experimentally reared worms must be regarded as a purely tentative attempt to differentiate the two species. It will be noticed, however, that it gains some extraneous support in the observations on the anatomy of *B. mansoni* quoted above.

In the males reared from *Bullinus,* the testes appear to number four or five almost constantly. They are also of fairly large size.

In males reared from *Planorbis,* the testes

number seven to nine, and appear to be relatively small. Differences between the two sets of males are noticeable in the shape of the anterior portion bearing the suckers, and the relative size of the suckers is probably also to be regarded as of specific account.

In females reared from *Bullinus,* the eggs are constantly terminal-spined, even in small young females. The ovary is smooth and situated near the middle of the body. The lateral branches of the gut are lengthy and the caecum correspondingly short. With this the range of the yolk glands which surround the caecum throughout its length is apparently short.

In females reared from *Planorbis boissyi* the eggs are constantly lateral-spined. Usually one, seldom two, and very rarely, four eggs, occur in the uterus at one time. This is due to the short length of the duct. The lateral branches of the gut unite early, and there is a very long caecum. The yolk glands surrounding the caecum have, therefore, a correspondingly long range. The ovary lying in the fork made by the union of the gut branches is elongated and is within a short distance of the uterine pore.

The difference in the point of union of the lateral branches of the gut in the two species is common to male and female. It is a very noticeable feature in the growing worms. The posterior portion of the young worm would seem to be a growing tissue, which, by its continued lengthening, changes the relative measurements of the various parts of the gut almost until maturity is attained.

The attainment of egg-production is more rapid in *B. mansoni* than in *B. haematobia.* In experimental infections from *P. boissyi* eggs were found after six to eight weeks, from *Bullinus* after nine to twelve weeks, depending on the intensity of infection and on the host.

The developing worms and coupled adults reared from *Bullinus* infections are illustrated in Plate 79. . . .

Reviewing the bilharzia problem in the Spring of 1912, in the light of Fujinami's experiments and the repeated failures to infect monkeys and other animals with the miracidia of *B. haematobia,* I concluded that the time had come to renew the attempt made by earlier workers to establish a molluscan transmission for this parasite.

In view, however, of the lack of success which had attended the previous efforts of Sonsino, Lortet and Vailleton, and others to follow the miracidia, a new method of approach seemed called for.

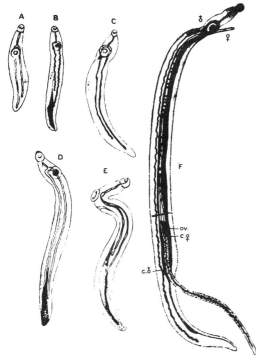

Plate 79. Bilharzia haematobia (s. str.), developed from cercariae discharged by *Bulinus* spp. *Figs. A–E.* Immature stages from liver showing delayed union of gut. *Fig. F.* Adults *in copula* from mesenteric vein, showing short cecum and corresponding changes. (ov) ovary; (c) commencement of cecum.

The occurrence of *Bilharzia magna* in *Cer cocebus fuliginosus* rendered it not improbable that by subjecting monkeys of this species to immersion in water containing the various cercariae, found in the endemic area, a positive result might eventuate. As *B. haematobia* occupied a peculiar habitat in man and did not naturally infect any other animals a negative result might follow. In any case such an empirical method would obviously involve the purchase, transport and maintenance of a large number of monkeys or necessitate an unusually prolonged investigation, for which the necessary financial support was not likely to be forthcoming.

The experiments of Fujinami and Miyagawa

appeared to me to open up a possibility that a morphological clue might be established by which the bulk of cercariae of unknown origin could be excluded microscopically; thus bringing the experimental use of monkeys within practical limits.

Was there any outstanding feature which distinguished the adult distomes from the adult bilharzia worms and which had, in all likelihood, persisted from the sexless cercarial stage? In the cercaria there are organs, like the tail, which are purely larval structures, and others, like the suckers and the gut, which persist from the body of the cercaria through adult life. In some cercariae, however, the gut has not yet formed although there is an oral sucker.

The suckers are, both as regards structure and position, very similar in distomes and bilharzias. The alimentary canal is, on the other hand, markedly different. The bulk of the distomes have a separate muscular pharynx. There is no pharynx in the bilharzia worms.

If this distinction were one which persisted from the cercarial stage then it afforded an easily determined morphological clue by which one could immediately exclude the vast majority of cercariae, which are distomes.

It might be that the pharynx, originally separate, became fused with the oral sucker in the adult as occurs in the amphistomes. Without definite evidence it was, therefore, impossible to come to a trustworthy conclusion regarding the absence of a pharynx in the cercaria of bilharzia.

Happily such evidence was now procurable as a result of the discovery of the "invasion forms" of *B. japonica* by Fujinami and Miyagawa. From the description of these bodies, which were said to possess oral and ventral suckers and a developed gut, it was evident that they were infecting cercariae, but there was no mention, in either paper, of the presence or absence of a pharynx.

It was obviously necessary to establish this point by actual observation, not merely by inference, if it was to be utilized as the basis for experimental work.

My plan then was, in 1912, to proceed to Japan, and by repeating the original experiments or by examining the original preparations to settle this question; to confirm the expected value of the clue by examining the molluscs of the district where Fujinami has conducted his immersions and which was known to be intensely infected; and thence to proceed to Africa. If one or more of the molluscs there was found to contain cercariae exhibiting this peculiarity, then it would be possible to attempt the experimental transmission of bilharzia to monkeys with every prospect of success.

These plans were, however, subject to other counsels and it was not until the summer of 1914 that I felt free to carry out my original scheme. This I was then enabled to do fully, thanks to the cordial cooperation of Professor Fujinami. Through him I was able to examine the "invasion forms" and to establish the value of my morphological clue by a visit to the rice fields of Katayama, where the ease with which the test could be applied to the molluscs in an endemic area was quickly demonstrated. With cercariae exhibiting this morphological peculiarity, mice were afterwards infected successfully with *B. japonica*.

In the meantime, however, Miyairi and Sudzuki, as related above, had succeeded by another method of approach in tracing the metamorphosis in a closely allied, if not identical, snail, in the South Island of Japan. My own observations therefore confirmed generally the results of these workers, apart from establishing my chief, ulterior object, which was to provide a simple and reliable means of attacking the complex problems of *B. haematobia*.

In regard to details, concerning which only the abstract by Kumagawa was available, I was unable to confirm the presence of "rediae" in the development of *B. japonica*. From my own observations I had concluded that the *B. cercariae* originate in sporocysts. I was not in a position, pending fuller information, to decide whether these "rediae" were actually developmental stages of bilharzia or of some other species with which the snails, experimentally infected with miracidia had been naturally infected previously.

On my return voyage, after the outbreak of war, I visited Egypt and found that though the results of the recent work on *B. japonica* were known there, it was still held that they gave no solution to the special problems presented by the *B. haematobia*.

Considering that the new facts derived from my own observations on *B. japonica* would enable me to overcome the experimental difficulties which had hitherto surrounded the Egyptian question and realizing the immediate importance of some simple and efficient prophylactic measures for the large bodies of troops then proceeding to Egypt, I sought and obtained the occasion for the investigations in Egypt related in this report. A study of the accounts given by Sonsino and Looss of the cercariae found by them in the course of their search showed that they had not seen and passed over the *B. cercariae*. The bulk of their cercariae possessed a distinct pharynx. In a few it was absent but in these there was merely an oral sucker without any development of oesophagus or gut. It was evident that these forms had still to undergo maturation before they could become infective to their definitive hosts and as some possessed a definite perforating spine and other peculiarities of forms that undergo encystment in fishes and other secondary hosts, these cercariae were readily excluded. It was therefore necessary to find further cercariae which had hitherto been overlooked. The search for this was made by the method of intensive study of a small heavily infected area. The fact that *B. japonica* developed in a genus of the family hydrobiidae was of no assistance. Indeed by those unversed in the bionomics of helminths this might have been taken, disastrously, as an additional and invaluable analogy. In point of fact the Egyptian bilharzia worms were found to infest two genera of freshwater mollusca belonging not merely to a different family but to a different order. In other words, *B. japonica* and *B. haematobia* were found in snails as distantly related in classification as are the lice to the mosquitoes. In its application to these new cercariae the morphological clue fully vindicated its use. Within three months no less than four *B. cercariae* were obtained by this method of exclusion. Two of these were selected, on epidemiological and other grounds, and with these two alone experiments were made on *Cercocebus fuliginosus* and other animals. These forms proved to be the infective stages of the two bilharzia worms which cause bilharziosis in man in Egypt. No experiments were made with any other cercariae.

Here I may well bring to an end a report that has been kept open much longer than was intended, and of which the earlier sections were written while experiments were yet in progress. Much material remains which, when elucidated, should add further to our knowledge of these and allied Egyptian parasites. Its description, however, scarcely comes within the terms of the present inquiry, which were "to investigate bilharzia disease in Egypt, and advise as to the preventive measures to be adopted in connexion with the troops." These objectives, I believe, have been fully achieved. A complete zoological study of the adult parasites, or of their development, has not been attempted. Such attention as has been given to their morphology and bionomics has been directed to those points concerning which an understanding was essential as a basis for prophylactic measures. The difficulties which beset the inception of the work in a strange country, with some elements critical and hostile, were quickly overcome. Sickness, however, almost wrecked the inquiry at its commencement. Within a month of our arrival Dr. Cockin had fallen sick, and was invalided home. Three weeks earlier I had been admitted to hospital with scarlet fever. It was not until the beginning of April that, foregoing my convalescence, I was able to start field investigations at Marg. Early in May the opening of the Gallipoli campaign, with its rush of wounded and the attendant excitement in Cairo, brought pressing local suggestions for the foreclosing of my mission. As on some other occasions, one found comfort in the aphorism of Huxley: "Surely there is a time to submit to guidance, and a time to take one's own way at all hazards."

But the pervading restlessness could not be wholly withstood. Later, in June, when it seemed advisable to transfer the work to London, my second colleague, whose assistance had been invaluable, decided to remain in Egypt for general service with the Royal Army Medical Corps. The position of the inquiry was full of anxious uncertainties, and I had still to complete many of the crucial experiments. The collections made in the field had still to be worked out, and the experimentally infected animals examined histologically. The extensive literature of Bilharziosis had to be overhauled. Finally, new experiments had to be made. These were the circumstances in which the preparation of the report had to be undertaken, and sole responsibility assumed for the conclusions arrived at and for the views herein set forth. . . .

CHAPTER 26

Schistosomiasis Japonica

AN ACCOUNT OF A JOURNEY TO KATAYAMA

Chugai Iji Shinpo, No. 691: 55–56, 1909 (published originally in 1847). Translated from the Japanese.

Daijiro Fujii [Pen name, Yoshinao]

Daijiro Fujii is credited with the first clinical description of Schistosomiasis japonica. It is known that he lived in Numakuma-gun, in the Bingo area, and that he wrote "Katayama Memoir"—an account of a journey to Katayama in the fourth year of the Kôka era which corresponds to 1847. This report was found in 1909 in the possession of Yaekichi Fujii who permitted its publication the same year by Kan Fujinami, professor of medicine at Kyoto Imperial University.

This is the first published clinical description of Schistosomiasis japonica.

To the south of the Sinpen town of Seibi (Nish-bin), there is a county called Kawanami (Sen-nan) village. There are two small mountains in the rice fields: Ikari (Yodo) Mountain and Kata Mountain (Katayama). The Kata Mountain is also known as Urushi or Lacquer Mountain. According to legend, a ship loaded with lacquer came to this place and was wrecked. Thus the locale has been so called ever since. It is said that the people who passed through this place were all poisoned by lacquer.

In the last two or three years, at the season between spring and summer, the native people who waded in the water to till the fields developed on their lower legs small papules which were extremely pruritic. A great number of people became infected. They thought it might be attributed to the lacquer; even the cattle and horses were not immune.

The clinical manifestations in severe cases—pallor, sunken yellow facies, night sweats with muscle wasting, a rapid and feeble pulse—were similar to those of consumption. Some people had watery diarrhea and some had tenesmus. Others had a bloody or mucoid diarrhea. Later wasting of the extremities occurred and the abdomen became swollen, like a drum. Below the breasts the abdominal veins were dilated and the umbilicus herniated outward. In advanced cases, the abdominal skin became shiny, even reflective; anasarca usually ensued and the patient died.

I examined these patients, but did not know what type of disease it was. It is not unlike consumption with respect to its onset, but in its terminal stage it is really an "abdominal swelling." The patients range from seven or eight years old to 40 or 50 years of age. The mildest form of disease, which does not require bed rest, may be cured within six months or a year. If the disease is severe, even the young adult cannot escape death. I tried treating them with several kinds of remedies [Because these medicines are proper names, it is difficult to understand and to translate them. From the characters, they are Chinese medicines made of powder or extract of plants, animals, or stones—effective symptomatically—Eds.]—medicine for poisoned people, medicine for difficult to diagnose, medicine for boosting spirits, medicine for four-times-rebellious disease, medicine for gastric diseases, medicine of "Kôtotô," medicine for spleen disease, medicine of various kinds— but without any result. About 30 people and more than 10 cattle died of this disease.

It is most prevalent in the Kata Mountain, with Ikari [The word means "anchor"—Eds.] Mountain having the next highest incidence. I am told that both Hei Valley and Yôrô Valley in that village also have such patients. Those two places are some distance from Kata Mountain, but the people from that area used to go there to work the fields. Currently a neighboring village, Senda, has one such patient. Is the disease actually due to lacquer? Had the lacquer infected the water of the rice fields? Being unable to identify the disease, I could not treat it. The native people sought the help of many other doctors, but I never heard of any good result. It is very disappointing.

First I thought that since the Kata Mountain is several miles from the sea, it must have been an island at some time in the past. Actually it was not; as can be found in an old book, the Seibi was also called Ana-seas. In fact, the people of the area found dried wood when they were drilling a well several yards deep into the earth. It was recognized as a mast of a ship. This is one of the proofs. What then is the nature of the poison? I don't know. I merely describe this to draw the attention of all doctors to the problem in the hope that they will solve it.

Dr. Fujii left another memoir.

"I recently read my manuscripts and found the script of the 'Katayama Memoir.' Thirty years have passed. Although the disease is gradually decreasing, it has not yet completely disappeared. Occasionally a case is fatal. It is still true that people are infected in fields of water during this season. Whether the patient is old or young, strong or weak, he develops a strange swelling below the chest. Natives call it 'Katayama disease.' Although the clinical picture is multifold, it starts merely with tiny papules on the legs. It is a serious disease. Medicine nowadays is highly developed. Many techniques and instruments are available. I heard that there is a technique of chemical isolation now develped in the West. Applying this technique, if the soil is analyzed, we can learn what kind of poison it is. By knowing, we can treat it. In this way, this mysterious disease which has existed for many years can be eliminated easily. This would be good for the people. So now I write again and publish, hoping that other people, when informed of this, can eliminate it at the earliest possible time."

A STRANGE CASE OF LIVER CIRRHOSIS CAUSED BY PARASITIC OVA

Tokyo Igakkai Zasshi, 2; No. 17: 898–901, 1888. Translated from the Japanese.

Tokuho (Naganori) Majima

Biographical material pertaining to Majima is not abundant, even in Japan. It is known, however, that in 1887 he found a strange parasitic egg later named Schistosoma japonicum.
This is the first description of S. japonicum *ova in the liver.*

Autopsy notes: A large man had generalized anasarca, with pitting edema especially on his back. The abdomen was tense and greatly distended, the abdominal circumference being 90 cm. Fluctuation and water sounds were present. The conjunctiva were slightly injected. The sclerae were icteric. There were no other noteworthy abnormalities.

When the abdomen was incised, the subcutaneous adipose tissue was fairly well developed. The thickness of the abdominal panniculus was 1 cm. The muscle was not pale, but was edematous and glossy. The stomach and transverse colon were greatly distended and edematous, occupying the upper half of the abdomen. The omentum was very fatty and retracted upward. Between the colon and the stomach the bladder was distended and the fundus reached to the fifth lumbar vertebra. The right side of the diaphragm was at the upper edge of the fifth rib, and the left side was at the lower edge. In the abdomen there was a large quantity (about 4,000 grams) of clear yellowish liquid which contained much protein and gave a positive reaction for bile.

The spleen was greatly enlarged, being 20 cm long, 14 cm wide and 4.5 cm thick; it weighed 880 grams. The capsule was thickened, white, and tendinous-hard. The parenchyma was slate-colored and was especially thickened on the periphery. The hilum was adherent to the pancreas and fundus of the stomach with fibrous connective tissue. Externally, there were scattered black spots. When it was opened, no extensive fibrosis was noted; simple passive congestion was present in the spleen.

The left kidney was 14 cm long, 7.5 cm wide, and 2.5 cm thick. The capsule was normal and came off easily. The renal veins were conspicuous and could be observed. But when the kidney was opened, the cortex and the medulla showed generalized hyperemia. The division between them was not distinct. There were no other abnormalities. The right kidney was 12 cm long, 8 cm wide, and 3 cm thick. It was the same as the left kidney in every respect, except that the hyperemia was greater in the latter.

As shown in Plate 80, the liver was shrunken and contracted. When measured, the right lobe of the liver was 14 × 12 × 5.5 cm; the left lobe was 14 × 12 × 3 cm. Its weight was 940 grams. The surface contained granular nodules the size of horse beans and small red beans. Between the nodules there were deep fissures which divided the surface of the liver into many sections. Glisson's capsule was hard, thickened, and white. The right lobe in particular had one area with scarlike formations. When the liver was cut open, it was hard and made a creaking (or rasping) sound. On the surface of the incision, as on the liver surface, small granularlike areas were observed among the thickened connective tissue. The scars consisted of completely contracted connective tissue. Because of the pressure from the connective tissue, most of the capillary vessels were diminished and the lumen of some were decreased. Similarly, the biliary ducts were dilated with bile because of fibrosis.

There was a small amount of dark yellowish bile in the gall bladder.

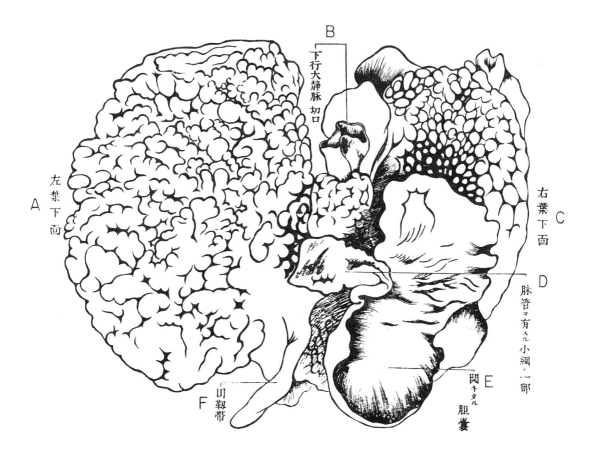

Plate 80. (A) The left lobe—inferior portion; (B) The cut-end of the portal vein; (C) The right lobe—inferior portion; (D) Vascular part of lesser omentum; (E) Opened gall bladder; (F) Hepatic ligament.

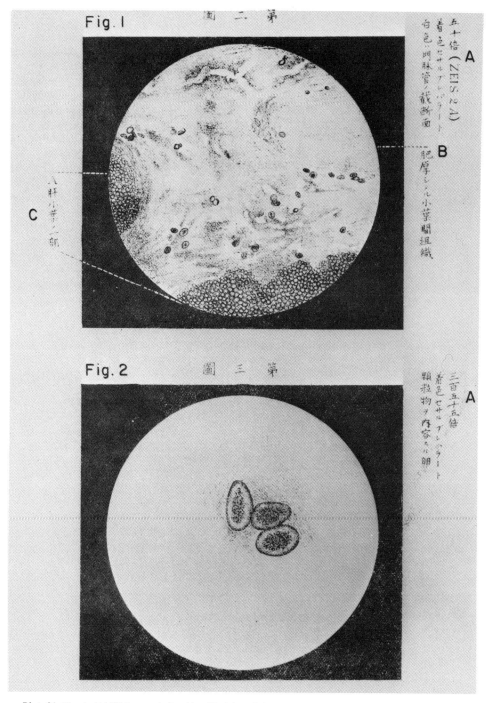

Plate 81. Fig. 1. (A) White area is the side of incision of the portal vein. Stained preparation; (B) Fatty tissue is part of small lobule; (C) A section of liver lobule. *Fig. 2.* (A) Stained preparation showing eggs containing granular material.

Microscopic Examination

When a transverse section of the liver was examined macroscopically, the interlobular tissue was found to be greatly thickened, as stated previously, and the lobules showed pressure changes. Now it was clear from the transverse sections that the liver lobules thus subjected to pressure had become convex and of unequal size, creating externally a granular surface, as already noted in the description at the autopsy. In order to clarify the relation of the fibrosis between the lobules and the borders of the lobules, it was assumed, before a microscopic examination had been made, that new connective tissue had spread into the lobules, restricting interlobular tissue.

When microtome sections were made and examined microscopically, it was found most surprisingly and unexpectedly that with the thickened interlobular tissue there were countless parasite eggs, and these were located only in the connective tissue; not one was observed in the lobules. None was found in any of the lobular tissue nor in the branches of the portal vein nor in the bile ducts—only in the thickened connective tissue (Plate 81, Fig. 1).

These eggs were oval (although there were a few round ones among them) in shape and varied in size from about 0.065 to 0.05 mm in length and 0.05 to 0.04 mm in diameter. The shells of the eggs did not possess small covers (opercula).

There were two kinds of eggs: the first type was pale yellow in color with contents of a granular nature streaked with a brownish-black pigment (Plate 81, Fig. 2). It was not clear whether this pigment was entirely within the egg or whether it was due to improper staining. Although a judgment on this matter was impossible to make, all the eggs of this first variety were oval, just as if their location in the greatly thickened connective tissue had caused them to be pressed into cylindrical shapes or bent to one side into hook shapes. The second type had only the egg shell with no contents and were, therefore, colorless and transparent. They showed various shapes, cylindrical or half-moon, and so on, with no characteristic one. Some were so twisted and bent that they lost all resemblance to eggs; some were square, and some were so atrophied that they were only granules.

All of these parasite eggs, both the first type and the second type, were in peculiar locations in the connective tissue, mostly with great numbers of eggs in large groups. Around the ends of these groups of eggs of the first type, however, a marked infiltration of round cells was observed, while around those of eggs of the second type there were lacunae formed by many eggs that seemed practically hollow; the many eggs in continuous contact formed a sort of rosette. It may be inferred that this was the arrangement of the parasite eggs within the vessels (portal vein and bile ducts) and that when the eggs assumed this position the vessels were blocked.

In one section, stained with hematoxylin and carmine and examined with the microscope, there were indications in various places of a new interlobular connective tissue; in these areas with increased interlobular connective tissue there was marked round cell infiltration as well as swelling and proliferation of the bile ducts. The contracted areas were all compressed in the same manner. However, these changes were limited chiefly to the interlobular tissue with little effect on the lobules and, because of the pressure by the new connective tissue, atrophy was seen likewise in a small number of liver cells.

In order to determine how the eggs described above came from the adult parasite, one part of the bile duct system and the duct leading to the gall bladder were opened in hope of finding the parasite, but not one could be found. Again, microscopic examination of the liquid contents of these ducts showed neither parasites nor parasite eggs. Exploration of the portal system yielded no better results. The feces excreted during the illness were not examined in this case; it was thought that parasite eggs might have been found if they had been studied. Therefore, it could not be determined how the parasite eggs in question came from the adult parasite. I have set down my experience in the hope that in a parasite-ridden country like Japan, a summary of the microscopic observations and the clinical record might be useful to students in the future.

THE ETIOLOGY OF A PARASITIC DISEASE

Iji Shimbun, No. 669: 1325–1332, 1904. Translated from the Japanese.

Fujiro Katsurada
(1867–1946)

The son of a samurai, Katsurada graduated from Ishikawa Prefectural School of Medicine and was licensed in 1887. He went on to become a student at the Tokyo Imperial University College of Medicine. Traveling in Germany for two years, he received the M.D. from the University of Freiburg in 1901.

In 1904, Katsurada returned to Japan to become professor of medicine at Okayama Medical College (1903–1914). From 1905 to 1906 he also served as a lecturer at the Fukuoka College of Medicine at the Kyoto Imperial University. Later he became director of the Seaman's Institute (Kobe) and director of the Hospital of Tropical Diseases.

In 1904 he found ova in the feces of patients afflicted with Katayama disease. He studied the infection in cats and dogs and was successful in obtaining both ova and the adult parasite which he described and named "Schistosoma japonicum."

This paper confirms the findings of Kawanishi and describes the adult parasite, S. japonicum, *for the first time.*

It is widely reported that in certain areas of Yamanashi, Hiroshima, and Saga prefectures, numerous people have been afflicted with an endemic disease which has caused many deaths and greatly decreased labor productivity. This endemic disease is a particular one whose symptoms are enlargement of the liver and spleen, anorexia, diarrhea occasionally accompanied by blood, general anemia, malnutrition, ascites, and peripheral edema. It appears that the disease is now spreading outside the boundary of these three prefectures and, furthermore, it is thought, with some reservations, that the disease exists throughout the entire nation without being recognized. Its etiology is not yet known; that is why I decided to embark on the study of the disease this spring—for the nation and as an interesting research project.

In April of this year I made a field trip to Yamanashi prefecture and examined 12 patients with this endemic disease, with the enthusiastic assistance of the director of Yamanashi Prefecture Hospital and his staff. During my examinations, I discovered eggs of a peculiar worm in the feces of five out of 12 patients. Until now, the eggs have been unknown to the medical world.

Convinced that they might be a clue to the cause of the disease, I made careful observations and recognized the following morphologic peculiarities.

Description of the Egg: The egg shell is usually oval, one end being a little narrower than the other. The average length of 32 eggs which I measured was 0.0797 mm and the average width 0.059 mm. The length of the largest egg was 0.09 mm and its width 0.0725 mm. The length of the smallest egg was 0.065 mm and its width 0.04 mm. The egg shell is yellowish or a light brownish-yellow and is very thin. The border is doubly refractile, and there is a lid (operculum). A thin, transparent membrane is seen inside the shell, and an occasional separation of the membrane and the shell is noted.

The content of the egg is variable, but a great number of eggs with miracidia were found in the feces evacuated with purgatives. The miracidium shows an irregular leaflike shape; its front end is narrow, tapering down to a beaklike point. It is covered completely and densely with cilia, especially in the front part. The development of any particular organs has not yet been observed in the body of the miracidium. However, in the vicinity of the border between the front third and the middle third is a mass of comparatively large yellowish granules. Besides this, in the middle and posterior parts, I observed the irregular distribution of numerous cells rich in small granules and of globular bodies of various sizes, consisting of a type of clear oil. The location of the front end of the larva of the above-mentioned morphology is not definite; sometimes it is in the broad end of the egg shell and sometimes in the narrow end. It has been observed that the membrane of the shell which surrounds the above-mentioned larva usually contains a thick liquid resembling clear oil. The content of those eggs in which the larva (miracidium) is not yet manifest appears as either a large granular or simple homogeneous vacuole; but the number of these eggs found in feces is negligible.

In an attempt to find eggs with morphologic characteristics similar to these, I reviewed every known parasite. I finally found the closest resemblance in the genus *Schistosomum* of the *Trematoda*. The *Distomum haematobium* discovered by Bilharz (*Bilharzia haematobium*) is found to be the closest morphologic relative. According to the description of *Bilharzia haematobium*, however, its ovum is from 0.12 to 0.19 mm long and from 0.05 to 0.073 mm wide. It is also recorded that the shell of the ovum of *Bilharzia haematobium,* residing in its host, has a spine at the side of its rear part. On the other hand, the shell of the ovum that I discovered is notably smaller in length and, when evacuated from the host, lacks any marks of ever having had a spinous process. True, regarding morphologic characteristics, I could not find much difference between the larva of my egg and that of *Bilharzia haematobium;* however, I have not been able to recognize in the larva of my egg the two large gland cells in the anterior part of the body discovered by Looss and noted as the unique feature of the larva of *Bilharzia haematobium.* Therefore, I cannot help but conclude that the egg which I discovered and that of *Bilharzia haematobium* are similar, but not exactly the same.

It is almost impossible to determine the location of adult worms simply by examining the stools. However, when I consider the fact that the ova are not found in the stool of every patient with the endemic disease, and that a comparatively great number of eggs are found in the purged stool, I cannot help but think that the adult worms do not reside in the gastrointestinal tract or any lumen directly connected with it, but live rather in the wall of the gastrointestinal tract and in the viscera directly connected with it. Thus, it may be inferred that eggs are delivered into the lumen from worms in the proximity of the inside of the gastrointestinal tract.

Post-mortem examination: Needless to say, autopsy is necessary in order to clarify the pathology and to ascertain the cause of the endemic disease. Unfortunately, I have not had an opportunity to perform an autopsy on a patient with the endemic disease. However, I did have occasion to examine minutely a portion of liver obtained from an autopsy performed in 1893 by Yosai Shimohira, director of Yamanashi Prefecture Hospital, and some of the liver and intestine obtained from an autopsy performed by Shuzo Muramatsu, former director of the same hospital. During my examination of these specimens, I observed the presence of a peculiar kind of ova. Many of the eggs showed various degrees of passive change; the normal ova were exactly the same as those which I had found in the patient's stools.

A great number of ova were seen in the inter-lobular connective tissue of the liver, and many of them were found between the branches of the portal vein. In another case, similar ova were seen in the intestinal wall and in the liver. In addition to my personal observations, there are published accounts that, in 1890, Professor Katsusaburo Yamagiwa of Tokyo Medical College autopsied the body of a person from Yamanashi prefecture and, by chance, discovered the same kind of eggs. Also, in 1898, Assistant Professor Tatsujiro Kanamori of Tokyo Medical College discovered identical eggs in a rectal tumor and the cirrhotic liver of a person from Yamanashi prefecture. From all this evidence, I have concluded that the eggs might be contained in the portal system, particularly in the distal region and the base, and that the adult worms might reside there as well. If, as I presume, the worms reside in the portal system, then it is most obvious that the eggs do not always reach the patient's feces.

Therefore, if I had had a chance to perform an autopsy, I certainly would have been successful in detecting the adult worms; unfortunately, I have not had an opportunity up to the present. Nevertheless, because of my conviction that the adult worm ought to be found in the bodies of cats and dogs, I killed a cat and two dogs that had been raised in the endemic district and autopsied them. From the autopsy of the dogs I gained nothing, but from that of the cat I obtained an important etiologic clue, as described below.

Autopsy of Cats

Cat No. 1—This cat had lived for 11 years in Ohkamada Village, Naka Kyoma County, Yamanashi prefecture (where the disease was endemic). It was killed on 9 April 1903 and was autopsied immediately. Marked changes in the liver were observed. Under the microscope two kinds of parasite eggs were found. One was the same as the eggs found in the feces of patients with the endemic disease and at three autopsies; usually they were found between the lobules and firmly fixed in granulation tissue.

The second kind of parasite egg had an extremely strange shape and was not found to have any relation to the cause of the endemic disease. As stated above, in the liver of this cat eggs identical to those discovered in the livers of patients with the endemic disease were found. At the same time white pieces of parasites were found in the large branch of the portal vein in the portal

520

SCHISTOSOMIASIS JAPONICA

system. After being suitably prepared, these worms were studied microscopically. They were males, probably of Bilharz' *Schistosoma haematobium* (or belonging to the same genus) and had not been seen in Japan before; that is my conjecture. My opinion, published in a medical journal (*Okayama Igakkai Zasshi,* No. 173), that the eggs found in the liver (the first kind of eggs) and these worms were directly related as a parent and its child, was disputed by a scholar of the subject. Therefore, I continued my studies by autopsying a second cat, over two years old, from the same region. The complete results are given below.

Cat No. 2—This cat was killed and examined on 25 July 1903. It was very scrawny and thin and had a distended abdomen. When the upper half of the portal vein and the first and second branches were cut, a total of 32 worms were discovered, 24 males and eight females, each with two suckers. Five males were holding females from whom they were not easily separated. In the cat's liver there were comparatively new foci of granulation tissue which contained eggs similar to the first kind found in the liver of Cat No. 1.

Description of the Adult Worm (Parasite): In general, the bodies of the worms were a dirty white; but in many females, because of the ovaries and the contents of the alimentary canal, the posterior half of the body was almost black. In both male and female worms the suckers were located anteriorly. The female worm was linear in shape; the anterior half of the body was narrower than the posterior half, but the posterior end was markedly pointed. The difference in diameter between the anterior and posterior halves of the body was not so marked in the male worm as in the female, but the greatest diameter seemed to be in the part a little posterior to the center of the body. In the male, both sides of the posterior part of the body, posterior to the ventral sucker, were folded almost into a tube (the "gynecophoric canal"); the posterior end was tapered but was not so pointed as that of the female. The measurements of the total body (length) are given below:

Female worms

Number	Length
1	12 mm
2	8 mm
3	12 mm
4	9 mm
Average:	10.25 mm

Male worms

1	12 mm
2	11 mm
3	10 mm
4	12 mm
5	10 mm
6	10 mm
7	7 mm
8	11.5 mm
Average:	10.43 mm

What should be noted, especially, is the fact that when the length of the males and females in the combined group was compared, both sexes were about the same, the females tending to be shorter.

In a 12-mm-long male worm, the length of the anterior body (in front of the posterior edge of the ventral sucker) was 0.8 mm, and the width of the anterior portion of the body, between the oral and ventral suckers, was 0.35 mm. The widest part of the body was slightly posterior to the central point (lengthwise) and measured 0.52 mm. The oral sucker was funnel-shaped with a diameter of 0.29 mm. The diameter of the ventral sucker was 0.32 mm, and this sucker had a conspicuous stalk. The greater part of the surface of the body and the suckers were covered with small spines.

In a female worm with a body length of 12 mm, measurements of the various parts were as follows: the length of the anterior section, in front of the posterior edge of the ventral sucker, was 0.29 mm; the width between the oral and ventral suckers was 0.067 mm; the width immediately posterior to the ventral sucker was 0.087 mm; the greatest width of the posterior half of the body was 0.29 mm. The diameter of the oral sucker was 0.0625 mm; that of the ventral sucker, 0.0737 mm. The latter had a stalk. The body of the female worm was smooth, but the suckers had small spines.

From the above description of the external morphology of the male and female worms it can be concluded that they belong to the same genus of trematode parasites as *Bilharzia haematobium*. However, in the *Bilharzia haematobium* described to date, the length of the male worm is 12-14 mm and the length of the female worm is 20 mm; the length of the worms that I discovered was usually the same in male and female; or else the female body was shorter than the male, but the difference was not sufficient to distinguish the two. The suckers in the parasites that I discovered differ in size from those found in *Bilharzia haematobium* and are of no value in differentiating the species.

As for the internal organs of thc parasites, a report on my studies is not yet finished. However, I can say first that the digestive system is the same as in *Bilharzia haematobium*. The conditions of bifurcation of the alimentary canal, especially in the male worms, were somewhat different from those reported up to the present as existing in *Bilharzia haematobium*. In cne male with a body length of 10 mm I found, after careful examination, that the length of the single alimentary canal (after two canals had joined to form one) was about 1.4 mm, filling the last fifth of the worm's body. Leuckart, an authority in this field, examined a male specimen 12 mm long and recorded his observation that the two alimentary canals joined slightly anterior to the center of the body (4.4 mm anterior to the posterior limit of the anterior part of the body). Moreover, he once described a case where the alimentary canals joined, then branched off again, and then joined once more. The relation of these alimentary canals cannot be considered as being sufficiently characteristic to differentiate both species. In general, no marked differences were observed between the reproductive organs of my worm and those of *Bilharzia haematobium*, but there are some peculiarities in the degree of development. In *Bilharzia haematobium* the yolk sac is developed enormously, occupying two-thirds of the entire body (according to Leuckart), and thus the uterus is comparatively short. In my parasite the ovary is located approximately in the middle of the body; since the yolk sac extends posteriorly from the posterior edge of the ovary, it occupies only about half of the total body length, while the uterus, being proportionately long, is present in half the body length. This relationship is one of the marked differences between *Bilharzia haematobium* and my parasite. In addition, the two parasites differ greatly in regard to the egg. The eggs found in the uterus of my parasite I had seen previously in the feces of patients with the endemic disease; they were exactly like the eggs found in the liver and other viscera during autopsy of patients who had died from that disease.

The differences between these eggs and those of *Bilharzia haematobium* have been discussed previously in detail; however, since these eggs are contained in the uterus and are pressed closely together within it, they are of many varying shapes. Now, out of the uterus, relieved of pressure, the proper shape is seen to be oval or possibly round. The eggs usually contained granules and leukocytelike globules; furthermore, no developing larvae were seen. As for the size of the eggs, I wanted to keep many complete worms. Only one female was destroyed, and among her eggs there were six of normal shape. On the average, they were 0.05875 mm long and 0.04916 mm wide. There is no doubt that the eggs in the uterus are the same as those in the patients, even though they are somewhat smaller when compared with the average size of the eggs found in the feces of patients with the endemic disease.

Results: For the time being, I want to call the parasite that I discovered, and which belongs to the genus *Schistosoma*, "*Schistosoma haematobium japonicum.*" Now there is no doubt that this very parasite is the cause of the dreadful endemic disease. However, when this parasitizes the human body, it is difficult to predict how completely it will develop and how many there will be.

SCHISTOSOMA CATTOI, A NEW BLOOD FLUKE OF MAN

British Medical Journal, 1: 11–13, 1905.

John Catto
(1878–1908)

After receiving the M.B., Ch.B. at the University of Aberdeen in 1900, Catto went to London, where he obtained the D.P.H. and was admitted to the Royal College of Physicians and Surgeons. In 1904, while he was working in the London School of Tropical Medicine, he examined some material he had brought back from Singapore and discovered a new trematode. Blanchard, who was visiting at that time, named it after him. Because of a delay in publication of Catto's findings, the description by Katsurada in 1904 gives Schistosoma japonicum *priority over* Schistosoma cattoi. *Nevertheless, Catto's paper in the* British Medical Journal *won for him the Cragg's Prize of the London School of Tropical Medicine. A lieutenant in the Indian Medical Service, he finally went to that country where he died of cholera at Imphal, Manipur.*

The following quotation is from Ernest Carroll Faust[1] "As has frequently been the case in many important contributions to science, several workers attack the same problem contemporaneously, but without knowledge of each other's investigations. Only the circumstance of time gives one the honor which the other quite equally deserves. Such is the case with Schistosoma japonicum *Katsurada, for had the publication of Katsurada's discovery (Dec. 1904) been delayed, the credit would have been given, no doubt, to Catto, who announced his discovery of the worm in January, 1905. Catto's material was obtained from an autopsy on a Chinese man from Fukien Province who died of cholera at Singapore. Whether or not the Chinese was a native of Fukien and had obtained his infection there remains in doubt. This investigator first confused the ova of the worms in the tissues with coccidia, but later corrected his error, although he was undoubtedly mistaken in thinking he found the adult worms in the mesenteric arteries as well as the mesenteric veins."*

Though out of the mainstream of Japanese science, this was the first report in English of S. japonicum.

While I was Resident Medical Officer at St. John's Island Quarantine Station, Singapore, cholera broke out on a passenger ship from China. Some four hundred coolies were quarantined. Amongst them was a Chinaman from the Province of Fukien who presumably had never been away from China before.

He died of cholera after three days' illness. He was plump for a coolie. During life it was found that the right lobe of his liver extended two fingerbreadths below the costal margin. The left lobe was a handbreadth below the sternum, and its percussion dullness merged into the splenic. The spleen was palpable 1 in. from the iliac crest, and its notch was in line with the anterior axillary fold.

A necropsy was made an hour and a half after death. The adipose tissue throughout the body was a prominent feature. The appearance of the peritoneum suggested repeated attacks of peritonitis. The appendices epiploicae were thickened, and in some places matted together. The recto-vesical pouch was almost obliterated. Encasing the large intestine was a coat of fat, most marked at the mesenteric attachment. The mesenteric tissues were all thickened and loaded with fat. The mesenteric and prevertebral glands varied in size from a bean to a golf ball, the largest forming a cluster near the duodenum. The liver was uniformly enlarged. Its surfaces were markedly nodular, its borders sharp and irregular,

the whole presenting the appearance of a very coarse cirrhosis. Its consistence was greatly increased, but its colour was not appreciably altered. The coats of the gall bladder were thickened, and a layer of fat almost completely encased this viscus, which was distended with clear mucoid, apple-jelly-like material containing several minute black gall stones. The colon was much thickened throughout. The mucous membrane was swollen, hyperaemic, and friable, presenting numerous small circular, superficial erosions and patches of necrosis. The outer coats were very tough, almost cartilaginous, and showed no tendency to ulcerate. The rectum was three-quarters of an inch thick all round, and was adherent to the bladder. It nearly filled the true pelvis. Where adhesions had formed the bladder wall was thickened, but elsewhere it was healthy, and nowhere was the vesical mucosa diseased. The sigmoid was uniformly thickened; in tracing the bowel upwards the thickening became less marked and more patchy. The coats of the caecum and appendix vermiformis were uniformly hypertrophied, the mucous membrane presenting small patches of ulceration and necrosis. The appendix was provided with a mesentery, and a distended lymphatic could be recognized running along its free surface. The liver and bowel cut gritty on section. The lower end of the ileum was thickened in patches, and the mucosa congested over corresponding areas. The enlarged spleen was pigmented. The stomach, pancreas, suprarenals, kidneys, heart, and lungs, showed no signs of coarse disease.

As the lesions above mentioned were peculiar, some of the viscera were preserved. Sections of the liver, mesenteric lymphatic glands, and bowel were made in Singapore by Dr. Finlayson, and at the Kuala Lumpur Research Institute by Dr. Daniels. Numerous small oval bodies having a smooth, stout capsule were found. Opinions differed as to whether these were coccidia or the ova of some unknown parasite, but the case was published in the Journal of the Malaya Branch of the British Medical Association as a case of coccidiosis in man. Subsequent examination in this country of sections of intestine showed ova and filariaform embryos in bundles in the mucosa and villi of the large intestine. These, along with other specimens, were shown at the Medical Research Club, London, but no definite conclusion regarding the nature of the oval bodies was come to. An eminent German authority, to whom pieces of tissue were kindly sent by Dr. Bulloch stated "that the oval bodies were neither coccidia nor the eggs of a trematode, but those of a nematode of unrecognizable species, etc." At Sir Patrick Manson's suggestion, to whom the specimens were shown, I devoted my whole time to working out the case at the London School of Tropical Medicine, where systematic examination and sections of all the preserved tissues were made. Soon after I commenced investigating, nematode embryos were found in smear preparations from the large intestine, and one was found in the vessel of a mesenteric lymphatic gland. These facts, coupled with the juxtaposition of ova—some empty—and embryos in the mucosa and villi of the large intestine, led to the suggestion of a nematode infection, but as no evidence of a differentiated embryo could be seen in any of the eggs, even in those lying in close proximity to the bundles of free embryos, one hesitated to adopt this conclusion. Subsequently, in sections of the mesocolon, I found adult trematodes, male and female, in the blood vessels, the ova in the uterus of the female corresponding in every particular with the oval bodies found in the various viscera. It was now clear that I had to deal with concomitant trematode and nematode infections; that the oval bodies were the ova of the trematode; and that their close association with the filarial embryos was merely accidental.

A preliminary paper was read and drawings with specimens exhibited at the meeting of the British Medical Association at Oxford. Later, on continuing my dissections, entire mature worms were found in the smaller mesenteric blood vessels (Plate 84). It was difficult to determine the nature of the vessels in which the mature parasites lay. They were manifestly blood vessels, but whether arteries or veins was not so evident. I submitted my preparations to several eminent physiologists and pathologists. Unfortunately, there was no unanimity among them as to the arterial or venous nature of the vessels. I am constrained therefore to admit that this important point is for the present unsettled. My own conviction, however, is that the parasites occur in both arteries and veins. (See Plate 84.)

Parental Forms

The male (Plate 83) is 9 mm long, less than half a millimetre broad, and, in my spirit prepara-

tions, of a light brown-yellow colour. The measurements are only relative as they are taken from spirit specimens. Three entire adult males, with fragments of others, were found. They closely resemble those of Schistosoma haematobium, having their lateral borders incurved ventrally, thereby forming a canal groove along the entire length—the gynaecophoric canal—in which the female lies. The anterior extremity is blunt, with a terminal sucker in which the mouth lies. The dorsal lip of the sucker is longer than the ventral. Behind the sucker the body is slightly constricted, forming a neck. The worm attains its maximum breadth at the posterior sucker, which lies ventrally in the gynaecophoric canal about half a millimetre behind the anterior sucker, whence the body tapers gradually to a truncated posterior extremity. The posterior sucker is oval and trumpet-shaped, its long diameter being transverse; it is larger and more muscular than the anterior. Both suckers are retractile.

The alimentary system consists of a mouth furnished with a sphincter, a strong muscular oesophagus, and two caeca joining posteriorly to form a terminal ampulla. The oesophagus, surrounded by small glands, is constricted at its middle, and divides, just anterior to the acetabulum on which rests the posterior sucker, into the two caeca which run along either side of the body. Three anastomoses of the caeca were made out.

The excretory system ends in an excretory pore which is subterminal and ventral. The nervous system has not been satisfactorily determined. The reproductive system consists of a lobular testicle or testicles, vesiculi seminales, vas deferens, and genital pore with its sphincter, opening centrally into the gynaecophoric canal behind the posterior sucker.

A distinctive feature of this schistosome is the absence of ciliated warts on the integument, the presence of which constitutes so marked a feature of the African worm. Minor anatomical differences are: (a) Smaller size of the worm; (b) its longer vas deferens; (c) the characters of the testes.

The female (Plate 83 B) is almost cylindrical (diameter 0.113 mm), longer, more slender, and darker than the male. The cervical constriction is quite as marked as in the male. The suckers, alimentary and excretory systems, correspond with those of the male, except that the excretory pore is terminal. Owing to excessive fragility of the spirit specimen it was found impracticable to mount an entire specimen of the female worm.

The reproductive system consists of a muscular, central, elongated uterus occupying the anterior half of the body, and opening near the posterior sucker. The ova are arranged irregularly in single or in double rows. At the posterior extremity of the uterus are the shell glands and opening of the oviduct with the vitello-duct. Behind this the body bulges slightly to taper subsequently to a sharply-pointed extremity. The bulging marks the position of the ovary; posteriorly are the vitellogene glands.

From the female *Schistosoma haematobium* the following differences have been made out:

(*a*) The posterior sucker is larger than the anterior; the converse holds good in the *Schistosoma haematobium*.

(*b*) The bulging in region of ovary is more marked.

(*c*) The arrangement of the yolk glands is different.

In both sexes minute, highly refractile spines are seen in the suckers and at their anterior extremities.

The eggs (Plate 82) are yellow-brown in colour, oval, measuring on an average 70 μ long by 40 μ broad. They vary between 60 μ and 90 μ in length and 30 μ to 50 μ in breadth. They have a stout, smooth shell on section. There is no trace of a spine or operculum. In the sections some of the ova were empty; others contained a central, circular mass which stained deeply; some contained cells staining at their periphery, whilst others had cells staining in the centre. These may or may not completely fill the ovum. In some cases the cellular contents were seen escaping from a ruptured ovum. In no one of the ova could distinct embryos be detected, although appearances suggestive of a developing embryo could be observed. The ova differ from those of *Schistosoma haematobium* in their colour, shape, size, and in the absence of a spine. The bilharzia ovum is of a brown colour, contains a well-developed embryo, and is larger, 0.19 mm (Looss). Moreover, its ends are more pointed, and it is provided with a spine.

The ulcerative lesions of the bowel produced by the new species differ from the corresponding lesions of the bladder produced by *S.*

haematobium in the entire absence from the former of the fungating masses so characteristic of the latter. Further, the new species does not give rise to the perihepatic nodules as described by Sandwith in bilharziosis.

In addition to the character of the ova and to the anatomical differences already noted, there are certain other points which serve to differentiate the species.

(1) The habitat of *S. haematobium* is reputed to be venous only, whereas the habitat of the new schistosome is mainly arterial; too much stress must not be laid on this point, seeing it has not been proved that the former cannot affect arteries or the latter veins.

(2) The ova of *S. haematobium* affect mainly the urinary system, and escape from their human host by this channel. In the new species the ova apparently exclusively affect the alimentary system, escaping by this route from their human host.

(3) In this case there is a much more general infection of abdominal viscera, for ova of *S. haematobium* have not been found in the pancreas and appendix.

(4) The geographical distribution differs, for no case of bilharziosis has yet been met with in China.

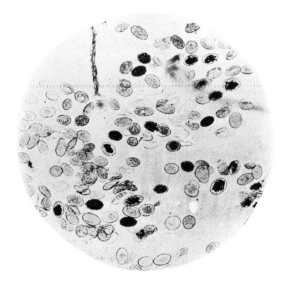

Plate 82. Ova.

Histopathology

The parent worms are found in small groups at the bifurcations of the smaller mesenteric vessels, and partially or completely plug the vessels. In one arteriole 0.621 mm in diameter two complete sections of the male and female are seen *in copula*. Blood cells are occasionally seen between the wall of the vessel and the parasites.

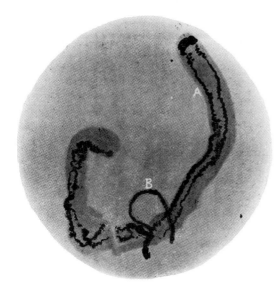

Plate 83. Male worm with a portion of female. (A) Male worm showing caeca; (B) Female.

Where ova accumulate they provoke at certain places a small-celled infiltration, which gives place later to a great proliferation of fibrous tissue. Pigment is seen in the liver and bowel. In the intestine from caecum to anus the ova occupy roughly two concentric layers—the one subperitoneal, where the ova are comparatively scarce; the other in the submucous coat, where they are innumerable, in some cases densely packed. Between these zones in the muscular layers ova with their long axes at right angles to the bowel lie in single or in double rows. Ova are plentiful in the mucosa, are more numerous in the necrotic areas, and are seen apparently in process of extrusion at the margin of an ulcer.

Of the intestinal tract, the rectum and appendix are most affected; the distended lymphatic vessel in the appendix already referred to is choked with ova. Everywhere throughout the small intestine ova were found, but only in patches and in relatively small numbers.

The obliteration of the rectovesical pouch was probably caused by the irritation produced by ova accumulating in vast numbers in the wall of the rectum. In many sections examined no ova were found in the vesical mucosa, though they were present in small numbers in the outer coats of the bladder.

In the liver the ova are plentiful, lying singly or in larger or smaller clumps embedded in the markedly hypertrophied fibrous connective tissue.

In many of the enlarged mesenteric lymphatic glands ova were found in the thickened trabeculae.

In addition to the localities already mentioned ova were found in the outer wall of the gall bladder, in the pancreas, liver capsule, fibrous coat of the larger mesenteric vessels, mesentery, pylorus, duodenum, jejunum, and ileum. Several sections were made of the round ligament of the liver and of the diaphragm without any ova being found.

Doubtless the life-history of the new schistosome corresponds with that of other trematodes, the geographical range of the intermediary host being the principal determining factor in its distribution.

That this case is unique is extremely improbable. When proper search has been made doubtless many additional cases will be found in the natives of the endemic districts. As a ready means of ascertaining the degree of prevalence and geographical range of the infection I would suggest systematic examination at *post-mortem* examinations of scrapings from the mucous membrane of the bowel, preferably of erosions or ulcerated patches. With a low power of the microscope only a few minutes are required to determine the presence or absence of the ova in such preparations.

The ova have probably been found many times in the course of ordinary microscopical examinations of faeces, but have been mistaken for the ova of *Ankylostoma duodenale*, which they closely resemble.

It is interesting to note the accumulation of filariaform embryos in the villi, probably in the lacteals, of the intestinal tract, and their presence in faeces. I am not aware of any similar observation.

Diagnosis

Sub Kingdom . . . . .Vermes.
Class . . . . .Plathelminthes
Order . . . . .Trematoda.
Family . . . . .Schistosomidae.
Genus . . . . .Schistosoma.
Species . . . . .Schistosoma Cattoi
                                (Blanchard) 1904.

Measurements given below are from specimens found in hardened tissues.

	Female.	Male.
Length	?	9 mm
Breadth	0.115 mm	0.447 mm
Breadth (near ovary)	0.134 mm	—
Diameter at neck	0.041 mm	0.180 mm
Gynaecophoric canal	absent	entire length of body
Shape and size of posterior sucker	0.061 by 0.047 mm	0.290 by 0.189 mm
	(long diam. longitudinal)	(long diam. transverse)
Shape and size of anterior sucker	0.51 mm circular	0.124 mm circular
Distance between centres of these	0.146 mm	0.552 mm
Genital pore	behind posterior sucker	behind posterior sucker
Excretory pore	terminal	subterminal
Tubercles and cilia	absent	absent
Spines in suckers	present but scarce	present

Habitat of Adults: Mesenteric vessels.

Ova: Oval with rounded ends and smooth stout capsule, destitute of spine and operculum.

Size: 0.065 to 0.090 mm. by 0.030 to 0.050 mm.

Found in intestinal tract and its appendages.

Number of Cases: One

Symptoms: Probably colic and dysentery.

Physical Signs: Enlarged liver and spleen.

Geographical Distribution: Province of Fukien, China.

Type Specimen: Museum of London Tropical School of Medicine. Mounted in xylol balsam unstained from preserved formalin tissue.

It is possible that the filariaform embryos above referred to also escaped into the lumen of the bowels from the ulcers, for on making smear preparations from various parts of the bowel these embryos were found. In one smear thirteen embryos were present but in many others none were found. These embryos had the following measurements and characters; these, however, cannot be taken as accurate as none were got in a fresh state.

Average length . . . . .0.300 mm
Greatest thickness . . . . .0.008 mm
Sheath . . . . .present.
Shape of head . . . . .truncate conical.
Shape of tail . . . . .sharp pointed.

(The sheath in many cases could not be seen, but embryos may discard it when in unnatural surroundings.)

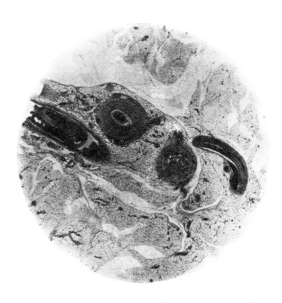

Plate 84. Section of mesentery. Worms seen lying in blood vessels in transverse and longitudinal section. Note difference in thickness of vessel walls.

Ova of *Trichocephalus dispar, Ankylostoma duodenale, Ascaris lumbricoides*, in numbers, were found in the smears. Adult worms of all these were also found in the bowel.

I am deeply indebted to Sir Patrick Manson for much encouragement and criticism; and also for his sending specimens to the International Zoological Congress at Berne, where they were examined by Professor Blanchard, Drs.Looss, Ward, Stiles, Grossi, Monticelli, and other zoologists, who all agreed that the parasite was a schistosoma and new to science. Professor Blanchard has done me the honour of naming this new helminth *Schistosoma cattoi*. To Drs. T. S. Kerr and E. E. Henderson the credit is due for the excellent drawings and photomicrographs.

[1]Studies on Schistosomiasis Japonica. The American Journal of Hygiene, Monographic Series No. 3, pp. 1–326, 1924.

A REPORT ON A STUDY OF THE "KATAYAMA DISEASE" IN HIGO-NO-KUNI

Tokyo Igakkai Zasshi, 18, No. 3: 31–48, 1904. Selections from pp. 31–34. 18, No. 4: 1–31, 1904. Selections from pp. 21–22, 31. Translated from the Japanese.

Kenji Kawanishi (Kasai)
(1868–1927)

Kawanishi came from a long line of physicians in the Nagano prefecture. In 1889, while studying at Tokyo Imperial University School of Medicine, he was drafted into military service as a medical officer during the Sino-Japanese War. Later, he returned to Kyoto Imperial University and graduated in medicine; he continued to serve in the army, traveling to Formosa, Manchuria, and Germany as a medical officer. In 1908 he received his M.D. degree. He was eventually appointed head physician of the South Manchurian Railway Hospital in Dairen, and later became the first director of the South Manchurian Medical School.

This is the first description of Schistosoma japonicum *ova in the stool and the first suggestion that Katayama disease might be parasitic in nature.*

During my student days at the Kyoto Imperial University, I was sent on an official trip to study the Katayama disease. I left the university on 4 June 1902 and returned on the 12th. In one week's time my primary endeavor was to learn about the clinical aspects of the disease; I also tried to determine its causes. However, my stay there was not long enough for me to gain much knowledge of the disease.

Having examined about ten patients, I returned to the university, hoping to come back at a later date. However, the government ordered me to return to the army, and I had no time off during the summer. I managed, eventually, to find a little time, and left on 12 October for a two-day stay. I re-examined the patients whom I had seen previously and noted the development of the disease. I was able to meet one or two new patients. However, I could not find anything that could be regarded as the cause of the disease.

In the meantime, one patient whom I had examined wished to enter the Kyoto Imperial University Hospital, and I encouraged him to do so. While he was hospitalized, his stool was examined and a new type of egg was discovered. On another trip to Higo-no-kuni on 23 March 1903, I found another patient with the same type of eggs. My purpose in making the following report is first to introduce the clinical symptoms

of the disease to those who study medicine and, second, to make the modest material available to those who will study about the disease in the future.

Katayama Area: Katayama is a village located on the southeastern foot of a small (80 meters high) mountain in Kawanaka-mura, Shinan-gun, Higo-no-kuni, Hiroshima prefecture; it is in the western end of Kawanami. The Takaya River flows by its western side and it (Katayama) borders Nakatsuhara village; the cultivated land is on the western side. The village has 36 houses and a population of 190. Its topography is high on the northern side and low on the southern side. Some land development has occurred at the foot of the mountain, and houses are built there. The soil shows the layer of rocks. The mountain is well forested and contains many old pine trees. The water in the north goes into the Bichu-no-kuni and to the Yakake River. The rivers south of the central area all flow into Katayama and Chida villages and then into the Ashita River.

The paddy fields of Katayama village are several feet lower than the level of the river, making it very difficult to drain the stagnant water, particularly during a prolonged rainy season. The Ashita, Kamo, and Takaya rivers together form swamp areas. It takes a few days, sometimes ten or more, for the swamp water to recede. Even after it is drained, bottom mud three to four inches thick settles there. Every summer, at ploughing time, brown-colored bubbles appear in the ditches and paddy fields. Persons who go into this mud immediately develop red rashes; the associated pruritis is said to be unbearable. The river embankment repair was accomplished in 1881, thus preventing the overflow of the dirty river water into the paddy fields. Just the same, anyone who went into the paddy fields developed rashes.

Geographical History of Katayama: There is no way of verifying ancient events; however, legend says that many, many years ago a commercial boat bringing lacquer to this area was wrecked by a storm and ever since, Katayama has been called the "lacquer mountain." It is said that those who pass by the mountain feel the "lacquer air." In modern times, the local people who enter the water to plough the paddy fields develop rashes on their legs. Cows and horses also are afflicted. The people say that the sickness is caused by the "lacquer air."

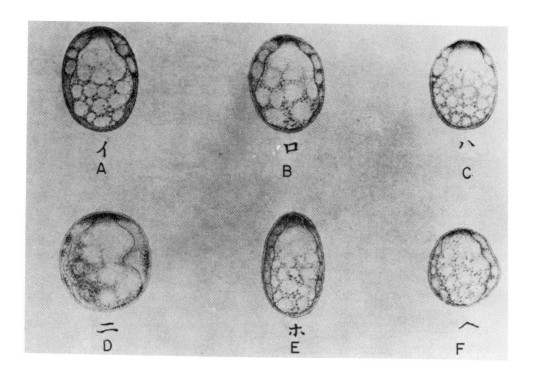

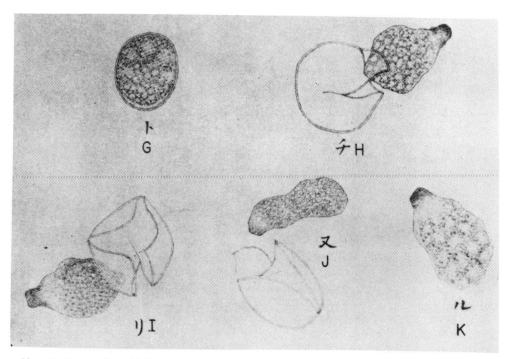

Plate 85. Figs. A, B, C. Medium large eggs. *Fig. D.* Large round egg. *Fig. E.* Long and slender egg. *Fig. F.* Somewhat small and round egg. *Fig. G.* Small egg. *Figs. H, I, J.* Larva coming out of egg shell. *Fig. K.* Slightly developed larva.

I read an old book which reported Seibi-rokkai dialect. According to this dialect, ''an-na'' was a hole (An-na-gun is in this region). In the years gone by the villagers dug a well. After having dug several *jo* [one jo equals 10 feet—Eds.] they found an old piece of lumber. A careful examination revealed that it was a ship's mast. There is no way of knowing whether or not this area was once a wide ocean.

The Beginning of the Katayama Disease: No one knows when the Katayama disease first appeared. Moreover, there is no oral tradition for it. I met a man over 70 years of age and asked him whether he had seen such patients when he was young. He remembered having had rashes on his lower legs when he was 15 or 16 years old, after having been in a paddy field. He occasionally saw men with ''abdominal dropsy.''

In other words, there is as yet no definite theory about the nature of Katayama disease. It is also difficult to find out when this disease occurs. Nevertheless, Dr. Fujii of Yamate-mura, Numakuma-gun, Hiroshima prefecture said, after having made the diagnosis and having treated several patients, that it is a regional disease of sorts. Because of this comment, people began for the first time (circa 1847) to pay attention to it.

History of the Studies on the Katayama Disease: Following the comment of Dr. Fujii, Dr. Jiro Kubota of Awane village of Fukayasu-gun, at the beginning of the Meiji era, gave his attention to regional diseases. Thereupon, the Katayama disease became a problem for the medical associations.

Between 1882 to 1884, the Hiroshima prefecture established a committee to study the Katayama disease. These men treated the patients with medicine and reported the results. . . .

Following is a report made by the author: ''Katayama disease'' is present in the Katayama region of Higo. The symptoms are enlarged liver and spleen, sometimes abdominal ascites, anemia, and bloody stools. In the stools of a patient with the disease, I found oval-shaped light brown colored eggs, 0.1-0.08 mm in length and 0.077-0.05 mm in width. As yet, the worm which produced these eggs has not been found. These are probably the eggs from a type of distoma which parasitizes the liver. . . .

The third time I visited the region, an examination of one patient's stools revealed the presence of elongated (distoma) eggs. The patient entered the Kyoto University Hospital. Other patients' stools were examined with the following results:

(1) Kishino Inoue—The same type of eggs were found.
(2) Aki Yokoyama—A small number of elongated distoma eggs and also young worms were found which resembled those found in the stools of the hospitalized patient.
(3) Natsumoto—Something like larvae were found.
(4) Sato—Something like larvae were found. The other three examinations did not reveal any of these.

The new parasite eggs have several shapes, but most of them are perfectly oval, have a thin shell, and seem to have two layers (doubly refractile). They are the color of pale yellowish tea, and an operculum is not found. These eggs vary in content; some are filled with what appear to be large, round granules. There is a very transparent substance. The content of the egg resembles primarily the shape of a wine bottle. This is a larva. Provided with a little warmth, it immediately comes out of its shell. (Plate 85.)

The size of the eggs varies. According to my measurements, the length of the egg is 0.109-0.081 mm and the width is 0.0765-0.0533 mm. The thickness of the shell is 0.0015 mm. Breaking of the shell may occur at one end or on one side and is very irregular.

When they first leave the shell, the larvae look like wine bottles. After one day they become larger and assume many different shapes. When present in the stool, the transparent larva is clearly distinguished and hence is easily detected.

In short, the characteristics of the new parasite eggs are as follows: When I see them, they have already developed into larvae. When the room temperature is a little warm, one can see immediately the rupture of the egg shells. Once, I was studying microscopically a large number of eggs in stool when the coldness of the room became intolerable. I then went into a room heated by a stove. When I looked at [the specimens] a few hours later, the young worms were outside of the broken shells. I noticed that the part which resembled the mouth of a bottle (the head of the worm) was moving faintly. . . .

A CASE OF DYSENTERY IN HUNAN PROVINCE CAUSED BY THE TREMATODE, *SCHISTOSOMA JAPONICUM*

China Missionary Medical Journal, 19: 243–245, 1905.

Oliver Tracy Logan
(1870–1919)

A native of Bethany, Illinois, and a graduate of Indiana Medical College, Logan was sent to China in 1897 as a missionary under the Cumberland Presbyterian China Mission and again in 1901. He was instrumental in having a modern hospital built and, in addition to his regular duties, he was visiting lecturer at the Nankow Medical School.

He became director of the American Red Cross Hospital in Vladivostok. After a furlough at home, he returned in 1919 to China where, while attending a battle-crazed officer of the revolutionary army, he was murdered by his patient. The three-day funeral at the behest of General Feng Yu-Hsiang was a testimony of Logan's life of uncompromising service.

This report in English was the first record of Schistosoma japonicum *infection in mainland China.*

I beg to report a case that, to my mind, is suffering of the disease caused by the blood fluke, *Schistosoma japonicum*. As this disease will likely be found often in the future, I would like to suggest that in the examinations of the fecal matter suspected to contain the eggs of this fluke, the smears be thin and free from vegetable fibers, so that the cover glass will lie flat, and furthermore that as little pressure as possible be used and that the illumination be slight. These rules will appeal to those who have done considerable of this sort of work. Unless one observes these simple rules he will be sure to overlook, not only the egg in question, but other eggs as well.

Cheng, Chinese, 18 years of age, male, reared in Changteh, Hunan prefecture. At the age of 12, while engaged as a fisherman's assistant, he first had bloody stools, which grew worse, until at 15 the disease had become well established and incapacitated him for hard work. Patient is only four feet six inches in height, has a cachectic look, but is not emaciated, neither is he of the bloated appearance one often finds in patients suffering of ancylostomiasis. The superficial veins over the upper part of the abdomen and lower part of the chest are much enlarged. Left lobe of the liver extends four fingers' breadth below the sternum and three inches to the left of

the median line. The right lobe is felt two fingers' breadth below the ribs. Spleen is slightly enlarged. The urine is clear, amber-colored, and the patient has never noticed any blood. Microscopic examination failed to show abnormalities in the urine, although it was slightly albuminous.

The patient complains that he has, several times a day, pain in the abdomen, which is followed by a bloody stool. He has an average of four stools in 24 hours. The two stools examined contained considerable blood, well mixed with mucus and the fecal matter. The microscope revealed a few eggs of the *Trichocephalus dispar,* the *Ancylostoma duodenale,* and a peculiar form of lumbricoid egg that we constantly find here, the characteristics of which are its elliptical shape, thin shell, globular yolk, and its comparative freedom from the albuminous coating that characterizes the typical *Ascaris lumbricoides*

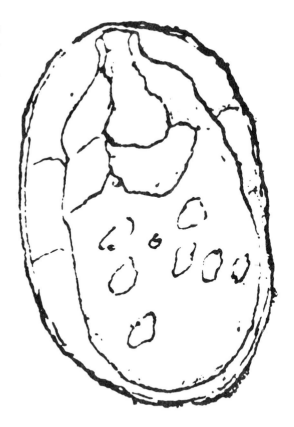

Plate 86. Embryo inside the egg.

egg. In addition to these I found eggs that are oval in shape, light yellow or clear in color, larger and more nearly round than the *A. duodenale,* and containing an embryo. The embryo is the shape of a melon seed, one end being more tapered and provided with a rounded protuberance, which is joined to the body by a short neck. By using an oil immersion lens and carefully focusing on the different planes, one is able to distinguish rapidly moving cilia on the neck and narrower part of the embryo. The rest of the body also is ciliated, but not so markedly, and there is no apparent motion in the cilia. When the embryo is in the shell (Plate 86), the cilia appear, not as rods but like pigment granules, such as one finds in the malarial parasites, especially the benign tertian. In two instances I was able, by slight pressure, to burst the shell of the egg and study the embryo. It comes out as a shapeless mass, but

soon assumes the characteristic shape. When out of the shell the cilia appear as rods which project from the body at different angles, depending on their location (Plate 87). I am not able to give a good description of the internal organs, as they seem very indistinct. Roughly speaking there seems to be a connection between the protuberance and the globules in the narrow part of the body. These globules seem to form a sort of a sac in some specimens. The globules in the middle and wider end of the body are coarser and not so refractile as those in the narrow end.

I was led to examine this patient more carefully on account of the reprints of papers by Dr. Catto and Professor Katsurada that appeared in the *Journal of Tropical Medicine.* As the eggs of the *Schistosoma cattoi* have not been reported to have been observed in the feces, and as none found elsewhere have contained an embryo, one is led to believe that the eggs I have described and made drawings of are those of the *S. japonicum.* The clinical symptoms tally closely with those described by Professor Katsurada, and his description of the embryo applies in its main features to those I have studied, and I may say that I have observed dozens of these eggs, all of which contained an embryo. It has not been our policy to take into the hospital cases of the sort described, and we have not examined the stools of many out-patients who have passed bloody stools. I do not recall other cases presenting the signs and symptoms of this one; still it is probable that similar cases will be found, now that we are looking for them.

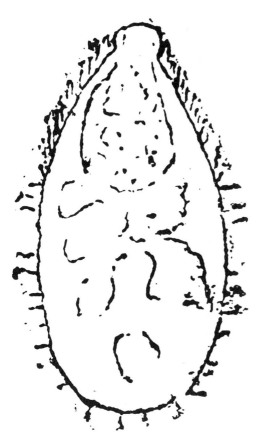

Plate 87. Embryo outside the egg.

KATAYAMA DISEASE IN HIROSHIMA PREFECTURE
Route of Infection, Development of the Worm in the Host and Animals in Katayama Disease in Hiroshima Prefecture (Japanese Blood Sucking Worm Disease—Schistosomiasis japonica)

Kyoto Igaku Zasshi, 6: 224–252, 1909 (extracted). Translated from the Japanese.

Kan Fujinami
(1870–1934)

The son of a physician, Fujinami was born in the Aichi prefecture of Japan. After receiving his medical education, he served as professor of medicine at Kyoto Uni-

versity. In 1896 he went to Germany for further study and to teach. He was awarded an Imperial Academy prize for his work on Katayama disease in 1918, and in 1923 he visited the United States at the invitation of the Rockefeller Foundation

Hachitaro Nakamura

Hachitaro Nakamura, a graduate of Kyoto University Medical School, was an assistant professor of pathology at the time this paper was written. He later became professor of pathology at Kanazawa University.

This is the first demonstration that infection with Schistosoma japonicum occurs by skin penetration.

Preface

The final report on Katayama disease, the endemic disease of Higo-no-kuni region in Hiroshima prefecture (the disease is in Shinan-gun and its vicinity) was made in 1907. Even after that report, we often made trips to the region and were able to obtain new research material with the help of the Shinan-gun Regional Disease Research Association.

The Route of Penetration of Japanese Blood-Sucking-Worm Disease, Schistosomiasis japonica

The route of penetration of this disease is uncertain; however, it can be speculated that the organism enters either through the gastrointestinal tract or the skin. The route of penetration probably depends on the habits of the farmer, but even this is speculative.

The main reason for suggesting that the gastrointestinal tract is a possible route of invasion is the presence of the worms in the veins of the intestinal tract. Dr. Kasita has postulated that the presence of the worm in the gastrointestinal tract is due to ingestion of contaminated water. Even though this is a reasonable speculation, there is no experimental evidence for it.

In contrast to this theory, it is apparent that the farmer acquires infection by placing his legs in the mud; therefore, another definite possibility is penetration through the skin. Further speculation along this line is based on the fact that the disease is most severe during the planting season. Accordingly, most physicians in the endemic areas believe that the worms can penetrate the skin as well as the gastrointestinal tract. The famous Looss had speculated that the young larvae penetrate the skin directly and enter the liver and there eggs develop into adults. We speculate, similarly as Looss, that the worms enter the body through the skin. Others have suggested that although the main route of penetration is through the gastrointestinal tract we still feel that we cannot eliminate the possibility of skin penetration.

This same speculation can be applied to our own Japanese blood-sucking-worm disease. Looss reported that even though a certain number of young larvae penetrate the skin, the majority of the worms enter via the gastrointestinal tract and penetrate the wall of the small intestine and reach the portal veins. Thus the large intestine is the location of egg deposition and yet not the site of larval penetration. While no one can deny the Looss skin-penetration theory, it is more reasonable to assume that the gastrointestinal tract is the main route of penetration

Dr. Kasita reported to the Tokyo Medical Society after the survey of the places where infection with this worm occurs and reported the following: even though there is no direct experimental evidence, it is quite possible that the Looss theory can be applied to the Japanese blood-sucking-worm disease.

Direct experimental evidence is required to make definitive conclusions.

Experimental methods. We used 20 cows initially for this experiment. Unfortunately only 17 completed the experiment, and these were divided into four groups. . . .

[The animals which were allowed into the river and mud became infected. Those fed contaminated water in feed lots did not become infected—Eds.]

The Length of Time Required for the Adult Worm of This Disease to Grow in the Body

From the following experiment we learned that the time required for the parasite to grow is comparatively short.

The calves were allowed to go into the river, muddy fields, and small ditches. Afterward, they were dissected and examined and were found to have adult parasites. A study was made on these calves. The number of days from the first day of the animals' exposure to the water (as mentioned above) to the day of examination by dissection are as follows:

Calves	Number of days
No. 15	26
Nos. 2 and 5	36

No. 4	39
No. 16	42
No. 3	52
No. 6	93 days

Not only were there time differences between the last day of exposure and the day of the autopsy, but also the exposure time varied. There were variations in the number of days required for the adult parasites to develop. Therefore, different stages, from small, immature worms to completely grown, mature worms, were present in the same animal (see Plate 88, Fig. 3, No. 1). From calf No. 15 we learned precisely the number of days required for parasite growth. The time required for infection was one day. Precisely 26 days from the day of infection, we were able to find 31 pairs of worms. Although still small, they were mature worms. The males were mostly 4 mm long, and most of the females were 4 to 5 mm. These measurements were made from fixed specimens. When they are alive, they are a little longer. (Plate 88, Fig. 3, No. 2 shows the actual size.) Among them, one pair was the male and female combination. However, no eggs were found in the uterus of the females whether they were single or attached to males. There were no eggs obstructing the liver.

Now we shall observe our dogs (see table). When the dogs were not outside, they were tied or kept in cages. Their food was cooked barley and powdered dry fish. During this period, their bodies did not touch contaminated water. As indicated in the table, on various dates they were released outdoors. From time to time, the dogs swam in the Takaya River, and on other occasions they were exposed in the small ditches and muddy fields. On occasion they drank the river water. The result of all these activities increased the degree of infection; this was evident at autopsy. However, up to the time of autopsy there were no symptoms of illness caused by these worms. Of all the dogs, No. 9 lived the shortest time (23 days) from the first day of exposure to the day of autopsy. This animal already had the small adult worms, although not a large number of them. The male worms were about 4 mm in length, the female not quite 5 mm. The reproductive organs were fully developed. There were already male and female pairs in copulation, but there were none with eggs in the uterus. Therefore, the longest period required for the worms to

grow—even if the dogs had been infected on the first day outdoors—was not more than 23 days. In other words, it definitely takes no longer than 23 days for worms to mature, although the bodies are small and they have not produced eggs. The experiment with the dog indicates that the shorter the time period between exposure and autopsy, the smaller the size of the worms present.

Good results were obtained from our experiments with rabbits. In our experiment, one rabbit was infected. It was learned subsequently that this animal had a predisposition to infection. On the 35th day from the day the rabbits went into the ditch, a rabbit was autopsied. The total exposure of this animal was 36 hours in 7 days. Ten pairs of completely grown, small mature adults were found. The length of the males was 4.5 mm–6 mm, and that of the female about 4.5 mm; there were other smaller ones. Among these there were three male and female pairs in copulation, including a male in joint copulation with two small females. It takes a very short time, according to these experiments, after the worms have entered the body, for them to become fully grown adults. Those dogs and rabbits which were exposed for a longer time and lived for a longer time before dissection not only had more worms, but larger ones.

Dog No. 1, dissected on the 54th day after the first day of exposure, had a large number of well-grown worms. According to the fixed specimens, the length of the largest male is 1 cm and that of the largest female, 1.3 cm (most of them are 1 cm). Calf No. 6 was in the small ditches and muddy fields 37 days, for a total exposure period of 106 hours and 32 minutes. The animal was dying on the 93rd day after the first day of exposure; it was sacrificed and dissected. The parasites were all large, the largest (male and female) being 1.8 cm; most of them were 0.8 to 1 cm. The total number of worms was more than 20,000.

As stated above, the adults mature in a comparatively short time; and even before they become fully grown, the reproductive organs develop. Furthermore, it is known that the male and female copulate very early. It does not take long for these early-mated worms to produce eggs. Eggs are found in the tissue of the bowel very shortly after the infection. Nevertheless, because of varied conditions, the process is never the same. It is impossible to state the exact number of

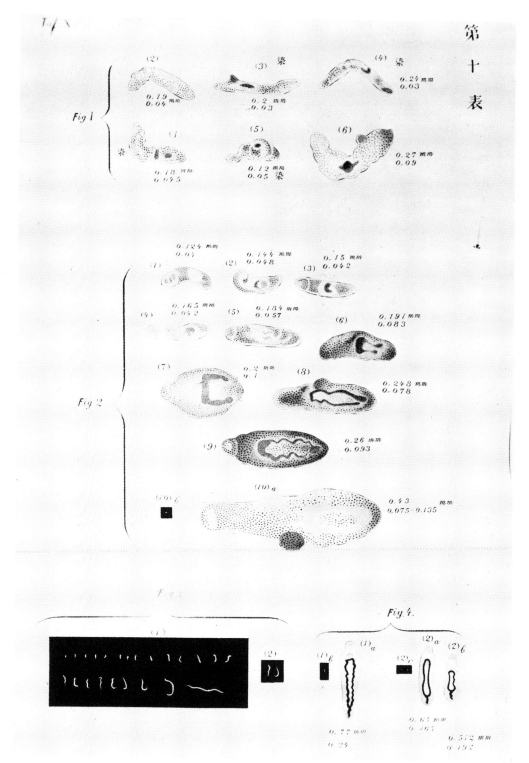

days before egg production, but the following facts provide some information on this question.

Dog No. 9. Dissected on the 23rd day from the first day of exposure. Eggs were not seen in the female.

Dog No. 8. Dissected on the 26th day from the first day of exposure. (The date of infection appeared to have been late, as the female worms were smaller than those found in No. 9.) No eggs were present.

Calf No. 15. Dissected on the 26th day from the day of infection. The date of infection is accurate. Neither the female in copulation with the male nor the single females had any eggs in the uterus.

Rabbit. Dissected on the 35th day from the first day of exposure and the 28th day from the last day of exposure.

Formation of eggs was seen in the females locked together with males. There were no eggs in the single females.

Calf No. 5. Dissected on the 36th day from the first day of exposure. There were eggs in the mature females.

Calf No. 4. Dissected on the 39th day from the first day of exposure. There were eggs in the mature females. A small number of eggs were seen in the liver.

Calf No. 16. Dissected on the 42nd day from the first day of exposure. There were many mature females, all of which contained eggs. There were eggs in the liver and in the feces.

Dog No. 1. Dissected on the 54th day from the first day of exposure. There were many mature females, and they all contained eggs. There were egg granuloma in the liver.

It was thus learned that the time required for the eggs to form, the resulting worms to reproduce, and their eggs to be found in the tissues or feces is comparatively short. (If I may dare say, roughly, the time period required would probably be about one month). . . .

Summary

This paper is the continuation of the report made two years ago on this Katayama disease. It describes the results of experiments conducted this summer and a few other matters.

One of the purposes of the experiments conducted this summer was to determine how the causative agent enters the body; and 17 calves were used for this experiment. The entrance of the causative agent of this disease is definitely from outside of the body. In the case of calves, ordinarily, invasion is not through the gastrointestinal tract, but this route cannot definitely be rejected. It is not clear whether invasion is through the skin or the mucosa. There is one case of a calf which was infected slightly through eating.

Generally, the conditions for infection are very simple. It is sufficient to immerse a leg in the contaminated water for several hours a day in order to stimulate invasion of the disease-causing worm.

A relatively short period of time is required for the disease-causing worms to infiltrate the host and grow into adults. The shortest time, counting from the first day the skin is soaked in the contaminated water to the day the adults are found at the time of dissection, is 23 days (this happened in a dog). However, the adults are small. Copulation and egg production all take a relatively short time.

Although the entire process of the development of the disease-causing worm is not yet clear, the stages of development from very small adults to the fully grown adult have been observed. The adults reside in the blood of the portal system. The shape of the smallest adult is very delicate; its length is 0.124 mm and its width is 0.04 mm; and it can be seen with the naked eye. The recognition of male and female, even as young worms, is not difficult.

The life cycle before they are found in the portal circulation is not yet known. The connection between the small worm (miracidium) which during the warm season leaves the egg shell which had been deposited in soil and water and the very young, immature worms in the portal vein must await serious study in the future. One or two experiments and tests concerning the eggs and small worms are included in the present paper.

The types of animals which are susceptible to the disease and their manifestations are also important matters for study. It is known that cows, dogs, and cats as well as horses easily contract this disease. This summer, it was learned that domestic rabbits, too, can contract this disease.

Plate 88. Fig. 1. The Japanese blood fluke from the portal veins of dog No. 9 in the early stage of development. *Fig. 2.* Same as above. From the portal veins of calves Nos. 4 and 5. *Fig. 3.* The Japanese blood flukes. (1) Obtained from the experimental calf No. 4. (2) Obtained from the experimental calf No. 15, 26 days after infection. These usually can be seen with the naked eye. *Fig. 4.* Small, young worms which can be seen with the naked eye.

Dogs	First exposure	Last exposure	Total exposure, days	Date of dissection	No. of days bet. first exposure and dissection	Results
No. 1	June 5	July 24	26	July 28	54	At the time of dissection there were: males 23, females 28; males & females together 2; extremely small ones 9. Some remained in blood vessels; approximate total 100.
No. 2	June 7	July 9	21	July 10	34	M 18, F 12; M & F together 1; mainly in small intestines in branches of thick mesentery veins and other veins of rectum and large veins of mesentery.
No. 3						Died of other disease.
No. 4	June 7	July 23	8	July 23	47	Very small ones 2. In portal vein.
No. 5	June 7	July 24	20	July 24	48	Comparatively large M 9; M & F together 8; very small M 2, F 5. Mainly in branch of mesenteric veins belonging to small intestines.
No. 6	June 7	July 9	12	July 12	36	Comparatively large M 3, F 1; M & F together 4. Very small M 2, F 4. One M in veins of spleen; others are in mesenteric veins belonging to small intestines.
No. 7	June 20	July 24	13	July 24	37	M 1, F 2; M & F together 1. They are in branches of mesenteric veins, belonging to small intestines and trunk veins of mesentery.
No. 8	June 18	July 9	7	July 13	26	Small M 2, F 1. Mainly in trunk veins of mesentery.
No. 9	June 18	July 9	8	July 10	23	Small M 2, F 3 (include M & F together). They are in large veins of mesentery, belonging to small intestines and trunk veins of mesentery.
No. 10	June 18	July 24	15	July 24	37	Small M 2, F 1. They are in branch of mesenteric veins belonging to small intestines and trunk veins of mesentery.

Table — Infection experiments utilizing dogs (Fujinami)

The important points in protecting against the disease are: (1) that feces which contain the eggs must be disinfected; (2) in order to prevent the growth of the causative agent, constructions on land and water must be renovated; (3) in order to prevent the causative agent's penetrating the body, contact with contaminated water should be avoided. Good, potable drinking water should be supplied.

ON THE ROUTE OF MIGRATION OF THE *SCHISTOSOMA JAPONICUM* FROM THE SKIN TO THE PORTAL SYSTEM AND THE STRUCTURE OF THE YOUNGEST WORMS AT THE TIME OF SKIN PENETRATION

Ueber den wanderungsweg des Schistosomum japonicum von der haut bis zum pfortadersystem und über die körperkonstitution der jüngsten würmer zur zeit der hautinvasion. Centralblatt für Bakteriologie, Parasitenkunde and Infektionskrankheiten, 66: 406–417, 1912. Selections from pp. 406–407, 415–416. Translated from the German.

Yoneji Miyagawa
(1885–1959)

A native of Aichi prefecture, Miyagawa graduated from Tokyo Imperial University in medicine in 1910 and presented his thesis in 1917. He worked in the Infectious Disease Research Institute (Kitasato) for a short time, then was sent to the United States, England, and Switzerland for further studies between 1918 and 1920. Subsequently he became professor of medicine at his alma mater and director of the Hospital of the Institute. In 1934 he became director of the Institute.

He described the etiologic agent of Lymphogranuloma venereum, *known at first as "Miyagawa's germ."*

Miyagawa's meticulous tracing of the developmental route of S. japonicum *from cercariae to the adult worm is recorded in these two papers.*

The mode of infection by *Schistosoma japonicum* is cutaneous, not oral, as has been determined for some years now by various authors. However, until now absolutely nothing has been known about the migratory route of these parasites from the skin to the portal system, where they usually lodge within the host, or about the body structure of the youngest worms at the time of skin penetration.

From May to October 1911, I stayed in the province of Yamanashi where schistosomiasis (the so-called "Yamanashi disease") is indigenous, in order to clarify this still obscure stage. At the beginning of this experiment I assumed that the migration of the parasite inside the host was neither through the lymphatic system nor between the tissue spaces, for example, in the nerve and vascular sheaths; because of other analogies, the venous blood stream seemed most probable. In contrast to the usual examination method of seeking the youngest worms in the skin sections, I endeavored to catch them in the middle of the migratory route; for that reason I examined the youngest parasites in the peripheral venous blood of the animal infected by immersion in brook water. During June and July of the previous year this procedure had enabled me to find some very young schistosome worms in the blood of the experimental animal. Shortly thereafter I was able to find and to identify the same worms in the skin of the same experimental animal and the same and still older worms (even almost completely developed parasites) in the portal blood.

The Examination of the Peripheral Venous Blood

For 3–8 days, 3–6 hours daily, I immersed numerous experimental animals, especially dogs and rabbits, in the brook water of the province of Yamanashi, where the disease is particularly rampant. At intervals of 2–24 hours after pulling the animals out of the water, I punctured the femoral or saphenous veins and examined the blood in the following way:

(1) I placed blood in a thick layer on the slide and let it dry; then I passed it twice through the flame and dipped it in sufficient distilled water. Thereafter, the blood pigment disappeared as a result of the hemolytic action of the water, and only leukocyte nuclei and the parasites were visible on the slide. In numerous preparations, with the aid of differential staining with borax carmine, methylene blue, and hematoxylin, I found some of the youngest worms.

(2) I poured 5–10 cc of venous blood into 50–60 cc of physiologic saline solution in a Petri dish and stirred it lightly with a rod. After about two hours a precipitate formed on the bottom of the dish which, with the aid of a pipette, I dropped onto a large slide and examined microscopi-

cally. In these large amounts of blood a few of the youngest worms could be found.

(3) Utilizing the same procedure with blood from the portal vein, I was able to find various sized worms and to compare two strains [sic] of the parasites and to identify them.

(4) In a similar process with the blood of three noninfected dogs and a rabbit I was unable to find the same forms microscopically. But after immersing the same animals in brook water the examination always had positive results.

(5) Into other healthy animals I injected, intravenously, the peripheral venous blood containing the parasite embryos; by so doing I hoped to see my microscopic findings confirmed experimentally. I sacrificed 11 animals for this purpose. With the aid of these examination methods I could pursue the migration of these parasites inside the host and determine their route. I was able to determine a few things about the development of these parasites by comparing many of the youngest worms at the time of the skin penetration with those from the portal vein blood. . . .

The Comparison of the Youngest Invading Worms with the Miracidia from Eggs

This study is very interesting and important, but unfortunately extraordinarily difficult. The investigation of the *modus vivendi* of the miracidium outside the egg will be made somewhat easier thereby, and it will become clear whether or not the schistosome has an intermediate host. It is necessary to describe very briefly and simply the structure of the miracidium.

In the fully developed miracidium, the buccal cavity, the esophagus with one celled glands, the stomach, and the intestine are already seen when inside the egg shell. The suction cup is never seen. At the posterior end of the body, the parenchyma is net-shaped, with small nuclei filled with structureless, homogeneous liquids and ganglion cells. The body wall is very thin, never doubly contoured. It has very long cilia, about three times as long as those of the invasive form, by means of which the organism can swim around very briskly in the liquid. After a single drying it becomes immediately immobile and disintegrates. If the miracidium is allowed to remain in water longer than 24 hours, it becomes inert and motionless and disintegrates gradually, while

from the parenchyma numerous granules appear at the anterior and posterior ends of the body. The miracidium which swims actively in the water is somewhat spoonlike with a broad front and tapered posterior end. Its shape is quite variable. For that reason, the determination of size is rather difficult, but it is about 0.1 mm in length and about 0.04 mm in width; within the egg shell it has a diameter of 0.06–0.03 mm.

From what has been said, it is apparent that the invasive form of *S. japonicum* is much smaller than the miracidium. It has much shorter cilia; distinct parenchymal organization; a thicker, at times doubly contoured body wall; stronger power of resistance against drying of the parenchyma and the body wall; peculiar aggregates of pigment; the rudimentary oral sucker is present, and there are indications of the ventral sucker. The results of all infection experiments with miracidia-containing water were negative.

From these facts I now want to conclude that the invasive form is not identical with the miracidium originating from eggs but is the product of an alteration of the miracidium in an intermediate host.

Summary

(1) Using three different examination methods of the peripheral venous blood of animals infected by immersion in brook water, I observed the youngest worms of the schistosomes at the time of the skin penetration.

(2) The so-called "invasive" form is longitudinally oval, somewhat flattened; it measures 0.040 mm in length and 0.015 to 0.02 mm in width and is provided with various primitive organs: a thinner, doubly contoured body wall with short cilia, a rudimentary buccal cavity, beginnings of the oral sucker and indications of the ventral sucker, a primitive intestine with peculiar, light brown pigment granules, and without sexual, muscular, or nerve tissues.

(3) The oral sucker seems to develop much earlier than the ventral one. From here, a cell cord develops which unites with the intestine to form the esophagus. The only indication of the ventral sucker is found as a tiny projection on the anterior third of the body.

(4) The primitive intestine is shaped like a horseshoe, closed anteriorly and open posteriorly in the anterior half of the body. Along this intestine

one sees peculiar light brown pigment aggregates which are perhaps identical to the pigment in the intestine of the adult, only somewhat fainter.

(5) I could distinguish the youngest worms seen in the peripheral blood from those in the portal blood; the latter, in part, looked much older or were almost fully grown.

(6) I found the same worms in the skin of experimental animals. The youngest worms penetrate, in part directly through the healthy skin and in part by way of the hair follicles, reaching subcutaneous tissue spaces and blood capillaries immediately. From there, they are carried through the larger veins to the heart, get into the main circulation, and finally enter the portal vein system. Whether they are carried also through the lymphatic system has not been determined definitely, but I consider it a possibility.

(7) On comparing the youngest described worms with the miracidia originating from eggs, I found a considerable difference. I assume, therefore, that *S. japonicum* very probably has an intermediate host.

ON THE MIGRATION OF *SCHISTOSOMA JAPONICUM* VIA THE LYMPHATIC SYSTEM OF THE HOST

Ueber den wanderungsweg des Schistosomum japonicum durch vermittlung des lymphgefässystems des wirtes. Centralblatt für Bakteriologie, Parasitenkunde und Infektionskrankheiten, 68: 204–206, 1914. Translated from the German.

Yoneji Miyagawa
(1885–1959)

Miyagawa's biography will be found with the preceding article in this section.

In my earlier work, "On the Route of Migration of the *Schistosoma japonicum* from the Skin to the Portal System . . . " I explained that the point of entry of *S. japonicum* is the skin of man and animals and that the migration proceeds via the venous bloodstream, right heart, lung, left heart, systemic circulation to the portal vein system. It is also clear to me from the position of the youngest worms in the skin that they penetrate actively through healthy skin and, like the *Ancylostoma* larvae, by way of the hair follicles to reach the lymph spaces or the blood capillaries in the subcutaneous tissue in order to proceed to the usual, much deeper, seat of habitation. In this study I found, in numerous lymph node sections from the infected animals, some younger worms immediately after skin penetration, but could not draw a definite conclusion about these findings. Thus I questioned the possibility that the youngest worms in the lymph spaces of the subcutaneous tissue could penetrate more deeply and reach the right heart via the lymphatic system. In order to answer this difficult question, I used numerous sections of the lymph nodes, especially the inguinal lymph nodes, of the experimental animal, but unfortunately with negative results. Nevertheless, it seemed very probable to me that the worms penetrate more deeply via the lymphatics: some remaining in the node, but the rest passing to the thoracic duct and the right heart. In the spring of 1912, I went again to Yamanashi, in order to solve this mysterious question.

The Method of Examination

For 5–6 hours daily for about seven days at various times during May and June, I immersed countless experimental animals, especially dogs, in the brook waters of Yamanashi, Nakakomagori, Ikedamura, and other provinces where the epidemic was particularly severe. At intervals of 1–2 hours after removing the animals from the water, I examined their lymphatic systems according to the following methods:

(1) The youngest schistosomes must enter, in part, through the lymph spaces of subcutaneous tissue, into the blood vessels, while others wander into the lymphatic system. In the lymphatic system some must remain in the lymph nodes and others pass through. At a certain time after that, they must gather in the thoracic duct in order to pass into the blood vessels. So that I might examine microscopically lymph containing the worms, I performed the following operation: Within the innominate vein at the left supraclavicular fossa, where the subclavicular vein and the jugular vein jointly enter the innominate vein, I sought the thoracic duct and removed blocked lymph by needle puncturing, after tying the blood vessel temporarily. Unfortunately, because of the difficulty of the operation, the venous blood kept mixing with the lymph, thus hindering my microscopic investigation. For that reason, I had to use

another procedure. I quickly opened the thoracic cavity of the dog and tied off the thoracic duct next to the aorta. For a short time the heart still beat strongly and, because of the blockage, the lymphatic ducts became more and more prominent. The lymph was removed from the swollen thoracic duct by needle puncture and placed in a thick layer on a slide and, after staining it with methylene blue, Giemsa solution, or picro-carmine solution, I found some of the youngest worms in numerous preparations.

(2) I fixed the lymph nodes, especially the inguinal lymph node of the experimental animal in 8 per cent formaldehyde, cut them into sections after placing them in colloidin, and stained them with hematoxylin-eosin or borax carmine for microscopic study. In numerous preparations I was able to find some worms in the hilus of the lymph node.

The Size and Body Structure of the Youngest Worms of Schistosoma Japonicum

The length of the youngest worms discovered in the lymph node averaged 0.040 mm, the width varied between 0.016 and 0.020 mm. The diameters of the diagonally cut worm ranged from 0.012 mm to 0.016 mm. The length of those discovered in the lymph of the thoracic duct varied between 0.035 and 0.052 mm, the width between 0.013 and 0.016 mm. (The size of the youngest parasites discovered in 1911 in the peripheral venous blood or in the main tissue was 0.040 mm in length and from 0.015–0.022 mm in width; thus, they were as big as those in the lymph system.) The shape was elliptical rather than round. The organism was widest anteriorly; the head was more rounded and the tail more pointed than in the 1911 study.

The double-contoured body wall consisted of a cuticulalike membrane and contained very short cilia.

Under the cuticular wall there was a series of very small cells. The body parenchyma was fine and netlike, with small, deeply stained cell nuclei. Distributed among the meshwork one saw very tiny granules deeply stained with hematoxylin or methylene blue. The worm discovered in the lymph node contained a rather clear indication of the oral sucker: behind it extended numerous small cell nuclei which, although initially in one row, soon bifurcated into two cords extend-

ing just beyond the middle of the mouth. Next to these cell cords were found the strangely stained pigment aggregates which I discussed in my 1911 publication. In the invasive form, the beginning of the oral sucker was seen only in outline. Like those mentioned above, the worms discovered in the lymph nodes or in the lymph have exactly the same size and structure as those found in the skin and in the peripheral venous blood.

Finally, I wish to remark here that, despite careful work and numerous preparations, I could find only very few worms in the lymphatic system. For that reason I suggest that the actual migratory route of S. japonicum from skin to portal vein system is probably not the lymphatic but rather the circulatory system.

THE INTERMEDIATE HOST OF SCHISTOSOMA JAPONICUM KATSURADA

Der zwischenwirt des Schistosomum japonicum Katsurada. Mitteilungen der Medizinischen. Fakultät Kaiserlichen Universität Kyushu, 1: 187–197, 1914. Selections from pp. 187, 189–197. Translated from the German.

Keinosuke Miyairi (1865–1949)

Miyairi, the son of a samurai, was born in Nagano Ken. He graduated in 1890 from the College of Medicine of the Tokyo Imperial University. He worked for a while in public health and then was sent by the government to Germany from 1902 to 1904. Upon returning to Japan, he was appointed professor of Hygiene at the Fukuoka College of Medicine of the Kyoto Imperial University. When the faculty was reorganized in 1919, he continued in the same capacity. In 1913, Miyairi had discovered that Oncomelania nosophora *is an intermediate host for* S. japonicum.

Masatsugu Suzuki (1884– ?)

Dr. Suzuki was Miyairi's assistant and co-author (on the following article). He graduated from Kyoto Imperial College of Medicine in 1911.

This paper completes the life cycle of S. japonicum *from ova through the development of the miracidia in the snail intermediate host.*

Today it is certain that the intermediate host of *Schistosoma japonicum* Katsurada is a small water snail. The entire life cycle of this strange animal has been pursued from the penetration of the miracidium into the water snail to maturity of the cercariae; infection experiments with mature cercariae penetrating the skin of the final host have been easily carried out and the results are beyond question. . . .

Experimental Infection of the Water Snail with Miracidia

Our investigative material was, almost exclusively, cow dung. We began our study with the question: What occurs in the endemic areas to animal and human excrement which are deposited in the open air? Therefore, we assiduously gathered excrement that was lying around and examined it microscopically. In this way we encountered a small, schistosoma-infected ox of a poor farm family which lived in complete isolation on the lonely dam of Chikugogawa. This little ox became the steady supplier of our investigative material.

A small amount of cow dung was mixed on a glass slide with a little well water and covered with a cover glass; after this, the preparation was ready to be examined microscopically for the eggs of the worm.

As a rule it took five to ten minutes until we encountered the first egg, and usually (May-June) the miracidium was more or less in motion (Plate 89, Figs. 1 and 2). The movement consisted primarily of a slight contraction of the animal's body; this occurred mostly near the head, although at times it was further back, and ran wavelike along the body.

Occasionally, one saw a jerky contraction of the whole body. The animal made quick, swinging motions with its anterior end. Even when the animal was motionless, there was a sign of life. The flame cells flickered constantly; there were two pairs of these, the rear one always attracting attention first.

The liveliness of this flickering movement clearly indicated an area of rapid metabolism. Also, with careful watching, one gradually noticed the germ cell masses as seen in *Schistosoma haematobium* by Looss. It was the recognition of the germ cell masses that repeatedly strengthened our conviction regarding the presence of an intermediate host.

The anterior pair of flame cells was located behind the poison [penetration] glands, somewhat toward the periphery. There was a particu-

larly lively movement when the hatching of the animal was imminent; this strengthened our belief that the animal would escape soon.

The hatching was begun by diffusion of the water, as Looss correctly recognized. One can easily be convinced of this by adding a drop of dilute neutral red solution at the edge of the slide, and in a few minutes the miracidium in the shell is colored slightly red.

After penetration of the water, the egg swells progressively and finally the shell bursts, always lengthwise. Usually the restless inhabitant spun around in the swollen egg, still remaining inside of the covering membrane; to free itself from this requires several seconds.

Once free, the miracidium swims away quickly; its body stretches and changes into a long cylinder (Plate 89, Fig. 3). The restless motion is literally as Leuckart described it to be in *Fasciola hepatica*.

The miracidium searches eagerly for its intermediate host. If it does not reach it within ten hours, not enough strength remains for the miracidium to penetrate the skin of the water snail.

We, therefore, arrange our infection experiments in such a way that the miracidia at birth are quickly able to attack their intermediate host. In order to remove food particles we stir the egg-containing feces in a sieve by moving it up and down on the water in a large glass sedimentation funnel.

In about ten minutes all eggs sink, together with the heavy particles. Thereupon the dirty supernatant is removed and clear water is added. Two minutes later the water which is clearing is taken off; three or four washings suffice.

Washed in this way, the residue with a little water is transferred to a large basin with hundreds of freshwater snails. Within one and one-half to two hours all snails are infected. However, it is advisable during this interval to look at the basin occasionally because most of the snails attempt to escape from the water as quickly as possible by crawling up the walls of the basin. They must be pushed back repeatedly.

In order to witness this ciliated animal migrating into the body of the water snail, one must remove some water from the basin and spoon it into a small, flat dish, about an hour after the washing was terminated. Under the magnifying

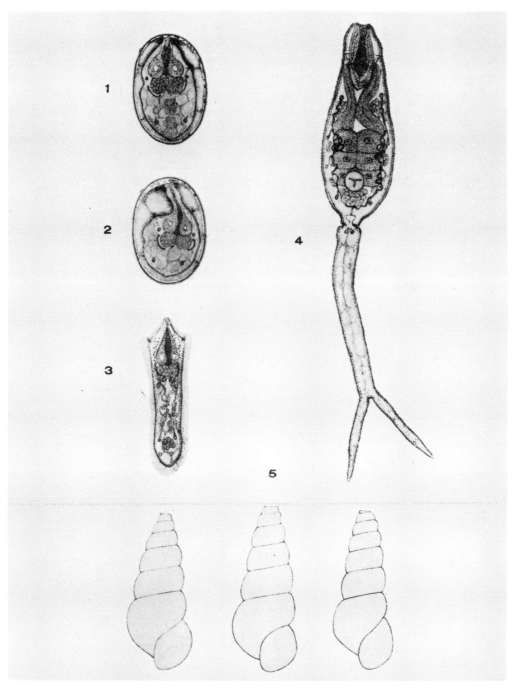

Plate 89. Fig. 1. Egg, miracidium at rest. *Fig. 2.* Egg, miracidium shortly before emerging. *Fig. 3.* Miracidium free. *Fig. 4.* Cercaria, not completely mature. *Fig. 5.* Shells of three kinds of water snails.

glass (about 10×) one will see little, whitish, ciliated animals swarming back and forth. Now, place a snail in the water and watch!

The observing eye does not need to wait long. Soon the miracidia are attracted to the snail. With the aid of the long extended head proboscis, the young worms attach themselves everywhere to the free body surface of the snails which, as a result of these attacks, become noticeably restless; they come out of their shells and move hastily, as if they wished to escape from the attacking parasites. But in vain. Already after a few minutes, feeler, head, foot, and shell edge are covered with embryos, as Leuckart describes it with *F. hepatica*. The picture cannot be drawn any better even in our case.

The actual penetration of the animal into the body of the snail can be watched only under the microscope. For this purpose we crush a water snail carefully between two slides in some water. The shell fragments are removed with a needle, and the whole specimen is covered with a cover glass. This naturally intimidates the miracidia. They drop off the snail and swim away. Shortly thereafter, they return eagerly and begin their work anew.

First, the animal makes its head sucker as thin as possible, pushes it between the snail's epidermal cells, and stretches its cylindrical body as long as possible. With a jerk it pulls itself together so that the base of the inserted proboscis cone and the epidermal slit becomes wider. Repeated efforts, alternate stretching and contraction of the body, push the cone further and further inside; after half of the body has passed inside, there is little further difficulty.

Once inside the tissue of the host, the animal still makes use of its ciliated covering. Its body is very soft and pliant. It stretches out completely in the tissue and seems to test whether any obstacle is in the way or whether it can proceed easily. Eventually it retracts and turns about. The animal is looking for a suitable place to settle peacefully for the formation of sporocysts. Such places are: the bottom of the buccal cavity, that is next to the cartilagenous plates, the coverings of the brain and foot ganglia, and the gills.

We have not been able to discover how the ciliary cover is lost. The animal stops and contracts, and the ciliary movement becomes less distinct, until finally the long-stretched-out worm transforms into a small oviform structure (about 0.05 mm long and 0.04 mm wide). The flickering of the posterior pair of flame cells remains unchanged or becomes even more lively. Shrunken glands can also be recognized by their color.

Development of the Sporocyst, Redia, and Cercaria

We now watch daily to see what becomes of this oviform structure, the developing sporocyst, and we welcome the fragility of the water snail which makes it especially favorable for examination.

We remove an infected snail from the aquarium with forceps and crush it gently between two glass slides. The crushed snail is again grasped with the forceps and is moved gently back and forth in water. All shell fragments usually drop off and what remains attached is the central shell core into which the shell muscle is inserted. The integument always remains attached, but then it does not need to be detached. However, the central shell core must be torn off; otherwise, the snail cannot be flattened evenly under the cover glass.

Thus prepared, the whole body of the snail can be examined easily and not a single sporocyst, no matter how small it may be, is overlooked.

In the beginning, the sporocyst enlarges slowly and the changes which occur at that time are difficult to explain. The appearance of fine granules is noticed initially. They are scattered over the entire organism, occasionally forming aggregates.

Gradually, the cytoplasm clears and the content of the sporocyst can be recognized as consisting of large, pale cells which, at the time, all seem to be similar in appearance. Four flame cells move vigorously.

As the sporocyst grows, the cells multiply, and the appearance of the various cells changes. Adjacent to the large cells with vesicular nuclei, numerous small ones are seen, divided into groups whose nuclear substance is generally rather compact. The groups of these small cells at first form round balls; in time they become longer and finally develop into rediae. We have counted over 50 such almost-mature rediae of the same age in a sporocyst. We saw the first free rediae on the 12th day after infection (at the beginning of August).

The redia is a strange animal which, in one movement, can stretch out and then again contract into an oval form. It is usually found in this tightly contracted state directly after preparation and shows many transverse folds and swellings. After it has recovered from this insult, it begins gradually to stretch out again. Its head is thickly covered with fine spines. The mouth is often wide open, as though the animal intended to bite something. Very little can be seen of the digestive tract. The entire abdominal content consists of rather large, pale cells which, in the course of time, divide to form large and small cell aggregates.

The rediae penetrate deep into the snail liver where they grow lengthwise. The exceptionally large, tortuous redia tube contains many cells of various sizes. The initially round cell group becomes elliptical and then, at one end, a budlike extension appears, the beginning of the caudal fin. At this time, six large gland cells appear in the middle of the posterior half of the body. The mouth apparatus and ventral sucker are also on the verge of developing.

We have seen almost mature cercariae (Plate 89, Fig. 4) only after seven weeks. It seems to us that development under natural conditions may progress even more quickly. The water snails normally feed on microorganisms which we are not able to get in sufficient quantity for them. Young snails (free of parasites at this time) thus are retarded in their growth in our aquarium. It is obvious that adults fare no better. However, we are surprised that, in spite of everything, the water snail is able to survive. Otherwise, we would not have been able to observe, even if only inadequately, the whole course of development.

Description of the Cercaria

The body of the mature cercaria is considerably more difficult to study than that of the less mature one; first because of the constant motion, especially the alternate stretching and contracting which the animal exhibits during its life; then, because of its poor affinity for stain in the fixed preparation, meaning the cercariae fixed in the redia tubes *in toto* (smear preparation).

A cercaria is provided with a powerful caudal tail and this is split, in its distal third, into two parts. The body and the caudal tail are thickly covered with spines. The oral pore is considerably larger than the ventral sucker. Almost the entire abdominal cavity is taken up by three pairs of very large glands so that the crowded genital cells have very little space left behind the ventral sucker.

Initially, the gland cells are round, but finally elongate and are found in threes on either side in the posterior half of the body. The ducts are very long and are not of equal width in all places; three equilateral ones are tightly attached to one another and run, irregularly anteriorly, ending at the outermost edge of the oral pore. Corresponding to these openings, four small spines can be seen on each side.

As far as the digestive tract is concerned, there is a rather spacious blind sac on the bottom of the oral pore. In the beginning, this is filled with numerous cells whose cellular organization gradually disappears with the formation of the tail and becomes a finely granulated mass. During movement of the oral pore, this mass is pushed forward and back again and stains intensively with acid stains.

Five pairs of flame cells are active. First the tail pair, close to the insertion of the tail; next to it the genital cell pair, the largest of all; then somewhat further anteriorly two gland pairs, next to the gland cell conglomerates close to the abdominal wall; and finally the anterior pair next to the nerve cell ganglion.

During the summer, most naturally infected snails contain all of the developmental stages simultaneously while some harbor nothing but mature cercariae. At the end of fall the latter are found only rarely. Those cercariae which are mature at this time seem to hibernate in the body of the host. In any case, in the middle of winter all stages are found simultaneously; namely, the small and large cell aggregates, the immature and the developing, and the completely mature cercariae together in one redia tube. Young rediae are not seen in winter. Formation in the redia itself, as is the rule in *F. hepatica* according to Leuckart, is not found here. The changes that occur in the snail body at the beginning of summer when irrigation ditches again start to carry water will have to be studied later. We only recognized this snail as the intermediate host of *Schistosoma* at the end of August last year.

Infection Experiments with Cercariae on Mice

We had not been successful in infection with cercariae from the laboratory. Since then we identified the morphology of *Schistosoma* redia and cercaria, and we began to use the naturally infected snails.

If we randomly gather 100 water snails (Plate 89, Fig. 5), we can count almost certainly on finding three or four infected specimens among them.

Experiment I. We place mice (not more than three animals; otherwise, they drown easily even in very shallow water) in a large basin, for one-half to two hours, with more than 100 water snails and a little water. The mice always become infected.

Experiment II. When we crush the water snails carefully, and examine them under the microscope to find the infected ones, then two infected snails suffice to infect the mice in an even shorter time, and more heavily than in Experiment I.

Experiment III. The shell is removed from an infected water snail and, with a drop of water, is placed on the skin of the mouse for about 30 minutes. The infection in most cases turns out to be so severe that the mouse sometimes cannot survive to allow maturation (around three weeks) of the very numerous intruders.

CHAPTER **27**

Clonorchiasis

ANATOMY AND PATHOLOGICAL RELATIONS
OF A NEW SPECIES OF LIVER FLUKE

Lancet, 2: 271–274, 1875. Selections from pp. 271–273.

James Frederick Parry McConnell
(1848–1896)

*Although McConnell was born in Agra, India, and
died in Calcutta, he received his medical training at
Aberdeen University and St. George's Hospital in
Scotland. After receiving his medical degree in 1869,
he joined the Indian Medical Service in Bengal, rising
to the rank of surgeon-lieutenant-colonel. He was
closely connected with the Calcutta Medical College,
serving as professor of pathology and resident physician at that institution and as compiler of the College
Museum catalog.*

    This is the first complete description of the adult
Clonorchis sinensis. *It should be noted that the patient
was outside the endemic area.*

On the 9th of September, 1874, I made a
post-mortem examination of the body of a
Chinaman, and found in the liver, obstructing the
bile-ducts, a large number of "flukes." A careful
examination of these, and comparison with other
known distomata, have convinced me that they
not only differ from the ordinary liver-fluke
(*Dist. hepaticum*), but constitute an entirely new
species. I desire therefore to describe the salient
anatomical characters of these flukes, then to
give a brief account of the post-mortem examination alluded to, and lastly to make a few remarks
upon the case.

The woodcuts which accompany this paper
will facilitate the description. Fig. 1 (Plate 90)
represents a few of these flukes drawn to natural
size. Fig. 2 (Plate 90) is one specimen enlarged to

about six times the natural size, showing the ventral surface. Fig. 3 represents the ova magnified. . . .

The individual from whose liver these flukes
were obtained was a Chinaman, aged 20, a car-
penter. He was brought into the Medical College
Hospital at midnight on September 8th, 1874, in
an insensible, moribund condition. The only history that could be obtained from the "friend"
who accompanied him was, that the patient had
been suffering from "fever" of a continued type
for about a fortnight. The insensibility was profound; the pupils were normal; the conjunctivae
looked pale. There was considerable dyspnoea; a
hard, tense, distended, and slightly tympanitic
condition of the abdomen; a hot skin, and an
almost imperceptible radial pulse. He never ral-
lied, but died, in much the same state, two hours
and a half after admission.

A post-mortem examination was made the next
morning, five hours and a half after death, a brief
summary of which is as follows:—Body fairly
nourished; pupils dilated; conjunctivae jaundiced;
rigor mortis strong in the lower limbs. The dura
mater yellow-stained; vessels of pia mater
everywhere gorged with dark blood, slight serous
effusion also into its meshes; cerebral substance
moderately firm; puncta large and bleed freely;
grey matter of both cerebrum and cerebellum particularly dark—a deep leaden hue, such as is met
with in many of the severe remittents of this
country. The large pulmonary vessels at the roots
of the lungs contained much fluid dark blood, but
the lung-substance everywhere else was rather
pale and anaemic—structurally healthy. One
ounce of deeply yellow-tinged serum was found

in the pericardial cavity; a few dark clots and fluid blood in the right chambers of the heart; the left were almost empty. The peritoneum was healthy, and no effusion was found into the abdominal cavity. The liver was large, swollen, and tense; superficially of a dark-purple colour, on section paler, more dingy or muddy-looking. Its parenchyma everywhere very soft. The large portal and hepatic veins were filled with fluid blood, and the bile-ducts particularly distinct from their large size, and distension with thick yellow bile. On incising the liver in different directions it was noticed that small, dark, vermicular-looking bodies escaped on to the table, and on more careful examination these were clearly seen to protrude from the bile-ducts, which, on being dissected, were found more or less obstructed by and containing them in large numbers, some lying free, others coiled up, and either solitary or in groups of twos or threes within the biliary ducts; all were dead. The gall-bladder was full; the cystic and cholodic ducts were patent. The bile in the bladder was of a very deep yellow (orange) colour, thick, and measured about an ounce and a half. No distomata were found in the gallbladder, nor were any ova discovered on microscopical examination of the bile and lining membrane of this sac. Numerous ova and shreds of epithelium were found in the biliary canals. (The weight of the liver after incision was 54½ oz.) Portions of this organ were hardened, thin sections made, and examined microscopically. A most remarkable and intense pigmentation of the parenchyma was observed—not mere staining, but a positive infiltration of black pigment, granular in character, and not confined or specially distributed in the interlobular tissue, but occupying the hepatic cells also within the lobules; the greater portion being disposed in the form of minute, very dark, granular depôts, from which smaller molecules radiated in all directions as from a centre. The pigment matter appeared to be biliary rather than haematoid. Many of the hepatic cells were also infiltrated with fat, and the nucleus in the majority was ill-defined or altogether indistinguishable. The spleen was found enlarged; its capsule stretched, slightly thickened, and opaque; its substance very dark and pulpy; weight 13¾ oz. The kidneys were moderately hyperaemic and dark. The small intestines were found deeply bile-stained; the large,

natural. The faecal contents of both—partly solid and partly liquid—were bile-coloured, but no distomata were found in them, although carefully washed and examined.

Remarks—The morbid anatomy of the liver in this case seems unequivocally to point to the presence of the flukes in its biliary ducts as the exciting cause of the acute and extensive structural degeneration of the proper structure of the organ, and of that cholaemic condition induced by the obstruction of the biliary channels which appears to have been the immediate cause of death. It is noticeable that the gall-bladder itself contained no distomata, nor exhibited any evidences of having been occupied by them, while the bile-ducts were found densely crowded. I must have collected at least thirty specimens in my dissections, and numbers doubtless still remain in those portions of the liver which I have preserved entire, for hardly any duct of medium size has not been found to contain two, three, or more of these parasites.

The discovery of this distoma may perhaps throw some light upon the pathology of those obscure liver enlargements and jaundices which every now and then, in this country at any rate, are presented to the practitioner; and although I never met with an analogous case, yet I can recall to memory a few instances during the past three years, of Chinamen especially, many of whom are settled in this city, who have applied to me in the medical out-patient department of this hospital for the treatment of obscure, hard, massive enlargements of the liver, with or without jaundice, and in whom I am now naturally inclined to suppose that a similar cause for the disease might have existed.

The Chinese as well as the Burmese are well known to be "filthy feeders," delighting in putrid messes of half-raw fish, &c.; they are bound by no caste prejudices (as the natives of India are) to abstain from any kind of "flesh, fish, or fowl"; they partake, moreover, of all kinds of "vegetable food." The sources from whence the larvae of such parasites may be derived are therefore not far to be sought. In the present instance, I regret to say, I have been unable to gain any information as to the antecedent history and habits of the deceased. The "friend" who brought him to the hospital never reappeared, and the body after death was "unclaimed." . . .

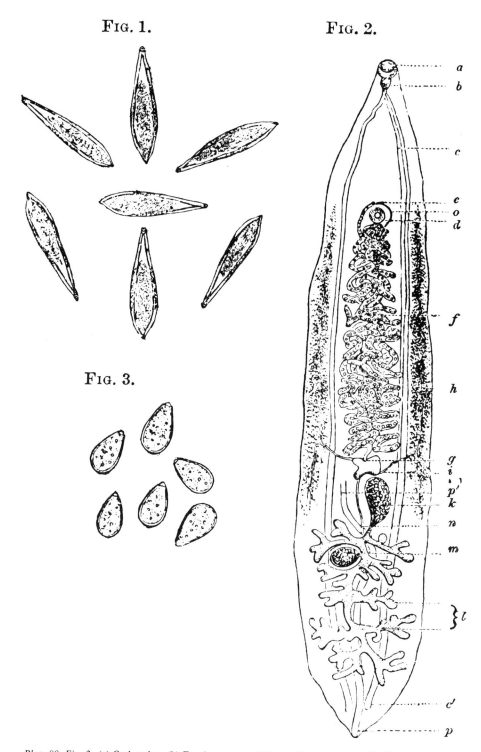

FIG. 1.

FIG. 2.

FIG. 3.

a
b
c
e
o
d
f
h
g
i
p'
k
n
m
l
c'
p

Plate 90. Fig. 2. (a) Oral sucker; (b) Esophagus; (c, c1) Right alimentary canal; (d) Ventral sucker; (e) Genital orifice; (f) Uterine folds; (g) Ovary; (h) Vitelligene gland (right); (i) Vitelligene duct (right); (k) Right testicle; (l) Receptaculum seminis (?); (m) Left testicle; (n) Vas deferens; (o) Termination of vas deferens; (p) Pulsatile vesicle; (p1) Water-vascular canal. Figures 1 and 3 are explained in text.

NOTES ON *DISTOMA ENDEMICUM*, BAELZ

Journal of the College of Science, Imperial University
(Japan), 1: 47–59, 1887.

Isao Ijima
(1861–1921)

*Born in Hamamatsu, Shizouka prefecture, Ijima
graduated from Tokyo University's Zoology Department in 1882. He proceeded to Germany for postgraduate study, returned to become professor of zoology at his alma mater, and was granted the Sc.D. in
1891. In addition to his university activities, he was
director of the Marine Experimental Station at Misaki,
Kanagawa prefecture.*

*Ijima is considered to be the father of Japanese
parasitology. His contributions to ornithology and to
our knowledge of porifers (sponges) are extensive. An
Outline of Zoology published in 1918 culminated his
work.*

The miracidium in the ova of Clonorchis sinensis
was first described by Ijima in this paper.

Since 1883 it has been known that in certain
districts of Okayama-Ken a species of Distoma
often infests the liver of the natives, causing de-
plorable diseases or even deaths. The parasite has
been described in no less than two papers, but not
quite satisfactorily, a fact which induced me to
apply to the Science Department of Tokyo
Daigaku for permission to visit infected districts,
in order to obtain an exact knowledge of the parasite, preliminary to an attempt at the elucidation
of its life history. Experiments for attaining the
latter purpose are being carried on. As I have
however no expectation of bringing them soon to
a close, I wish to fulfill my duty in submitting the
following report to the authorities of the Imperial
University. I venture to believe that my notes will
put the characters of our Distoma in a clearer
light than heretofore and hope that they may be of
some service for future investigations by our
naturalists and physicians. . . .

I wish here to express my thanks to the medical
staff of Okayama hospital, especially to Messrs.
Yamagata and Matsuwo, for giving me every
facility in collecting information. The last named
gentleman kindly supplied me with a number of
Distomes from two sources. Those from human
liver could easily be identified as Dist. endemicum Baelz, while those from the liver of cat
showed slight differences inasmuch as they possessed very fine spines in the skin (=cuticula)
and were of smaller size than the former. Perhaps

this cat distome from Okayama is to be considered as a distinct species, but I firmly believe that
in Tokyo, Dist. endemicum does sometimes inhabit the liver of cats. During December of last
year I have had occasion to dissect three cats. In
one of them, I found the gallbladder and hepatic
ducts unusually enlarged. They were almost filled up with Distomes, which agreed in every respect with Distoma endemicum for Okayama. I
counted over 600 of them. In the second cat, the
gallbladder and hepatic ducts were of normal appearance and only a single specimen of Distoma
was found within. It is probable that some more
were left undiscovered. The third cat did not
seem to be at all infested.

It thus stands beyond doubt that Dist. endemicum infests not only the human liver but also
cats. This fact affords a great convenience in experimentally ascertaining its life history, since
the mode of infection must be the same in both
cases. Again, it is clear that conditions requisite
for the development of Distoma endemicum do
also exist in Tokyo, the cats examined having
been reared up in this city or in its environs. But
as yet no one has ascertained the occurrence of
our Distoma in the inhabitants of Tokyo. Notwithstanding, the possibility or even the probability of its occurrence is not to be denied. Perhaps it
may be that the parasitic worm owing to some
local circumstances, does not become introduced
into the human body in a number enough to cause
any calamitous influences, and thus passes unnoticed. Baelz also assumes the occurrence of
human liver distome elsewhere than in
Okayama-Ken, since he met with cases in Tokyo,
analogous to the Distoma disease of the above
mentioned Ken. Recently some cases of Distoma
disease have been reported from a certain district
in the neighborhood of Lake Biwa.

According to Kiyono and his colleagues there
are no less than 21 localities in Okayama-Ken
and one small village in Hiroshima-Ken where
the Distoma disease has been observed. I could
visit only a few of the infected villages in
Kojima-Gōri about seven hours' voyage on
steamer from Kōbe and about eight miles distant
from the town of Okayama. Amongst them a
small village by the name of Nakaune was
pointed out to me as the place suffering most
from the disease. On the authority of Dr.
Yamagata and of a local physician there are about
10% of inhabitants affected with the disease

(Baelz gives as much as 20%). The nature of the locality and its situation has been described by Kiyono etc. and also by Baelz. It is a strip of low land along the seashore, lying beneath the sea level during high tide. The sea water is kept out by means of a dam constructed some 60 years ago. The land is traversed by a broad ditch with sluggishly flowing water. The villages in which the Distoma disease occurs are all situated along this ditch. There is no well in the whole strip of land and drinking water is brought from the adjoining hills. The ditch water is drunk, according to the information I received, only in exceptional cases, if ever it is so taken. Its main use is for washing purposes. It is important to mention however that amongst other things kitchen utensils, vessels of all sorts, and vegetables to be eaten half-raw are always washed in the ditch. Moreover this ditch water is usually resorted to in watering vegetables growing on farms and also in irrigating rice fields which remain dry during uncultivated seasons.

It is a settled fact that the eggs of Distoma endemicum are discharged like those of other Distomes together with the feces of patients. In those villages as in other parts of Japan, human excrements are used for manuring purposes. I frequently observed farmers transporting manure in boats on the ditch and unrestrainedly cleaning their manure tubs in the water. Here are undoubtedly chances enough for millions of Distoma eggs to reach the ditch water, in which ciliated embryos would hatch out. Indeed it admits of hardly any doubt that the ditch water stands in intimate relation with the development of our parasite; and one can not be going too far in asserting that the establishment of a new system of water supply would ensure the annihilation of Distoma disease, so far as the above mentioned villages are concerned.

The question into what animal those ciliated embryos next find their way must remain unanswered for the present. After the analogy of those Distomes whose life history has been worked out, I naturally fixed my attention on molluscs. I found in abundance Limnaea japonica Jay, Melania libertina Gould, and a small species of Paludina. Less abundant were the large species of Paludina, and species of Planorbis, Cyclas, Corbicula, and Anodonta. Land snails were said to be exceedingly rare. Notwithstanding the spe-

cial search made, I failed to discern any trace of Sporocyst, Redia or Cercaria in any one of these molluscs. Dr. Kiyono informed me that some years ago he found Sporocysts or Redias, whichever they were, in almost all Melania of the same locality that he examined. Unfortunately I was unable to verify this fact myself. It is less probable, although the possibility should not be excluded, that the ciliated embryo should first enter into some other invertebrates. At any rate it requires no comment to assume that somehow broods of Cercaria would finally be formed. As to the way in which these Cercariae become introduced into the human body, one might think of four alternatives. Firstly, they may enter it together with water that is drunk. Baelz does not hesitate to assume this as *the* way of infection; but I am inclined to put some doubt on this point, for the ditch water, as I have already said, does not form the usual drink of the natives. A number of patients whom I saw assured me of never having drunk the ditch water. I do not mean however to exclude all chances of infection directly from the water. Secondly, they may be taken in together with the host in which the Cercariae have developed. In this case the Distoma would have but one intermediate host. In this connection I should mention that Paludina and Corbicula are eaten, but never in a raw condition. Oysters are abundantly cultivated in the neighborhood, but they are clearly above suspicion since most of them are sent to markets in Okayama where the Distoma disease is unknown. Thirdly, they may be eaten together with vegetables in an encysted condition after the manner of Distoma hepaticum. I did not observe any edible plants in the ditch, but the fact that the ditch water is often used for watering vegetable farms must not be forgotten. Fourthly, they may enter the human body together with the second intermediate host. In this respect shrimps and small miscellaneous fishes as well as molluscs fall under suspicion. Eels and Carassius vulgaris are sent to Okayama markets and are probably harmless. If the words of villagers are to be trusted, symptoms of the Distoma disease generally manifest themselves late in Summer or at the beginning of Autumn. This is suggestive of the fact that the immigration of young Distoma broods takes place about that time. In the case of sheep rot, it is known that symptoms appear in the interval from July to September in consequence of the immigration of young Dist. hepaticum, which attains maturity in 2–4 months. . . .

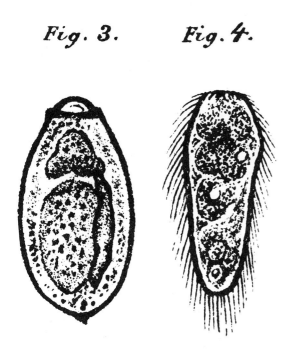

Plate 91. *Fig. 3*. An egg containing an embryo. *Fig. 4*. An embryo, examined in weak acetic acid.

It remains yet to say a few words about the eggs. They are unusually small, measuring 0.028–0.03 mm in length and 0.016–0.017 in breadth. In those eggs contained in the hind end of the uterus the shell is colorless and transparent. Each encloses an egg cell and a number of yolk cells, the nuclei of which can easily be demonstrated by coloring. In the anterior portion of the uterus, where the egg shells have assumed a dark brown or dark olive color, embryos are already formed. Such an egg is represented in Plate 91, Fig. 3. . . . In the interior three distinct bodies beside some yolk granules are seen. One of these bodies is a granular mass of triangular or irregular shape. Behind this body, away from the operculum, there is a second mass of larger size and clearer appearance. The third body lies mainly on the side of the second and has the form of a rod, slightly curved and often showing constrictions. This elongated body does not form a

part of the embryo; it is probably the remnant of yolk matter.

Embryos can be forced out of shells by a sharp tap on the coverglass. In Plate 91, Fig. 4, I have drawn an embryo as examined in weak acetic acid. It has an elongated oval shape, measuring 0.025 mm in length. The body slightly tapers toward the hind end. I believe I have seen an indication of head papilla. The delicate skin is covered all over by cilia, which are turned posteriorly. The anterior portion of the body is made up of a few large cells with granular contents. The hind portion contains small cells of clear appearance, probably germinal cells. These two groups of cells apparently correspond with the two granular bodies that we have seen within the egg shell. There are no eye spots.

Embryos artificially pressed out remain perfectly quiet. Only once I saw an embryo moving slowly by means of its cilia, after a preliminary pause.

Eggs from the gallbladder and intestine of a cat have been kept from December last until this day for over five months, but I observe no changes in them. Nor did the artificial warmth of an incubator enhance the hatching out of embryos.

THE INTERNAL ORGANS OF *CLONORCHIS SINENSIS* OVA AND THE MORPHOLOGY OF THE MIRACIDIUM

Tokyo Igakkai Zasshi, 12: 579–587, 1898. Selections from pp. 579, 581, 583–586. Translated from the Japanese.

Seiichiro Saito
(1873–1960)

Born in Akita prefecture, Saito graduated from the Okayama Medical College in 1898. He went to Germany in 1904, studied at Würzberg (internal medicine, pharmacology, physiology, and the like), and received his M.D. degree in 1905. After one year in Berlin, he returned to Japan. For many years he was a professor in the section of internal medicine at Okayama Medical College.

This is a more complete description of the miracidium of Clonorchis sinensis *than that given by Ijima.*

The writer is going to report the results of his research regarding the contents of the *Clonorchis sinensis* ova and the morphology of their miracidia, since it is believed that this report will contribute greatly to present knowledge regarding the growth of the distomal family and to the diagnosis of the distomal diseases.

Shells of the Ova

Although the reports on the external appearance of the ova by Drs. Leuckart and Otani are satisfactory, nonetheless, the shortcoming of Dr. Otani's report pertains to the following: instead of having said, "there was a tiny lid like the crystal of a wrist watch on the slender edge of the ovum," he should have explained more fully that "at the narrow edge, there was a tiny lid like a *jingasa*[1] and a small protuberance along the line of contact. This protuberance was formed by the adherence of the processes which projected outward along the edge of the shell lid and the mouth brim of the ova shell."

The Embryo's Growth within the Ova

As in Dr. Leuckart's theory, the growth of the ova begins in the uterus. The youngest ovum was found near the ovary, and the greater the distance from the ovary, the more mature the ova. According to the theories of Drs. Otani and others, it has been thought that no mature miracidium was found in the uterus; even those ova found in the stool have been deemed immature eggs. In fact, however, it is the mature miracidia that are observed in the ova in the uterus as one approaches the genital pore. In other words, those eggs, the contents of which researchers had reported as consisting of three elements, actually were the mature, transparent miracidia. The present writer could always obtain the mature miracidia by the following methods.

The youngest eggs: The ova were almost colorless; on the edge of the operculum (though often in the central part or on the other edge), there were large, homogeneous, transparent, glassy, foamy spots which had comparatively small granular nuclei. These were the cells of ovarian origin. In addition to these cells, there were variously sized fatty drops which were light-refractile; various sizes of irregular granules were scattered through the cytoplasm. The inside of the egg was generally less dense, yet there was no egg yolk similar to those found in the hepatic distomal (*Schistosoma japonicum*) eggs. The component which corresponds to the egg yolk (vitellaria), the nutritional source for the growth of the ova, seemed to be primarily thick liquid. The eggs in the uterus were examined separately by gradually removing them from the ovary. The examination revealed a cell which had a nucleus which was the largest one of the granules at the point of the previously mentioned foamy spots. The ova were either in the process of gradually splitting from that point or massing gradually to form the miracidia. . . .

The Observations on the Miracidia

To allow the miracidia to move out of the shell, it is necessary to choose the uterus section near the genital pore, examine it with considerable care, and remove extraneous particles. The individual eggs must then be arranged in a line under the microscope so that they will not overlap. The cover glass and the slide must adhere cleanly and evenly. After this, the eggs are placed under the immersion lens, and the ocular moved with the fine adjustment toward the mature eggs; then, the fine adjustment must be moved, giving a light pressure to the eggs. This process can completely express the miracidia from within the shells. If a thicker slide and cover glass are used, one can still observe the relationship between the miracidia's mode of exit from the ova and its contents; however, it is seen more clearly when the thinner slide is used.

However, since this method for expressing the miracidium is artificial, the pressure tends to be exceedingly strong, thus crushing all the miracidia and their contents which may be altered as they are expressed out of the shells. In any case, it is important to manipulate the fine adjustment dexterously up and down, in order easily to observe the contents.

Even though the time interval from the laying of the eggs to the escape of the mature miracidia from the ova is not yet known in detail, the mature eggs in the uterus can move out by themselves whenever the opportunity presents itself. The writer examined the adults microscopically the day after he removed eggs from the region of the genital pore; applying the foregoing method, he observed that the eggs taken from near the vagina had active miracidia. He observed them further and found that the motion of the miracidium pushed the operculum open; and then it pushed its head out of the shell in an effort to free itself from the shell. The miracidium looked just like a silkworm when it is trying to escape from the cocoon.

Having moved out of the shell, the movement of the miracidium's cilia became more active, and the miracidium quickly moved across the field of vision. The contents could be observed only when their movements were slowed. If this was the state of the new eggs in the uterus, so much more would it be in the case of the eggs in the stool. When one patiently watches the miracidium exit spontaneously from the shells using the foregoing method of expression, he will be likely to find it. Is this possibly because of proper light intensity to the area?

Morphology of the Miracidia at the Time of Exit

The miracidium was leaf-shaped. On its anterior edge, as Dr. Ijima has reported, there was a papillary process. This process was often not clearly observed in the hatched miracidium, but it was seen when the miracidium was about to get out of the shell. No light-sensitive organelles were seen, as other reporters have already stated. The miracidium could be divided into parietal section and somatic cavity. The former was colorless and transparent, and its width increased toward the posterior edge. The somatic cavity was located centrally and was somewhat dark. Anteriorly, a mass of granules could be seen from the outside of the shell. However, it was not clear whether this was a single mass or several small masses of granules. Furthermore, the existence of the nuclear granules inside the mass was not confirmed, although others have observed this at times. Perhaps this might have been what Dr. Ijima had reported with the expression, "a couple of granular-size cells." However, the writer does not quite agree with Dr. Ijima's opinion. Rather, he wonders if these were not the foamy, transparent bodies that were seen; he observed that they looked oval from the outside of the shell, and the granules which occupied the posterior portion of the body were found and existed greatly massed or scattered. Inside of the body, there often appeared a nucleus.

In the middle of the body on one side, there were rod-shaped or roundish triangular masses of granules which corresponded to the so-called rod [cephalic penetration glands—Eds.]. In the case of hatched miracidium, these masses did not always appear on the sides. Rather, they were often seen in piles together with the roundish granular body mentioned above. This was confirmed by high-power examination. In addition, five or six transparent, foamy bodies (Dr. Ijima's so-called germinative cells) were observed posteriorly, but the true number of them was far more than that. The rest of them might have been covered with the operculum. The cilia, most of which were long, coarse, and bent posteriorly, grew thickly on the surface of the parietal portion.

Conclusion

In the foregoing sections, the writer reported the results of his investigation on the growth changes of the contents of the *Clonorchis sinensis* ova, on the miracidia artificially expressed from the shell, on the method of expressing them, and on the spontaneously hatched miracidia. Particularly the writer has described the contents of the mature ova and has demonstrated that the rod, which had been deemed the residue of the egg yolk in the shell, actually is a component of the miracidia and is composed of tiny granules.

---

[1]A strong wooden headpiece or camp helmet used by premodern Japanese soldiers.

ON THE LIFE HISTORY AND MORPHOLOGY OF *CLONORCHIS SINENSIS*

Centralblatt für Bakteriologie, Parasitenkunde und Infectionkrankheiten, 75: 299–317, 1914. Selections from pp. 299–303, 307, 314–317.

Harujiro Kobayashi
(1884–1969)

A graduate of Kyoto Imperial University, he studied schistosomiasis japonicum *while at the Infectious Disease Research Institute at the University of Tokyo. Then he went to Korea in 1916, where besides observations on* Clonorchis sinensis, *he reported on malaria,* Paragonimus, *and* Trichostrongylus. *He published several texts of parasitology, including an authoritative text on parasites of Korea. Kobayashi's initial studies on* C. sinensis *were published from 1910 to 1912 in the Japanese literature.*

In addition to clarifying that C. sinensis *represented one species, the fish was demonstrated to be the intermediate host in this study.*

Introduction

Since the discovery of the liver Distome, *Clonorchis sinensis* (Cobb.), in Japan, several investigators, such as Baelz, Ijima, Leuckart, Inouye, Katsurada have made quite extensive studies regarding its morphological as well as pathognomical features. Their efforts to clear its life-history, however, have so far been futile. Engaging in the study of the liver distome for several years the author was rewarded with the discovery of the intermediate host of the parasite. The main result was published in the form of a short note in May of 1911. The present paper embodies detailed description of the results obtained. It may be admitted, that gaps still remain in the life-cycle of the liver distome that will be filled by future investigation.

Experiments on the Source of the Liver Distome

Two hypotheses have hitherto been proposed regarding the source of the liver distome in Japan: viz. (1) the water theory, and (2) the fish-mollusk-theory. The former ascribes the cause to unhealthy water due to insufficient drainage of the region, where liver distomiasis prevails endemically, e.g., Okayama prefecture, and is held mostly by medical authors, while the latter has been advocated by the natives of Miyagi prefecture.

While engaging in the study on the trematodes parasitic in the fresh water mollusks, fish and others, I was fortunate enough to find out not only many species of cercariae and young encysted distomes from numerous localities in Japan, but also the fact that the geographical distribution of one kind of young distomes encysted in the muscle of some fresh water fish coincide exactly with that of human distomiasis, and moreover that they strikingly resemble the liver distome in Japan. The flesh containing the young distomes was therefore, given to 30 cats, one dog, 20 rabbits, 40 guinea-pigs and 50 rats. In the case of cats and dogs especial precaution was taken to submit them to repeated examinations of their faeces to exclude the possibility of previous infection. Within several days in all these subjects employed in my experiments were found typical *Clonorchis sinensis*. I arrived, therefore, at the conclusion that the encysted distome is a young stage of the human liver distome.

Further study has revealed that following fishes are found to be infested with the young *Clonorchis sinensis*:

> *Pseudorasbora parva* (Schlegel)
> *Leucogobio güntheri* Ishikawa
> *L. mayedae* Jordan et Snyder
> *Sarcocheilichthys variegatus* (Schlegel)
> *Pseudoperilampus typus* Bleeker
> *Paracheilognathus rhombeum* (Schlegel)
> *Acheilognathus lanceolatum* (Schlegel)
> *A. limbatum* (Schlegel)
> *A. cyanostigma* Jordan et Fowler
> *Abbottina psegma* Jordan et Fowler
> *Biwia zezera* Ishikawa
> *Carassius auratus* (Linnaeus)

Pseudorasbora parva and *Leucogobio güntheri* are infested most numerously, especially so in the former. It is not seldom that the number of larvae found in a single specimen of *P. parva* may be several hundreds. In the liver of a cat, to which six *P. parva* were given, were found three thousands of distomes! In other kinds of fishes only a small number of the larvae is found. *Carassius auratus* has very seldom the larvae of liver distome.

Structure of the Larva encysting in the Fish

Distribution of cysts in the host—The encysted distomes are present abundantly both in the subcutaneous tissue and in the muscle of the host. They are more numerous in the superficial part than in the deeper. The myocommata have nothing to do with their distribution in the muscle. . . .

The cyst in fish can be found throughout the year, though the younger ones are met with most abundantly in the months of August, September and October.

Experiments on the tenacity of life of the larvae—As above mentioned, the wall of the cyst is not thick yet it resists against various external conditions. To test this I made some experiments on the cat and the rabbit trying Japanese method of eating fish one after another. It should be mentioned that the fish employed for the following experiments were examined beforehand microscopically and the presence of the parasites was ascertained.

Experiment I. Several of *Pseudoperilampus typus* and *Pseudorasbora parva* were roasted over live charcoal and were given to three cats. After 4, 10, and 78 days the cats were dissected but none had the parasites.

Experiment II. Six of *Pseudorasbora parva* after cooking in boiling water for 15 minutes, were given to two cats, that were dissected after 12 and 47 days. One cat had no distomes at all while the other had one.

Experiment III. Six *Pseudorasbora parva,* after boiling in the water of 100° C for 15 minutes were given to a cat and as many to a rabbit. Both were dissected after 80 days and no distomes were found in them.

Experiment IV. Two *Pseudorasbora parva* were cooked in the water of 70° C and 50° C for 15 minutes, and were given to two cats. They were dissected after 23 and 19 days respectively. A number of distomes were found in them.

The fishes which were employed in above four experiments, were roasted or boiled as a whole.

Experiment V. Three *Pseudorasbora parva,* that had been cut up into several pieces and soaked in vinegar for 15 minutes, were given to a cat. After an elapse of 17 days numerous distomes were found in the animal.

Experiment VI. In the muscular tissue of the fish soaked for 5 hours in vinegar larvae were alive and found moving.

Experiment VII. Three *Pseudorasbora parva* were cut up into pieces and were soaked in soya-sauce for 15 minutes, and were given to a cat. The result was the same as Experiment V.

Experiment VIII. The encysted larvae in the muscle of the fish soaked for 5 hours in soya-sauce did not move, but when the soya-sauce was replaced with tap water the larvae began to move even after 12 hours.

From these experiments it may be concluded that the larvae are killed by heat (100° C or approximately so), while they retain their vitality at lower temperature, at least 15 minutes and in vinegar and soya-sauce as long as 5 hours. It may be added that the larvae live at least for several days in the fish kept in the refrigerator. If the fish is kept at room temperature, they soon die as their host putrifies.

Development of the Young Distome in the Final Host

The route by which the parasite enters the host—In order to ascertain the route of entering of the parasite into the host, the cats were fed with the fish meat containing encysted distomes and were dissected at various intervals. Three hours after taking in of the cysts some of them were found to be empty in the half digested food mass. The liberated distomes were creeping about very actively with the aid of both suckers. In two cats dissected after 15 and 24 hours respectively free distomes were found both in the gall bladder and in the bile duct. It is quite natural to infer that after they reach this part they go into the hepatic duct and in it they cease to travel and grow.

The cyst remains for some time undissolved after the occupant is out. And it is very probable that the distome comes out bursting the wall of the cyst by its own exertion not through the action of the digestive fluids of the stomach or the intestine of the host. In this connection it is interesting, to note the following instance. The crushed meat of the fish containing the cysts was soaked in the water for several hours; many cysts were isolated from the muscle fibres and a day or two later all of the distomes were out of the cyst and found dead. . . .

Habitat—The hosts of the liver distome hitherto described are man, the dog, the cat and the pig. I succeeded in rearing the larvae into the adults in the rabbit, the guinea-pig and the rat. Probably because of its small size the development of the parasite is slower in the rat than in other hosts. Moreover in the animal only a small percentage of the larvae becomes adult, while the remaining ones retain their larval condition. The following instance seems to attest this statement. A rat which had been fed several times with the infested fish (*Pseudorasbora parva*) containing several hundreds of encysted larvae in the muscle and after some three months it was found that only six mature distomes were in its liver; they moreover were not fully developed, measuring 6–8 mm in length. Another rat dissected after two months from the feeding yielded some 60 small distomes from 4–4.5 mm in length; their uteri were filled in part with the eggs. In other animals used for experiments the distomes grew just as well, provided that approximately the same number of the parasites were in.

The usual seat of the distomes is the hepatic ducts, the gall bladder and the bile duct. When numerous parasites are found the larger part of them are in the fine hepatic ducts and only few in the gall bladder. In several instances the pancreas and the duodenum contained a few specimens which were apparently in good condition. . . .

The First Intermediate Host

Taking the life history of allied species into consideration, it is highly probable that the larvae of our distomes encysted in fish come from cercariae parasitic in some mollusks, the first intermediate host. I have made careful search after the cercariae and found several species of them in the districts where the liver distomiasis occurs endemically. But none of the cercariae has been identified with certainty as that of the liver distome. One kind of them which bears a close resemblance in its structure to the young encysted larvae of our *Clonorchis* is found in several species of *Melania,* especially *Melania livertina* Gould. The fact that *Melania* infested with the cercariae is very abundant in the rivers and swamps of those regions where liver distomiasis prevails endemically, makes us to think that this may be the first intermediate host. A more detailed description of this subject will be published after the completion of my experiments, which are now going on. . . .

Specific Identification of *Clonorchis*

When Baelz first discovered the liver distome in Japan, he distinguished two species; viz., *Distoma hepatis endemicum sive perniciosum* and *Distoma hepatis innocum.* Soon it was found that Baelz's distomes are identical with *Distoma sinense* Cobbold and Leuckart amalgamated Baelz's two species into one since he could not detect a specific difference between them. In 1907 Looss wrote a paper based upon the specimen kept in the museum of the School of the Tropical Medicine at Liverpool. He could recognize Baelz's two species among them and established a new genus *Clonorchis* for the two. These species have been accepted by other authors. Verdun and Bruyant, however, maintain that they are not good species at all but varieties. Are there any actual specific differences between Looss's two species, *Clonorchis sinensis* (Cobb.) and *Cl. endemicus* (Baelz)? Looss distinguished these two species from the following characteristics:

(1) *Clonorchis sinensis* is larger than *Cl. endemicus,* being 13–19 mm and 10–13 mm in length respectively.

(2) Ordinarily in the larger form the vitellaria are discontinuous, interrupted by several undeveloped portions, while the smaller has the continuous vitellaria.

(3) Larger ones commonly contain yellowish or blackish pigment in its parenchyma, while the smaller are free from it.

(4) In the larger form the egg narrows more distinctly anteriorly and its lid is higher and has a more sharply projected rim than the smaller.

In the first place as to the size of the liver distome Katsurada thinks that the size of the liver distome depends upon the size of the host and also on the number of parasites in one host. Regarding this Looss disagrees with Katsurada stating: "I have for several years paid special attention to this question, but all my experiences tend to show that every species of parasites has a size of its own . . . as a rule, their size is very much the same, whether they live in a large or in a small host." The reader is begged to refer to one of the preceding sections where I expressly mentioned that the size of a liver distome can vary according to the space and the nourishment available to each individual. So I shall not go into the argument here.

Secondly as to the interruption of the vitellaria and the pigmentation. The description of the following six specimens will be added here in order to show that there is no constancy on these points.

These clearly show that it is not difficult to find intermediate forms between Looss's two species. However, as he correctly observed, the larger forms generally contain pigment but have discontinuous vitellaria, while the smaller ones lack pigment but have continuous vitellaria. This may be due to the age, larger ones naturally being old, and partly senile forms as previously mentioned. If that is really so, the proposed specific differences lose their significance.

Thirdly and lastly as to the shape of the egg shell. I have noticed in many eggs just the reverse of what Looss mentions as specific: an egg from a specimen (length 10 mm) obtained from a cat had the shell considerably tapered at one end and provided with a more vaulted lid while another egg from a specimen (length 14 mm) obtained from a man had a shell less tapered anteriorly and a relatively flat lid. The cases like these have been obtained by myself too repeatedly to be taken for exceptional.

Taking all the above facts into consideration one cannot escape the conclusion that we have in Japan only one species *Clonorchis sinensis* (Cobbold) and not two.

Host	Length mm.	Breadth mm.	Vitellaria	Pigment
I. cat	18	3.5	continuous	no
II. man	11	2.7	continuous	abundant
III. man	9.5	3	1 interruption on one side	abundant
IV. man	11.5	2.5	2 interruptions on both sides	no
V. cat	14	2.5	1 interruption on one side	no
VI. cat	7.5	2	several interruptions on both sides	abundant

Summary

(1) Liver-distomiasis in Japan is caused by *Clonorchis sinensis* (Cobbold). The natives in the district where the disease is prevalent are infested with the parasites through eating fresh water cyprinoid fishes raw that are the intermediate hosts.

(2) Experimentally the following twelve species are ascertained to be the intermediate hosts of the distome:

> *Pseudorasbora parva* (Schlegel)
> *Leucogobio güntheri* Ishikawa
> *L. mayedae* Jordan et Snyder
> *Sarcocheilichthys variegatus* (Schlegel)
> *Pseudoperilampus typus* Bleeker
> *Paracheilognathus rhombeum* (Schlegel)
> *Acheilognathus lanceolatum* (Schlegel)
> *A. limbatum* (Schlegel)
> *A. cyanostigma* Jordan et Fowler
> *Abbottina psegma* Jordan et Fowler
> *Biwia zezera* (Ishikawa)
> *Carassius auratus* (Linn.).

(3) The encysted larva in the fish grows and reaches maturity in the cat, the dog, the rabbit, the guinea-pig and the rat.

(4) In the final host the cyst ruptures and the larva is set free.

(5) During the development in the final host, the spines of the ''cuticula'' enlarge and then disappear. The size relations of the oral and ventral suckers are reversed.

(6) The final shape and position of the testes and the ovary are attained in seven days and the egg formation begins in 12–15 days. The parasite matures in 23–26 days.

(7) Yellowish or brownish pigment of the adult is probably degenerated shell material contained in the yolk cells.

(8) Senile degeneration is found in larger specimens, in which the vitellaria are partly or wholly disappear, the pigment is present and the uterus is empty.

(9) The liver distome in Japan constitutes a single species *Clonorchis sinensis* (Cobbold).

ON THE PRIMARY INTERMEDIATE HOST OF *CLONORCHIS SINENSIS*

Chuo Igakkai Zasshi, 25, No. 3: 49–52, 1918. Translated from the Japanese.

Shochi Muto
(1886–1967)

A native of Yamanashi prefecture, Muto graduated from Aichi Prefectural College of Medicine (now Aichi University of Medicine) in 1913. He studied pathology in Kyoto in 1916 and eventually became professor of pathology at Aichi. He was awarded many national prizes for his contributions to parasitology.

The role of the snail (Bulimus) as the primary intermediate host was presented in this paper to complete the life cycle of Clonorchis sinensis.

Since last year, I have been doing research on the growth of *Clonorchis sinensis* [In Muto's original text he uses *Distoma hepaticum*—Eds.] and on the prevention of the disease caused by this parasite. I was fortunate to be able to identify the primary intermediate host of *C. sinensis*, and I reported this finding at the general session of the Eighth Japanese Pathological Association and at the Third Subcommittee of the Fifth Convention of the Japanese Medical Association held in April of this year.

After numerous studies on the primary intermediate host, I came to the conclusion that the river snail (*Thiara libertina*) mentioned by Mr. Kobayashi as the primary intermediate host of *C. sinensis* had been so established without solid grounds. However, as I reported previously, the *T. libertina* is, without any doubt, also the primary intermediate host of *Metagonimus yokogawai*.

With the above-mentioned fact in mind, I did further research. I happened to obtain a species of the snail from Lake Biwa, Koshu, and discovered in it the existence of three species of cercaria. I presumed one of the three species to be the cercaria of *C. sinensis*. The snail was identified as *Bulimus striatula* (var. japonica pilsbury) by Mr. Kawamura at Otsu Rinko Laboratory, the director of Kyoto Hirase Kaikan, and as *Bulimus striatula* japonica pilsbury by Mr. Iwakawa. It is called "mametanishi" in Japanese.

I. Experiment

I have successfully infected some fish (*Pseudorasbora parva*) with one species of cercaria from the snail; these fish were previously known to have been absolutely uninfected with any species of cercaria. In this regard, it should be noted that in most cases, no matter where they are from—rivers, lakes, or swamps—fish are the host to some kind of encysted larvae. This fact has been pointed out in my paper, "On the Primary Intermediate Host of *Metagonimus yokogawai*," published in the *Kyoto Medical Journal*, No. 1, vol. 14, January 1917. Therefore, it is a prerequisite that the fish used in my experiments be absolutely free of parasitism by various encysted larvae. This experiment of infecting the fish with cercariae was carried out in August of last year. By February, this year, I obtained positive results from my experiment of the *Pseudorasbora parva* on animals. The results are shown on the following chart. The control experiment shows no parasitism by *C. sinensis*.

The results of my experiment confirmed the presence of *C. sinensis* both in the two dogs and the two guinea pigs fed on *P. parva* which in my experiment, was host to the cercariae of the snail. In the dog fed on the *P. parva* raised symbiotically with the *T. libertina* as control, only

Metagonimus was found. (I conducted this kind of experiment more than ten times when I was investigating the primary intermediate host of *Metagonimus,* and I repeated the same experiment several times after that. In every experiment, only *Metagonimus* was present. This fact probably led me to the conviction that *T. libertina* is not the primary intermediate host of *C. sinensis*.) The two guinea pigs fed on the uninfected *P. parva* have shown no evidence of parasitism. Needless to say, prior to the experiment, special care was taken to see that the animal used was free of any kind of trematode.

Recently, I obtained the miracidium of *C. sinensis* and with it infected the snail. Upon examining the snail approximately three weeks later, the existence of a sporocyst was confirmed. This corroborated my conviction and the results of my experiment.

II. Summary of the Experiment

I collected a species of snail ("mametanishi") from Lake Biwa and discovered three species of cercaria in the shell. I succeeded in infecting uninfected *P. parva* with one of these species. After a certain period, I fed the *P. parva* to small dogs and guinea pigs and confirmed the existence in these animals of parasitism by *C. sinensis*. In this way, I proved that the primary intermediate host of *C. sinensis* is "mametanishi,"—*Bulimus striatula* var. japonica pilsbury.

III. Relationship between the Incidence of the Disease Caused by Clonorchis Sinensis and the Distribution of "Mametanishi"

The snail used in this experiment was from Lake Biwa. It was necessary, then, to relate the distribution of the snail and the incidence of the clonorchiasis in some other area. (The relationship between the two has a great bearing upon the validity of my experiment.) Therefore, last March I made field trips to Senoo-machi, Okayama prefecture, and to towns such as Fukudamura village, Kojomura village, and Fujidamura village in the vicinity of Senoo-machi.

The incidence of clonorchiasis is high in these areas. With the assistance of two gentlemen, in addition to Mr. Takejiro Ojima, who is devoted to the prevention of the disease in Fukudamura village, I searched for snails of the variety used in

Animal No. and Type, Date Exp. Begun	Materials for experiment (All fed thru mouth)	Result of feces examination	Days prior to feces examination	Results	
				Clonorchis sinensis	Metagonimus
1. Small dog 8 Feb.	Two *P. parva* have cercariae of *C. sinensis*	One or two eggs of *C. sinensis* on 18th day	21	Obtained approx. 500 worms	(−)
2. Small dog 8 Feb.	,,	A few *C. sinensis* eggs on the 20th day	40	Obtained a great number of worms	(−)
3. Small dog 8 Feb.	Three *P. parva* raised with the river snail, *T. libertina*	Found *Metagonimus* eggs on the 10th day	15	(−)	(+++)
4. Guinea pig 20 Feb.	One *P. parva* having cercaria of *C. sinensis*		15	(+++)	(−)
5. Guinea pig 20 Feb.	,,		15	(+++)	(−)
6. Guinea pig 20 Feb.	Two *P. parva* (control)		15	(−)	(−)
7. Guinea pig 20 Feb.	,,		15	(−)	(−)

Chart: results of animal experiments [Adapted—Eds.]

my privious experiment. The search resulted in the discovery of a large number of snails in the rivers and ditches of the area. I collected a number of snails, and upon examining them, found five species of cercaria. Three species were identical to those found in the shells from Lake Biwa, and one species was exactly the same as that of the *C. sinensis* in my experiment. Recently, I made a field trip to Sayamamura village along Shimo-Ogura Lake in the Kyoto prefecture and found the same snails. Upon examining them, I recognized the existence of cercaria. This recent field trip was made with deliberate purpose, for, as stated in my other treatise, it was clearly manifested by my experiment that several species of the fish from the area have the encysted larva of *C. sinensis*.

At the end of April this year, I made a field trip to Shimekiri Swamp and its vicinity in Yanaizu-machi, Motoyoshi-kori, Miyagi prefecture, which is widely known for the high incidence of clonorchiasis, and I discovered quite a number of snails identical to those used in my experiment. A few of the same snails were also found in the vicinity of Toyoma-machi, Toyoma-kori in the Miyagi prefecture. I have also heard that they are widely scattered in Korea and Taiwan. In Japan, however, the area of the snails' distribution to date is, according to Mr. Kawamura and Mr. Hirase, the Saga prefecture, Okayama prefecture, Osaka prefecture, Shiga prefecture, Chiba prefecture, Ibaragi prefecture, Kyoto City, and a few others. The incidence of the disease of *C. sinensis* is documented for these areas.

It is clear from the above description that there is a close relationship between the incidence of the disease caused by *C. sinensis* and the distribution of the snail called "mametanishi."

In conclusion, I would like to mention the relation between the drinking water and cercariae. Experiments were attempted to determine whether the cercariae grown in the primary intermediate host ("mametanishi") could undergo development in the final host, without entering the secondary intermediate host. This was an attempt to see whether, as certain scholars maintain, the secondary intermediate host is necessary only to maintain the mature cercaria in the primary intermediate host and, therefore, it has no significance in the developmental stages of cercariae. In other words, an experiment was designed to see what would happen to cercariae grown entirely in "mametanishi," when they entered, with water, into a mammal's stomach, which is the ultimate host of *C. sinensis*. For this purpose, I floated cercariae on the water and then made an animal (a domestic rabbit) drink it. However, I could not find parasitism of *C. sinensis* in the rabbit. I concede that this experiment is not complete yet, but on the basis of experiments done to date, it appears that cercariae, as in the case of *M. yokogawai,* cannot grow to the adult stage when they enter the body of a mammal directly, but must first achieve their complete growth in the fish for a certain period. A full report will be submitted upon completion of the experiment, for this question is of great importance in preventing the disease caused by *C. sinensis*. . . .

CHAPTER **28**

Fascioliasis

THE GOOD SHEPHERD

Le bon berger ou le vray régime et gouvernement des bergers et bergères: Composé par le rustique Jehan de Brie le bon berger (1379). Paris: Isidor Liseux, 1879. 160 pp. (Reprinted from the edition of 1541.) Selection from p. 93. Translated from the French.

Jean de Brie

Though not a physician, de Brie had a reputation of being one of the best breeders of cattle and sheep in all of France. According to Reinhard, he was commissioned by Charles V of France to write a treatise on wool production and the proper management of sheep. Le bon berger was completed in 1379; from it we have the benefit of his accurate description of the manner of acquisition of Fasciola hepatica *in the sheep and its damage to the liver.*

Flukes which resembled in shape both fish, especially flounders, and leaves, such as Ranunculus *sp. or spearwort, were called in Anglo-Saxon "floc" meaning flounder and in French "la dauve."*

. . . The good shepherd should be extremely careful in the month of March not to lead his animals to pasture in marshy regions that are low and damp. For there grows a very dangerous herb with a small, round, green leaf that is called *la dauve*, which the sheep like very much to eat, but which is very harmful and damaging to them because, as soon as the sheep have tasted it and swallowed it down into their entrails, *la dauve* is of such nature that it adheres to and lives in the liver of the sheep or other beasts. And this bad herb does not rise, does not return to the throat of the animal as do other herbs. But from *la dauve*, by its corruption of the liver, is produced a type of worm which by putrefaction does eat and destroy the entire liver of the animal, which is killed by infection of *la dauve*. After the sheep has eaten it, one can detect it because the animal drinks more often and in greater quantity than it does when it is healthy. The malady of *la dauve* can remain hidden for a year or more, but finally the sheep dies because *la dauve* destroys the liver, and the liver is one of the three principal places where life lies, after the heart and the brain, and therefore, the sheep cannot live. Thus the shepherd should take care not to lead his sheep near marshy places where *la dauve* grows all summer long. . . .

WHAT THYNGES ROTETH SHEPE

A Boke of Husbondrye. A newe tracte or treatyse moost profytable for all husbandemen: and very frutefull for all other persons to rede. 1523. 65 pp. Selection from pp. 24–25. Reprinted in the original Middle English. (Plate 92).

Anthony Fitzherbert (1470–1538)

An early English judge and barrister, Fitzherbert was one of the commoners who negotiated the "pacification" of Ireland. His La Grande Abridgement *was the first important attempt to systematize the English law.*

Sir Anthony had plenty of opportunity of learning about the different methods of farming in use in various parts of the country as he traveled the judicial circuit. Farming was one subject in which everyone was interested in his day and he would also have ample opportunity of practicing the art during the very lengthy vacations which were the privilege of his profession (G. E. Fussell, The Old English Farming Books from Fitzherbert to Tull 1523 to 1723. *London: Crosby Lockwood and Son, 1947).*

The opening paragraphs emphasize the importance of the ecology of Fasciola hepatica, *which was explored in* extenso *450 years later by the Royal Agricultural Society. The last sentence of this article as-*

561

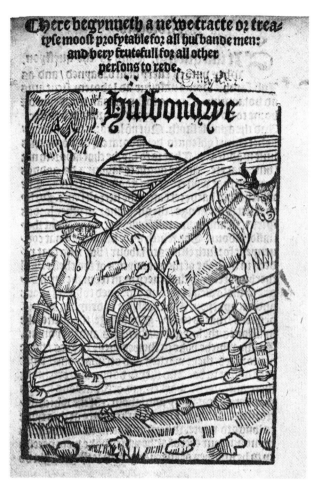

Plate 92. The title page from *A Boke of Husbondrye.*

sociates *ascites, jaundice, liver disease, and the presence of "flokes"* (= flukes).

. . . It is necessary that a shepherde shuld knowe what thyng rote shepe: that he might kepe the the [sic] better. Ther is a grasse called sperewort and hath a long narow lefe like a spereheed and it wyll growe a fote high and bereth a yelowe flour as brode as a penny: and it groweth alway in lowe places wher the water is used to stade in wynter. Another gras is called penny grasse: and groweth lowe by the erth in a marsshe grounde and hath a lefe as brode as a penny of twopens and never bereth floure. All manner of grasse that the lande flode ronneth over is yll for shepe: bycause of the sand and fylth that sticketh upon it. All marres grounde and marsshe grounde is yll for shepe the grasse that growth upon falowes is nat good for shepe for there is moch of it wede and oft tymes it cometh up by the rote and that bringeth the erth with it and they eate both. Myldewe grasse is nat gode for shepe and that shall ye knowe two wayes: one is by the leves on the trees in a mornyng aspecially of okes. Take the leaves and put thy tong to them and thou shalte fele lyke honny upon them: and also there wyll be many kelles upon the gras and that causeth the myldewe. Wherefore they may nat well be lette out of the folde tyll the sonne have domynacion to drie them away: also hunger rote is the worst rote that can be: for there is nother good flesshe nor good skynne and that maketh for lacke of meate. And so for hunger they eate suche as they canne fynde: and so wyll nat pasture shepe for they syldome rote but with myldewes: and than wyll they have moche talowe and flesshe and a good skyn. Also whyte sneles by yll for shepe in pastures and in falowes. There is another rote is called pelt rote: and that cometh of great weate aspecially in wood countre is wher they can nat drie. . . .

To Knowe a Rotten Shepe Dyuersmaner Wayes whereof Some of Them Wyll Natte Fayle

Take both your handes and twyrle upon his eye: and if it be ruddy and have reed strynds in the whyte of the eye than he is sounde. And if the eye be whyte lyke talowe: and the strindes darke coloured than he is rotten: and also take the shepe and upon the wole on the syde and if the skynne be ruddy colour and drie thane is he sounde: and if he be pale coloured and watry than he is rotten. Also when ye have opyned the wole on the syde: take a lytell of the wole bytwene thy fynger and thy thombe and pull it a lytell and yf it stycke fast he is sounde and yf it comes lightly of he is rotten. Also whane thou haste kylde a shepe his belly woll be full of water yf he be sore rotten: and also the fatte of the flesshe woll be yellowe if he be rotten and also and thou cut the lyver therin wyll be lytell quykena lyke flokes and also the lyver woll be full of knotts and whyte blysters yf he be rotten. . . .

OBSERVATIONS CONCERNING LIVING ANIMALS WHICH ARE FOUND IN LIVING ANIMALS

Osservazioni di Francesco Redi . . . intorno agli animali viventi che si trovano negli animali viventi. Florence: Piero Matini, 1684. 244 pp. Selections from pp. 132–134. Translated from the Italian.

Francesco Redi
(1626–1697)

Redi's biography will be found in the chapter on Basic Science.

In 1684 he published the monumental tome Osservazioni intorno agli animali viventi che si trovano negli animali viventi, which is one of the earliest and best works on parasitology. This volume has received as much praise for its lucid style as for its scientific value.

In the following extract, Redi describes the cysticercus of the Taenia pisiformis *and, apparently,* Fasciola hepatica *in a rabbit. Since the fluid in the bladderworm did not coagulate when boiled, he concluded that cysticerci could not be the eggs of the flukes. Hoeppli reminds us that this is one of the earliest helminthologic experiments carried out with the purpose of determining the nature of a parasitic worm. Also included is his drawing (Plate 93) of* F. hepatica *from* Esperienze intorno alla generazione degl' insetti *(Naples: Giacomo Raillard, 1687. p. 167).*

I noted that, between the membranes, the mesentery of a hare was disrupted with certain vesicles, transparent hydatids, in the shape of melon seeds and filled with very clear water. They were of different sizes; some no larger than grains of millet, and some the size of grains of wheat; others were as large as watermelon seeds. Thus they are located between the membranes without being attached to them at all. It is not only the mesentery that is filled with hydatids; many of them nestle underneath the first membrane external to the alimentary canal, and many, many were as self-contained "animals" free and loose in the great cavity of the lower stomach, and many were enclosed in the membrane which covers the liver. Still many others were grouped in heaps and joined together, hidden deep within the liver. Those within the liver were the largest of all, among them some were bigger than any large gourd seed.

The shape of the gall bladder of this hare was much different from normal (resembling a pear with its stem intact). Here, instead of a bladder, could be seen in the liver two large, long, and extensive ramifications filled with bile in which were swimming 18 of those worms whose shape resembled somewhat the fish called "sole." As I indicated in *Observations about the Generation of Insects,* these are not infrequently found in the livers of sheep and castrated rams; the Florentine butchers call them "Biscioule." Because of this I began to wonder whether the aqueous swellings, shaped like the seeds of a melon or gourd, could possibly be the embryos, so to speak, of the worms which dwell in the bile, and whether they, upon growing and perfecting themselves, became such. However, I could not affirm this with certainty, nor have I ever been able to clarify the matter for myself in spite of the fact that I have observed the above-mentioned vesicles in many other hares, and I was quite diligent in order to learn with greater certainty what they were and what the water was with which they were filled. I took a considerable quantity of the fluid and boiled it for a long time in well water. However, the water of the vesicles never coagulated on the application of heat, as serum, which separates itself from the blood and congeals on heating, and as the water of the eggs found in ovaries of quadrupeds congeals. This conforms to my observation of the ova of horses, bears, cows, oxen, mules, does, and hinds, and of other animals— all quadrupeds.

The water of the vesicle remained always fluid, as does that water or fluid which purging medicines bring forth from human bodies. This has been proved many times, and many times I have made experiments concerning this. . . .

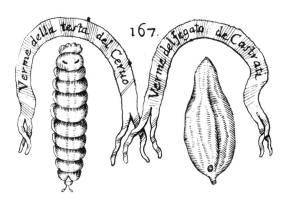

Plate 93. Left: worm from the head of a deer. Right: worm from the liver of a castrated ram.

OF AN ANIMALCULE OR SMALL LIVING CREATURE WHICH IS SOMETIMES FOUND IN THE LIVERS OF SHEEP AND OTHER BEASTS

A letter to Mr. van Leeuwenhoek from G. Bidloo dated 21 March 1698. *In* The Select Works of Anthony van Leeuwenhoek Containing His Microscopical Discoveries in Many of the Works of Nature. Translated by Samuel Hoole from the Dutch and Latin Editions of Works Published by the Author. London: Henry Fry, 1798.

Godefridus Govert Bidloo (1649–1713)

Born in Amsterdam, Bidloo studied in Leyden and later became professor of anatomy and chemistry in the same school. His medical expertise brought him the appointment of physician to William III of England.

Bidloo is perhaps best known because he was the victim of a scientific fraud. The 105 superb plates by the artist Gerard de Lairesse, which illustrated Bidloo's Anatomia, *originally published in Amsterdam in 1685, were plagiarized by the English anatomist and surgeon William Cowper, who reproduced them without credit in his* Anatomy of Human Bodies, *published in Oxford in 1698, a book which is original only as to the text and nine perfunctory illustrations. Bidloo scolded the plagiarist in a paper published in 1700 in Leyden and bearing the scathing title, "Guglielmus Cowper, criminis literarii citatus."*

Bidloo's detailed and exaggerated drawing of Fasciola hepatica *seems quite realistic, even though it does have human eyes.*

To make my observations on this subject the more intelligible, I shall place them in the following order: First, as to the shape and make of this animalcule; Secondly, the part of the intestines where it is found; Thirdly, its numbers, and the manner of its propagation; and Fourthly, how these creatures, and other animalcules of a similar nature, by fixing themselves in the liver and other internal parts of the body, can produce certain diseases, and their fatal consequences.

First, as to the shape and size of this creature, and its similitude to other known animals; it bears a near resemblance (in miniature) to our sole or flounder, as appears by Fig. A (Plate 94) which represents it of the size it is commonly found; this figure shews the back or prominent side; and Fig. B, the belly, or flat side of it. C is one of the young of the same species, shewing the back, D the belly of the same; E and F are figures of the same creature somewhat magnified, and shewn in the positions before mentioned.

These animals are not often seen alive, because the disease they produce does not always shew itself by outward tokens, and the beast afflicted with them, sometimes seems fat and in good health, and then the liver is not perhaps examined till sometime after the beast is killed; and these creatures cannot endure cold, but if by being exposed to it they are deprived of motion, they will revive, if the liver be held in a warm hand or put into warm water. Their motion is undulating or wriggling like that of the fishes before mentioned, their colour a yellowish brown, the belly quite flat, and much paler coloured than the back, the skin rough and covered with prickles or points, and so transparent, that the bowels and vessels may plainly be seen on both sides. The head (which is shewn considerably magnified, at letter G,) is of a pointed form, planoconvex, that is, rounding above and flat below, the mouth projecting, open, and of an oval shape, nearly in fashion like a carp. The eyes, which are pictured separately at H and I, are very prominent, and surrounded with a cartilaginous or gristly ring, which is shewn at K, and they are placed, as we see in many flat fishes, both on one side of the back, with a division between them.

The heart is so near to the head, and the bowels so closely conjoined to the heart, that I question whether there is any thing properly to distinguish the head from the rest of the body, which yet in most animals are separate and distinct. From the heart arise two vessels spreading over the whole body, with a wide space between them, extending almost the whole length of the back, as represented at letter L, and between these vessels are many smaller ones, as shewn at M, which are so minute that no moisture can be discovered within them. I observed in the larger vessels two sorts of juices, namely, in some a yellowish brown, and sometimes a kind of purple; in others a pale green, both of a glutinous or flimsy nature, and yet flowing in the vessels (even after the death of the animal,) towards the heart, if held up by the tail, and back again, upon the head being raised.

The excretory duct, or passage of the bowels, is in an unusual place, being on the right side of the body, close under the head, for which reason the intestines are as it were, crowded together in an heap. There is a small protuberance at the beginning of the bowels, which I take to be the liver, and between this and the bowels, I find in all of those animalcules which I have examined, an innumerable quantity of oval particles, hundreds of which, taken together, are not equal to

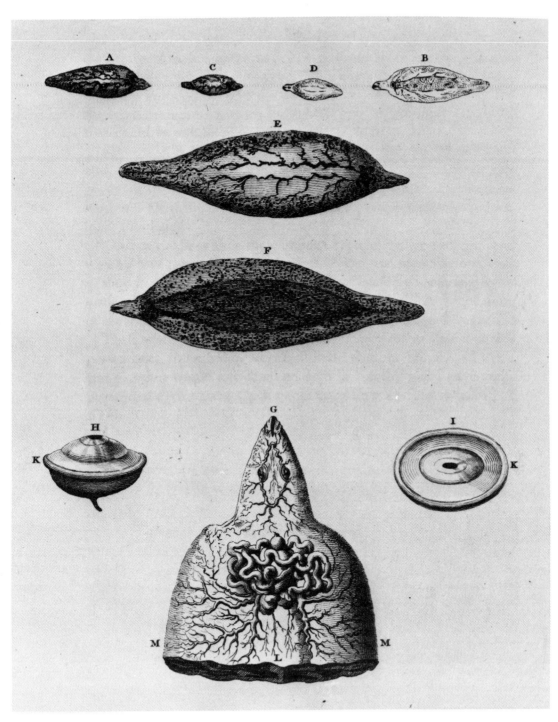

Plate 94.

the size of a grain of sand. They are of a pale red colour, and I take them to be the spawn or eggs. Notwithstanding my most diligent examination of these creatures, I never could discover any difference of sexes; and it seems to me most probable, that they are of that species called Hermaphrodites, or every one equally prolifick; at least, none has ever fallen into my hands which appeared plainly to be a male. The tail, though of the same texture with the rest of the body, is much tenderer, breaking or tearing upon the slightest touch.

The parts in several animals wherein I have hitherto found these creatures, are only the vessels, tubes, and channels wherein the gall is formed and collected, though most commonly in the liver and here they may be said to swarm, producing grievous swellings, callosities, contorsions, and sinuses in the part; and cavities which will be often found an inch and an half in diameter. In these parts these noxious animalcules are found in heaps, and the places where they lie become hard and cartilaginous. In the small gall-ducts they lie longitudinally, and sometimes rolled or curled up together; and I believe that many persons have hereby been led into a mistake respecting the shape of them, describing them to be oblong, round worms; but in truth, however closely they may be thus rolled up, they will spread open again, even after they are dead, upon being thrown into warm water, for then they recover their flat shape, but at the same time they become rather of a paler colour than they originally were.

These creatures are commonly found in great numbers, though in this particular they vary much, as it depends on their having had more or less time to propagate; I have taken out of one liver, 870 in number, besides many fragments, and exclusive of those which were cut in pieces or destroyed in opening the liver. And in another liver I have seen but ten or twelve.

They are found in many different kinds of beasts. I have been informed by Hunters, that they have found them in Stags, wild Boars, and other kinds of game, both great and small. I myself have seen them frequently in Calves, and once in a young Bullock. Sheep are infested by them even from the womb of the parent, and Lambs of a year old and upwards, as well as aged Sheep.

As to the production and propagation of these animalcules, I consider as idle tales, what some writers assert, of their being generated by putrefaction or decayed substances, immoderate wet or heats, and other equally senseless imaginations; and I lay it down as a certain truth, that these, as well as all other small living creatures, are produced from their like, by the means of eggs, seed, or spawn, according to the nature implanted in them at their first creation. And it seems to me most probable, that these animals, with their eggs, find their way into the bodies of Sheep, (and which we may suppose to be the case also with other insects and their eggs,) in the following manner; namely, that in wet summers and autumns these animalcula, which originally bred on the surface of the earth, may, with the water in which they live, be swallowed by the Sheep; and I have been confirmed in this opinion by conversing with Countrymen, Huntsmen, and Butchers, on the subject. But I am not of the opinion that after being swallowed, they do themselves force their way out of the stomach and bowels into the gall-bladder; I rather conclude, from reason and my own experience, that their spawn or eggs may, with the oily part of the chyle in the infected beast be carried into the vessels of the gall bladder, and there fix themselves; forasmuch as these vessels are lined with a slimy and tenacious substance, and also because the gall is not like the blood, in continual circulation, but is retained in its vessels, or emitted, as the calls of the animal economy require. Again, they are found swarming in the liver, where they produce tumours and callosities, and cause the colour of it to change. And it seems to me not at all surprizing that these animalcules should live and be nourished in the juices of the gall, for every living creature has a situation and species of food peculiar to itself. Seafish die in fresh, and river-fish in salt water. A worm cannot live in the air, and a fowl expires in the earth. What wonder is it then that the creature of which we are treating, when introduced into the body of another animal, should find its peculiar place of life, growth, and increase in the vessels of the gall, and in the gall itself?

In the last place, like as we experience, that many living creatures are found in the human body, producing disease, pain, and death itself; so it is my opinion, that the animalcules of which

I have been treating, and which are sometimes found together by thousands, may produce the following mischievous consequences:

First, the extraordinary distension of the parts where they harbour, as well by the growth and increase of their own bodies, as by the multiplication of their species or brood.

Secondly, by their biting or gnawing the parts they infest, so as at length to break or destroy their texture; and thus wholly, or in part, render them incapable of performing their functions.

Thirdly, by forcing their bodies into the small tubes, and vessels, whereby the delicate frame of those tender parts is torn asunder.

Fourthly, by obstructing the passages in the vessels, whereby the circulation of the juices is prevented, and an inflammation ensues.

Fifthly, by devouring and consuming the nutritive juices, whereby the adjacent parts are deprived of their support and nourishment.

Sixthly, by clogging the vessels with their excrements, their eggs or spawn, and the bodies of such of the animalcules themselves as die, whereby the motion of those parts being impeded, the most fatal consequences follow.

There are many other ways in which these creatures may prove noxious to animals, but those which I have here enumerated may be sufficient to give an idea of the rest.

He, then, who can find out and practise a method whereby, without injury to the parts of the body where these vermin harbour, can prevent their gnawing the parts, their creeping about in the intestines, and what is worse, their dying there; or rather, can discover how to expel them while alive out of the body, will in this respect bid fair to effect a cure. It is laid down as a truth, that a distemperature of the blood and juices, whether proceeding from an ill constitution thereof, or from an interruption in the circulation, can cause many diseases and their ill consequences: but must it therefore be deemed unreasonable to attempt proving, that animalcules being found in the juices, or even in the more solid parts of the body, may also produce diseases? The first of these points is mere matter of theory or argument; of the second, more certain proofs can be brought; consequently, it seems more rational, that those persons, who altogether rely upon their experience, should, in their enquiries, diligently investigate the reasons on which they found their opinions.

I forbear to say any more on this subject, forasmuch as what I have written is only for the improvement of medical knowledge, and as an incentive to the laborious enquirers after new discoveries in science, the field of which is indeed indefinite.

Addition by the Translator [Samuel Hoole—Eds.]

It is proper to inform the Reader, that the preceding Essay has not Mr. Leeuwenhoek for its author, but is taken from a letter written to him on the subject by G. Bidloo, a professional Gentleman at Leyden, under date of the 21st March 1698, and published in the Dutch Edition of Mr. Leeuwenhoek's works, though it does not appear in the Latin Version; but as the subject is interesting, and probably this Essay has not before appeared in any other than the Dutch language, the Translator thought that it might be acceptable to the English Reader.

Since the perusal of this Essay, the Translator has had opportunities of conversing with several judicious Gentlemen, who are conversant in the grazing of Sheep, from whom he has collected the following particulars:

That in very wet seasons, particularly towards the latter end of the year, a species of gras springs up in the low and wet lands, by feeding on which the Sheep are supposed to contract the distemper called the Rot. That if the rains do not abound until after the winter frost has been experienced, the Sheep are not then obnoxious to this disease, but otherwise, if a wet season precedes the frost; and lastly, that Sheep infected with this disease, do for a time appear fat and healthy, but when the disorder gets to a heighth, they fall away rapidly.

These particulars seem to prove, that the disease called the Rot in Sheep, does in fact proceed from the animal described in the preceding Essay, which being bred in the water, and adhering, with its eggs, to the gras growing in watery places is swallowed by the Sheep. And it is probable that when the frost precedes a wet season, the animalcules and their eggs are killed by the frost, and consequently the Sheep escape; we may also conclude, that while this noxious animalcule is in an infant state in the bowels of the Sheep, it may not be particularly injurious, but when it arrives at a size to prey upon the liver, first a sicknes, and wasting in the animal, and afterwards death must ensue; and the Translator has been informed by a gentleman's Gamekeeper, that he has frequently found Hares dead of this disease, and that upon opening them, hundreds of the animalcules were found in their livers.

These particulars the Translator thought proper to notice, leaving it to those who are qualified, to exercise their medical skill in the discovery of a remedy for this fatal distemper.

The animalcule before described is called in some countries a Fluke, in others a Loop, but most generally a Flounder, probably from the resemblance it bears to the fish of that name.

ON THE HISTORY OF THE DEVELOPMENT OF THE LIVER FLUKE

Zur entwickelungsgeschichte des leberegels. Zoologischer Anzeiger, IV: 641–646, 1881. Translated from the German.

Friedrich Rudolf Leuckart
(1822–1898)

(Leuckart's biography will be found in the chapter on Onchocerciasis.)

Leuckart's work on the life cycle of Fasciola hepatica *coincided with that of A. P. Thomas.*

Between 1881 and 1882, Leuckart published a series of articles on the life cycle of F. hepatica; *this is the first article of the series.*

The question of the life and developmental history of the *Distoma hepaticum* has occupied me for many years. Again and again, I attempted to infect indigenous snails (at least those most frequently encountered) with the embryos of *D. hepaticum*. All attempts were in vain until the late summer of 1879 when I introduced into my breeding vessels a number of small *Lymnaea* which, on a visit to the Dresden Botanical Gardens, I had found there in the water containers. On Rossmässler's statement that the locality concerned harbored *L. minutus (L. truncatulus)*, I added this species which I had not used previously for my experiments. After only a few days I found, to my pleasant surprise, that some of the snails were covered with small parasites. These were without a doubt related to the embryos swarming around the snails. They were found mostly deep in the breathing cavity, sometimes singly, sometimes in large numbers, next to one another. They appeared as small, sharply defined tubes without cilia with two eye spots more or less far apart, and with a head sucker; these characteristics indicated their origin without a doubt. The content of the tubes consisted of clear cells beginning to proliferate and at times had already changed into larger cell aggregates.

Prior to this time, I thought that my findings indicated that the embryos of *D. hepaticum* became sporocysts after their migration into *L. minutus* and then brought forth young distomas. I had expressed myself along these lines several times to close colleagues. As simple as it seemed to me in the beginning further to pursue the development of this parasite after determining the intermediate host, I was soon to learn otherwise.

The *Lymnaea* which I collected were quickly used up, and the material sent to me several times by Professor Drude furnished only sparse observational matter, since almost all the snails remained free of parasites, although the opportunity for infection, as compared to previous experiments, had not been diminished in any way.

The year 1879 passed without my being able to augment my experiences significantly, and the following year was even less fruitful since the breeding material, which I could only obtain in small amounts, perished before the embryos emerged.

In the meantime, however, I began to doubt whether my experimental animal had really been *L. minutus*. A comparison with the young forms of other *Lymnaea* finally led to the conviction that I had experimented with *L. pereger*. I had used this species several times before for my infection experiments. However, at that time, I had used mostly half-grown or completely mature specimens, without success, as I already mentioned above. Since I subsequently remembered the circumstances under which I found the parasites—mainly, in the smaller and smallest specimens of my young forms—the thought gradually occurred to me that the embryos of this distomum might find only in the younger snails the proper conditions for their migration and metamorphosis; that the development of the liver fluke, therefore, like that of the coenurus, might be associated with the young of the intermediate host.

This supposition was fully confirmed. During

the summer in which I resumed my experiments, I was able to infect many hundreds of young *Lymnaea* (naturally, *L. pereger*) with my embryos and was able to pursue their further development. The younger the snails were, the surer and more massively the infection succeeded. Frequently I have discovered, in specimens the size of a pinhead, several dozen embryos. Half-grown and older animals were always spared, and the majority of the larger young forms also proved to be immune. The same holds true for the rest of the *Lymnaea* species (*L. palustris, L. auricularis*) with which I experimented. Now and then I noticed in young snails, especially of the first kind, undoubted signs of infection; however, the invasion was consistently sparse, and further development failed to take place, since the parasites quickly perished—a frequent happening also with *L. pereger*.

It is not my intention to give here a complete report of my investigations or to describe fully the development of the *D. hepaticum* so far as I know it because my observations, even now, are not without gaps. This I will report shortly in another place. Nevertheless, it might be of interest here to point out briefly the important results obtained.

First, as far as the embryo is concerned, it already contains a full complement of germinal cells on emergence from the egg shell. These occupy the posterior portion of the abdominal cavity, while the anterior portion is filled with a granular substance which one might justifiably consider the rudiments of a digestive apparatus. The germinal cells themselves are probably of mesodermal origin. At the boundary of the anterior and posterior portions, one sees, deep in the abdominal wall on the right and the left, a ciliary funnel (I have already described this in the supplements to the first volume of my work on parasites, 1863). The epidermis consists of a few large cells which are arranged very regularly in two rows in the posterior portion of the body and have numerous cilia.

In several aspects, the whole structure of the embryos [miracidia] resembles so strikingly the *Girard orthonectides* that one can hardly resist the thought that the latter are nothing but trematodes which, in spite of their sexual maturity, have not developed beyond the embryonic state of the distomas.

The first change to occur in these embryos [miracidia] after invasion of the host is desquamation of the epidermal cells. As a result of this, the organisms lose their earlier mobility and their body shape. They pull themselves together into an oval or spherical mass and begin to grow so quickly that the x-shaped eye spot, belonging to the deeper layers of the abdominal wall, which continues distending, falls apart into two dot-shaped halves. The germinal cell mass participates in this growth. It grows to such a degree that in a short time it displaces the rudimentary intestine and fills the entire inside of the tube. Some of the cells, especially anteriorly, have become sizable cell aggregates by repeated division and show the first traces of the later brood.

It is remarkable, however, that these cell aggregates do not change into young distomas or cercariae but into redias which by the second week are characterized plainly as such; toward the end of the second week they break through the wall of the mother tube, one by one, as they develop. The number of these offspring may average between five and eight in the various tubes. Their bodies are cylindrical and, as in the majority of the species, initially are thin posteriorly with two cone-shaped projections which are turned ventrally and serve for support during locomotion [locomotor appendages]. The head cone, which projects from the middle of the body by a muscular thickening of the cuticula, has great mobility stemming mainly from the contraction of internal muscles which are attached to the pharynx. The mouth edges can spread, cuplike, and thus permit tight and powerful suction.

The internal organization of the redias resembles that of the embryos except that the individual organs, and especially the digestive gland, have reached a higher level of specialization. This is particularly true regarding the germinal cells which are not, as one usually assumes, derived from the abdominal wall but have their origin from the rest of animal's organs; these then develop into mature organs. The germinal cells arise from the mesoderm which forms, when the germinal sphere has become a gastrula, between the ectoderm and the entoderm. Behind the pharynx the redias have a two-lobed ganglion and, in the body wall, slightly ahead of the locomotor appendages, a ciliary funnel on each side.

The germinal cells begin their development soon after the release of the redias which, at that time, measure about 0.5 mm. They probably produce a brood of tailless distomas which remain at their place of birth and are delivered, with the snails which harbor them, to the definitive hosts of the liver flukes. I say "probably" because, unfortunately, it has been impossible for me, up to this time, to pursue the development of these germinal granules to maturity, since all the *Lymnaea* infected by me—and in all of my experimental series—perished during the fourth week, just at the time of the development of the distomas.

I am justified in the assumption that the brood of the redias belongs to the tailless distomas; not only by the massive occurrence of liver flukes in sheep and cattle but also by the finding of, among others, a redia in mature specimens of *L. minutus* which I owe to the kindness of Mr. Clessin—a redia which, according to the nature of the tailless distomas contained in it, probably belonged to the developmental cycle of the liver fluke. The young brood already had the spiny coverings of the mature *D. hepaticum*—though naturally less than full size and development. They still had a single, forked intestine as, according to Joseph, is also the case in the younger liver flukes of sheep.

If my assumption is valid, then it is the two small *Lymnaea* indigenous here, *L. pereger* and *L. minutus (L. truncatulus),* which we must consider as the intermediate hosts of the liver fluke; two kinds which, even if in somewhat different distribution, have great similarity to one another with respect to their occurrence and their way of life.

Unfortunately, I have not yet had the opportunity to use the *L. minutus* in my breeding experiments, due to the fact that this species has not been found in Leipzig or its vicinity. Since I plan to resume my experiments next year, I take the liberty here of closing my report with a request for shipments of living (and particularly young) specimens and perhaps also of the spawn of *L. minutus* in amounts large enough to enable me to complete my observations. In this way, I hope to add to the solution of a problem whose clarification reaches far beyond the boundaries of mere scientific interest. I shall also gladly receive reports on recently occurring liver fluke epidemics.

REPORT OF EXPERIMENTS ON THE DEVELOPMENT OF THE LIVER FLUKE (*FASCIOLA HEPATICA*)

Journal of the Royal Agricultural Society of England, 17: 1–28, 1881. Selections from pp 1–7, 13, 16–19, 22–25, 27.

Algernon Phillips Withiel Thomas (1857–1937)

A. P. Thomas, as a 23-year-old graduate of Balliol College, Oxford, fortuitously received a grant from the Royal Society of Agriculture to investigate sheep liver rot, which was devastating the herds of the British Isles. His mentor, George Rolleston, had been approached first; however, his poor health precluded his undertaking the task, and he recommended his prize student. Shortly after completing this monumental task, Thomas became the first professor of biology and geology at Auckland, New Zealand, and remained in that position for 30 years. Prior to his death at 80 years of age, he was knighted for his achievements as an educator.

Thomas completed the life cycle of Fasciola hepatica *independently of Leuckart. This was the first complete description of a life cycle of a digenetic trematode.*

The Egg and Embryo of the Fluke. The eggs of the liver fluke occur in very large numbers in the contents of the bile-ducts and gallbladder of the infected animal. They give a dark-brown colour and sandy appearance to the bile, and in some of the smaller terminal ducts often form a stiff brown mass completely plugging up the lumen. They pass with the bile into the intestines, and may be found abundantly in the droppings of rotten sheep. . . .

The number of eggs produced by a single fluke is exceedingly large, and its fecundity has been under-rated. Leuckart has estimated that the oviduct can contain as many as 45,000 eggs. In one case I obtained 7,400,000 eggs from the gallbladder of a sheep suffering from the rot, and as the liver contained about 200 flukes, this gives an average of 37,000 eggs to each fluke. And these eggs were found in the gallbladder alone; the liver must have contained at least as many more, and eggs had been passed copiously by the sheep for some months past. The number of eggs produced by a single fluke may be safely estimated at several hundred thousands.

When the egg has just been laid, the contents are formed by a number of spherical masses of a clear substance containing many granules. These spheres consist of secondary yolk, and are physiologically equivalent to the white of the fowl's eggs; they are often slightly polygonal from mutual pressure, and between them are a few bright yolk-granules. Surrounded by the secondary yolk-spheres and near the anterior end of the egg is a heap of pale nucleated cells with indistinct outlines which represent the future embryo, and have been formed by the cleavage of the primitive ovum in its descent through the oviduct. The development of the embryo does not proceed beyond this stage whilst within the bile-ducts of the sheep; it can only take place out of the body of the bearer of the adult fluke, and at a lower temperature. Eggs kept in water in an incubator at the temperature of the mammalian body do not make any progress, whilst other eggs kept at a lower temperature complete their development in a few weeks. The necessary conditions for development are moisture and a certain moderate degree of warmth; light I have found to exert no influence. Eggs taken from the gallbladder and placed directly with water into an opaque vessel, develop as soon as similar eggs exposed to the light, but otherwise kept under the same conditions. A temperature of about 23° C to 26° C is most favourable, and with this degree of warmth the embryo is formed in about two or three weeks. At a lower temperature development takes place much more slowly, and with an average warmth of 16° C occupies two or three months. During the winter no progress is made.

All the eggs under the same conditions, however, do not produce embryos in the same time; a certain number are hatched out on every successive day for some weeks or even months, and at the end of this time some of the eggs may remain in the same condition as when just laid. No explanation can be discovered in the eggs themselves of the very variable time required for the development of the embryo, but the fact is of much practical importance, for eggs scattered over any damp ground will render it more or less dangerous for a longer period than one year.

The body of the embryo is formed by the growth of the inner cellular mass at the expense of the secondary yolk-spheres which surround it. The outlines of the yolk-spheres become more distinct and their contents less granular, whilst the granules are often aggregated at one side of the sphere; they become more fluid, and their remains gradually coalesce and lie on one side of the egg. The body of the embryo elongates and comes to occupy the whole length of the egg. A papilla appears at the anterior end, and behind this two annular furrows, between which a quantity of dark-brown pigment is produced, forming the eye-spot. Wave-like peristaltic contractions pass along the body from the anterior to the opposite end. In the last stage when the embryo is nearly ready to emerge from the shell, it lies slightly curved upon itself at one side of the egg, the remainder of the space on the opposite side being occupied by the fluid remains of the coalesced yolk-spheres. At the anterior end, just beneath the operculum, is a quantity of viscid mucus, which forms a sort of lining or cushion at this end of the egg. Around the body of the embryo may be distinguished a bright border, which is formed by its covering of cilia; these cilia, however, can only in exceptional cases be seen in motion before the animal quits the egg.

The embryo is now ready to come forth; its movements become more marked, and at length a more vigorous extension of the body causes the operculum to fly open as if moved by a spring. The cap of mucus pours out, the embryo thrusts a fore part of its body out of the shell, the cilia begin to move instantly the water touches them, and the animal after a short struggle succeeds in drawing the whole of its body through the narrow opening of the shell, and glides away with ease and rapidity through the water. Although light has no influence in accelerating development, the embryo itself is sensitive to it. I have repeatedly observed that on removing a vessel of eggs from the darkened incubator in which they were being hatched, only two or three embryos could be seen, but that after it had stood in a window for 20 minutes, the water was quite nebulous from their presence. . . .

In water the average duration of the embryo's life is only about eight hours, though occasionally one may live over night. The motion then becomes gradually feebler, and at length ceases; the embryo assumes an oval or elliptical shape; the ciliated cuticular cells absorb water, and swell up into round vesicles, and the whole body disintegrates. In mucus the embryo will live rather longer, and in a feebly alkaline solution of peptone I have been able to keep them alive for three days. The cilia were not lost, but their motion after the first day became very sluggish; the embryos increased a little in size, but no advance in organization took place, except perhaps that the cellular parenchyma became arranged into rather more definite spherical masses.

Further Development of the Embryo. What is the ultimate fate of this embryo? By what stages is it connected with the adult fluke as found in the bile-ducts of the sheep? Its instinct evidently prompts it to bore its way into some object, and its organization is so simple, and its resemblance to the embryos of other *Distomidae* whose life history has been made out is so close, that there is little reason for supposing its further development to depart from the ordinary type among the *Distomidae:* that is, we should expect to find it make its way into some animal—most probably a mollusc—and then, losing its cilia, be metamorphosed into a brood-sac or sporosac, from which, in the first or later generation, larval cercarian forms will be produced by internal gemmation; and after a period of quiescence these cercariae will, if they gain access to a suitable vertebrate host, give rise to adult sexual flukes. The embryos of *Distoma nodulosum* and *Distoma trigonocephalum* are very like that of *Fasciola hepatica*; the former gives rise to a sporocyst in *Bithynia tentaculata*, and the latter to a redia in certain species of *Paludina.*

This intermediate host will most probably be a mollusc, for very few instances are recorded of the occurrence of the sporosac form in any other than a molluscan host. There may indeed be more than one bearer for the brood-sac of *Fasciola*, for although some larval forms of trematodes are restricted to a single host, such as the *Leucochloridium paradoxum* of *Succinea amphibia*, others are less particular, and may be found in several different molluscs; thus the rediae of *Cerc. echinata* occur in *Paludina vivipara, Limnaeus stagnalis* and *Planorbis corneus*, and the sporocysts of *Cerc. armata* in the two last.

Assuming that there is an intermediate molluscan bearer, the question still remains, In what form does the fluke enter the sheep? In what way? Does it enter with the food? Or with the drink? Or by some other method? In the case of other *Distomidae* the migration into the ultimate host is, so far as is known, always passive, and the parasite is taken up with the food. The cercaria, when fully formed, makes its way out of

the sporo-sac which has produced it, and encysts itself either in the same mollusc, or more frequently it passes out into the water, and after a short free life encysts itself in another snail of the same species, or it may be of a different species. But with all aquatic cercariae an encysted stage seems to be necessary, and no instance is known of direct development of the cercaria into the mature form without the intervention of a period of quiescence. When *free* cercariae have been given to the animals which form their natural abode in the adult state, these cercariae have always failed to develop further. . . .

Judging from the analogy with other flukes, it is most probable that sheep pick up the young liver-flukes whilst in the encysted state with their food. It is not likely to be taken up with the water drunk by the sheep, for free cercariae would perish. Moreover, rabbits are exceedingly liable to flukes—I have found as many as 50 in a single rabbit's liver—and sportsmen deny that they ever drink. It has been conjectured that the sheep takes up the fluke by eating the mollusc which harbours the larvae. Sheep and many other animals are passionately fond of salt, and might possibly eat snails intentionally on account of their saline taste. Mr. C. Spence Bate, F.R.S., says that "as a rule, farmers encourage the snails, as they say that the sheep are fond of them." But other observers have come to the opposite opinion, and it would seem more probable that the molluscs, if eaten at all, are swallowed accidentally, being mixed with the food. In this case of course any large mollusc could not be taken up.

Or, infection may be produced in another way. The cerceria of *Fasciola* may encyst itself at the moist roots of plants, and then be taken up when the sheep is grazing. In examining the contents of the paunch of recently infected lamb, I found numerous portions of the roots of grasses. This view has much to recommend it, and in accordance with it is the opinion of farmers that the fluke is especially taken up when the sheep graze closely, and that the better the biter is, the worse are the chances of escape. . . .

Experiments have been made to determine which mollusc or molluscs act as host to the conjectured sporosac form of *Fasciola hepatica*; and here the number of molluscs which need concern us was indicated by their geographical distribution and by that of the fluke itself. . . .

Experiments with Embryo. [Experiments were done with *Arion ater, Limax agrestis, Arion hortensis, Limax cinereus, Planorbis marginatus, Succinea amphibia, Limnaeus pereger,* and *Limnaeus truncatulus,* all of which proved negative. See second report.—Eds.]. . . .

The failure of infection experiments in the hands of different observers leads us to inquire whether the development of the liver fluke deviates from the type usual among the digenetic Trematoda with which it is always classed, or whether there is any cause for failure in the line of experimentation. . . .

Investigation of "Sheep-rotting" Fields. The problem of the development of the liver fluke may be attacked from another point, viz. by visiting the scene of actual infection, examining the conditions of the ground, and the circumstances which favor the contraction of the parasite, studying the fauna and examining it for larval forms of Trematodes. With this view a large number of farms have been visited in the neighbourhood of Oxford, where the outbreak of the disease was very serious in 1879–80, and some of the more interesting and important observations will be briefly noted. In these investigations I am especially indebted to valuable assistance from Professor Rolleston.

Wytham. There was here a well-marked case of upland infection, and it appeared to be so free from sources of error, that numerous visits were paid to it, both by day and by night, and the fauna thoroughly investigated at the time which is supposed to be most dangerous for the contraction of the fluke-disease.

Rot first appeared upon this land in the autumn of 1879; the tenant had held the farm for over 40 years, but had never had a single case before. He lost more than 40 sheep, and even his cattle suffered from the fluke. None of the neighbouring farmers had any rot amongst their flocks. The sheep had been kept entirely on five fields, situated on the side of a hill, and quite above the reach of any floods; they were not turned on to arable land, but some hay and clover was brought to them, and their water they got in the fields. The ground on the whole appeared fairly good, most of it distinctly sloping, but it lies upon the Oxford Clay, and in places there are depressions which remain moist, or even a little marshy, in dry weather. The summit of the hill is covered

with woods containing much game, and rabbits were seen about these fields in considerable numbers, and are said to have suffered severely from flukes. The disease was very likely introduced by them, as their droppings containing eggs would be spread all over the fields. A small rivulet rises in the wood above, and flows down through these fields; troughs are placed in its course, and it was from these troughs that the sheep drank. Its waters were searched for molluscs, but none found except in a single minute specimen of *Cyclas* and two equally minute specimens of *Physa fontinalis.* . . .

Here two or three small specimens of *Limnaeus truncatulus* and some aquatic larvae were found. These contained no cercariae, but in another *L. truncatulus* found at the same spot a month later, an interesting form of cercaria occurred. . . .

One of the conditions most necessary for the prevalence of rot is moisture; and whilst lowlying ground is thus naturally more exposed to it, rot may occur on upland (as at Wytham) if there be sufficient moisture to allow the egg of the fluke to develop; that is, any heavy or ill-drained land may give the rot. In the neighbourhood of Hampton Poyle and Bletchington, north of Oxford, the rot has followed the geological character of the ground very closely. All fields upon the Oxford Clay have been dangerous, whether exposed to floods or not. On the other hand, floods on low porous ground or on gravel appear to do no harm, unless the water stands for a long time. All this is easily intelligible when we remember the necessity of moisture for the hatching of the embryo. Winter floods are not necessarily dangerous because warmth is required as well as wet.

Surprise is sometimes expressed at the way in which the rot breaks out in a wet season suddenly in isolated flocks. The eggs of the fluke must be present on the ground or rot cannot occur, but the distribution may take place in many ways, as by floods or running water or in manure. Rabbits also have much to answer for in distributing the parasite. Everywhere about Oxford the same account is given of the way in which these animals have suffered from the rot, and in some neighbourhoods they have almost been exterminated. I have received livers of fluked rabbits and have found them to contain as many as 40 or 50 flukes. Wherever they go, and they often wander far from home, the eggs of the fluke are distributed in their droppings, and the first condition for the existence of rot is satisfied.

Practical men seem to have come to the conclusion that the rot is particularly due to close grazing, and that those animals suffer most which can bite the nearest to the ground. A sheep can graze where cattle or horses can get nothing (indeed, it can graze closer than any other animal except a kangaroo), and some farmers ascribe to this cause the special liability of sheep to fluke disease. "Hog-jawed" sheep are known to escape the rot when all the rest of a flock take the infection. Lambs suffer more than older sheep, and this may be due to lesser digestive power, which does not enable them to digest the germs of the fluke; but one good observer has told me that at Michaelmas of the year in which a lamb is born, it can graze closer than an older sheep, quite down into the roots of the grass, and would do fairly well where an old ewe would starve. Hence he attributes the liability of lambs to rot partly to their grazing so closely. This generalization, if true, indicates that the germ of the fluke is picked up close to the damp roots of the grass. . . .

Growth of the Fluke and the Duration of its Life. A lamb's liver was received on September 24th from Stratton Audley. The surface was of the normal color, except where it was marked with red inflamed spots and with white ragged bits of connective tissue which are considered by those who have had much experience in slaughtering to be extremely characteristic of the earliest stages of the rot.

This liver was said not to contain any flukes, but did contain over 200, all immature, the largest only one-third of an inch in length. Many flukes were obtained from the surface, some projecting from holes, others visible immediately beneath the peritoneum and from openings on the surface a red ooze containing a young fluke about one to three lines long could be pressed. When a cut was made into the liver, the surface had a mottled appearance, due to a solid yellow substance, and to small spots where the substance was inflamed or destroyed, and reduced to a red ooze. The bile ducts could hardly be said to be enlarged, and no flukes of any kind could be found in the larger ducts. By far the largest

number were in the smaller branches of the bile ducts or in centers of destroyed hepatic tissue. They occurred especially near any surface of the liver. The young fluke on entering the liver by the bile duct appears to push its way onwards into the smaller ducts where some remain whilst others penetrate the walls of the ducts and crawl forward to the surface, causing the destruction of the parenchyma as they proceed. Arrived at the surface of the liver they may pass along beneath the peritoneum, as may be seen from the long inflamed tracks which they leave behind them, or they pierce the peritoneum and set up perihepatitis and the consequent adhesion gives rise to the ragged patches of connective tissue visible on the surface of the liver when this is removed from the body. The flukes may also be found in the peritoneal cavity of the animal, as I have seen them in a rabbit. In another case, where all the flukes present were of full size, and atrophy of the hepatic parenchyma had made some progress, several flukes were found at the thin free edge of the liver, with the anterior part of the body projecting into the peritoneal cavity. The power of the fluke to wander within its host seems to be greater than is generally supposed. Mr. A. H. Cocks informs me that on examining a Welsh ewe which had died from the rot, he found several flukes in folds of the mesentery, and others in the uterus.

Conclusion. The necessary conditions for the existence of rot in any given locality where sheep are kept are (1) the presence of the eggs of the fluke, (2) water or wet ground during the warmer months to enable the embryo to hatch out of the egg, (3) the presence, it is believed, of slugs or snails upon the ground to secure the further development of the embryo and the production of the cercarian form which eventually enters the sheep.

If any one of these conditions be not satisfied, there can be no rot. Very little attention is paid to the eggs of the fluke, but these, like the eggs of all entozoa, should as far as possible be rigorously destroyed; if we can effect this we shall prevent the rot. The eggs are present in immense numbers in the droppings of infected animals, and hence are distributed wherever such animals are kept. Unless sheep are very valuable it may be better to kill them instantly they are known to be infected; for we shall thus prevent the produc-

THOMAS
575

tion of more eggs and the propagation of the fluke. The cure of the sheep, if cure be possible, will probably cost more than it is worth. If rotted sheep are kept in a yard, the manure should be collected, and never spread upon damp ground. The eggs may be hindered from developing by adding a little coal tar oil to the manure, and keeping it for some time before it is spread on the fields. Or, the manure may be spread on dry, well-drained ground. Above all, livers of fluked sheep should be destroyed, for if every egg succeeded in producing one fluke a single liver might contain sufficient eggs to destroy a flock of 50,000 sheep. Fortunately the chances are immensely against any egg giving rise to an adult fluke, but we should do all we can to increase these adverse chances.

With regard to the second condition for the existence of rot, the obvious remedy is that the land should be thoroughly drained. The third condition is the presence of slugs or snails. It has not been possible as yet to prove the presence of the cercaria of the liver fluke in one or more particular slugs or snails, but for reasons already given, there is no ground for doubting its existence. Hence all slugs or snails on sheep-rotting fields should be destroyed. A dressing of lime will destroy both the eggs of the fluke and the snails or slugs. . . .

SECOND REPORT OF EXPERIMENTS ON THE DEVELOPMENT OF THE LIVER FLUKE (*FASCIOLA HEPATICA*)

Journal of the Royal Agricultural Society of England, 18: 439–455, 1882. Selections from pp 439, 442, 446–447, 451–455.

Algernon Phillips Withiel Thomas
(1857–1937)

Thomas' biography will be found with the preceding article in this chapter.

My experiments on the development of the liver fluke were continued during the summer and autumn of last year, and other experiments have been performed during the present year, or are still in progress.

Renewed search was made for the intermediate host of the liver fluke, and I again endeavored to infect molluscs with the embryo. These experiments have been almost entirely confined to fresh water snails. From the consideration of the geographical distribution of the liver fluke, and of the various species of mollusca, I was led to strongly suspect *Limnaeus pereger* of being the host of the long-sought larval form. The only two fresh water snails found in the Faroe Islands, where the liver fluke is very common, according to von Willemoes-Suhm, are *L. pereger* and *L. truncatulus*. The only aquatic pulmonate in the Shetland Islands where the fluke also occurs is *L. pereger*. If then the bearer of the larval form of *Fasciola hepatica* is a fresh water snail, there is a strong case made out against *L. pereger*. . . .

Experiments with Limnaeus truncatulus. On obtaining the snails I had so long been searching for, I exposed a number to infection by placing fluke eggs and free fluke embryos in the vessel with them. The snails were speedily found to have afforded a suitable place for the further development of the embryos, and of those examined up to the present time all have proved to be infected, often containing as many as 80 embryos. Indeed, the infection was too successful; for about the tenth day, many of the snails began to sink and die simply because they were exhausted by the excessive number of parasites, so that at the end of the fourth week I had only two left alive out of the 80 that had been infected. . . .

Two points which I was enabled to make out during these experiments have a bearing upon the development of other species of trematodes besides the liver fluke. In the first place I found that the snails swallowed the eggs of the fluke contained in the aquaria in large numbers. I had already observed that various species of slugs devoured eggs strewn on their food without injuring them. But in the case of these water snails, the large numbers picked up from the bottom of the aquarium showed that the snails do not swallow the eggs accidentally, but intentionally, no doubt mistaking them for food. The eggs and the contained embryos are uninjured by their passage through the digestive tract, and may be swallowed over and over again. Such being the case, eggs will undoubtedly be often hatched during their passage along the digestive tract; and if the embryos are not killed by the action of the digestive juices, they have only to pass through the walls of the intestine or up the bile ducts into the liver (an organ very frequently infested with sporocysts or rediae) to find themselves, if in a suitable mollusc, in a favorable place for further development.

That the embryos hatched out in the intestine may escape injury from the digestive juices of the snail, I have been able to observe directly in the case of the embryo of the liver fluke. An embryo of this species was seen escaping from an egg in the intestine of a small *L. pereger,* and during the three hours it was under observation it remained alive and active, although bathed in the fluid contents of the intestine. In this case, the embryo was prevented, partly by the pressure of the coverglass, and partly by the presence of other eggs, portions of undigested food, etc., from escaping from the intestine. But in another example of the same species of snail, an active embryo was found free in the body cavity, and as the digestive canal had not been ruptured, it must have bored its way through the walls of the intestine, which contained very numerous eggs.

It is clear, therefore, that those snails which have this habit of swallowing the eggs may be exposed to infection with trematode larvae. The species in which I have more especially noticed the habit are sufficiently numerous (viz. *Limnaeus stagnalis, L. pereger, L. auricularis, L. palustris, Plamorbis marginatus, P. carinatus, Bithynia tentaculata,* as well as three slugs, *Arion ater, Limax agrestis,* and *L. cinereus*) to allow us to assume that it is very generally prevalent amongst our land and fresh water molluscs. . . .

Another of the rediae found in *L. truncatulus* appears to be the same as the one I had already met with in the same snail on infected fields at Wytham. The cercariae produced with it are characterised by the presence of a lobed lateral organ, composed of coarsely granular cells. Leuckart does not consider that this cercaria has any connection with the liver fluke, partly because he did not detect any spines upon the cuticle. I have seen the same larval trematode since writing my former paper, though not in sufficient quantity to allow me to try feeding experiments, and I am able to say that the cuticle of the oldest cercariae is beset anteriorly with spines; in the less mature cercariae they could not be seen. It appears to me that this form is to be regarded with suspicion for the following reasons: (1) Its

anatomical characters are not contradictory to the idea that it may prove to be the larva of *Fasciola;* the cuticle of the anterior part of the body is finely spinose, and the oral and ventral suckers are of nearly equal diameter, the ventral being sometimes a little the larger. The lobed lateral organ I regard, for a reason already given, as merely a passing larval character. (2) The rediae show a greater resemblance to the young rediae descended from fluke eggs, as I have observed them, than do those containing tail-less distomes. The resemblance indeed is very striking. (3) The cercaria has the suspicious habit of encysting itself upon water plants, grass, etc. Moreover, I have twice met with this cercaria in the course of my investigations—on one occasion in almost the only mollusc that could be found on the scene of an outbreak of the liver-rot at Wytham, whereas I have never found the tail-less larval form mentioned by Leuckart. Experiment must decide whether this, or the tail-less form in question, or some other cercaria, is the juvenile form of the liver fluke. . . .

Addendum

Since the above report has been in type I have carried my researches further, and have been enabled to complete the cycle of forms which occur in the life history of the liver fluke.

In a *Limnaeus truncatulus* dissected on the 31st day after the first exposure to infection, I found that the rediae of liver fluke had much increased in size. The largest was 1.12 mm long, and .23 mm broad across the middle of the body. The larger rediae contained nearly a score of germs in various stages of development. The smaller were still spherical; the larger ones, situated more anteriorly, were of an irregular oval shape, with a smooth surface, and enclosed each in a loose and delicate pellicle. The largest germ was .116 mm long by .073 broad. But there was no clear evidence as to the form these spores would assume.

In another snail dissected at the beginning of the seventh week after infection, I found rediae containing cercariae, and although the latter were not quite perfectly mature, they were still far enough advanced to enable me to determine the character of the cercaria. I have mentioned above that Professor Leuckart found tail-less distome—larvae in a redia in *L. truncatulus,* and that, inferring simply from the anatomical character of the larvae, and notwithstanding that the form of the redia was unfavorable to such conjecture, he considered himself entirely justified in assuming, until further results, that these belonged to *Fasciola hepatica*. But I have already shown that the characters of the redia and larvae furnished me with reasons for gravely doubting the correctness of this conjecture, and from my further researches I am now warranted in asserting that this tail-less form does not belong to the liver fluke, for the true cercariae descended from the embryo of the fluke has a tail of considerable length. The body of the cercaria is about a quarter of a millimeter in length, and oral and ventral suckers are of nearly equal size (.05–.06 mm), the ventral sucker being situated just behind the middle of the body. The pharynx is quite distinct, and the digestive tract is simply forked, the two divisions reaching to the end of the body, but not showing any of the numerous branches so characteristic of the adult. Around each cercaria and germ is a loose delicate pellicle.

The rediae containing the cercariae still shows the characteristic ring running round the body a little behind the pharynx, and at the hind end are still visible the two short lateral processes, now, however, more stumpy than in the younger rediae. The digestive tract was short, being only .24 mm long in a redia of four times the length.

There can be no doubt that the cercariae I found really belong to the liver fluke. The rediae in which they occurred were closely similar to those I have found throughout in the examination of the snails I have infected with embryos, and in the same snail with these rediae was a sporocyst, still recognisable by the eye-spots and papilla as belonging to *F. hepatica*. Moreover, *all* the specimens of *L. truncatulus* which I infected have proved to contain larval trematodes, clearly belonging to one and the same zoological species, and as a preliminary precaution a number of snails of the same gathering as those submitted to infection were examined, and all were completely free from larval trematodes.

In the same snail I found also rediae producing not cercariae but other rediae, which we may term daughter-rediae. Indeed I have not been able to prove as yet whether the rediae forming the second generation in the series of forms belonging to the liver fluke ever produce cercariae. In many cases, at any rate, the cercariae only appear as the fourth generation, and it may be that this is always the case. The rediae generating the rediae appear to have a larger pharynx and intestine, and to contain fewer germs than those producing cercariae. I saw as many as three well-formed rediae in a single parent-redia in addition to several smaller germs. The ring behind the pharynx is well-developed, and in one parent-redia I found it so large that the diameter of the body was nearly doubled at this point.

I reserve further details as to the structure of the cercaria and redia for a subsequent paper. I may, however, mention that the existence of as many as four generations gives rise to a great increase in number whilst within the snail; so that a single fluke egg may well give rise to over 1000 cercariae.

The one point remaining that I have still to elucidate is the manner in which the cercariae are transferred to the sheep, and this I hope very soon to accomplish. This may be effected either by the sheep eating the mollusc containing the cercariae, or the cercariae may pass out of the snail and encyst upon grass, etc. The presence of a tail is certainly in favor of the latter view. Leuckart is inclined to believe that the larval flukes are swallowed with the snail containing them, principally on the ground that when flukes are found in an animal, they are usually very numerous. But a stroll around the Oxford meat market is quite enough to convince one that sheep often contain a very limited number of flukes. The bile ducts of the liver are then opened, the flukes removed, and the livers sold for food. Moreover, I have often had livers sent me which contained a very small number of flukes, on one occasion only a single fluke, on another occasion seven.

ON THE LIFE HISTORY OF THE *DISTOMA HEPATICUM*

Zur lebensgeschichte des Distoma hepaticum. Zentralblatt für Bakteriologie und Parasitenkunde, 11: 783–796, 1892. Selections from pp. 791–796. Translated from the German.

Adolfo Lutz
(1855–1940)

Rio de Janeiro was the birthplace of this Brazilian of Swiss ancestry. In 1880 he received his Doctor of

Medicine from Berne, traveled in Europe visiting other medical clinics, and then returned to Brazil to practice clinical medicine. He returned to Europe in 1885 to study the microorganism causing leprosy in the laboratory of Professor Unna of Hamburg. As director of the Leper Hospital in Honolulu from 1889 to 1892, Lutz described the juxta articular nodes of leprosy. He returned to Brazil as assistant director of the Bacteriology Institute and shortly thereafter, he became director. He was a recognized authority on hematophagic arthropods. Under his aegis, the epidemic diseases of cholera, typhoid fever, and diphtheria were studied by the Bacteriological Institute. He made numerous contributions to mycology, parasitology, herpatology, and entomology besides those recorded here.

In spite of the extensive studies of Thomas and Leuckart, many gaps in the complete description of the life cycle of Fasciola hepatica *remained. Experimental proof that animals acquire* F. hepatica *by swallowing the encysted stage is found in this article.*

. . . I had the impression from the literature that the mature cercariae passively emerge from the host animal. For this species, however, I must absolutely deny this phenomenon. The cercaria certainly can slip out of the genital opening of the redia, but then it remains inside the tissue of the host, relatively quiescent and without taking on solid food, until it is liberated either by the death of the animal or by breaking of the shell. *Every undamaged snail, therefore, still contains the complete number of the previously produced cercariae.* If one pulls a heavily infected *Lymnaeus* from its shell (and this is rather easy to do), one can look completely through the superior end of the visceral sack filled with parasites and observe the slow movements of the mature cercariae, while the mature rediae, especially their neck parts, still appear rather mobile. If one adds some water, the cercariae do become a little more lively, but only reach their full activity when the abdominal wall of the host is torn and the water touches them directly. The tail then begins to move so vigorously that one can see its contours only on both ends of the trajectory in the form of an "8." I can only see herein an expression of dislike for the new medium; this is followed very soon by formation of a cyst. The production of the cyst material, however, can only occur when the organism has found a support, for which a longer period of swimming is often necessary. When this has happened, no time is wasted in forming the cyst, and soon the larva becomes

apathetic, in marked contrast to the spasmodic movements of the free cercaria.

As the cercaria migrates from the undamaged and living *Lymnaea* (resp. the Melania), so it may encyst on it. This can only occur if the upper end of the shell has been damaged. The latter, however, occurs more easily, since very frequently the first shell windings seem eroded (probably by calcium-dissolving microorganisms). After contact with the water, even immature or poorly mobile cercariae encyst. One recognizes their outer coat by the much more roughly granulated material; frequently it remains incomplete, and in any case useless since such premature cercariae soon perish. The redia, too, first becomes immobile under such circumstances and then dies gradually.

Kept in a larger vessel the cercariae encyst on the surface as well as on the bottom; it is true, plant parts are utilized readily, but are not noticeably preferred. In the aquarium one not infrequently sees other *Lymnaea* with cysts on the shell; in nature, of course, this will occur much less frequently. I have found encysted *Distoma* still alive after two months; however, some of them perish probably for the same reasons as the offspring. This happens particularly when the water is not replaced frequently; in running water their life span might be very considerable.

If the cysts are attached to plant parts which gradually decompose, the former detach themselves gradually and sink to the bottom. But the adhesion to the base is loosened in time, especially if this is smooth, so that currents in the water are sufficient to detach the cysts. Most of the cysts are found in the sediment of the waters where they can easily rise due to their slight specific weight. In this way they can easily get into the stomachs of animals while they are drinking, especially when the animals first wade into the shallow water. Anyone who has ever observed the procedure knows that during drinking, large quantities of sediments are lapped up by the larger animals. Therefore, I consider this method of infection by far the most frequent and, for some of the places examined by me, the only important one. Snails surely are swallowed, even if not particularly frequently, but it is highly questionable whether an infection can be caused in this way. In any case, unencysted cercariae are also swallowed most easily by drinking.

As far as the eating of plants covered with

cysts is concerned, this can occur at the drinking place; it was my experience that cabbage leaves thrown into the water for catching snails were eaten by the cattle. However, as is known, the grass growing in swampy places is usually spurned by the cattle, and in flooded pastures the cysts quickly perish when the water level drops. In individual cases such conditions might occur; for instance, in epidemics among rabbits. However, it is probably unproved that rabbits do not drink water. The food which they find outside probably is not as juicy as that which my rabbits eat, and yet they do not scorn to drink water at all.

The influence of wet years upon liver epidemics is sufficiently explained by the facile development of the *Distoma* eggs; the spread of the *Lymnaea* is also favored. In contrast, the place and mode of infection are hardly influenced.

The experiment which has been cited by Leuckart (Friedberger and Frohner's *Manual of Spec. Pathology and Therapy of Domestic Animals,* Stuttgart, 1886) on the feeding of grass snails from a suspected sheep pasture proves nothing without details, and the designation "grass snails" is hardly applicable to *Lymnaea.* By the way, I hope to experiment soon with infected *Lymnaea.*

For examination purposes the cercariae encyst on glass plates or in dishes, in which thin sheets of insoluble gelatin have been placed. For experiments I take a piece of paper on which the date is written and I place it, folded filterlike, in a porcelain dish or, flat with folded-up edges, in a photographic cup. The cup is filled with water, and the snail is placed in it after its shell has been cut open by a scissor from the upper end of the opening to its point. In this way, all the cysts are collected on the paper and stained, if desired; after rinsing, they are free of foreign particles. They can be kept in water as long as desired; scraped from the softened paper without damage after some time; or cut out with manicure scissors and mixed with the food or drink. (On silk paper they are even suitable for microscopic examination.) Plant parts are recommended only for early use.

I now turn to the results of my transmission experiments. Up to now, they have been made on three guinea pigs, a kid, and a piglet. My first results, which are probably the first ones in this field, were produced on a guinea pig which was not previously known as host of the liver fluke; at least for the first stage it proved a favorable experimental subject. The kid died accidentally, probably as the result of too early weaning, 20 hours after the feeding of some hundred older cysts. In the stomach and the biliary passages, in spite of careful examination neither cysts nor their contents were found; these probably passed completely (perhaps because of insufficient digestive activity) or went through the intestinal tract without hatching. In the piglet, which in the course of a week had at various times received numerous cysts of different ages, no young *Distoma* were found; unfortunately, the stomach was completely full in spite of prolonged fasting, and with the already considerably large liver an absolutely exhaustive search for the one-millimeter-long organisms was impossible.

After reporting these failures, I now come to the positive results. The experimental animals were two grown guinea pigs and a very young, half-grown guinea pig. The cysts were given partly on greens and partly on wet bread. One could assume from the one-week-old and otherwise well-preserved *Distoma* cysts that the majority of the larvae reached their destination. The two larger animals died of the infection; the smaller one was sacrificed.

The first guinea pig was given on 23 and again on 24 December about 20 older cysts; on the 27th it received about 20 which were a week old. Some loss in the feeding of the first portions was expected since they had been scraped from the walls of a glass container; the later ones were encysted on grass which had been kept in water with the roots. Some of both types may have been lost during feeding. This experimental animal was found dead on 23 January 1892 and showed the following autopsy findings:

The abdominal cavity was filled with free blood which coagulated soon after opening. There was a considerable serous extravasation, which was slightly mixed with the blood. The surface of the liver was normal only in certain parts of the right lobe; otherwise, it was hyperemic, finely granulated, and covered with a fibrinous exudate. Under the serosa there were many small cavities filled with blood and in the parenchyma numerous small, worm-shaped blood clots. In one of the cavities a *Distomum* about 8 mm long was found without difficulty; it contracted actively, thereby changing its shape considerably. Its branched intestine was filled with a brown liquid which flowed back and forth during the contractions but was soon largely excreted. Excretory vessels and spiny scales were very evident, the latter particularly anteriorly.

Since the large biliary passages (including the bladder) proved to be empty and the finer biliary passages could not be followed because of the smallness of the worm, the following procedure was employed in the examination.

The liver was kept in lukewarm water while one lobe after the other was examined; finally, about one-quarter of the whole mass was placed in alcohol for later examination. The individual lobes were cut into pieces which were crushed between glass slides. In this way the whole liver (except for the lobe mentioned) was carefully scrutinized under light and all *Distoma* were collected; a number of specimens were also retrieved from the water which had come out during the sectioning of the liver. The total count was 29 *Distoma;* the smallest was about 4¾ mm long with a greatest width of about 1½ mm; the measurements of the largest were 9½:2½ mm. Dead parasites or those stiffened by cold were also measured, thus the differences in the individual specimens were clearly apparent. In any case, however, significant differences in size exist which were probably not to be explained only by the difference in age, since other conditions also must have contributed. A small nodule in the lung might have contained a lost parasite.

The examination of the other organs was more casual and revealed nothing abnormal; the liver itself was so carefully examined that probably not one specimen escaped.

The next day the other guinea pig also died of serous peritonitis and liver hemorrhage. The liver showed exactly the same condition; here also the right lobe was somewhat less involved and the left lobe was very extensively invaded; the surface of the liver was covered with a fibrinous exudate.

In this instance, about 20 older cysts had been given 32 days before death. Eighteen flukes were found, of which only one was in the liver, while the other 17 were dispersed throughout the peritoneal cavity. Their size was more uniform; however, there were considerable variations.

The third, very young, guinea pig was killed after it had received, 44 days previously, a few older cysts and, nine and eight days before, many two-week-old cysts. About 20 flukes, approximately 1 mm long were found, in addition to a larger one, in the fibrinous exudate of the surface. The flukes were very difficult to find and were so delicate that only a few could be found undamaged. The liver was permeated by a mass of winding passages with walls apparently infiltrated by pus. These infiltrates were considerably thicker than the diameter of the parasites and evidently did not correspond to normally existing channels.

From these experiments, I have drawn the following conclusions:

In the guinea pigs (and the same probably holds true for other small rodents) the invading flukes soon go to the periphery of the liver and when the normal bile passages have become too narrow, they burrow further, independently, through the soft parenchyma. Having reached the surface, they perforate the capsule and thus can reach the peritoneal cavity where they live perhaps for some time, but probably do not reach full development even if the host survives this emigration. (Here, perhaps, lies the explanation for the negative results of Leuckart's experiments on rabbits.)

As far as these flukes observed by me were concerned, there is no doubt that they came from the cysts which were fed, since they correspond completely to the descriptions of Thomas and Leuckart, and my guinea pigs otherwise have never shown liver flukes. . . .

The spiny covering and the excretory system seem completely developed at a very early stage. In my smallest specimens the intestine (observed full) seemed to show only convolutions and yet no clear ramifications; however, the latter soon appear and also quickly become complete. In the young flukes the ventral sucker is prominent and is probably important for locomotion. Of the sexual organs, the cirrus pouch and shell gland appear first, then the uterus, the testes, and the vitelline apparatus follow. The recognition of these structures, however, is quite difficult since the first stages have little that is characteristic, and the parenchyma, in place of the later vesicular formations, shows only tightly compressed, small round cells. The earlier young forms also seem capable of great liveliness and considerable strength. . . .

NEW FACTS ON THE BIOLOGY OF THE *FASCIOLA HEPATICA*

Neue tatsachen über die biologie der Fasciola hepatica L. Zentralblatt für Bakteriologie und Parasitenkunde, Sec. 1, 74: 280–285, 1914. Translated from the German.

Dimitry F. Ssinitzin
(1871–1937)

Ssinitzin was born in Symferopol, Crimea, in 1871. He did his undergraduate work at the University of Warsaw, then part of Polish Russia, and received his doctorate in zoology from the University of St. Petersburg.

At the time he presented the new details of the life history of Fasciola, *he was a professor in Shanjasky University in Moscow and had already won a reputation among parasitologists for his important studies on the trematodes of frogs and fishes. He subsequently held academic positions of high rank and was president of Nijny-Novgorod University between 1918 and 1919. For political reasons, he was forced to escape from Russia in 1923. Taking refuge in the United States at the age of 52, Ssinitzin lived for some time in abject poverty and then commenced a new career. First obtaining employment as a technician at the American Museum of Natural History, he later became associate zoologist in the Bureau of Animal Industry in Washington, D.C., and finally moved to California where he engaged in private research. Ssinitzin described his experiments as might a novelist who imagines how one of his characters would act. (D. F. Ssinitzin,* Methods I have Followed in My Research. J. Parasitology, 13: 84–86, 1926).

"I am now a cercaria which has just emerged from its cyst and has found itself in the intestinal tract of a sheep. On me are poured smart, biting fluids from the digestive glands and I wish nothing more than to escape this horrible place. . . . What am I to do? If I were smaller, I should penetrate into a blood vessel but I am too big for that; Dr. Leuckart advises me to look for the opening of the gall duct in the duodenum, but while I am listening to him I am transported far behind this opening and how can I, in such a spacious hollow filled with moving food, find that commended spot? I do not accept this advice; I hasten to conceal myself any place; I work my way into the bottom, between the folds of the epithelium and penetrate through the intestinal wall.

"The picture is finished. The work of the imagination is over. Now the experiment: I feed a rabbit encysted cercaria; after a lapse of time I open its abdominal cavity, pour in cold water and then rinse out the water into a glass cup and at the bottom of it I find the young Distoma *or liver fluke. The experiment is over!"*

Our knowledge of the life cycle of Fasciola hepatica *was completed when Ssinitzin demonstrated that the young flukes migrate through the intestinal wall into the abdominal cavity and then penetrate the liver.*

Leuckart's and Thomas' investigations of the liver fluke are rightly counted among the classic ones, since in them, for the first time, the complicated history of the transformations of the trematodes has been pursued almost from beginning to end. Nevertheless there are gaps in these observations, and not all conclusions drawn by these investigators appear to be proven by experimental facts.

They have unquestionably established that the eggs of *Fasciola hepatica* need water for their further development; the miracidium emerges and penetrates the mollusc, *Limnaea truncatula*, and this produces a generation of parthenogenetic females, sporocysts, and redias. Further, it has been proved that the cercariae of this type do not encyst in the body of any intermediate animal host, but on grass. Regarding later phases, namely the manner in which sheep and horned cattle are infected by this *Distoma* and how the young *Distoma* reaches the liver of its host, we only have assumptions because Leuckart's experiments attempting to produce an infection with the cysts of the liver fluke had negative results. In addition, there are certain facts which Leuckart explained inadequately; for instance, that distomiasis occurs frequently in regions where *L. truncatula* is not found; that the animals grazing on wet meadows are not more (and sometimes even less) infected than those grazing in dry and more highly situated places; that a number of cases are known where *F. hepatica* has been found in men who under no circumstances had eaten grass and the like. This suggests that Leuckart's and Thomas' observations are not always complete and that many important data have been disregarded by these investigators.

In order to correct and complete those data, I instituted in my laboratory a series of observations on the liver fluke which occurs frequently within the territory of Moscow. The work began only recently, and it is difficult to determine when it will be finished; however, facts have already emerged which essentially supplement Leuckart's investigations and which, it seems to me, could be of significant value in devising a practical method of combating this parasite. For this reason I have decided to publish some of our observations in preliminary form, prior to their completion.

From our own observations and data gathered by an inquiry among the inhabitants, I can state that the Moscow area is widely infected by *F. hepatica;* however, this cannot be said of the host of its parthenogenetic generation, *L. truncatula.* During a five-month search I succeeded in discovering this mollusc in only a few areas around Moscow and only in small numbers. I found none in the meadows flooded by high waters where distomiasis is generally less prevalent. Instinctively, one arrives at the supposition that, in addition to *L. truncatula,* some other mollusc can serve the liver fluke as primary host. However, after further investigations, I have concluded that *L. truncatula* is the only carrier of the parthenogenetic generation of *F. hepatica* and that consequently this part of Leuckart's and Thomas' observations remains unchallenged. How does one explain the disparity between the limited spread of *L. truncatula* and the exceptionally large one of *F. hepatica?* This question was to be answered by investigating the life cycle of the cercariae and their cysts, since only these two unite the two periods of the life cycle of the liver fluke. The results fulfilled my expectations.

In the free state, cercariae of the liver fluke last a very short time, as Leuckart also pointed out; as soon as they have left *L. truncatula* they encyst by attachment to any immovable object. This encysting process needed closer study, and this was started by my pupil, Mr. M. Domontovich. Among other things he determined the height, with respect to the surface of the water, up to which these cercariae encyst; his observations on the vertical distribution of cysts of *F. hepatica,* more than 2,000 in number, have been summarized. . . . [Diagram omitted—Eds.].

The largest number of cercariae (66 per cent) encyst ½ cm below the surface of the water; the rest either deeper (about 24 per cent) or higher (about 10 per cent) than the surface of the water.

Most interesting is the fact that about 6 per cent of the total cercaria mass in the free state encysts directly on the surface of the water. . . . The cercariae react to a membrane of surface tension as to a solid body; they attach themselves by suction and begin to encyst. First they produce the outer covering which from one side has the appearance of a round disc indented in the center; this indentation faces the water. On the other side the covering is shaped like a semispherical arch which hangs downward freely. Then the cercaria produces a second covering which directly surrounds its body. As can be seen from this description, the outer covering serves as a swimming apparatus; in fact, these cysts maintain themselves very well on the water. If one attempts to push one down with a pin, a bubble of air appears in the described indentation which brings it again to the surface as soon as the pin is removed. If this experiment is repeated several times, it is finally possible to make the air bubble leave the cyst, which sinks to the bottom since it is heavier than water.

From this observation, the following practical conclusions can be drawn.

(1) If the cercariae of *F. hepatica* can form sessile cysts as well as those that swim, then infection of sheep and cattle is possible not only through grass but also through water.

(2) An infection of the animal can occur not only in regions where cercariae develop, especially where *L. truncatula* lives, but also in places reached by water from these points; that is, in all brooks, ponds, puddles, and other sources of drinking water for animals which are supplied from there.

(3) An infection with the liver fluke can also occur in man, if he drinks such water.

(4) If there are some regions where *L. truncatula* infected with *F. hepatica* are found, then an infection with the liver fluke is possible wherever drinking water is obtained from these places and if, as a result of rain or flooding of rivers, the water overflows beyond the usual boundaries, the infection appears then in new, unaccustomed places—an epidemic starts.

Another observation which I want to discuss here relates to the manner in which the young *Distoma* gets from the intestine into the liver of the host.

Leuckart attempted to infect a rabbit[1] by feeding it with cysts of the liver fluke, but he was not successful. However, he gave a very definite description, reasonable and natural, of the migrations of the young *Distoma*. He maintained that the young *Distoma,* after it becomes free of its cysts in the host's intestine, begins its migration, searches for an opening in the biliary passage, penetrates it, and thus reaches the biliary passages of the liver. Leuckart and other investigators found the very youngest *Distoma* in the peripheral parts of the liver and more mature ones in the central part. Leuckart further describes the migration of the young *Distoma* in the following way: having reached the gall bladder, it continues migrating in the biliary passages until it reaches the peripheral parts of the liver, where it stops and remains for a time before gradually returning to the gall bladder.

Such a migration of the young *Distoma* seemed to me unnatural from the beginning and not very probable. It is difficult to imagine how, in relation to its microscopic size, a weak, young *Distoma* just recently escaped from the cyst, could move into the immense space of a sheep's intestine, undertake getting to the duodenum, and find the tiny opening of the biliary passage. Furthermore, it seemed improbable to me that such a weak *Distoma* should be able to overcome the current of the bile stream and wander through this stream from the intestine to the gall bladder.

The migration of the young *Distoma* from the gall bladder to the periphery of the liver and back again was also untenable to me.

When I began to doubt the correctness of Leuckart's conclusions, I started to infect rabbits experimentally, assuming that the penetration of the young *Distoma* into the liver could take place every other way, but not through the biliary passage. I have made several series of experiments which, to date, have furnished positive results without exception, and I have obtained young *Distoma* of different ages; namely of 1, 2, 3, 4, 7, 10, 14, 17, 21, 24, 32, and 39 days.

In order not to exceed the boundaries of a preliminary report, I will omit all details regarding the arrangement of my experiments and my observations and limit myself to a report of the final results.

The young *Distomas* free themselves from the cyst from two to three hours after they have reached the intestine of the rabbit. Then they penetrate the intestinal wall into the body cavity, crawl around there from four to 14 days on the various organs, including the liver; then they attach themselves by suction to the latter, bore in, and penetrate further every day by means of the biliary passages. The strong mouth suction cup and the hard, pointed spines which are found on the mature ones, instead of the scales, and which cover the body of the young *Distoma* in regular rows, make penetration of this microscopic organism through the intestinal wall easily comprehensible. With this apparatus the young *Distoma* nourishes itself in the body cavity the same way the mature one nourishes itself in the liver; namely, with blood corpuscles, which it takes from the capillaries found on the surface of the various organs lying in the body cavity. Of all these organs, the liver, because of its loose tissue and rich blood supply, is the most suitable place for such nourishment. Hence the *Distomas* gradually gather one after the other on the liver. However, I found, as late as the 14th day after infection, a few specimens of young *Distomas* in the body cavity which differed markedly in their nutritional state from their brothers in the liver. In the first four days I did not find young *Distomas* in the liver of an infected rabbit. They were still in the body cavity. It is now understandable why the results of Leuckart's infection experiments on rabbits were negative. In reality, the experiment probably succeeded, but he looked for the *Distomas* in the liver at a time when they were still in the body cavity.

I must add to this that, when the young *Distomas* penetrate the liver, they leave behind openings from which blood seeps. Consequently, after an attack by numerous *Distomas,* a large hemorrhage occurs, and considerable blood accumulates in the body cavity; the liver becomes bloodless, contracts, and the animal dies. It is thus permissible to assume that the epidemic of sheep deaths stems not only from the causes pointed out by Leuckart but also from a large hemorrhage of the liver.

---

[1]The rabbits and hares are infected by the liver fluke to the same degree as the horned animals; therefore, hunters observe an epidemic among hares at the time of a severe distomiasis epidemic among sheep.

CHAPTER **29**

Fasciolopsiasis

ON DISEASES OF THE LIVER

In: George Budd's On Diseases of the Liver, 2d ed. London: John Churchill, 1852, 486 pp. Selections from pp. 484–485.

George Busk
(1807–1886)

Born in St. Petersburg, where his English father was a successful merchant, George Busk was sent to England for the typical preparatory school education of a member of the upper middle class. During this period, he acquired a passion for natural history which he never lost despite the fact that he became a physician, receiving his training as a student of the College of Surgeons and later at St. Thomas' and St. Bartholomew's hospitals. During service as surgeon on board the Seamen's Hospital (the famous Dreadnought*) Ship at Greenwich, he studied the pathology of cholera and made important observations on scurvy. After retiring from his naval post, he settled in London and devoted himself to scientific pursuits, principally to the microscopic investigation of the lower forms of life and especially the Bryozoa. He was also interested in paleontology and did significant scholarly work in that area.*

Busk recorded here the first description of the parasite which Lankester later named Fasciolopsis buski.

In the winter of 1843, 14 flukes were found by Mr. Busk in the duodenum of a Lascar [an East Indian sailor or native artilleryman—Eds.] who died in the *Dreadnought*. There were none in the gall bladder or gall ducts. These flukes were much thicker and larger than those of the sheep, being from an inch and a half to near three inches in length. They resembled the *Distoma hepaticum* in shape, but were like the *Distoma lanceolatum* in structure; the double alimentary canal, as in the latter variety, being not branched, and the entire space between it toward the latter part of the body being occupied by a branched uterine tube. Two of these flukes, which were given me by Mr. Busk, are in the museum of King's College and from one of them, which is

584

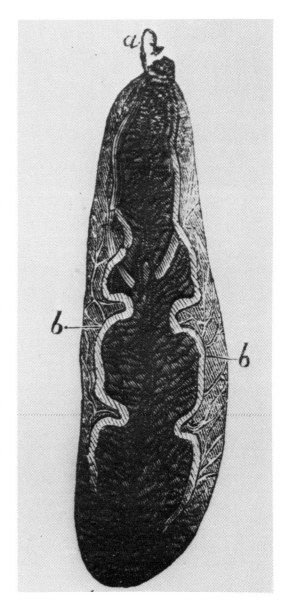

Plate 95. A fluke from the duodenum of a man, injected. (a) ligature round the neck; (b) alimentary tube.

injected with size and vermilion, the annexed woodcut (Plate 95) was made.

ON THE LIFE CYCLE OF *FASCIOLOPSIS BUSKI*, LANKESTER

Kitasato Archives of Experimental Medicine, 4, (2): 159–167, 1921 (Extracted).

Koan Nakagawa
(1874–1959)

A graduate of the Department of Medicine, Fourth High School (predecessor of the Kanazana Medical College) in 1894, he practiced medicine in Tokyo until 1904, when he entered the medical service of the Taiwan Government General. He rose rapidly and by 1926 was the chief physician of the Taiwan government and director of the largest hospital. He held many public offices, yet was a productive investigator in parasitology and medicine.

This is the original description of the life cycle of Fasciolopsis buski. *Nakagawa's article was printed in English. As his English is so much better than our Japanese, we have not altered the few grammatical errors which are evident.*

Introduction

Fasciolopsis buski is a human parasite found extensively in the Far East, especially in China. Though this worm has hygienic importance in that region, little is known about it. In Formosa it is very frequently found in pigs, but no human cases have as yet been reported there.

Ever since 1915, when I discovered some new facts about the lung fluke, my attention has been directed towards the investigation of the life cycle of this fluke.

Since the morphological features of *F. buski* bear a close resemblance to those of *Fasciola hepatica*, I conjectured that they may take a similar course of development. Consequently it might not be a difficult matter to trace the life history of the former. When I began the study of this worm, I soon met with a great difficulty in obtaining the material. The facts that are dealt with in the present paper is the fruit of my study during the past five years.

Methods

The specimens that had been obtained from the pigs were washed thoroughly with water. They were allowed to lay eggs in water. During sum-mer season, they hatched into the miracidia in 2–3 weeks. They swam about freely in the water. These miracidiae were kept in the water with several species of water snails to see which snails they prefer to infest. It was my plan to trace the further development of the miracidia in the intermediate host till they encyst, and then to give the final host the encysted larvae so that to get full grown flukes. Since I did not follow the above mentioned method of investigation, I failed to identify any of 17 different forms of cercariae found at Shinchiku, Formosa.

Intermediate Hosts

I have seen that miracidiae of *Fasciolopsis buski* penetrate into the four species of water snails, *Limnaea pervia* Mart(?), *Pl. compressus*, Hutton, *Pl. coenosus* Benson and *Segmentina largillierti* Dkr. I thought at first that *Limnea* serves as the intermediate host of *Fasciolopsis buski*, but it was not the case; for by repeated experiments I failed to make the miracidia develop further in the water snail. It was the same with *Pl. compressus*. In the present investigation, therefore, I have employed only two last mentioned species of snails, *Pl. coenosus* and *Segmentina largillierti*. It should be mentioned that water snails collected from brooks and the ditches failed to live long in the aquarium; of all the scores of snails artificially infested and kept in confinement, only two or three were found to be alive after a few months. In the surviving individuals cercariae were found. These cercariae have a tendency to encyst at the bottom of the water. Since the cercariae could not be identified to any that I have ever seen, I considered that they would surely be those of the species under question. I then gave to a cat the encysted cercariae liberated by crushing the snails (September 1917 at Shinchiku). This experiment turned out to be a failure. Afterwards, it was found that this was due to the fact that the cercariae were too young. The results of the experiment thus having been proved negative, I could not at that juncture obtain any notion about the identification of the cercariae. I, therefore, tried another series of experiments. This time I considered it necessary to employ the water snails free from any species of cercariae. But trouble was that such cercaria-free snails can never be obtained from their natural habitats. I, therefore, tried to artificially raise the snail in the aquarium from the eggs. After several trials, I finally succeeded in cultivating *Pl. coenosus* and *Segmentina largillierti* from the eggs. These snails absolutely free from cercariae were infected with the miracidia of *Fasciolopsis buski* and in these snails I was fortunate enough to obtain all the stages of development of the fluke. I also succeeded in obtaining the full-grown flukes from those encysted cercariae. Thus it may be concluded that the intermediate hosts of *Fasciolopsis buski* are *Pl. coenosus* Benson and *Segmentia largillierti* Dkr. in Formosa.

Development of *Fasciolopsis buski* in the Intermediate Hosts

Pl. coenosus and *S. largillierti* raised from the eggs strewn into aquarium in which numerous miracidia of *Fasciolopsis buski* had been swimming, were soon found covered by swarming miracidia which tried to bore into the head, foot, tentacles, mantle etc. They left their ciliated coats as they penetrated into the snail. In the tissues of the host, they ceased to move and turned into elliptical sporocysts (0.08 mm × 0.07 mm). In five days from the infection they grew considerably (0.17 mm × 0.1 mm). The flame cell could still readily be seen. In seven days from the infection, the rediae were found in the sporocysts (0.2 mm × 0.1 mm). By this time, they migrated as far as the mantle or into the walls of the alimentary canal. The rediae of the ninth day were doubled their sizes, the largest ones measuring 0.42 mm. in length and 0.17 mm in breadth. They had a broad pharynx measuring 0.08 mm in diameter. The intestines were very wide and filled with a dark brown substance. In the anterior part of the body of the redia and just posterior to the pharynx was a ring shaped protuberance. In the posterior part of the body, there were also two lateral protuberances. They moved about fairly briskly. In ten days some of them reached already the liver.

In 14 days, the largest redia measured 0.5 mm in length and 0.17 mm in breadth. The lumen of the alimentary canal had narrowed. The contents had turned into deep black. Several germ cell masses were present and had grown larger.

On the thirty-fifth day, young cercariae developed in the rediae. There were seen a number of cases, in which young redia developed in the [parent] redia. On the fortieth day, the redia measured 1.0–1.5 mm long and 0.23 mm wide.

The body walls of the redia became usually light brown. The cercariae in the redia, would gradually grow and measure 0.23 mm long by 0.13 mm wide. The cercaria had a long tail measuring 0.4–0.5 mm. In the cercaria, the cyst forming cells were found and gave a dark appearance. At this period, a few coarse granules appeared near the lower ends of the limbs of the excretory organs. Each redia contained some 4–7 cercariae.

The fully grown cercariae has less pigment granules than in the younger ones, owing to the excretion of the cyst forming substance. They measure 0.21–0.23 mm in length and 0.12–0.15 mm in breadth. The tail is long, and measures some 2–3 times the length of the body. The general form of the cercaria is flat and appears like a tadpole. The oral sucker is situated on the abdominal surface, having a diameter of 0.04 mm. The pharynx is situated immediately posterior to the oral sucker. It assumes a spherical shape, having a diameter of 0.02 mm. The intestinal canal soon bifurcates, but it is very difficult to observe. The limbs of the excretory organ are long and take a tortuitous course along the lateral sides of the body. They are very conspicuous due to the presence of a coarse granular substance which is remarkably refractile. The excretory vesicle is very small. It has an elliptical form. The abdominal sucker is situated a little posterior to the middle of the body and anterior to the excretory vesicle. It is 0.03 mm in diameter. Soon after liberation, the full grown cercariae attach themselves to the grass on which they encyst.

The encysted cercaria is disk shaped, having a diameter of 0.13–0.135 mm. The excretory organ filled with the coarse granular substance is peculiar to this species and is a reliable differential character. The wall of the cyst consists of two layers, the thickness being 0.007 mm. Around this cyst is attached the residue of the cercaria which is faintly yellowish.

The above described developmental changes were observed in the water snails experimentally infected with the miracidia on April 19, 1920. The cercariae obtained from the water snails that were already infested on May 15th of the same year, developed very rapidly and in 38 days the full grown cercariae were already found and the cysts had been formed.

The cercariae like those described above were seen in April 1918 in the water snails collected at a small pond situated in Ronnansho village near Shinchiku. My attention was then especially directed to that region because of the abundance of pigs infected by *F. buski* there.

Animal Experiments

Since I found out that the encysted cercariae of *F. buski* are on the water grass, some series of animal experiments were performed to get full grown flukes. The droppings of the experimental animals were examined several times. The animals that had been diagnosed to be free from the infection alone were employed for experiment. During the entire course of the experiments, they were fed with nothing but thoroughly boiled food.

Experiment I: Puppy:—The animal was fed on June 19, 1920, with 40 specimens of the encysted cercariae and then on June 22, it was again fed with 50 encysted cercariae. On July 16, 1920, the puppy was killed for examination. The intervals between the feeding and the killing of the animal were 24 and 27 days, respectively.

Post mortem examination:—The small intestines were taken out and cut open. Numerous small distomes were found squirming in the duodenum and jejunum. I collected 59 specimens in all. The spleen and the gall bladder were found to be free from the worms.

The distome is grayish white in color and measures 2–3 mm in length and 1–2 mm in breadth (in formalin). The oral sucker is ventrally situated, having the diameter of 0.25 mm. The pharynx is spherical, the diameter of which is 0.12 mm. The intestine bifurcates quite close to the pharynx. Each limb running along the side of the body ends near each other. Towards its terminal portion the intestines take a zigzag course. The abdominal sucker is large and conspicuous, measuring 0.6 mm. in diameter. It is situated remarkably anteriorly. The reproductive organs are not well developed. The genital pore is situated immediately anterior to the abdominal sucker. The cirrus sac is a long thread-like tube running posteriorly along the median line. The uterus is a simple tube attached to the posterior end of the cirrus sac. The shell gland is at the posterior end of the uterus. The ovary is represented by a group of cells situating lateral to the shell gland. The vitellarium is not yet developed. The testes lie still posteriorly to the ovary, being

two branching cell masses lying behind the other. The excretory vesicle is very small and opens at the posterior end of the body. Both the limbs of the excretory organ commence at a level just below the oral sucker and run straight along the side of the body and go into the excretory vesicle. The skin is provided with short spines, which are scattered here and there.

Experiment 2. Young pig:—On June 15, 1920, 45 encysted cercariae were given to a young pig. On June 19, 45 and June 22, 70 cercariae were again given to the same animal. It was killed on July 17, i.e. 25, 28 and 33 days from feeding with the cercariae.

Post mortem findings:—Nourishment good. 74 specimens of the worm were collected from the intestines.

In the physiological saline, the worms move about rather briskly in a leech like fashion. Some of the elongated specimens measure 10 mm long. The largest specimens are somewhat reddish. In formalin, they measure 2–4 mm long by 1–3 mm wide. Differing only in sizes, they have the morphological features agreeing perfectly with the ones found in the dog.

Experiment 3: Young pig:—The animal was fed with a small number of the encysted cercariae on June 19, 1920 and 29 cercariae on June 22. On September 20, the eggs of *F. buski* were found in the droppings. The animal was killed for examination on the same day, i.e. 90–93 days after the feeding of the cercariae.

Post mortem findings:—Nourishment fairly good. From the small intestines (mostly from the coecum) 23 specimens of *F. buski* were found. In formalin, they measured 13–15 mm in length and 6–8 mm in breadth. None was found either in the liver or the gall bladder.

Living specimens are foliacious and red. The elongated one measures 20 mm long by 10 mm wide. The oral sucker is 0.4 mm in diameter. A globular pharynx measuring 0.5 mm in diameter is situated close to the oral sucker. The intestine bifurcates immediately behind the pharynx, and each limb runs along the side of the body and after taking a winding course each ends near the posterior end of the body. The abdominal sucker is shifted remarkably toward the anterior end of the body. It is quite large, having the diameter of 1.0 mm. The genital pore opens near the anterior margin of the abdominal sucker. The cirrus sac runs along the median line of the body. It has a long cylindrical shape on the whole, having an uneven surface. The ovary and the shell glands are situated nearly at the middle of the body. The testes lie posterior and the uterus anterior, to the ovary. The ovary is bifurcated and appears something like the antlers of a deer. It is situated right to the midian line. There are two testes, one lying behind the other. Each testis still further branches and presents a fine dentritic form. The vitellaria occupy the whole space near the lateral margins and the posterior end of the body. The ovum has a lightly yellowish brown color, measuring 0.12–0.13 mm in length and 0.08 mm in breadth. The specimens, though small, are mature and agree in every respect with *Fasciolopis buski.*

From what has been said it will be seen that my premise that the life cycle of *F. buski* resembles that of *Fasciola hepatica* turned out to be true. From the eggs that found their way into the water, the miracidia come out which go into the water snail, the first intermediate host. In the water snail, they develop into the sporocysts, rediae and cercariae. The cercariae again get in to the water and there they attach to the water plants or the like and encyst waiting a chance to be devoured by the final hosts.

Mode of Infection and Its Prevention

The mode of infection of *F. buski* is very simple. The only means of being infected is to eat raw water plants, which carry the encysted cercariae or to drink the water containing them.

The preventive measures, therefore, are to prohibit the eating raw water plants and drinking the water without boiling. The fresh water fish and molluscs sometimes contain the encysted cercariae, and the eating of them, uncooked, must also be prohibited. The washing of the table utensils and vessels in the water from the ditches and rivers is better to be avoided.

In order to eradicate the worm, the disinfection of the faeces containing the eggs and the hygienic disposal of the infected domestic animals, and the destruction of the intermediate hosts should be enforced.

Summary

The results of the study on the development of *Fasciolopsis buski,* which I have hitherto attained may be summarized as follows:

(1) In Formosa, *F. buski* Lankester has been found only in the pigs, but not in man.

(2) From the eggs of *F. buski* hatch out the miracidia in 2–3 weeks after they have been put in the water during the summer time in Formosa (chiefly in the districts of Shinchiku and Taichyu).

(3) The intermediate hosts of *F. buski* in Formosa are *Planorbis coenosus* Benson and *Segmentina largillierti* Dkr.

(4) The cercariae of *F. buski* develop in the intermediate hosts. The characteristic feature of the cercariae is the conspicuous limbs of the excretory organs, which is provided with coarse granules. The encysted cercariae that are found attached to the water plants also have this characteristic.

(5) By feeding the dog and the pig with the encysted cercariae, fully grown *F. buski* were found in the small intestines.

(6) The mode of infection of *F. buski* is very simple, i.e., the infection takes place from eating raw water plants or drinking water without boiling.

(7) The preventive measures against being infected by this parasite is to prohibit the eating raw water plants, molluscs, fishes, and also drinking the river or pond water without boiling. It is also important to take special care of the infected animals and to destroy the intermediate hosts.

I deem it proper here to express my sincere thanks to Prof. Miyajima, in the Kitasato Institute for Infectious Diseases, for his kind suggestions which he gave me regarding the present work.

THE LIFE CYCLE OF THE HUMAN INTESTINAL FLUKE *FASCIOLOPSIS BUSKI* (LANKESTER)

American Journal of Hygiene, Monographic Series, No. 4. 1925. 93 pp. Selections from pp. 1–2, 7–8, 12, 17, 25, 32–33, 35, 38, 41, 45, 49, 53–54, 58–59, 60–66, 68–69, 86, 98.

Claude Heman Barlow
(1876–1969)

This unorthodox researcher in tropical medicine studied several self-inflicted parasitic diseases including malaria, fasciolopsiasis buski, and schistosomiasis haematobium. A native of Michigan and a graduate of Northwestern Medical School, he worked in China as a Baptist missionary from 1908 until 1928. He joined the

International Health Division of the Rockefeller Foundation in 1929 and served on it for 21 years. He worked on snail control in schistosomiasis in Egypt and other parts of Africa. He retired to Trumansburg, New York, where he died at the age of 93.

Barlow demonstrated the incubation period and the clinical disease associated with F. buski *on himself.*

Introduction

The present study was made not only as an addition to pure science, but because of the intensity and severity of fasciolopsiasis in the area surrounding the Shaohsing Christian Hospital, located at Shaohsing in Chekiang Province, China, and the fact that the author's work is in this region.

Little seems to be known about the pathogenicity of the parasite outside of this region, although the parasite is found in many other localities. In the Shaohsing region, the disease is more severe and occasions greater economic loss than do hookworm and schistosome infestations put together. From 40 to 50 per cent. of the patients of the Christian Hospital harbor the parasite, and in some villages, where routine examinations have been extensively made, 100 per cent. of the people examined were found to be infested. For a short summary of cases from the Shaohsing hospital records the reader is referred to Sweet (1921). Fasciolopsiasis is widely disseminated, being reported from many parts of China, as far north as the Yangtse Valley and as far west as Chengtu and Suifu in Szechuen province and throughout the southern provinces. It has also been reported from India, Assam, Siam, and the neighboring Malay Archipelago. It would not be strange to find it in the Philippines and in the Hawaiian Islands, because of the migration of Chinese to those parts in large numbers. However, it is a subtropical disease and is found to the greatest extent in China. The Shaohsing area, which is the most heavily infected endemic center, covers an area of about 1,600 square miles. . . . In this area the disease profoundly affects the life of between a million and a million and a half people, reducing their efficiency and causing great loss of life. Nearly all of the cases come from a district lying north of the southernmost limits of the city of Shaohsing and extending out in a fan-shaped area to the east and west. Hardly any cases have been reported from the south of the city. This may be explained by the drainage conditions obtaining here. Three rivers rise in the hills to the south and flow through the city out into the canal system of the plains of silt to the north. The parasite develops best in quiet water, and the intermediate hosts do not live in rapidly flowing streams which probably explains this phenomenon. . . .

Ova

In diagnosing fasciolopsiasis there are only two pathognomonic signs: the finding of ova in the stool and the vomiting of live flukes. Only in cases of massive infestation does the latter occur, while it is almost impossible to overlook ova in the stool when but one fluke is harbored because of the large number of ova discharged by one adult. From counts made of weighed specimens of stool from a patient known to harbor but one fluke, from ten to fifteen thousand ova per stool were estimated.

The literature of *Fasciolopsis buski* is replete with disputes about the size and shape variations of the ova and specific differences have been claimed, based partly on these variations. The reason for these different findings lies in the fact that the variations do exist and to a greater degree than has been previously pointed out. . . .

In freshly passed stools the ova may be nearly colorless or a faint tinge of yellow, or they may be as dark yellowish-brown as ascaris or trichuris eggs. The cause of this difference was well demonstrated, in the author's case, by change of diet. If a rich protein diet was indulged in and vegetables were restricted, the stool became constipated, the number of eggs increased in each stool, and the color became quite dark. If vegetables were largely eaten, the stool became mushy and the eggs took on the usual, characteristic, pale-yellow color. For a week a strict milk diet was adhered to and the eggs became greatly increased in each stool and were almost colorless. There were, also, fewer non-fertile eggs than before. These were recognized by their finely granular contents and lack of either yolk-balls or germinal area. In fertile eggs the germinal area and yolk balls show up plainly. The germinal area in freshly passed eggs averages 23.9 microns in diameter. When aspherical, which often happens, they average 28.1×24.3 microns. The yolk-balls average 19.9 microns in diameter and are spherical except when they are crowded by the miracidium and become irregularly polygonal. They contain minute fatty globules which measure, on an average, 4.5 microns in diameter.

The ovum is enclosed in a shell which is thin, frangible, dialytic, and transparent. It is quite resistant to the action of chemicals engendered in the bodies of animals. Snails eat the ova and pass them seemingly unaffected. Man and animals may do the same. Such eggs develop and hatch readily.

They are operculate eggs, having the operculum attached at one point and sealed down around its circumference with a substance which is resistant to outside influences, but which is probably dissolved by the secretion of the head glands at the time of maturity of the miracidium. In many instances, the opercula of eggs which had hatched two years previously and which had remained standing in water, were still attached to the shell. The shells do not disintegrate under any conditions which have been observed. . . .

As development of the embryo proceeds, excretions from the miracidium pass out through the shell, rendering the surface sticky. Such eggs are found with little particles of stool detritus adhering to them. They are readily cleaned with glass rods spun out in flame to the finest filament and the end knobbed. Unless the end is knobbed, the filaments of glass pierce the shells spoiling the egg. Cleaning may be avoided by pipetting out ova before the embryo begins to form, when the egg-shells are smooth and do not collect dirt. . . .

After the development has gone but little past the morula stage, and before the miracidium has taken definite form, a light clear zone appears at the opercular end of the egg. These two zones are slightly yellow and much more refractile than the fluid contents of the egg. After these two oily zones appear at the poles of the egg, another mass makes its appearance and the oily masses are displaced to the ant-opercular end of the egg with the developing miracidium between. This mass is denser, less refractile, slightly granular, and translucent. It lies always at the opercular end and seems to serve the purpose of protecting the operculum from the action of the secretions of the miracidium. The chemical nature of this mass has not been determined and, for lack of a better term, it is called a *mucoid plug*. It is almost inflexible and lies like a convexo-concave lens,

with its concavity facing the miracidium. Later on, when the miracidium is nearly developed, the mucoid plug becomes rigid and distinctly thinner than when it first made its appearance.

The oily masses at the poles of the egg stay separated, but are freely movable with the movements of the miracidium. There are never more than two after the miracidium is well developed, and they never coalesce, no matter how much pressure is put upon them by the miracidium during its growth, which is considerable during the later stages. They even withstand a pressure, sufficient to kill the embryo, without joining. They serve a definite function in keeping the diminishing number of yolk-balls held closely to the body of the miracidium, where perhaps they may be readily assimilated. As soon as the cilia appear, the miracidium may turn about a good deal, having the oily masses now on one and now on the other side or lying between the two. It may drive them first to the opercular end and then to the other, but in no instance does the miracidium escape far from the yolk-balls and granules. The miracidium lashes the yolk-balls with its cilia and they break up, setting the granules free. These, in turn, are swept forward along the body of the miracidium to be used as food. In breaking, the yolk-balls set free the granules and then show as circular rings of fatty material which may possibly coalesce with the oily masses, to augment the size of the latter, though this has never been observed. These oily masses, when the miracidium is full grown, occupy either one side or the other of the shell holding the miracidium close against the opposite side, and lying one above the other. . . .

The Activities of the Free-swimming Miracidium

As soon as they hatch, the miracidia become wonderfully active, swimming here and there, seeking a suitable host. They sometimes hatch by thousands during a period of a few hours in the morning. During its free-swimming life the miracidium is quite versatile in its movements, now darting restlessly here and there and again spiralling along a steady course. Quite a common motion is for it to hang suspended from the surface of the water and to spin on its long axis, or it may stand on its posterior end at the bottom of the dish and spin. It swims more below the surface of the water than at the surface, because the snail, for which it has a predilection, is thoroughly aquatic in habit. It swims with rapidity and with the utmost flexibility. Contraction and extension occur even while swimming at top speed. In motion, the anterior end of the body is larger than the posterior, but it may even contract posteriorly, while enlarging at the head end. The miracidium varies its progress by periods of swimming in circles, with the head as the center of the revolution. While swimming with this pinwheel motion, the body is always in contraction. As soon as it extends itself, the miracidium darts off at a greatly increased rate of speed. The shape, when at rest, is not unlike the outlines of the old-fashioned nipple of a baby's nursing bottle, with the big end pointing forward and the head retracted into it. The miracidium may take on a cylindrical shape, with almost square ends or it may suddenly elongate while swimming. It swims counterclockwise.

The miracidium is a sporocyst with cilia and does not change its essential features after losing the cilia, but develops them. There is little change discernible looking at the sporocyst through the snail's tissues, and in observing the miracidium through its egg shell. Almost immediately after the miracidium finds the snail, it begins its entrance, the initial steps of which have already been given. When the head has come into contact with the epithelium and by the very force of its cilia, which increase in vibration, especially during extension, at which time there would be a tendency to be forced away, the miracidium keeps itself in contact with the snail's epidermis. It is probable that the head-glands eject an erosive fluid which dissolves an opening sufficient for the ingress of the head. When the head is through the epidermis, it bulbs out on the inside and acts as a point of traction by which, in a succession of intrusions and extrusions of the body contents, the miracidium is partly pulled into the snail. The backward-pointing spines of the head also assist in holding the head in possession of occupied territory and of advancing it into new positions at each muscular contraction of the snail, as well as of itself. As the head advances through the tissues inside of the epidermis, it becomes evident that there is a fluid issuing from the anterior tip which is of different specific gravity from that of the lymph of the snail. This is shown by the little waves preceding the mouth, which look like convection currents. During intrusion of its body contents through the little ring of epithelium of the snail, the miracidium keeps the part already inside in broad contraction in order to get as much purchase as possible for pulling itself past the ring. During extension, either free end of the worm is larger than the part constrained by the ring, thus conserving every advance. This constriction by the ring is essential to entrance, as is proved by killing the snail which relaxes its tissues and widens the ring. In this case the miracidium lodges right where it lies and is unable to go in or to back out. This resistance on the part of the snail in an effort at self defense, spells its own doom, in aiding the parasite. Every contraction of the obstructing tissues of the snail, makes each successive extension and contraction of the invading miracidium another decisive step forward into the snail's body. Once through, and into the lymph system, the miracidium follows these vessels instead of piercing tissue. . . .

If many miracidia are allowed to enter a snail, the skin becomes excoriated and thus open to attacks by cyclops and water fleas. If many enter, they sometimes make the snail so sick that it crawls up out of the water, withdraws into its shell and dies. The fewer miracidia are allowed to enter, the stronger the resulting infection and the sturdier the parthenitae become. This provides for optimum infestations. . . .

If we consider the miracidium as merely a ciliated, immature, sporocyst, then the sporocyst stage begins properly with its entrance into the snail and the discarding of its cilia. . . .

In my material the early sporocyst stages remain very much like the miracidia and never become immobile even up to the time of discharging rediae. The digestive tract becomes larger and functionally more active as the sporocyst grows in size. This may be observed with ease through the shell of the snail. Sporocysts have been seen to move along the lymph spaces in the neck and mantle till they came to lie well within the body of the snail before the rediae were born. . . .

Sporocyst Stage

. . . The redia feeds upon the juices contained in the sporocyst, which in turn, gets its nourishment from the snail. The growth, from the entering of the snail by the miracidium, till the expulsion of the mother-redia, is very rapid, occupying only nine or ten days. In some cases the expulsion is slower than in others, so that there is a marked difference in size and development of mother-rediae at the time of expulsion. In but one instance was expulsion seen, and it seemed to be by rupture of the sporocyst.

Mother-redia Stage

Eight days after infection of the snails, one sporocyst had given off a mother redia, which could be observed lying in the lymph spaces around the heart. This redia was from a miracidium which had penetrated the pulmonary chamber at its inner end. From eight days on to as high as 254 days, mother-rediae were being born in snails infected on the same date as this one. It was not ascertained whether they all came from one generation of mother-rediae or not. Probably not. . . .

At any one time of observation of the rediae, they were found to contain large and varying numbers of germ-balls as well as well developed daughter-rediae. . . .

Daughter-redia Stage

In some respects the daughter-rediae are more interesting than the mother-rediae, because they give rise to the final larval stage of the fluke and also because of the question whether or not this stage is a constant generation. . . .

The daughter-rediae are easily picked out by the shape and size of the gut, which in the mother-rediae is larger and broader in proportion to their length than in the daughter-rediae and susceptible to fewer variations in shape. . . .

Cercaria Stage

In from 25 to 30 days after infestation of the snail, cercariae begin to emerge from the daughter-rediae, but they do not come, at once, out of the snail, as they are not fully matured, and they pass hours, or oftener, days in the snail to complete their development. They leave the daughter-rediae, one at a time, and usually stay awhile in the liver region before beginning their migration down the lymph spaces to an exit from the snail. In this migration they spend some time, lingering in spots favorable to growth and offering easy exit. One of these spots, which seems to be agreeably sustentative, is the lymph-space about the heart. They lie in this space long hours in relative inactivity, being moved to and fro by the heart beat. When the impulse to leave the snail finally comes, they move rapidly down the serous spaces of the pulmonary chamber and make their exit either through the mantle or out through the pulmonary orifice. . . .

Usually the snail, from which the cercaria is escaping is feeding on some plant and the contact with the plant may be direct on the part of the cercaria. If so it immediately sucks onto the plant with its mouth and ventral sucker and begins to encyst. If it moves along the plant surface, it does so with a measuring-wormlike movement.

The whole period of free life is exceedingly short.

Metacercaria Stage

The cercaria may creep about on the plant with which it comes in contact for a few minutes and then it begins to encyst. The first step in encystment is the extrusion of the round-celled cystogenous gland material, which exudes from all over the surface of the body, at once coming out along the muscle rugae and giving a hazy outline to the cercaria (Plate 96, Fig. 1). . . .

It turns itself freely from end to end, forward and backward, and side to side until it is completely surrounded by the sphere of transparent chitinous cyst wall. So it comes to lie within two covers of cyst material, the outer one very friable and the inner one so tough that it cannot be broken without great effort. Crushing it under a cover-slip always results in the destruction of the metacercaria. . . .

The whole time of encystment may be from one to three hours. The outer wall is sticky enough to adhere firmly to glass. Pushing it with a camel's hair brush quite vigorously will dislodge it, but would be apt to rupture the outer wall. In order to get them off without breaking them, a piece of bamboo shaved to a transparent edge on one end was used. This would slip under the edge of the cyst and lift it off whole. Even while using this amount of care many of the cysts were ruptured on the outer surface of the outer cyst wall. This shows how well adapted is the cyst for ingestion by the definitive host. . . .

The caltrop (Plate 96, Fig. 15; Plate 97, Fig. 4) is a most acceptable feeding ground for the snails. It has a broad, soft, spongy leaf on a gibbous, cellular petiole, and the root-stalk is spindle-shaped and cellular. The air cells keep the plant supported on the water, and the rootlets get their food largely from the water, although there is a root which is sent down to the bottom, even though the depth may be 12 to 15 feet. These plants are usually alive with the little snails, feeding on the tender skin of stems, petioles, leaves and nuts. It is not unusual to find more than 20 on a single nut (Fig. 15). This obliterates distance for the emerging cercariae and brings encystment where it is most efficacious and dangerous. . . .

The cysts are not very resistant to drying and would not withstand one day's hot sun. For this reason vegetables, dry-grown near the ponds where there are many infected snails, are not found to be infected. Many examinations of the cabbage fields shown lying between the ponds (Plate 97, Fig. 3b) never gave any positive results.

Other plants may be implicated later, but it is unquestionably true that the water caltrop is the one most involved in the transmission of fasciolopsiasis in the Shaohsing endemic area.

Experimental Infestations

Experiments on man were carried out with the two-fold purpose of keeping the experiment human and of obtaining more intimate knowledge of the clinical and symptomatological aspects of the disease.

Experiment. In order to compare results with those obtained by Nakagawa (1922) in his experimentation with the pig-fluke, an infestation was kept up for the same length of time as that recorded in his experiment with pigs. November 27, 1922, the stools were carefully examined and found to be ova-free. Just before the noon meal, November 27, 1922, 96 cysts were swallowed. These cysts were collected from the red-water-caltrop fields near Shiao Shi Tsong. The following day 36 cysts from aquarium-reared snails were ingested, making a total of 132 cysts. December 28, 1922, ova appeared in the stool, but

unaccompanied by noticeable symptoms. January 12, 1923, symptoms of a mild nature were noticed, such as epigastric pain and hunger preceding meals. This continued for a few days and then subsided, to be renewed with increased severity. February 2, 1923, the hypogastric pain became severe and lasted from four o'clock in the morning till food was taken. It was griping in nature and continued for half an hour after eating and then subsided entirely. It was of daily occurrence and came on only in the early morning. There were periods of diarrhoea, lasting for a day or more, followed by two or three days of well-formed stools which showed quite hard fecal masses at the beginning of defecation and ended in a mushy stool. Such stools would continue till diarrhoea began again. There was some mucus in the stools.

February 13, 1923, a severe diarrhoea, with six movements during the 24 hours, began and lasted till the 20th of February, with from four to six movements daily, accompanied with severe griping pain which was irregularly intermittent all day long. The pain was confined to the hypogastrium and seemed to be caused by an increased peristalsis and a large quantity of gas. The gas passed was of an offensive nature and generated in large quantities. The pain was so intense that lying on the abdomen was the only way to get relief. During the periods of diarrhoea there was marked aversion to food. From February 20, 1923, the diarrhoae ceased and did not return, but there were regular well-formed stools twice daily, accompanied with an almost uncontrollable desire to defecate just prior to going to stool and considerable griping at the time of defecation. February 26, 1923, little was eaten except fruit juices with sugar. At night a teaspoonful of Cascara Evacuant was taken without results. On the morning of February 27, 1923, 90 minims of carbon tetrachloride were taken in water at 7:30. At 8:00 A.M. one soft stool was passed containing a mucous cast, making up about half of the stool. There was marked nausea but no vomiting. After sitting quietly in the laboratory till 11:30 A.M. a desire to defecate was followed by a large loose stool at 12 o'clock noon, containing 20 specimens of *Fasciolopsis buski* and one ascarid. There was a constant and nauseating eructation of carbon tetrachloride gas and the whole treatment

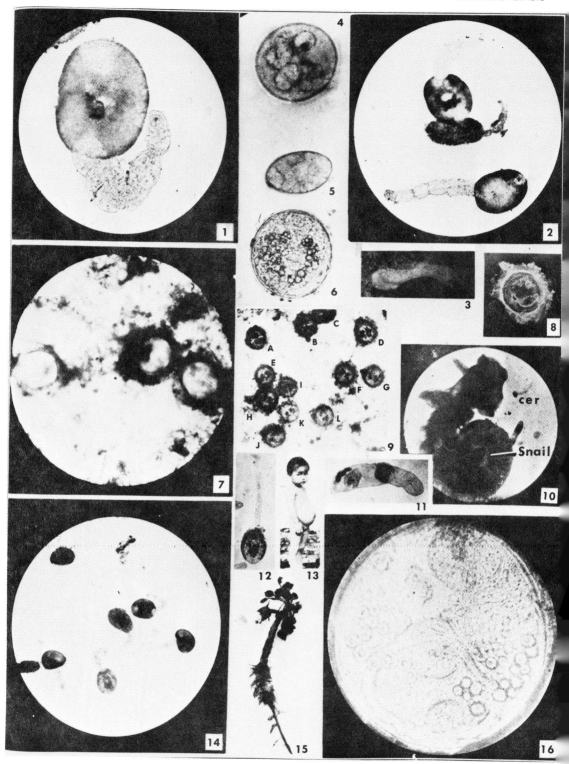

was accompanied by weakness, dizziness, nausea, and tinnitus aurium. There was no rise in temperature, the pulse stayed at 74 and the respirations at 15 a minute. The progress of the drug could be followed through the digestive tract by the presence of a slight burning pain. It made me decidedly ill, but, after four stools, this feeling subsided and a comfortable night was passed. At 12:30 P.M. 24 flukes were passed, and at 6:10 P.M. 32 more were passed. Then half an ounce of magnesium sulphate was taken, and at 8:10 P.M. 17 more flukes were passed. At 9:45 P.M. one more stool, very small and all liquid, was passed, but no flukes with it. February 28, 1923, there was still some aversion to food, but breakfast was eaten as usual and no abdominal pain was felt. In this respect carbon tetrachloride is superior to beta-naphthol for, following the administration of the latter, there was pain of a burning nature for several days. Following carbon tetrachloride there was no mucus in the stools, while with beta-naphthol there was considerable and it continued for several days. February 28, 1923, at 8:50 A.M. there was one stool with 20 flukes, at 11:20 A.M. one stool with 2 flukes and one at 10:00 P.M. containing 9 flukes. For three days all stools were saved and screened and searched for shreds of flukes, but none were found. Washed stools were examined March 11 and March 18, 1923, and found to be ova-free. . . .

Growth of the Adult Stage in the Definitive Host

The adult stage has been described by various authors, but much remains to be done to determine the rapidity of growth and the actual life activities of the worm, especially the biochemistry as related to itself and to its host. There is every reason to believe that the symptoms of the disease are caused by the excretory products of the worm, because it lives free in the lumen of the intestine and does not feed on the tissues or on the blood. They probably do not wander far from one spot in the intestine. Those which have been observed were all in the duodenum and all fastened to the mucous membrane by their ventral suckers or were buried in mucous secretion. None were loose in the bowel. There is a typical life-shape which is quite unlike the death-shape. The head is very much attenuated, running out in a slender, almost thread-like extension from the shoulder. They may remain attached to the mucosa till little reddened spots appear which persist in post mortem findings. During life in the intestine there is an almost constant contraction and extension of the head and body, the one being independent of the other in its movements. The body is sometimes in contraction, while the head is thrust out in a slender tube; the head and body may both be extended or contracted at the same time, or the head may be solidly contracted, while the body is greatly extended and curled ventrally upon itself. Progression has been observed in the pig's intestine, but never, in even the most active flukes, after being passed. In saline, warmed to 99° F., the movements more nearly simulate life activities, but even so one does not see life activities duplicated.

It is probably true that all stages from adult to metacercaria are spined, the redia stage less so, perhaps, than the other stages. That only the ventral surface and head of the adult are spined is because it lives inside a viscus and does not progress through tissues. It always faces the peristaltic wave and the scales, pointing away from the wave, give firm anchorage to the fluke while feeding. Constantly bathed in the intestinal juices, the adult fluke, like the redia, probably feeds through the skin as well as by mouth. The

Plate 96. Fig. 1. Cercaria showing general extrusion of round-celled cystogenous material. Tail still attached subterminally. *Fig. 2.* Three cercariae, the centre one showing the extrusion of round-celled cystogenous material in a marked degree. *Fig. 3.* A daughter redia filled with cercaria germballs. Taken through the tissues of the snail. It lies extended. *Fig. 4.* Cyst, showing excretory tubules filled with concretions. *Fig. 5. F. buski* ovum for comparison. *Fig. 6.* Same cyst as Fig. 4, showing oral and ventral suckers, pharynx and the bifurcation of the intestinal cecum. The concretions show plainly. *Fig. 7.* The first 3 cysts found on the skin of the red water-caltrop. *Fig. 8.* The cyst in both its coverings. *Fig. 9.* Appearance of 12 out of 21 cysts found on a piece of skin of the red water-caltrop nut. *Fig. 10.* Cercaria, broken out of a snail, showing comparative length of tail. *Fig. 11.* Showing that there is no definite orientation of the cercariae within the redia. *Fig. 12.* Cercaria, showing the hoof-like appearance of the body. *Fig. 13.* The appearance of a child with fasciolopsiasis in not very severe form; oedema and ascites present. *Fig. 14.* Swimming positions of cercaria. *Fig. 15.* Red water-caltrop showing part of the 8-foot root-stalk and a nut with 22 *Segmentina nitidellus* snails on it and an adult *Planorbis schmackeri* snail to the left of the nut. *Fig. 16.* Cyst, showing digestive tract of the contained metacercaria.

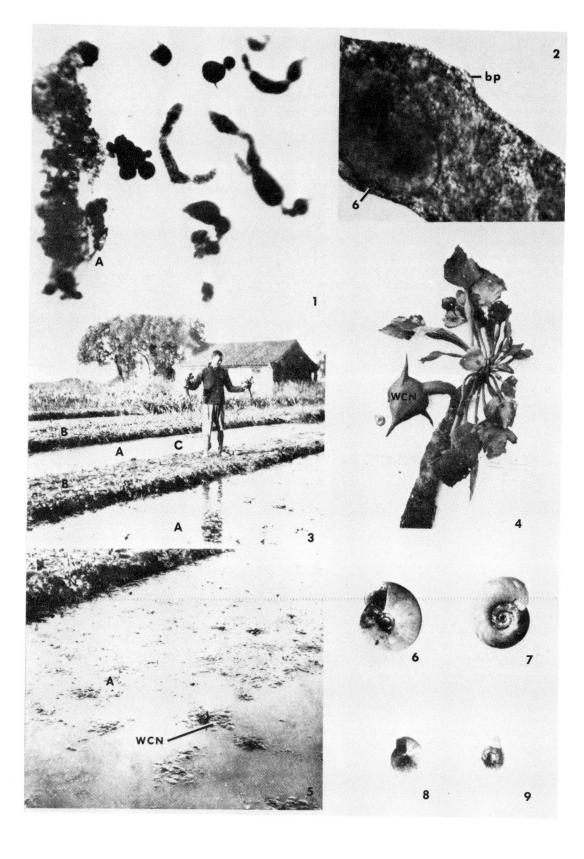

1

2

bp

6

3

B

A   C

B

A

4

WCN

A

5

WCN

6

7

8   9

parasite sometimes buries its head in the mucosa of the intestine, as added anchorage, and is then assisted by the spines with which the head is covered. This is not the feeding posture, however.

The color of the adult, while in the intestine of experimental animals, is exactly the color of normal fresh blood, but in older specimens it may be darker in hue. In some specimens which were probably many years old, which were obtained alive from hospital patients, the color was a dark brownish-red, but no light red specimens were observed in experimental animals. . . .

One, possibly, might say that there is a period of growth or development extending from infestation to a size sufficient to produce an amount of toxin which would cause apparent injury. There is a direct escape of the metacercaria and attachment at the site of its future habitat. The attachment probably takes place within a few minutes after the metacercaria leaves its cyst-shell. Then, too, development is steadily progressive, with concomitant symptom accompaniment, on to adulthood. There are no migrations, no resting stages, and no moults which might produce such a period. The whole onset of clinical manifestations is in a gradually increasing scale of severity, as would be expected from an infestation due to growing parasites which progress to maturity without intermission.

The size of the parasites varies greatly in different patients. . . . Very much seems to depend upon the physical and financial status of the patient. Poor people are unable to provide the parasites with so good or so varied a fare as are wealthy ones. Perhaps another influence which tends to inhibit the growth of the parasites in massive infestations, is the presence of the large amount of excretory material produced by and affecting the flukes themselves. It is true that massive infestations usually run smaller in size than do infestations of a few dozen or hundred. The largest flukes recorded have come from small infestations. This observation does not take into account the factor of time of infestation, because this is not known and is only to be approximated by the case history, which depends upon the appearance of symptoms and is never very reliable. But symptoms usually develop within 30 to 60 days after infestation, especially in massive infestations. More study of the effect upon size, of such factors as time of infestation, individual development, environmental changes, is needed before one may speak with certainty. That there is a variation in size in flukes living in the same environment, developing with equal opportunity, and coming from an infestation dating from the same hour, is certain. It is possible that the extreme ends of the small intestine may give quite different environments to these worms. That they are only found in the small intestine seems likely, because, though they have been found in the stomach, intestine, and the bowel as low as the rectum in post mortem examinations, it is probable that the conditions previous to death may have caused the dispersion.

Oedema is present within 20 days of infestation in case the patient is small or undernourished and the infestation is massive. In most fatal cases there is a marked oedema with ascites (Plate 96, Fig. 13) and an extensive anasarca. However, there seems to be little or no anemia and no primary anemia at all. One may say that it is not a constant symptom in any series of cases, but appears because of the asthenia produced by the intoxication. The apparent anemia is largely due to viewing the blood stream through an overlying oedema. As soon as the oedema subsides "it is astonishing how rapidly the anemia disappears, once the intestines are cleared" (Goddard, 1919). This is due to the fact that primary anemia does not exist, rather than to the clearing of the intestine. The oedema never involves the lung and probably not the chest cavity at all, even in advanced cases. Photographs of many individuals suffering from the disease show a definite demarcation of the chest and an exceptional freedom there from any oedema. The period of oedema (Goddard, 1919)

Plate 97. Fig. 1. The destruction of the rediae by the snail. (a) The last stages in the formation of the little inclusion cysts. Note the bands of tissue at the lower end of the liver tissue at (a). *Fig. 2.* The birth-pore of a mother-redia, showing its relative position to the gut. *Fig. 3.* Caltrop ponds (a, a) and cabbage fields (b, b); (c) shows the root-stalk of a caltrop plant. *Fig. 4.* Caltrop plant and nut with a *P. schmackeri* snail to the left of the nut. *Fig. 5.* Water caltrop pond (a) and cabbage patch (b), as in Fig. 3, showing the growth habit of the caltrop. The nut, lying on the patch of leaves, was put there for comparison only, as the nuts all grow beneath the surface of the water. *Fig. 6.* Ventral surface of shell of *Planorbis schmackeri* Cless; *Fig. 7.* Dorsal surface of same. *Fig. 8.* Ventral surface of shell of *Segmentina nitidellus*, Mts. *Fig. 9.* Dorsal surface of the same.

may come much sooner than is suggested, and it may not be present at all in fatal or in advanced cases. Also there may not be diarrhoea at all in the course of the disease, and at best, it is not a constant symptom, but usually alternates with periods of constipation. The stool is not noticeably offensive at any time, but there may be an odor of oysters in a very liquid stool in a massive infestation.

There is but one pathognomonic sign of fasciolopsiasis and that is the finding of the egg in the stool, though fluke-harboring individuals are easily recognized on the streets after one has seen many cases clinically. The eggs are found in largest numbers in formed or constipated stools and in the first part of such stools rather than in the aftercoming and softer part, while in diarrhoeic stools there are only about half the number, per slide, to be found when using Stoll's method (1923) for egg counting. They are found most plentifully in the feces of such stools and not as much in the mucus. . . .

In the autumn of 1910 in Shaohsing, the author was surprised at the large number of ova appearing in the stools of patients entering the Christian Hospital. Fully half of the in-patients harbored the parasite. Later on, while doing out-patient work at Ko-Chiao, a small town ten miles to the northwest of Shaohsing this surprise was increased at the great number who harbored the parasite. Beginning a cursory geographical survey it was found that En Tsong, a little town to the northeast of Ko-Chiao seemed to be the endemic centre of the infection, and that from 95 to 100 per cent. of the people were infested. One man named Wang, from this village, brought in his wife and family all suffering from the disease. The daughter, Wang Da-gu, a girl of nine, was nearly moribund and the others were all very sick. On examination of the stools of these four I was struck with the enormous number of ova and their marked variation in shape from the classical egg of *Fasciolopsis buski*. . . . In the stool of the daughter were literally millions of ova, and they could be sedimented and observed in a mass at the bottom of the sedimenting graduate. As the stools were watery it was easy to collect the ova from them by sedimentation. She had marked oedema and beginning anasarca, but no anemia. On receiving treatment with beta-naphthol, she passed 3,721 flukes, which is the largest number

of these flukes which have ever been counted from one patient. This number has been incorrectly reported by both Goddard (1919) and Sweet (1921) as being 3,328, but the case was on my own service and the worms were all counted and measured by myself. They were remarkable because of the stage of growth which they showed. . . . The wash-water, containing thousands of immature flukes, not much past the metacercaria stage, was mistaken by the laboratory assistant for waste and was thrown away. These forms have been searched for in hundreds of cases since then, but have never been found in just the stages which this case exhibited. The father of this family passed 2,273 flukes, the mother 1,024, and the little son 604, but in none of the other cases did these immature forms appear. . . . [Barlow includes measurements of 113 out of 124 *F. buski* passed by him after treatment with 90 min. of carbon tetrachloride, 92 days after he swallowed 132 cysts. The average length of the parasites was 18.34 mm and the average width 9.57 mm—Eds.]. . . .

Snail Hosts

The intermediate hosts are two dextral planorbids (Plate 97, Figs. 6–9), *Planorbis schmackeri* Cless and *Segmentina nitidellus* Mts. In habits they are very much alike, but *P. schmackeri* lends itself much more desirably to the study of the parthenitae because of its thinner, flatter, and more transparent shell. . . .

The *possibility* of control is fairly simple and easily accomplished. With laws effective, living conditions regulated, and customs subordinated, the disease could be blotted out in one season. That this may be the case is forcibly demonstrated by the ease with which any one of the links in the chain of the life cycle of the parasite may be destroyed. With things as they are, looking with optimism upon the problem of control, one may predict that it will take from ten to 20 years to reduce the disease to the point at which it will cease to be a menace, and 50 years or more to stamp it out completely, unless Chinese officialdom and the common people cooperate in a common plan with the control-man to eradicate it. This is a desideratum hardly to be contemplated. What more could be asked of a parasitic disease to make the problem of control easier or simpler than obtains in fasciolopsiasis, viz.

(1) A limited endemic area.

(2) A complete knowledge of the life cycle of the parasite.

(3) Ease of diagnosis, because of the large egg.

(4) Effective and cheap anthelminthics.

(5) Non-resistant larval stages of the parasite.

(6) Restricted and tender intermediate hosts.

(7) Cheap and intrinsically valuable agents for the destruction of intermediate hosts.

(8) Known and easily controlled infective agents.

(9) No animal-host-reservoir complications. The case would be complete, if we could but add

(10) *Cooperation* on the part of the people, the hospital, and the local government. . . .

CHAPTER 30

Heterophydiasis

A CONTRIBUTION TO HUMAN HELMINTHOLOGY

Ein beitrag zur helminthographia humana. Zeitschrift für Wissenschaftliche Zoologie, 4: 53–76, 1852. Selections from pp. 62–64. Translated from the German.

Theodore Bilharz
(1825–1862)

Bilharz' biography will be found in the chapter on Schistosomiasis.

Another of the contributions of Bilharz from his sojourn in Egypt was the description of Heterophyes heterophyes.

From the letters of Dr. Bilharz in Cairo to Prof. C. T. von Siebold in Breslau, with comments by the latter.

Distomum heterophyes Siebold

I gave the name *Distoma heterophyes* Sieb. to a small trematode which Bilharz called to my attention in his letter of 1 May 1851, in the following way:

"A short while ago, on 26 April, I discovered, in the intestine of a boy's cadaver a large number of small red dots which, under the microscope, proved to be a beautiful fully developed *Distoma* 1 mm in length and 0.3 mm in width. The red color was due to the red-brown mature eggs which were visible through the body of the worm. The outline of the body of these *Distomas* is oval; posteriorly, more rounded, anteriorly, more pointed. The oral sucker is small and funnel-shaped; it opens more toward the under surface than toward the front. Behind it begins the narrow, membranous throat which, after a short distance, turns into an oblong, muscular pharynx; from there the narrow esophagus extends backward and then divides in front of the ventral sucker in the usual way into two intestinal tubes which extend downward laterally and terminate blindly at the rear end of the body. The extremely muscular ventral sucker is 12 times bigger than the oral sucker and is situated somewhat anterior to the middle of the abdomen. Behind it is a formation similar to a sucker which, however, I consider to be the cirrus sac. The latter exhibits on its surface a circle of many small, peculiarly shaped rods seemingly of a horny substance which, toward one side, possess three little branches attached at an acute angle. In the rear end of the body lie the two round testes; between these and the cirrus sac in the middle is a small round organ (ovary) and behind this a blind tube (seminal vesicle). The spaces between these organs are filled by the twisted oviduct, and, posteriorly, ramified 'vitellaria' were visible. On the middle of the posterior portion of the body, a secretory organ opens up to excrete the characteristic calcium corpuscles. The skin is covered with small spines, pointed backward; these occur abundantly and distinctly, particularly on the front end of the body. I have gathered a few hundred of these parasites but had to leave the majority of them in the intestine of the cadaver because of lack of time. I have never found this parasite again."

According to a later communication, Bilharz saw this *Distoma* only once more. He convinced himself, by another examination of this small trematode, that the organ he considered to be the seminal vesicle showed a lively swarm of spermatozoides; further, he was able to count on the cirrus sac 72 horny rods and not three, as he had thought earlier, but five equally long side branches lying one after another. In the specimens of this *Distoma* sent to me by Bilharz, I have still been able to recognize plainly the peculiar, so far as organization and position are concerned, cirrus sac. I have been reminded, by the horny rods, of the lobster pot arrangement of the horny rods of the cirrus sac of polystomum and octobothrium (see my textbook on comparative anatomy of invertebrates). [See Plate 72, Figs. 16 & 17—Eds.].

CHAPTER 31

Paragonimiasis

CONTRIBUTION TO THE KNOWLEDGE OF TREMATODES
(A preliminary communication)

Zur trematoden-kenntnis. Zooligischer Anzeiger, 1: 271–273, 1878. Selections from pp. 271–272. Translated from the German.

Coenraad Kerbert
(1849–1927)

Kerbert studied in Amsterdam and eventually under Leuckart in Leipzig, where he wrote his dissertation on reptile skin in 1876. In 1877 he was appointed assistant of the Zoology Laboratory in Amsterdam, which was founded in the same year. He was subsequently active as a lecturer in the University of Amsterdam and became chief curator of the Aquarium. In 1890 he succeeded Professor C. F. Westerman as director of the Royal Zoological Society, "Naturae Artis Magistra," a position he held until his death.

This is the original description of an adult Paragonimus *from a tiger in the Amsterdam Zoo. Nakahama, while studying with Leuckart, compared Kerbert's specimens of adult lung flukes with those found in autopsies in Japan and found them to be identical, as reported by Leuckart in 1889.*

As I have been occupied lately with investigations on trematodes, I take this opportunity to report to my colleagues some of the primary results of these investigations.

During the autopsy of a royal tiger that had died in September 1877 in the Zoological Garden in Amsterdam, *Distomas* were found in the lungs; through the kindness of the director, Dr. C. F. Westerman, these were submitted to me immediately for further examination.

These *Distomas* were found, always in pairs, inside rather thick, fibrous capsules which, because of their somewhat blue color, were noticed immediately on the outer surface of the lungs. Since *Distomas* had been found previously by Cobbold in the lungs of *Viverra mungos* and by

Natterer in the lungs of a *Lutra brasiliensis*, it was assumed that the trematodes found in the lungs of the royal tiger might belong to one of these two species. This, however, was not so. On further investigation, our trematodes turned out to be representatives of a still undescribed species. I feel justified, therefore, in introducing this unknown worm to the zoologists as *Distoma westermanni*, n. sp.

In zoological classification: the body of our animal is oval, swollen, anteriorly somewhat pointed, posteriorly rounded and dark gray. The dorsal surface is convex and the ventral surface somewhat flattened; length 7–10 mm; width 4–6 mm; thickness 2–3 mm.

The oral and ventral suckers are about 2 mm distant from one another, of equal size, with a diameter of .78 mm. The cuticula is covered with dense transverse rows of fine spines.

A muscular pharynx extends directly from the oral sucker. The esophagus is forked after a short distance and forks into two appendices which have a tortuous course. They do not branch any further, and occasionally they show localized enlargements. Only the central portion of the excretory organ has been observed, which is sometimes rounded and swollen.

With the exception of the two vitellaria (these extend over the entire length of the body and also beneath the layer of a skin muscle and entire dorsum of the body), the remaining reproductive organs are limited to the central portion of the body. In the middle lies another gland, the *Schalendrusen*, which is irregular in form and consists of cells in a "ray" formation.

Into the *Schalendruse* terminate the following: (1) a heart-shaped excretory duct of the two transverse ducts of the vitellaria; (2) the excretory duct of the lobulated ovary (I counted six larger ones); (3) Laurer's canal.

Laurer's canal can be followed from its beginning in the *Schalendruse* to its termination at the dorsal surface of the animal, and it clearly shows a rounded, thick-walled appendage, the receptaculum seminis.

Laurer's canal communicates with the *Schalendruse* and the receptaculum seminis.

In the egg chamber of the *Schalendruse* the seminal threads of one individual come into contact with the eggs from the ovary through Laurer's canal.

A direct connection between the testes and the female sexual organs of the same individual does not exist.

The uterus has its origin in the egg chamber of the *Schalendruse,* and its brown convolutions are situated in the middle of the left half of the body and occupy relatively little space. The testes, like the ovaries, are lobed glands which are situated beneath the back behind the transverse axis of the vitellaria.

The vas deferens unite on the level of the *Schalendruse* to the left of it into an ejaculatory duct. The uterus, as well as the ejaculatory duct, finally lead to a sac-formed antechamber which one can designate as the sexual cloaca.

The external surface of this antechamber, the genital pore, is located at the ventral surface about 2 mm behind the ventral sucker. The penis I have not seen. The oval eggs which are placed together in a yellow shell and cover were heaped and adherent to the winding uterus—.75 mm long and .04 mm in width.

I soon hope to be able to publish a more extensive description of the structure of this worm with a consideration of other species of trematodes as well as their relationship to trematodes and cestodes.

ON PARASITIC HEMOPTYSIS
(Gregarinosis pulmonum)

Ueber parasitäre hamoptoë (Gregarinosis pulmonum). Centralblatt für die Medicinischen Wissenschaften, 18: 721–722, 1880. Translated from the German.

Erwin Otto Eduard von Baelz
(1849–1913)

Baelz, the son of an architect, was born in Bietigheim, Germany. He entered Tübingen to study medicine. La- *ter, in order to study clinical medicine under Wunderlich, he transferred to Leipzig, where he was graduated in 1872. In 1876, at the request of the Japanese government, he went to the newly created medical department of Tokyo Imperial University. He succeeded Wernich as chief of internal medicine and trained more than 800 physicians before his retirement in 1902. Baelz made original observations on beriberi, leprosy, and paragonimiasis. He was much decorated and much loved by the Japanese people. In 1905 he returned to Germany with his Japanese wife, and he died in Stuttgart in 1913.*

A superb clinician, Baelz described in this article the ova of Paragonimus *and its relationship to endemic hemoptysis. Nakahama was a medical student under Baelz at the Tokyo Imperial University at the time of this discovery. He obtained the adult worm of* Paragonimus *from autopsies at the Okayama Prefectural Hospital and sent them to Baelz, who described them in April of 1883 in* Berliner Klinische Wochenschrift.

In Japan, there exists a disease which has not yet been described and which is still unknown even to the native physicians. The disease manifests itself in that otherwise completely healthy individuals cough up blood-containing sputum for a long time, very often for many years, either frequently or intermittently. The sputum is not related either to tuberculosis or to any physically demonstrable lung infection; even in cases where the disease has existed for ten years, the patients show absolutely no symptoms except for occasional throat irritation and a completely untroublesome cough.

This disease must be of great incidence; I have observed 19 cases up to now, 12 of which occurred last year alone. Probably thousands of Japanese suffer from this disease. The illness has been observed so far only among young persons between the ages of 15 and 25 years. It is found throughout the entire Japanese empire; that is, over ten degrees of latitude. However, it seems to occur more frequently in the south.

The sputum is very viscous and has a characteristic dirty-red color. The red color is due mainly to the blood content. In some cases the color is a dark red; at other times, but less frequently, it is a very pale red. More often, however, the color depends on the presence of specific parasites. These are found in two forms: (1) As intensive yellow-brown, oval bodies, 0.13 mm in length and 0.07 mm in width. They have a transparent, sharp, doubly refractile shell, 0.02 mm thick, which shimmers greenish or reddish at different settings of the microscope. At the blunt end a kind of cover is often found; here, the cyst or "egg" opens. The contents consist of a viscous gelatin in which three to five (most often, four) lumps are embedded. Each lump consists of (a) a very sharply contoured colorless ball, twice the size of a white blood cell, the contents of which are in constant motion; surrounding this body lies (b) a coarsely granulated yellow substance, loosely dispersed in the gelatin, in which molecular motion is often observed. For some time after they have left the shell, the balls exhibit the aforementioned motion; then they surround themselves with the granulated substance as a shell and seem motionless. (2) These motionless balls are of the exact same nature as the countless granulated, round-to-oval, colorless or yellow-brown blood cells; having no shell and measuring 0.01 to 0.04 mm in diameter, these are most often the chief component of the sputum.

The larger oval bodies are psorosperm cysts; the smaller, unshelled balls are immature psorosperm [probably epithelial cells—Eds.] which are identical to those from the intestine and liver of mouse and rabbit that Waldenburg and Eimer have illustrated. Since, according to the findings of the above-mentioned investigators and others, the name psorosperm represents only a developmental step of the gregarines, and since the name gregarine well describes this kind of organism, I therefore wish to name this disease *Gregarinosis pulmonum* and the parasite *Gregarina pulmonalis,* or perhaps also, because of its color, *Gregarina fusca.*

I shall discuss all details in a complete paper which is soon to follow.

DISTOMA RINGERI

Medical Reports for the Half Year Ended 30th September 1880. Published by order of the Inspector General, Shanghai; Imperial Maritime Customs (China). Special Series No. 2, 20th issue: 10–12, 1880.

Patrick Manson
(1844–1922)

Manson's contributions to tropical medicine were many. His biography will be found in the chapter on Malaria. Independently of Baelz, Manson described the etiology of endemic hemoptysis.

The list of parasites inhabiting the human body is gradually becoming a long one; another addition—the latest, I believe—has been recently made by Dr. Ringer, of Tamsui, Formosa. The following notes embrace all that is yet known of the new parasite.

Some time ago, 6th November to 18th December 1878, I had in hospital here a Portuguese suffering from symptoms of thoracic tumour presumed to be an aneurism. He improved with rest and treatment, and returned to Tamsui, whence he had come and where he had resided for many years. He did not live long after his return, and died suddenly (June 1879) from rupture of an aneurism of the ascending aorta into the pericardium. Dr. Ringer made the postmortem examination, and, knowing I took an interest in the case, kindly wrote me the particulars of the examination. Besides describing the immediate cause of death, he told me he had found a parasite of some sort in making a section of the lung, and promised to send the animal to me for inspection. He wrote:—

After making a section I found the parasite lying on the lung tissue—it might have escaped from a bronchus. Whilst alive a number of young (microscopic) escaped from an opening in the body. There were some small deposits of tubercle, no cavities, and, if I remember aright, slight congestion of the lungs.

Last April a Chinaman consulted me about an eczematous eruption he had on his face and legs. The eruption had been out for some time, and had its origin, he believed, in an attack of scabies. Whilst he was speaking to me I observed that his voice was rough and loud, and that he frequently hawked up and expectorated small quantities of a reddish sputum. At that time I was making examinations of lung blood in connexion with another subject, and as this man's sputum afforded a favourable opportunity for examination, I placed a specimen under the microscope. The sputa, which to the naked eye appeared to be made up of small pellets of rusty pneumonic-like spit, specks of bright red blood, and ordinary bronchial mucus, contained, besides ordinary blood and mucus corpuscles, large numbers of bodies evidently the ova of some parasite. These bodies were oval in form, one end of the oval being cut off or shut in by an operculum, granular on the surface, blood-stained, measuring on an average $1/300'' \times 1/500''$ (Plate 98, Figs. 1, 2, and 3). Firm pressure on the covering glass caused them to rupture and their contents to escape, the shell being left empty and fractured at the opercular end (Figs. 4, 5); though empty, the shell had a pale brownish-red colour. No distinctly organised embryo could be made out in the uninjured ovum, but when the contents were expressed they resolved themselves into oil masses, and granular matter having very active molecular movements. A delicate double outline could be made out in most of the ova. They were so numerous that many fields of the microscope showed three or four of them at once.

Two days afterwards I again examined this man's sputum, and found it full of ova as on the previous occasion. I asked him to come again and to supply me from time to time with sputum, but he did not return, and has left the neighbourhood, I believe. I hoped to attempt successfully the hatching of the ova, as has already been done in the case of other distomata, but his disappearance and my failure to get another and similar case oblige me to postpone the experiment.

At his first visit I obtained the following particulars of his case:—

Tso-tong, male, aet. 35; native of Foochow; a secretary in the Salt Office; resident in Amoy about one year.

He was born on Foochow city, and lived there till he was 21 years of age; he then went to Tecktcham, a town in North Formosa, about two days' journey from Tamsui, and resided there for four years; then he returned to Foochow for a year and a half. He was again sent to Tecktcham for a second service of four years. He returned again to his native town for a year, and was then sent for six months to Henghwa. Afterwards he lived successively in Foochow, one year; Amoy, a year and a half; Foochow, four months; and, again, Amoy for one year, where he is at present stationed. A year after his first arrival in Tecktcham, when he was 22 years of age, he first spat blood. Every day for 19 days he brought up from an ounce to half an ounce of blood; he emaciated slightly, but had very little cough. Haemoptysis returned about six months later, smaller in quantity, but, as in the former attack, the blood at first was pure, unmixed with mucus, and of a bright red colour; this second attack lasted for a few days only. Since then he says he has spat blood for two or three days at a time, in small quantities, every second or third month. He has never had much cough, and he says the blood is always mixed with mucus after the first mouthful. Once during two years he had no blood-spitting. Though rather thin, he enjoys good

health. I could discover no signs of lung disease on auscultation. His father is dead, but never had a cough; his mother had a cough and died 10 years ago. He has had two brothers and two sisters; they are all of them alive and in good health.

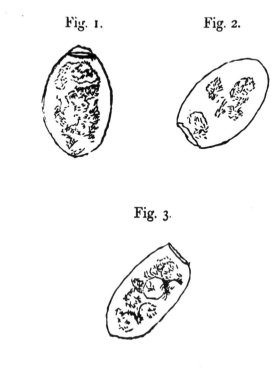

Fig. 1.   Fig. 2.

Fig. 3.

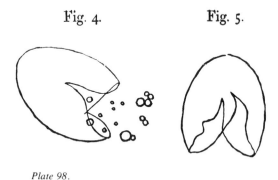

Fig. 4.   Fig. 5.

Plate 98.

When I discovered the ova in this man's sputum I recollected Dr. Ringer's parasite, and that the Portuguese in whose lungs it was found had also lived for many years in North Formosa; and I came to the conclusion that this Chinaman's lungs probably contained a similar parasite, and that it was the cause of his blood-spitting. At my request Dr. Ringer sent me the solitary specimen he had found a year before. It was preserved in spirits of wine. I placed a little of the sediment in the spirit under the microscope, and found in it several ova of the same shape, colour, and dimensions as those I some time before found in the Chinaman's sputum. Most of the ova were ruptured; a few, however, were still perfect (See Plate 99, Figs. 6, 7, 8). The parent parasite was of the shape, size and outline represented (Fig.

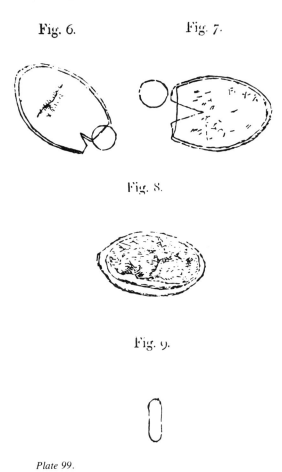

Fig. 6.   Fig. 7.

Fig. 8.

Fig. 9.

Plate 99.

9). It was of a light brown colour, firm, leathery texture, and measured $14/32'' \times 5/32'' \times 1/32''$. It was evidently a distoma; but, not feeling sure if it was a new species or not, I sent it to Dr. Cobbold, who has pronounced it to be new, and has

named it Distoma Ringeri, after the discoverer. Referring to the specimen, he says:—

I satisfied myself that the fluke was new to science and accordingly I propose to call it Distoma Ringeri, after the discoverer. Though mutilated, the oral sucker was well shown, as also were traces of an organ I regarded as the remains of the ventral acetabulum. When flattened on a glass slide, the capsules of the vitellarium were well seen, and occupied fully four-fifths of the body, lying deep under the dermal surface. The worm reminds me very much of *distoma compactum*, which many years ago I detected in the lungs of an Indian ichneumon, but it is much larger and evidently a distinct species.—*Journal of the Quekett Microscopical Club,* No. 44, August 1880.

We are as yet not in a position to say much about the pathological significance of this parasite. I do not think it common in this locality, but when practising in South Formosa I recollect seeing many cases of chronic and oft-recurring blood-spitting without apparent heart or lung lesion, and it is just possible that the haemoptysis in many of these cases was caused by distoma Ringeri. My patient told me that blood-spitting was a very common complaint in Tecktcham.

The intermediary host or hosts, the geographical distribution, and the mode of entrance of the parasite into the lungs offer a very interesting field for future investigation.

ON THE ROUTE OF MIGRATION OF *PARAGONIMUS WESTERMANI* IN THE DEFINITIVE HOST

Taiwan Igakkai Zasshi, No. 152: 685–700, 1915 (excerpted). Translated from the Japanese.

Sadamu Yokogawa (1883–1956)

Yokogawa was born in Okayama prefecture and graduated with honors from the Medical College in 1908. He continued to work in Okayama after graduation, then went to Taiwan as lecturer in pathology, rising to professor of pathology in 1918. His thesis presented at the Kyoto Imperial University described his discovery of Metagonimus yokogawa.

Considered by many to have been the greatest of all Japanese parasitologists, Yokogawa defined the migration of Paragonimus westermani *metacercariae in the definitive host in this paper.*

. . . The problem of *Paragonimus westermani* on Taiwan Island has always been studied in the vicinity of Shinchiku and its environs because it was believed and expected that the solution to this problem would come eventually from research in this area. Dr. Koan Nakagawa of the Shinchiku Hospital, the successor to Dr. Matsuo, has been engaged in research on this subject, collecting all the necessary data and examining the freshwater fish and shellfish which have been known as the intermediate hosts among the general class of trematodes. He made repeated field investigations of the simple living conditions of the aborigines of Taiwanese communities which are heavily infected by the parasites we are discussing, and thus he was able to bring an auspicious event to our world of scholarship last February through the publication of an article which summarized his research on this subject.

Dr. Nakagawa has proved that this trematode, *P. westermani* had the same intermediate host as other distoma, in general, and that its secondary intermediate host was *Thelpusa* sp., a kind of *Potamon* (*Geothelphusa dehaaani,* White). Here, it was proved that the route of infection of the trematode was by mouth, thus it seemed possible to find the route of migration of this worm in the definitive host.

In February of this year, through the kindness of Dr. Nakagawa, I received several crabs from this area. I then separated the small encysted larvae from the crabs, and thus transferred the larvae orally to mice in order to trace the route of migration. I experimented several times in this connection with animals killed at various stages and with different time intervals after feeding the larvae.

The experiments on the infected mice showed that the encysted larvae did not migrate, and there was no evidence of parasitism by *P. westermani* found in those mice which had been infected with larvae for 30 days. Accordingly, it was concluded that mice were not proper experimental animals. It was decided, thereafter, to use animals which were larger than mice. It was clear, however, that the larger the experimental animal, the more difficult it would be to trace the route of *Paragonimus'* migration. In addition, it was difficult to carry out the experiments with a small number of encysted larvae.

Therefore, I brought several dogs from Taipei

on 1 April of this year and went into the area under the jurisdiction of the Sinchiku Provincial Government. An adequate number of encysted larvae were given to these dogs, which were then sacrificed at various time intervals. I then examined them microscopically, studying the various internal organs systematically, and thereby attempted to define the route of migration of the metacercariae. I also attempted to find a way of preventing this disease caused by the worms.

I plan to elucidate the route of migration of *P. westermani* in the definitive host, and request the valuable suggestions of readers of this article, even though I delay the final report on the route of migration of the worms for another time.

I. *First Experiment. Experimental Dog A.* On 3 April, Dog A was fed 98 of thè encysted larvae at 1:00 P.M.; an additional 90 larvae were fed at 4:00 P.M. On 4 April, 100 larvae were given to the dog at 10:00 A.M. Using chloroform, the dog was then sacrificed and dissected at 11:00 A.M. on 5 April. Therefore, the dog was fed a total of 288 encysted larvae with various time lapses (46, 43, 25 hours, respectively) until its dissection.

Results from examination of the dissected Dog A. The experimental animal was secured to a wooden board. Examination of the abdominal cavity revealed that the surface of the serosa of the intestine was somewhat congested; generally speaking, it was a light pink color, and numerous fine blood vessels were seen. Judging from the results of the preceding investigation, it was my impression that the larvae most probably caused some kind of damage to the wall of the intestine. The thorax was dissected and examined, but no remarkable change was noted. I did not, of course, neglect the possibility of the route of migration of the larvae through the blood vessels or lymphatics; therefore, I ligated all the blood vessels, large or small, to stop the escape of blood when removing the internal organs, and then I immersed them in formalin.

II. *Second Experiment. Experimental Dog B.* On 4 April, Dog B was given 68 encysted larvae at 11:00 A.M. and 90 at noon the next day; on 6 April it was given 114 at 5 P.M.; and on 8 April, 107 at 9:00 A.M. The animal was sacrificed and dissected at 9:00 A.M. on 12 April. Dog B, therefore, was fed with a total of 379 encysted larvae, with various time lapses (96, 136, 165, and 190 hours, respectively) until it was dissected.

Results from examination of the dissected Dog B. Examination of the abdominal cavity showed that the surface of the serosa of the intestine was not "bloodshot" as in the case of Dog A, except for several petechiae on the intestinal wall. In contrast to these findings, a large amount of slightly turbid serum could be observed in the abdominal cavity. At this point, I compared the results of the present experiment with those from the preceding one and concluded that the present findings indicated that the larvae caused a slight peritonitis due to irritation of the intestinal wall as they migrated to the abdominal cavity.

I, therefore, stopped the dissection and took the serum from within the abdominal cavity and placed it in a clean glass dish. Subsequently, I examined the thorax and found a small amount of pleural fluid bilaterally, similar to that which was found previously in the abdominal cavity. After removing this fluid to another clean glass dish, I examined the surface of the pleura, but could find no gross surface changes. However, several petechiae could be seen within the membranous portion of the diaphragm and also near the border of the membranous and muscular regions. Furthermore, countless petechiae of light brown-pink color, as big as a half-grain of rice, could be found on the surface of the lungs (which were light pink in color). In removing the internal organs, similar precautions were taken as in the first test, and the internal organs were immersed in formalin.

Examination of serum found within the abdominal cavity and thorax. The examination of the serum in the abdominal cavity and thorax (mentioned above) revealed white specks which seemed to be quivering lightly. These specks were examined further microscopically, confirming that they were metacercariae. These metacercariae within the abdominal cavity and thorax varied in size; the big ones 0.8–1.0 mm and the small ones 0.5–0.6 mm.

The entire form of a metacercaria had a strong resemblance to a mature *P. westermani;* therefore, it was easy to distinguish the young forms of the *Paragonimus.* Furthermore, no difference in the degree of development between the ones found in the thorax and those found in the abdominal cavity could be observed. The degree of

growth was directly proportional to the time interval after the larvae were fed. . . .

III. *Third Experiment, Dog C.* . . .

IV. *Fourth Experiment. Experimental Dog D.* On 5 April this dog was fed 50 encysted larvae at noon, 70 at 6:00 P.M. the following day, and 127 at 4:00 P.M. the next day, 7 April—a total of 247 larvae. On 21 April, the dog was dissected at 10:00 A.M. Therefore, this dog was dissected after 389 hours (approximately 16 days) from its first feeding, or after 352 hours (approximately 15 days) from the time of its second feeding, or after 320 hours (approximately 14 days) from its last feeding, respectively.

Results from examination of the dissected Dog D. Examination of the abdominal cavity showed a light pink intestinal serosa, with few petechiae. The greater omentum and the mesentery had a few petechiae, yet there was no gross change. Yellowish-pink thick fluid was found in the abdominal cavity. This fluid was examined, but no larvae were present. In order to confirm the existence of the metacercariae which entered the abdominal cavity, the intestines and viscera were washed with warm saline; the solution was then examined and several metacercariae were found.

Examination of the dissected thorax showed a small amount of slightly thick light pink fluid, and several metacercariae were found. The pulmonary visceral pleura was slightly elevated, giving a vacuolated appearance. Some petechiae were present. Some metacercariae in the process of migrating through the visceral pleura were found after washing the thoracic cavity with the warm saline. However, the only lung nodules were one in the right lung and two in the right lower lobe. No larvae were found in the soft tissues of the cervical region and mediastinum. The whitish area was seen in the middle and anterior portion of the tendinous section of the diaphragm which was removed with the thoracic organs; two additional small white areas were found at the border between the tendinous and the muscular portions. Therefore, the diaphragm was stretched on a wooden frame and examined through the dissection microscope. The white spots in the tendinous section were, without a doubt, metacercariae, since the intestinal tract (with its peculiar dark gray color) was recognized on both sides, and their appearance was just like the encysted metacercariae and actively moving. At the same time, it was noted that the dark gray intestinal tract moved slightly.

V. *Fifth Experiment. Experimental Dog E.* The dog which had been given to us by Dr. Nakagawa on 24 March of this year was fed with seven crabs from the aborigines of Taiwan. The number of encysted larvae fed to the dog was not known. The dog's nutritional status was excellent, and it took food well even on its dying day. It died suddenly at 4:00 P.M. on 24 April, 31 days after the dog had eaten the larvae. The abdominal cavity was opened; no pathologic changes were obvious to the naked eye, except petechiae on the surface of the greater omentum, the mesentery, and the intestinal serosa. The serum in the abdominal cavity was very scant, and no larvae were found on it. Therefore, after the intestines were covered with gauze saturated with saline solution the thorax was dissected, and a large amount of a slightly thick yellowish-pink fluid was found. Several metacercariae as big as half a kernel of hemp were found therein. The visceral pleura of the lung was granular and contained countless tiny vacuoles, some of which were lightly adherent to the parietal pleura with a fibrinous exudate.

Further investigation of the peculiar tiny cavities on the surface of the lungs showed that metacercariae were alive and were moving in a certain number of the vacuoles. Yet, it was very difficult to determine the presence of the tiny metacercariae on the gray-pink surface of the lungs, for the wide intestinal tract peculiar to the metacercariae was a similar dark gray color; therefore, it was hard to distinguish between them. These larvae under the visceral pleura did not move into the parenchyma immediately, but most of them formed tunnels under it, or moved out to the surface of the outer pleura. Noting this, I picked up 27 metacercariae that moved out to the surface of the visceral pleura and thoracic cavity. Those larvae which penetrated the parenchyma formed peculiar nodules, three in the right lung and six in the left lung, respectively. This number was extremely small as compared with those existing separately under the visceral pleura and in the thoracic cavity.

Examination of the pericardium and mediastinum demonstrated metacercariae wriggling in the tissues of the anterior mediastinum. Further, on examining the soft tissues of the cervical re-

gion, the same type of metacercariae were found in the fatty tissue behind the superior portion of the sternum. On removing the soft tissue of the cervical region, two metacercariae in the loose connective tissue around the arteries and veins on the left cervical area were in contact with each other and were moving upward together. This phenomenon was really sensational to the investigator. If it were possible to fix this phenomenon *in situ* and make a specimen out of it, it would have been the masterpiece of the world. [In these experiments, Yokogawa was obviously seeking the explanation for the pathogenesis of human cerebral paragonimiasis, which was first described by Otani in 1887 (Cysten Otani, S., Cysten des Gehirns mit Eiern von Distomen sonst in der Leber, Darmevand, Peritoneum, Lymphdrusen; Zeitschrift Medicina Gesellschul Tokyo 1: 8–9, 1887)—Eds.]

However, the investigator stripped the vessels of that region carefully and found that the metacercariae moved under the thin sheath around the left jugular veins, either by providence or merely coincidence. At this moment, the investigator felt that all questions about larvae were solved immediately. Even though he had not doubted and believed that the larvae would move up into the cranial cavity along the soft tissue of the anterior cervical region, he had never expected that the route of migration of the metacercariae was formed so conveniently in this manner.

After adequately dissecting this unusual specimen, the examiner further studied the inside of the orbit and cranial cavity by cutting the cranial cavity from the anterior cervical region to the bottom of the cranium. No larvae could be seen in this region.

Since the larvae's route of migration to the brain has already been proved, anyone who takes a look at this specimen would clearly understand the answer to this subject. The diaphragm was examined after all of the internal organs of the thorax and cervical region had been removed. One larva in the anterior section of the central tendinous portion of the diaphragm was found wriggling under the pleura. I was about to stretch the entire diaphragm on a wooden frame; however, by then the sun had already set and I had to take the time to turn on the lights. When I returned to the autopsy table to put the diaphragm into the fixative, the larvae had already penetrated the thin pleura and had reached the surface of the diaphragm. I proved under the electric light that the metacercariae had infiltrated fairly deeply into the surface of the peritoneum in the central tendinous portion of the diaphragm. Again I examined the inside of the abdominal cavity and found several metacercariae that were attached to the surface of the greater omentum and the peritoneum.

Several larvae were also found within the greater omentum. However, no metacercariae were found on the surface of the liver, even though some petechiae and ecchymoses were seen on the liver capsule. Two live metacercariae were found under the capsule on the spleen. This may have been a new, previously undescribed discovery. Further, several metacercariae were found also in the gastrolenic ligament and in the lenophrenic ligament. These larvae were similar to those in the greater omentum.

A metacercaria was found under the capsule in the central part of the superior pole of the left kidney; fatty white spots surrounded it. Also, under the capsule of the right kidney, several metacercariae were found, and their appearance was similar to those found under the splenic capsule. Two metacercariae were found under the *transversalis fascia* of the abdominal wall. One of these two larvae was comparatively large, and a white fibrotic area as large as the high-power lens was found around it.

VI. *Sixth Experiment. Experimental Kitten F.* This kitten was fed 228 encysted larvae at 2:00 P.M. on 8 April. Its condition was normal for 10 days after it was fed. However, its vigor waned somewhat after that, and its appetite distinctly decreased until the kitten's death; it took almost nothing on its last day. The kitten died the night of 26 April and was dissected on 27 April. Therefore, 18 days and some hours had passed since the initial feeding.

The results from examination on the dissected kitten F. Examination of the dissected kitten revealed marked wasting, with absence of subcutaneous fat. The skin was extremely loose. Examining the abdominal cavity, no particular change was noticed except that petechiae were seen on the greater omentum and the mesentery.

There was very little fluid in the abdominal cavity, and no metacercariae were found in it.

The intestine was covered with gauze and the dissection of the thorax begun. A small amount of somewhat thick yellowish-pink fluid was found in the thoracic cavity; no larvae were found in this fluid. Instead, several metacercariae were seen adhering to the surface of both the visceral pleura and the thoracic wall. Two larvae were found in the tissues around the right internal mammary artery near the manubrium. Also under the pleura of the chest wall, at the level of the rib on the right side, larvae were found.

Examination of the soft tissues in the anterior cervical region, by careful dissection, revealed the following: under the fascia, of the left sternoclavicular muscles, near the edge of the clavicle, migrating metacercariae were found. No larvae were seen in the connective tissue around the vessels in the anterior cervical region. In the lungs there were tunnels and tiny vacuoles on the surface of the visceral pleura formed by the penetration of the metacercariae. However, these changes were not as distinctive as those found in the case of Dog E. This resulted probably from the fact that the larvae examined were comparatively smaller than those found in Dog E; therefore, the visceral pleura was less involved. This difference was so small that it might not be noticed unless a careful comparison was made with Dog. E.

Regarding the pathology (that is, the peculiar nodule in the pulmonary parenchyma), only six or seven nodules were found in both lungs. Metacercariae were found under the pleura in the central tendinous portion of the diaphragm, and several were found in the mesentery and the greater omentum. Again, some metacercariae migrated under the liver capsule from the upper part of the hepatic duct near the portal fissure to the right lobe of the liver; others migrated into the hepatic parenchyma. Several metacercariae were found, which had migrated into the connective tissues of the uterovesical pouch. Besides these, some metacercariae were found under the *transversalis fascia* of the abdominal wall.

VII. *Seventh Experiment. Experimental Cat G.* On 10 April, at 4:00 P.M., this cat was fed 120 of the fully matured encysted larvae; it was subsequently kept in an animal cage. Its activity decreased, and its appetite diminished after 10 days. It was killed and dissected on 23 May, 42 days from the initial larvae feeding.

The results of examination on dissected Cat G.
The cat was of medium size and poorly nourished. Exceedingly purulent, thick, pink fluid was found in the abdominal cavity (approximately 100 cc). Although the thick turbid fluid looked almost half purulent, no leukocytes could be observed microscopically; however, a large number of red blood cells and their fragments were seen. Even though the surface of the liver was generally glossy and smooth, several petechiae and some areas of membrane rupture were seen. On the surface of the spleen, there were several subcapsular petechiae, and two areas similar to the nodules previously described were noted. No particular change could be seen with the naked eye in the greater omentum or the mesentery. Again a metacercaria that had gotten into the greater omentum re-entered the abdominal cavity. On the lower portion of the peritoneum, there were irregular petechiae and ecchymoses and several irregular, rough-edged scars. Thirteen metacercariae were gathered from the exudate in the abdominal cavity. The fluid in the thorax was similar to that which was taken from the abdominal cavity, and the quantity was quite large (approximately 50 cc in each side of the thorax, respectively). The surface of the lungs was covered with granules the size of a grain of rice or a hemp kernel and with dry flaky material.

There was only a small nodule which was considered a parasitic cystoma, near the anterior edge of the upper part of the left lung. In the parietal pleura, there were irregular forms of scars with gray-white color as seen in a map. Nine metacercariae of almost the same size were found in a search of the anterior mediastinum, on the surface of the lungs, in the chest wall, and in the exudate from the thorax. The examination of the diaphragm, after the thorax and the internal organs of the abdominal cavity were extracted, demonstrated that the irregular petechiae and white-gray linear scars appeared in the muscular and tendinous portions of the diaphragm. . . .

X. *Tenth Experiment. Experimental Dog I.*
The dog was fed 176 of the fully matured metacercariae at 3:00 P.M. on 19 June and then with 50 additional larvae at 10:00 A.M. on the next day. It was killed and dissected at 4:00 P.M. on 20 June. The time that elapsed between feeding and death ranged from 6 to 25 hours.

Results of examination of dissected Dog I. The dog was of medium size and in a good state of nutrition. In general, the surface of the intestinal serosa was intensively hemorrhagic, and the fine vessels of the mesentery and intestinal serosa were numerous. No serum as seen in the abdominal cavity. However, since the investigator presumed that the metacercariae might already have left the wall of the intestine and moved into the abdominal cavity, he washed off the intestine with the saline solution and took the fluid. He found two metacercariae in the solution. However, no unusual serum was seen in the thorax. The surface of the lungs was light pink, but no petechiae were found. As a trial, the organs of the thorax were washed with the saline solution and the solution examined, but no metacercariae were found. No petechiae were noticed on the diaphragm. . . .

Here, it would not be too presumptuous to say that the metacercariae's route of migration in the definitive host was almost perfectly proved by the foregoing series of investigations. These experiments showed that the metacercariae which enter the intestine of the definitive host become excysted by the action of the digestive fluid; thereafter, they push aside the villi of the intestine, thereby penetrating into the mucosa (as Mr. Yokogawa's proof of the larvae of *Metagonimus'* infiltration into the villi). However, the young metacercariae in the mucosa of the intestine were more round than those of *Metagonimus*; the larvae found in the villi of the intestinal mucosa of Dog A at the first test were oval-shaped on cross-section. Apparently, it was more difficult for them to penetrate, and thus they appeared slightly distorted in the villi of the intestine. Accordingly, it is difficult to conclude that the metacercariae's passage from the intestine into the abdominal cavity is always the same. In our tenth experiment, on Dog I, we found that the metacercariae got into the abdominal cavity earlier (within 24 hours) although in the first test with Dog A, with time lapses of 25 to 45 hours after feeding of the larvae, they were still in the intestinal mucosa. In such cases, with time lapses of from ten to several scores of hours after ingestion by the experimental animals, metacercariae penetrated the digestive canal to the abdominal cavity, passed through the diaphragm and entered the thorax where they stayed for a certain number of hours, and then moved from the visceral pleura into the pulmonary parenchyma. Here, they form their peculiar parasitic cysts. Through microscopic observation it could be proved that the metacercariae penetrate the lungs via the surface of the lungs.

The migration from the abdominal cavity into the thorax depends entirely upon the random locomotion of the larvae, and the route of migration was considered to be along the blood vessels or lymphatics; therefore, there is no definite direction to their motion.

Consequently, the larvae's movement from one place to another takes varying amounts of time because they take a circuitous route to the lungs by way of the intestine, liver, spleen, mesentery, and so on, in the wide abdominal cavity, or pass through them. Some of the larvae lose their way and accidentally get into the fatty tissue of the greater omentum, mesentery, spermatic cord, or abdominal wall. There they form the parasitic cysts and remain forever. The oral route of infection of the metacercariae is the rule. The route of migration from the intestine to the lungs is proved completely. The preceding experiments explain the presence of metacercariae in different sites. Here, the investigator believes that the route of migration of the metacercariae being found in the brain, in the orbit, and in the eyelids, which was previously unknown, is now fully proved.

Since the larvae have an affinity for movement in the loose connective tissue of the host, it was presumed that their presence in the brain meant that their journey began in the connective tissue of the anterior cervical region; however, it was not certain from which point they would initiate their movement. But it was possible here, to prove, by the studies of the Dog E, that the natural course of migration is by ascent through the connective tissue around the internal carotid arteries and jugular veins. Here, these larvae ascending along the internal jugular veins can enter the cranium directly from the foramina of the jugular veins, while the other way, via the internal carotid arteries, is to proceed upward along the connective tissue around the arteries, thereby entering the cranium. However, it is possible to assume, in view of anatomy and the amount of distortion between the arteries and veins, that the latter course is obviously more difficult than that of the former course of ascending in the connective tissue around the internal jugular veins.

As for the route leading to the orbit and eyelids, the larvae may possibly move first into

the cranium along the internal jugular vein or the internal carotid artery and from there move further into the orbit, along the external carotid artery. On the other hand, the larvae may pass directly into the orbit along the internal carotid arteries which are the branches of the external carotid artery. At any rate, it is a definite fact that the route of migration of the metacercariae to the cranium is guided by the connective tissue around the great vessels of the anterior cervical region.

The subject of the action of the metacercariae on the lungs is also very interesting. The results from the examination of Dog E will well explain this. It has been questioned why the metacercariae could not be found—in spite of the examination of several hundred sections of petechiae which were deemed peculiar to Dogs B and C. I now feel as though I understand this problem. That is, the metacercariae parasitize not only the lungs of the human body and animals, but all the connective tissues as well. Even though the metacercariae move into the thorax, they don't instantly penetrate the parenchyma, but rather they penetrate the visceral pleura; from that point, they form the tiny vacuoles or tunnels. Even if they move into the parenchyma, their young larvae penetrate freely into the tissues of lung and form petechiae in many places there. Thus one can accept this phenomenon as evidence of penetration of the larvae into the lungs. Consequently, the investigator believes it valid to say that these metacercariae parasitize not only the lungs but the connective tissues in general.

This is the plain fact judging from the results of a series of animal tests. They are able to live and grow in connective tissue such as the mediastinum, the greater omentum, subcutaneous connective tissue, orbit, eyelids, the scrotum, and brain. They don't have means of discharging eggs or of ovulation. What is more, a mechanical stimulation causes suppurative inflammation in the area, thus the larvae might be destroyed by lack of nutrition. In contrast to the above fact, those parasites which reside in the lungs easily produce ova when the nutrients are provided; thus, they stay there longer and produce those symptoms which initially attracted my attention to them as parasites.

Since the route of migration of the metacercariae within the body apparently begins in the connective tissue, those cysts of these metacercariae found in the subcutaneous tissues of the thigh or abdominal wall were generally caused by the migration from the connective tissue such as the intramuscular connective tissue, *fascia lata,* inguinal canal, and the like, and not by those metacercariae moving directly into that region breaking through the muscle. The passage of the metacercariae into the thorax from the abdominal cavity must, most frequently, be through the central tendinous region of the diaphragm.

It is also believed that the metacercariae can penetrate the thorax, penetrating the muscle, as it enters into the wall of the intestine, judging from the numerous petechiae in the muscular region and the linear or irregular scars in this region. However, we must not forget that these scars are caused by tunnels formed by the metacercariae which penetrated under the pleura of the diaphragm or under the peritoneum. These relations have been confirmed by the fourth, fifth, and sixth experiments, respectively. Besides, the above-mentioned migration is also accomplished by way of natural openings such as the esophageal hiatus, *lacuna vasorum,* or by way of lumbocostal triangle and sternocostal triangle tightly contracted between the parietal pleura and the peritoneum in the case of the human body.

In conclusion, I wish to express my thanks to the Taiwan Research Society of Local Epidemic Diseases for its kindness, rendered directly or indirectly to the writer, and to Dr. Koan Nakagawa for offering part of his invaluable materials to me.

THE MODE OF INFECTION IN PULMONARY DISTOMIASIS
Certain Fresh-water Crabs as Intermediate Hosts of *Paragonimus westermanii*

Journal of Infectious Diseases, 18: 131–142, 1916. Selections from pp. 131–132, 134–135, 137–138.

Koan Nakagawa
(1874–1959)

Nakagawa's biography will be found in the chapter on Fasciolopsiasis.
Several distinguished Japanese parasitologists studied the life cycle of Paragonimus *at about the same time. First the parasite, then the secondary intermediate host, and finally the primary intermediate host were recognized. Although Nakagawa intimates that*

the Melania sp. *is the primary intermediate host, he did not confirm his hypothesis until late 1915.*

Paragonimus westermanii Kerbert, the distome of the human lung is rather widely spread in the Far East. Ringer was the first to discover it, in 1879, in the lungs of inhabitants of the city Tamsui in Formosa. Since then it has been found in the various parts of Japan proper. In some places the distomes affect so large a number of the inhabitants that pulmonary distomiasis assumes almost an endemic nature. Consequently, the distome has been very carefully studied by various Japanese investigators. Altho it is now over 30 years since the discovery of the distome, the developmental stages of the worm, except its miracidia, have not as yet been clearly understood. For 10 years I have been carrying on an investigation of pulmonary distomiasis in the locality of Formosa, where the disease is most prevalent, and finally I have been fortunate enough to discover the second intermediate host of the lung distomes. Recently the mode of infection has been experimentally determined. . . .

Investigation of the Second Intermediate Host of Paragonimus Westermanii

Appointed head of the Public Hospital at Shinchiku in 1912, I was placed thus under favorable conditions for carrying out an investigation of the lung distome. My attention was first directed to the search after the second intermediate host of the distome so that I might trace its developmental cycle. When I started the investigation, all that was known of the life-history was contained in Nakahama's and Manson's observations, that the miracidia hatched from the eggs begin to swim in about 4 weeks from the time of entering the water after they come out of the patients. As to what becomes of them afterwards, nobody had any idea.

Collecting as many fresh-water molluscs as possible from the streams or ponds in the region where distomiasis exists as an endemic disease, I made careful search after the cercariae. I succeeded in obtaining 17 different kinds, but I could not distinguish the cercariae of the lung distomes from others. So I put various molluscs into the water in which miracidia of the lung distome were kept, to see what kinds of molluscs the miracidia would infest. It resulted that they infested Melania libertina Gould and M. obliquegranosa Smith most abundantly. From this it may be assumed that these two species of fresh water molluscs are the first intermediate hosts of the lung distomes. Notwithstanding the utmost care taken in keeping the molluscs infested with miracidia alive in an experimental pond, all of them died within a few weeks. They were found to contain no grown cercariae. Altho this experiment turned out to be a failure, I found that a certain kind of cercaria is found in all M. libertina living in the rivulets and creeks of the mountainous regions where the aborigines are infected in an enormous percentage.

The cercaria has a tadpole-like appearance, the body being 0.12 mm long and 0.09 mm wide, with a tail 0.054 mm long. Attached to the oral sucker (0.036 × 0.032 mm) are 2 pear-shaped bodies, the apices of which point towards the median plane of the body. The sucker has spines, each provided with a ring along its anterior edge. The ventral sucker is much smaller than the oral one, being 0.018 mm in diameter. Within the parenchyma are 3 pairs of poison glands. The excretory vesicle is heart-shaped. Besides this kind of cercaria, the liver of the molluscs contains a good many sporocysts. Some melaniae have a number of half-grown cercariae. From the fact that M. libertina is found abundantly in the region where distomiasis of the lung prevails most widely, it may not be unreasonable to conclude that these cercariae are those of the lung distome. However, we have not as yet any experimental proof.

Encysted Larvae of the Distome of the Human Lung in Crabs

Kobayashi's interesting work on the discovery of the encysted larvae of Clonorchis sinensis Cobbold in certain fishes gave me an impulse in the study of the question of the second intermediate host of the distome of the human lung. At first I selected a region of the Shinchiku prefecture where patients are abundant and made several difficult excursions to collect all molluscs, fishes, amphibians, and insects that I could. My microscopic examination showed that M. libertina Gould only has a certain kind of cercaria. In September, 1914, I captured in the rivulet in Kalapai Village a kind of crab which had not been caught before. My microscopic examinations were rewarded with the discovery

of numerous encysted larvae in the liver. They were all half grown, but they were unmistakably larvae of certain trematodes. At first I had no idea that they were the young distomes of the human lung. However, as the result of further investigation I found in the gills full-grown ones with all the morphologic structures peculiar to the distome of the human lung. Furthermore, I observed that the encysted larvae, when they were introduced into certain animals by mouth, grew into Paragonimus westermanii.

The young encysted larvae infest chiefly the liver of the crab, while the farther advanced ones are found in the gill. Sometimes they penetrate the muscle. The young encysted larvae are round, 0.2 mm in diameter. The young distomes in the cysts lie straight. They have a conspicuous, large, black excretory vesicle and comparatively large oral (provided with a spine) and ventral suckers. They do not have a distinctly developed alimentary canal. The encysted larvae found in the gill are well developed, measuring 0.3 to 0.4 mm in diameter. The young distome in the cyst has a short and thick body and lies straight, unlike others, which are contorted. The oral sucker has a spine, and is 0.08 to 0.11 mm in diameter. The short esophagus is connected with the bifurcate intestine. Each branch of the intestine is thick and undulating, running parallel to, and outside of, a long, thick excretory vesicle. The ventral sucker is a little larger than the oral one, measuring 0.07 to 0.12 mm in diameter. The entire surface of the body is provided with short spines. The wall of the cyst is 0.01 mm thick—a characteristic feature of the species. The young distome rotates sluggishly in the cyst. The full-grown encysted larvae sometimes reach 0.5 mm in diameter, and to the naked eye look like a white speck. Sometimes they assume an elliptical shape, 1.0 mm long and 0.4 mm wide. They can readily be removed from the gill. Twenty percent of larvae thus freed were observed to float on the surface of the water. Under natural conditions the full-grown larvae would leave the crab's gills, get into the water, and be taken up by the dwellers on the banks of the lower stream.

Fresh-water Crabs with the Larvae of Paragonimus Westermanii

Potamon obtusipes (*Stimpson*)—''Red crab.'' This was the first of the three species of crabs in which the encysted larvae of the human-lung distome were found. The carapace is coarse, flat, and provided with teeth along the lateral margins; the pterygostomian region is granular; the dorsal surface is a deep-chestnut color; the abdomen and legs are somewhat reddish. One large specimen has a carapace over 38 mm in diameter. The native name of this crab is "shahoi" or "chahoi," which means red crab. Sometimes it is eaten. This species has never been found in any place in Japan other than the mountainous region in Formosa. I have found that the crab is most abundant in rivulets or creeks running through the mountainous regions of Shinchiku Prefecture. The number of encysted larvae in the gills increases in correlation with the number of cases of distomiasis of the lungs; for instance, in the region where 30–50% of the inhabitants are found to harbor the parasites in their lungs, 100% of the crabs carry the encysted larvae, while 5 miles down the river, where comparatively few patients are met with (I have had no opportunity to make sure of the percentage), only 11% of the crabs have the encysted larvae. In the crabs of Sansaka region no encysted larvae were found.

Potamon dehaanii (White).—This species occurs in the same locality with the species mentioned, but not so abundantly, and it is a little smaller in size. The carapace is somewhat round and smooth. There are no teeth on the lateral margin. The pterygostomian region is smooth. The dorsal surface is grayish-black, or sometimes slightly reddish. The ventral side and the legs are grayish-white. This species also occurs in the rivers of the mountainous regions in Japan proper. The natives, who call it "sai-hoi" (dung crab), do not eat it. Encysted larvae of the distome of the lung were also found in this species, tho less numerously than in the former.

Eriocheir japonicus De Haan.—Unlike the other two species, this one never occurs in the streams of the mountainous region, but occurs in the rivers flowing across the plain. This species can easily be discriminated from the other two by its chelae, which are provided with a thick growth of hair. Very big specimens have a carapace over 76 mm in diameter. The native name is "mon-hai," or "mun-hai" (hairy crab). This crab is eaten by the natives. The encysted larvae were found in only 2 out of 330 specimens (300 large and 30 smaller ones) which I collected and examined. I am not certain whether or not the attachment to the crabs is merely an accident. The solution of the problem awaits further investigation.

In conclusion I may say that of the three species of fresh-water crabs the encysted larvae of the human lung distomes are found in the first and the second species, the occurrence in the third being problematical. In view of the fact that the second species occurs outside Formosa, this may be the second intermediate host of distomiasis in Japan proper. . . .

CHAPTER 32

Taeniasis

LUMBRICUS LATUS, OR A DISCOURSE READ BEFORE THE ROYAL SOCIETY, OF THE JOYNTED WORM, WHEREIN A GREAT MANY MISTAKES OF FORMER WRITERS CONCERNING IT, ARE REMARKED; ITS NATURAL HISTORY FROM MORE EXACT OBSERVATIONS IS ATTEMPTED; AND THE WHOLE URGED, AS A DIFFICULTY AGAINST THE DOCTRINE OF UNIVOCAL GENERATION

Philosophical Transactions, 13: 113–144, 1683. Selections from pp. 113–114, 124, 127–131, 136, 138–141. Reprinted in the original English.

Edward Tyson
(1650–1708)

Tyson's biography appears with his description of the anatomy of Ascaris lumbricoides.

In this paper, Tyson demonstrated that the tapeworm had a head.

The consideration of Insects, and their manner of generation, as it is a subject of curious speculation; so of late hath been much illustrated by the laborious researches of many inquisitive persons: whose travels therein, tho' they have much advanced the doctrine of univocal generation; and bid very fair for the exploding of that, too easily received, and common error, of their production from putrefaction, yet one great difficulty still remains with me, how to account for several of those, that are bred in Animal bodies not such as we may suppose to be hatched from the eggs of the like kind, that are received with the food or other ways; but of whom we cannot meet with a parallel, or of the same Species, out of the body, in the whole world as is known besides. I shall instance onely in two, the *Lumbricus latus,* and *Teres.* Of the former I shall give at present onely these remarks; wherein its difference from any other does more remarkably appear: (1) being

flat; (2) joynted after a peculiar manner; (3) the great disproportion of both extreams; (4) the vast length 'tis often of; (5) the head so remarkably beset with hooked Spikes; (6) what has never that I know of, been remarked of this, or any other Insect or Animal in the World besides; the great number of Mouths it hath; more than the Poets fain'd Briareus had hands, or Argus eyes, viz. in every Joynt one; (7) that any part of the body being broken off from the rest, should still remain alive, and thrive.

All which particulars, besides what others may be added, if duely considered, will render it difficult to give an instance of the like out of the body, from whence, or from the seed of the same, it may be any ways thought, this may be propagated here. . . .

The head of Nile does not seem to be more perplex't, and obscure to the Ancients, than that of this Worm, which has created as many Controversies among Anatomists of late, as that has with Geographers of old. And those too who have had the advantage of observing vast quantities of this Worm, after their most strict enquiries, and most diligent research thereinto, have at last been forced to confess, that they are still at a loss and know nothing certain of it; and what they propose, they deliver rather as a conjecture at random, than any thing as an established truth. And many, as most of the Ancients, are utterly silent in it. . . .

Indeed I must confess that account I had from the women who first observed it, and the Patient who voided that Worm I mentioned to have by me eight yards long; and was given me by my worthy Friend Mr. Houghton, an Apothecary, seemed agreeable to this, tho when I first saw it I could take notice of no such thing; and therefore am apt to think 'twas onely some Thrumbs of the inward coat of the Intestine, which might stick to the hooks here, which might make this figure. For in the heads of all I have had yet an opportunity of seeing; I could never observe any such thing.

I shall therefore now deliver my observations of the heads of this Worm as I have seen them, in three several ones I have taken out of the bodies of Dogs upon dissection; and it being so, makes me to be something more at a Certainty; where I know I have them whole. And altho all three, did exactly agree; yet there being some circumstances, which attended the one, who not the others; yet being very material to our purpose, I shall recount them here. And it was in a Dog I opened at our private meetings, at the Anatomical Theater of the College of Physicians, where I observed this Worm alive in the Ilion; not lying streight, but in many places winding, and doubling. Having taken notice how the Joynts were, I traced it up, by carefully opening the Intestine, to the smallest Extream; where I expected the head to be; and which did lye towards the Duodenum; whereas the broader end was downward towards the Rectum; and this broad end was free, and did nothing adhere; whereas that small extream did so firmly stick, and had fasten'd itself to the inward coat of the Intestine, that it was not without some trouble, by gently raising it with my Nail, that I freed it from its adhesion. Having lifted it up, I carefully viewed it; and did observe neither that Biceps in Tulpius's first figure, nor the head like a Tricoccos as in Mich Fehr, but a very slender body; which being alive, it would sometimes shoot out a considerable length; at others retract it in again, and so very much alter its figure, by becoming broader. But whilst I was doing this, by its wrigling its body, it happening to fall off my finger; it presently took hold again, and gave me as much trouble to free it a second time from its adhesion, as at the first. Other observations I then made of its motion, and of the two single Joynts which were broken off, which I shall mention in my last particular: as also of those Orifices at the sides, which I shall discourse of in my next; and for the present I put it into Spirit of Wine, that I might more carefully view it with a Microscope at home. And in doing this, making use of some extraordinary good ones, it very plainly appeared as is represented in my 11th Figure (Plate 100) thick beset with two orders of Spikes, or Hooks, whereof the larger did arise from the Center or Middle spreading themselves over the edges of the circumference; the other which were lesser issuing out about the middle from the Center, and were shorter, as is seen in this Figure, and are represented sideways in the twelfth. I could not upon my strictest Enquiry and with extraordinary Glasses too, inform myself of any Orifice here, which we may suppose to be the mouth; onely a little indenting there was, in the Center, occasion'd by the issuing out of the Spikes thence. This end was not perfectly flat, but a little globous, and I could perceive by the swelling a little below on the neck, and wrinkling of the Skin, as in the figure; how it did shoot out, and contract its neck, as I observed it when alive: For some little space here, I could not observe with the glasses any Joynts at all; but after, very thick set, and small, and gradually increasing in length, as they descended towards the Tail.

The heads of the other two Worms exactly appeared the same in the Microscope, as this described. And afterwards by carefully viewing them by my naked eye, I could observe these hairs or Spikes. . . .

It was objected by some ingenious persons, who had been acquainted with what I observed concerning this head, whether these spikes, or hairs might not be like the small feet of the tick or Ricinus for its fastening itself the better to help its suction. And indeed were it blood it lived upon, the case were plain; but since 'tis Chyle what service they could do it in this, I do not see; for when they fasten, the head is deep immerged in the inward Coat of the Intestine; and so may be thought for that time, to get but a very inconsiderable soop, if any; and nothing in proportion to what is requisite for so vast a long body; and what it is often observed to be Turgid with. Upon the whole, what seems most agreeable to me, and to be the true use of this part we call the head is this; that by means of these hooks, and Spikes it might fasten itself, and so prevent, its too easy ejection out of the body. For it being so very long, and large too, and its body in many places winding, and convoluted, the descent of the feces upon all occasions would be apt to carry it out with them; had it not this hold, which is so fast, that rather than loosen itself, parts of the body are sooner broken off, which we frequently see in the stool. When it penetrates the coat of the Intestine it contracts its hooks in, and draws up its head to a point; then expands them, and takes firm hold of the Membrane, by darting its several poniards into it, which excites those intolerable pains, which those that are troubled with them, so much complain off; that I have known it to that extremity, that some have been scarce dissuaded from offering violence to themselves, to free themselves, as they thought, from a great misery, and hence it is that this Worm is of so difficult a cure; that though by Medicines, and Purges, vast quantities at times may be brought away; yet some can hardly get a perfect cure all their life time; as I know of one who for above 20 years has been afflicted with it; that has had the advice of several able, and eminent Physicians. And indeed all,

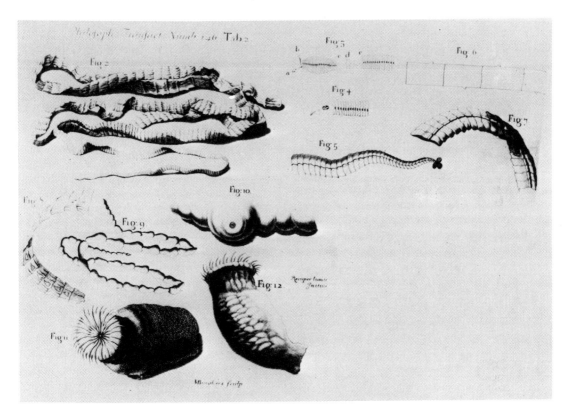

Plate 100. Fig. 2. Represents the worm I took out of a dog I dissected in the College Theater, which was about 5 feet long; and was alive. The small end shows the head as it appeared then to the naked eye, and is represented magnified by the microscope in the 11th and 12th figures. The protuberances at the sides are the mouths. The broad end, the tayle, as in the 5th figure.

Fig. 3, 4, and *5* represent the figures of the head of this worm, which are given us by Nich. Tulpius and Jo. Mich. Fehr. *Fig. 3.* Represents the two heads, which Tulpius in the former edition of his *Observations*, gave to this Worm, where he makes it a biceps. *Fig. 4.* Is the picture of the head of this worm which Tulpius gives us in the latter edition of *Book of Observations. Fig. 5.* Shews the Head of the Worm, as tis delineated by Jo. Mich. Fehr. which appears like a Tricoccos.

Fig. 6. This figure I met with in Franc. Sanchez which tho rude and plain, yet very well represents those Orifices which I take for the several Mouths of this Worm. The Figures 7 and 8 are those of Adrian Spigelius, and Gul. Fabricius Hildanus; where the Mouths seem to be placed on the flat, not in the Edges of the Worm, I have observed them so in some, but those by me, being dry and so not fit for an accurate draught, for the present I have made use of these. *Fig. 7.* A piece of this Worm as delineated by Spigelius. *Fig. 8.* A part of the same Worm as tis Pictured by Fabricius Hildanus.

Fig. 9. Is the figure of this worm in Cornel. Gemma. The following figures represent parts of this worm as viewed by the microscope. *Fig. 10.* Represents the protuberance or papilla about the middle of the edges; and in it the orifice which I take for the mouth of this worm. *Fig. 11.* Is the head of this worm as it appeared in the microscope, in three several ones I took out of the body, upon dissection, wherein is observable, a double order of spikes or hooks; the longer arising from the center; the other more towards the edges, which at pleasure it can contract in or protrude, and with them, part of the neck too, as does appear by swelling out a little below, as it is very curiously delineated, as likewise the other figures by my most ingenious friend and accomplished gentleman, Rich. Waller, Esq. *Fig. 12.* Is a side prospect of the head and the hooks in it of the same worm.

who have wrote of this Worm, do make the same Prognostick of it; that the Story of Hippys Rheginus in Aelian is not insignificant, where he tells us; that a Woman being troubled with this Worm, and the most skilful Physicians despairing of helping her, she went at last for a cure to the Temple of Aesculapius at Epidaurus; but the god being absent, his servants there advised her to sit in the place, where he used to do his Cures; and then cutting off her head, one of them thrusting his hand into her belly, pulled out a huge Worm, and then endeavored to place her head on again, but could not; but the god by this time being returned, he severely check't them, for rashly attempting what Art nor Human power was able to do; and having set it on himself, he dismist the woman perfectly cured; But since in this head we find no mouth; we must seek it somewhere else, and I come now to discourse of it, which is my sixth Particular. . . .

But I find that those who admit this Worm to be alive, have several of them very different thoughts of it; and many there are, who do assert, that 'tis not one, but many Worms linked together. . . .

I met . . . in a Dog in the College Theater, whilst alive, and in my hand, a joynt or two fell off; but I could no way observe any Membrane hanging to the foregoing joynt, out of which it might slip, but it broke off entire. And although there were two Single Joynts which I found in the Intestine, upon the first opening it, yet there was nothing I could see affixt to the last, which might include them. And indeed the setting on of the Joynts here is such, that seems to me sufficiently to shew, that this Worm cannot be a continued membrane, articulated only by the several *Cucurbitini* included in it, since there is so large a protuberance of the lower Extreme of the foregoing joynt, over the upper part of the following; which I plainly perceived in this Worm. If only a Membrane, why constantly, and thus regularly a difference of both extremes, as to their length and breadth? How happen the hooks at the head? How are those orifices formed at the Edges, or on the Flat of the Worm? And if it was so, as Gabucinus imagined, I cannot think but I must have perceived something of it, in those several pieces of this Worm, which I have observed: and

especially in that eight yards long, where I opened several joynts, and could find no such thing. That Mucous matter, therefore, which is observed to be voided, by those, troubled with them; which he tells us the women there, take for the beds of this Worm, may be better accounted for; it being likely in a great measure to be but the Mucus of the Intestines themselves, or a slimy Spolium cast off from these worms. Thus Leeches I have observed being put into water do cast out a slime, which covers their bodys which afterwards they slip off, and is found in the bottome of the Glass in the form of a mucous Coat. So Earth-Worms do void a large quantity of a mucous liquor, at several parts of their body, so Snailes, etc. of which more in my *Anatomy* of those Animals. Upon the whole, I see nothing why we may not justly ascribe that life, we find here, to the *Lumbricus Latus* itself, and not to any Animals, we may fancy it pregnant with. And what I do give to the Whole, I must attribute likewise to the several parts of it, even when separated from the rest of the body; and can't but think that they do live likewise. Not that I think those *Cucurbitini,* are to be reckoned as the partus of the Latus. . . .

But they are onely the Joynts or pieces broken off from the Latus, and when they are voided in the Stools, are a sure sign of a Joynted Worm. And the cure must accordingly be adapted. But that all these single Joynts whilst in the body do live, besides those considerations I have already delivered to prove that in every joynt there is a mouth for receiving the food; and no doubt answerable Organs for the digestion, and distribution of it; so I am the farther induced to believe it; because it has been often observed by myself, and others; that both single Joynts, and oftener larger pieces have been voided alive; and where vast quantities of this Worm too have been voided at the same time; in abundance of pieces, I have observed them almost equally turgid, and alike filled with Chyle in proportion to the magnitude of the parts. Now I cannot think that in voiding it can always be broken into so many pieces; and if it be done sometime before, and they lye dead in the body; they must be emacerated, and different from what they appear. But that observation, I have already often mentioned of that Worm, I met with in the Dog, I dissected in the College Theater; does furnish me with something apposite to our purpose. For here about the middle of the Worm, as it lay in the Intestine about a foot and a half from the Tayle, or lower Extream, I observed two single Joynts, about ¾ of an Inch long; alive, and which continued their motion briskly for ¾ of an hour, or more in warm water. That these were broken off from the Tayle I nothing question; being in all respect so like them. And that it must be done sometime before, I am apt to think, because they were so remote from it. For they could not otherwise easily, being but single Joynts, make so great an advance, being upon all occasions liable rather to be driven down, not being able as I could observe any ways to fasten themselves, and so resist the force of the descending feces. Which is the reason when broken off, they are so frequently voided.

Upon the whole I have been sometimes apt to think, what Analogy there may be between this Joynted Worm, and knotted Plants; of which each Joynt can so easily propagate itself. And whether it may not be thought an Animal Plant-Animal or Zoophyton bred in Animal bodies, since so large, and frequent detruncations of the body, does not destroy the life of the whole. Which I think can scarce be instanced in any Animal besides.

But my design here, is not raising of any Hypothesis, but the enquiring into the truth of those of others. It being much easier to spy others faults, than to avoid them ourselves. In what I have said I have done the former; but can no ways secure myself as to the latter. But in the whole, if I have not hit the mark; I have fairly aimed for it, and it may be some help, and direction to others in prosecution of this subject. And what I have laid down I think I have made out, how different this sort of Worm, bred in Animal bodys, is from all others hitherto observed out of it; from whence or any Seminal matter of it, it may be supposed to be propagated.

And how strange soever what I have here related of the head; of the many mouths; of the great length; and other particulars of this Worm may seem to others; who will be presently apt to censure it, as Romance and Fable; I shall onely add that Saying of Pliny, "Careful observation of the nature of things persuades me to think of nothing as beyond belief."

VESICULAR WORMS OR HYDATIDS IN THE OMENTA OF GOATS, AND PUS IN THE LUNGS OF ANOTHER

Miscellanea Curiosa Sive Ephemeridum Medico-Physicarum Germanicarum Academiae Naturae Curiosorum Decuriae II. Annus Quartus Anni MDCLXXXV [1685]. Observatio LXXIII. Nuremberg: Typis Johannis Ernesti Adelbulneri, [1705], pp. 152–157. Selections from pp. 152–154. Translated from the Latin.

Philip Jacob Hartmann
(1648–1707)

Hartmann, who was born in Pomerania, near East Prussia, first studied theology and philosophy but then turned to medicine, receiving his degree in that discipline in 1678 at Königsberg. He pursued further studies in France, Holland, and England, finally returning to accept a professorship at the University of Königsberg. Although well known in parasitology, he was primarily an anatomist.

Hartmann demonstrated conclusively in this work that cysticerci are separate, independent animal life forms when separated from the host.

(1) As soon as a large goat had died of disease, he was cut open; the remains of the membrane of the omentum were very thin, lacking fat.

(2) At the branching of the larger vessels, hydatids as they are commonly called, or more properly vesicular hydatids (watery worms of the urinary bladder) were found, the largest of which was greater than a chicken's egg.

(3) I noticed that each possessed its own skin; therefore, when I had made a small incision in the whole, I extracted many others unharmed.

(4) A small appendage was examined at the other extremity which, when incised in a circle, allowed gas to escape and revealed an empty space around it. Using a stylus, I attempted to find out how this had been introduced; if there might be some route which would allow liquid to pass into the bladder. When it was not possible to find a passage for this humor, I gently pressed that white globular appendage to find out why the empty space might exist. I turned that small particle inside out, and the rounded tail of a protruding intestinal worm became evident. I thought I noticed some movement (see Plate 101, Figs. XXV and XXVI).

(5) In order to ascertain this, I placed it in a small container of warm water: indeed, when it was submerged and clinging to the bottom I saw

not only the proboscis but also the vesicular body begin movement in a marvelous manner: it moved with a singular form of undulation, exhibiting contraction and expansion with the rising and falling of its parts, just as occurs in the case of silkworms. . . ; but because the fibers of its very thin skin were moved not only up and down, but also laterally with the same motions, the appearance of the water enclosed within the sac was amazing, for in one place it rolled, in another it broke, and in a third curled, in the same manner as water swells in its flow; several others demonstrated similar phenomena (see Fig. XXVII).

(6) When the sac was cut, it yielded a very clear, very liquid lymph; no trace of sediment was found. In certain corners a certain broad, small bit of fat was found, somewhat worn to a point.

(7) About the structure, the sac showed nothing organic beyond parallel lines, nor any other surface than that of the thin membrane was immediately encountered; the sac was very smooth without and within. When it moved beneath the water, certain very fine fibers seemed to extend from its neck, as if it were stimulated in these undulated motions by these fibers.

(8) Seeking to confirm this, I intentionally pulled out the center of the head (see Fig. XXVIII b), and the sacs then settled into the water without movement. However, a part of the center was thinner; close to the sac, more globose and glandular (see Fig. XXVIII).

(9) The common skin, which was that of the omentum, had no fibers and no ducts leading into the sac or the body of the worms.

(10) On the day after the worms had been examined, another goat was brought in which had died so recently it was still warm. Since I had no time, the animal was given to my pleased students, Master Thormann and Master Litius, *Med. Cand.,* to dissect; this goat had similar bladder (vesicular) worms, along with many others. They demonstrated clearly very similar movements when the membrane of the enclosed omentum was still adherent.

(11) The color of the fluid contained in the sacs varied in these respects; it was reddish with blood, diluted, more or less aqueous.

(12) Those with bloody fluid presented a noteworthy sight when they agitated their bodies under water; the small white head shining from the water made the reddish sac glitter like madder [an Eurasian herb producing a deep red dye—Eds.], with a surging motion.

(13) These were observed to be bound more closely by blood vessels. . . .

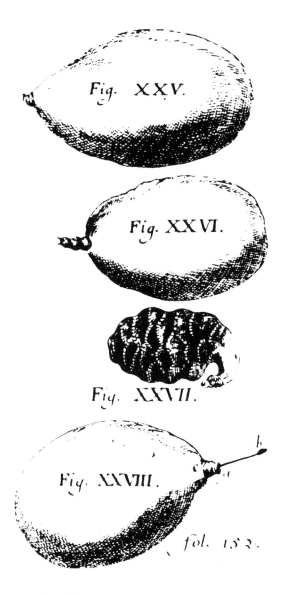

Plate 101.

STUDY OF THE NATURAL HISTORY OF THE INTESTINAL WORMS OF ANIMALS
Main class of intestinal tapeworms in man

Versuch Einer Naturgeschichte der Eingeweidewürmer Thierischer Körper. Blankenburg: P. A. Pape, 1782, 471 pp. Selections from pp. 278–284, 287–288. Translated from the German.

Johann August Ephraim Goeze
(1731–1793)

A native of Ascherleben and educated in theology at Halle between 1747 and 1751, Goeze was pastor of St. Blas' Church in Quedlinburg when he acquired a microscope. He became know for his research on insects, small aquatic animal life, and the fauna of Europe. He made many original entomologic descriptions as noted by his friend Linneaus. In 1786 he was appointed Dean of the Cathedral of Quedlinburg and died there 27 June 1793.

Although Goeze believed that tapeworms were inherited, he published 44 excellent drawings and an advanced system of classification in this first German work on parasitology, the most complete text of the eighteenth century, which he dedicated to Peter Simon Pallas. This excerpt is the first reference to differentiation, although not always completely clear, of Taenia solium *and* Taenia saginata *on the basis of their morphology. He clearly described the presence of* Taenia *eggs and suggested the hermaphrodite nature of* Taenia.

. . . I know and possess two species of intestinal tapeworm; the first is well known—long, with long, thick, fattened segments which I shall call *Taenia cucurbitina, grandis, saginata.*

The second seems to be a variety of the first, which under all circumstances remains the same and is found in my part of the country more frequently than the former; I call it *Taenia cucurbitina, plana, pellucida* [*Taenia solium*—Eds.].

Of the first species, I possess seven incomplete specimens without heads and two complete ones with intact heads.

The first measuring 3 to 4½ feet came from a cook from Braunschweig. The second, third, and fourth, each about five feet in length, came from a four-year-old girl from Hamburg. The fifth, measuring 6½ feet with well-fattened segments, came from a nursing child with a centipede which passed from the child at the same time; she was from Laubach in the German Empire. The sixth, eight feet in length, with a narrow head of which

not much can be missing . . . came from a man, unknown to me, from the same place.

The seventh, 5¾ feet, came from a young scholar who did not know previously that he had a tapeworm; it was sent by the late Wagler who reported the following additional circumstances: "The young scholar from whom these pieces of such an extraordinarily fattened tapeworm came felt little distress from what was still left, except when he heard music. Then he had to run away out of fear or had to ask that one would stop the music. Otherwise, he was healthy and had great strength. I have seen anxiety and unpleasant sensation from music in several cases of taeniasis. For that reason they feel sick in church from the organ. This reminds me of the assertion by Dr. Langens in Lüneburg that one could cause removal of the worms in man by the oscillation of a Jew's harp."

It is truly amazing to compare the pieces of this fattened tapeworm with others. The most mature lower segments are not as long as in the flat, transparent variety, but are much thicker. Some have the thickness of ½ line [1 line = 1/12 inch—Eds.] and are all marked with little lines lengthwise on the surface. In a section of worm more than 1 ell [ell = 45 inches—Eds.] in length, the marginal openings are set in each segment, one on each segment, some right, some left. In these segments there is still a yellowish egg pulp which dissolves in water into granules.

In the next 3½ feet of this specimen, the segments are much narrower and almost pushed one on top of the other and thereby give a considerable thickness. In this section the marginal openings have a completely different order. First two and two right, then left in the following segments two and two; then again one right and one left. But then on the right in one section six in a row; on the left six again, followed by two and two. This way it continues until the tract loses itself toward the thinner end in shorter and shorter segments and the marginal openings disappear as well.

On the mature lower segments the marginal openings in part project so far that the protrusion and the indented osculum can be seen with the naked eye. I inserted a horse hair, and afterward I pulled off the surface with fine instruments until I saw with pleasure under the magnifying glass that the hair was in the transverse canal which led to the ovary.

These mature lower segments were attached in such a way that the whole edge of one segment does not completely join the edge of the other, but the junction of the two joined segments is more toward the center; on both sides, however, the edges of the following segment protrude about ¼ of a line. I have torn some of these segments slowly out of their groove, and on each side of every segment I noticed two small openings which I could see even without the magnifying glass; they were openings of the two side canals because they showed themselves just where the canals run along lengthwise; under the magnifying glass I could pursue the small canal like a crystal tube, if I pulled some of the tissue away.

The two complete specimens have the threadlike neck and the button about which there has been so much discussion. The first I owe to Court Councillor Wickmann in Hanover, the second to Dr. Kliptsch in Magdeburg. They are both about 3 to 4½ ells long; the lower segments are longer, but not as thick as the previous one. All marginal openings in both, *oscula solitaria,* right and left, are single up to the point where the segments start to become shorter and then the openings disappear. . . .

The order in the position of marginal openings, which is hardly ever the same, still remains very puzzling and yet it cannot be without purpose. . . .

The worm from Councillor Wickmann was removed from a child. "I have," writes this excellent man, "in my practice, only one other parallel to this case, where a three-year-old child likewise passed a worm in pieces and probably, according to the mother's description, already had it in her second year."

In the first specimen the head is not flat and ribbonlike but round, ascarislike; in the latter, however, it is flatter. I am only adding that the head end of both these specimens is completely different from the head end of the notched, segmented tapeworm from the cat, as mere observation shows. In the first, however, one cannot see, as in the cat's tapeworm, the suckers and hooks with the naked eye, and the segments only start after a very narrow neck.

As far as I was able, I have examined the shape and composition of the eggs of every kind of tapeworm because in this way the difference of some otherwise very similar species can be determined. [Goeze now turned to a description of *Taenia cucurbitina plana pellucida (Taenia solium)*—Eds.]

The second kind of the long, segmented human intestinal tapeworm I call the flat, transparent variety (*Taenia solium*). That this is not an immature species of the first is clarified: (1) by the fact that it remains the same in all segments, from the head to the mature terminal segments and is very flat and transparent; (2) because all segments which I possess from children and old persons have one and the same size, shape, and form; (3) because this species is found more frequently in our part of the country around the Harz Mountains than the first one; (4) because the dendritic figures in the mature terminal segments appear in no other kind as plainly as in this one; (5) because this kind is much more resistant to the remedies used against it than the first, which probably stems from the flat segments which adhere more tightly to the intestinal mucosa.

A few years ago, Dr. Bremer of Berlin sent me such a tapeworm with complete head from the Charity Hospital, expelled by gumm. gutt [guttaperclia] and asafetida. A sexton's wife in Eisleben suffered many years from it. At times she passed pieces an ell long. She had used almost everything possible and made the worm so restless thereby that she had the most violent epileptic attacks [sic]. After a rest of four weeks, without the use of any medicines, the worm was removed by Wagler's remedy; but it was scalded by the extremely hot water placed under her.

On 28 March 1778, a farmer from a neighboring village came to the pharmacist in a drugstore here and complained that, for some years, his stepmother of 42 years had had the "mother's plague," that she had passed and torn off a piece of the intestine which he had with him in a glass of water. I recognized it immediately as a piece of the flat, segmented variety, but it was mostly putrescent and unusable.

The man received a laxative of rhubarb, some jalap, and mercur. dulcis. After a few days he came back and reported that after the use of this remedy a long piece of this worm had been expel-

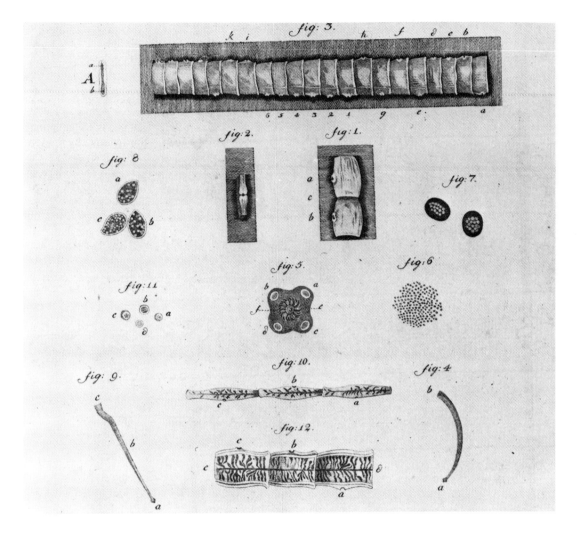

Plate 102. Fig. A. The high edge of a torn-off, mature lower segment. (a, b) the two openings of the lateral canals which one can see in every torn-off segment.

Fig. 1. A pair of the most mature lower segments of the long segmented human tapeworm. (a, b) the marginal openings; (c) the kind of junction of these segments. *Fig. 2.* One such marginal opening with bulge and lateral pore on the high edge. *Fig. 3.* A piece of the thick segments pushed on top of one another. (a) a marginal opening, torn from the preceding segment of this side; (b, c, d) three right; (e) one left; (f) one right; (g, h) again the same, then left 1–6; (i, k) two right, etc.

Fig. 4. The round head end of the long segmented human tapeworm. (a) the projecting head; (b) the neck and continuation, on which nothing segmented is seen with the naked eye. *Fig. 5.* The surface of the head. (a, b, c, d) the four suction openings; (e, f) the double hook crown. *Fig. 6.* Eggs pressed out of a mature terminal segment. *Fig. 7.* Two of the same. Actually every ball is an ovary filled with eggs. *Fig. 8.* Not mentioned in text.

Fig. 9. The head end of the flat, long-segmented human tapeworm. (a) the head; (b, c) the beginning delicate segments. *Fig. 10.* Three rear segments with dendritic figures of extraordinary length. (a, b, c) the marginal openings. *Fig. 11.* Four eggs from the most mature rear segments. (a, b, c, d). These round balls, actually ovaries in which the extremely small eggs can be seen. *Fig. 12.* A piece of the widest segments of the flat, long segmented tapeworm from the three-year-old boy, with the finest dendritic figures. (a, b, c) the marginal openings; (d, e) the longitudinal canal. The eggs exactly like those from Fig. 11.

led by the patient. Also, she had had the feeling as though a lump which had been in the rectum had gradually retracted.

When I placed this piece in a black vessel with lukewarm water, it was greatly tangled and much mucus came off. I cleaned it by brushing, put it in clear water, and undid the knots. I noticed also the joint where the remaining worm was separated. This was not in the groove of the segment but a good line away from it, with a half-moon cut out, torn transversely through the segment. The length of the worm was 34 zoll [zoll = 1 inch—Eds.] and 9½ lines [34¾ inches—Eds.]. The longest individual segment was 8 lines long and 2 lines wide.

The marginal openings were quite visible and protruded slightly. The order of these openings is quite peculiar starting from the bottom. First they appear singular to alternate sides then followed by six to the right consecutively then again two to the left and then two to the right then again seven in a row to the left. What can one say about these variations? How can these marginal openings have sexual function when their order is so variable? The entire section of the worm contained 68 segments.

The dendritic figures of the most developed segments were defined and visible. Each segment had a main central trunk connected by a fine membrane to many lateral branches, some being thicker than others. There was a clearly visible transverse canal leading to the marginal opening of each segment. In the central trunk there were innumerable eggs which looked like small peas under No. 1 Tub. A. At the periphery of the eggs there was a black circle as if possibly the young worm were curved within the black circle.

Thereafter, Wagler's medication was administered to a female patient together with the proper directions to the surgeon. . . .

One hour later the whole worm was passed together with five large *Ascaris,* and the patient had no aftereffects from the treatment. There were (1) 31 individual segments; (2) three individual sections one of two segments, one of three segments, and one of 8½ segments; (3) the largest section with a head measured 3½ ells. In two places it was thickened and each thickening grasped the intestinal mucosa and stretched it [sic].

The large section as well as the individual segments and section were soft and pulpy. As the worm lay in the water an oily substance rose to the surface. This is definite proof that this ingredient of Wagler's medication causes the worm to become weak and, therefore, unable to withstand the purgative, it leaves the host.

The head of the worm is like a small box and not round. At the four corners of the head there are four suckers and a superior rostellum which can be seen through the microscope.

I must cite here another curious case of this species. Two ells of a tapeworm were passed spontaneously by a local three-year-old boy. His voracious hunger could not be satisfied. The physician was consulted and prescribed jalap and rhubarb and a 3⅓ ell section of worm was passed. Some time later a 4 ell section was passed, and the boy refused to cooperate further.

Longer and wider segments of a tapeworm I have not observed. The longest was 1 zoll and frequently 1-2 lines longer than that; the width of the widest segment was 5½ lines.

The marginal openings were in a most unusual order, single, in pairs, in fours, and in one section five in a row. The ovaries were distinctly visible where at the point where one segment entered the next there was a fold as though there was a slight overgrowth. The eggs were similar to those in Figure 11 (Plate 102). . . .

How do the eggs mature in the tapeworms and how do they get into the most mature segments? Since all kinds of tapeworms of animal bodies propagate by means of eggs, what holds true for one holds true for all. One of my most important observations in the examination of the tapeworm has been that in every kind, from man and other animals, I found this unchanging phenomenon. . . .

How does fertilization of the tapeworms take place? I have not found a single tapeworm which did not have eggs. Are there, therefore, two sexes among them? Or is every tapeworm sufficient to itself and does it fertilize its own eggs? How are the organs for this purpose constituted and where are they? Finally, if only one tapeworm has lived in man for many years, where did it first come from? How was its egg fertilized? Why do not several tapeworms develop in man at the same time, since the number of eggs is infinite? . . .

CONTRIBUTION TO HELMINTHOLOGY

Helminthologische beitrage. Archiv. für Naturgeschichte. 1: 45–83, 1835. Selections from pp. 82–83. Translated from the German.

Carl Theodor Ernst von Siebold
(1804–1885)

Siebold, who established the class Protozoa, *was born in Würzberg, studied at Göttingen and Berlin under Rudolphi, and received the M.D. from the latter university in 1828. After some years in private practice, he went to Danzig, where he devoted much of his time to zoology and to insect and helminth collection. In 1836 he discovered the ciliated epithelium in man while examining an extirpated nasal polyp.*

In 1840, Siebold went to Erlangen as professor of zoology, comparative anatomy, and veterinary medicine. From 1845 to 1849 he worked in Freiburg and then succeeded Purkinje as professor of physiology and director of the Institute of Physiology in Breslau. In 1853 he went to Munich as professor of physiology and comparative anatomy, and three years later a chair of zoology was established especially for him. His influence as a teacher is evidenced by a roster of distinguished pupils, including Bilharz, Ferdinand Cohn, Ehlers, and Metchnikoff. One of the most distinguished biologists of the nineteenth century, Beneden, referred to Siebold as the "prince of helminthologists."

Siebold demonstrated for the first time that Taenia *eggs contained a larva with three pairs of hooks (hexacanth larvae).*

. . . I point out here that the remaining classes of helminths offer no less surprising phenomena in their evolutionary history. I shall soon publicize what my investigations about this have taught me already. I was especially interested in finding that in all kinds of *Taenia* which I have examined up to now (there is a whole series of them), the eggs and their egg shells, which vary in the most wonderful way in number and form, are already developed in the uterus; also that the embryo in most cases is similar to a round, unsegmented body and moves in the egg. Every embryo without exception is provided on its frontal end with six hooklets which are placed in a circle and which it extends and retracts in a lively manner. . . .

Clearly, I saw these embryos provided with hooklets and moving in the egg of *Taenia ocellata percae cernuae* in the fall; of *Taenia infundibuliformis phasiani Galli, Taenia engulata*

Turdi musici, Taenia lanceolata and *setigera* of the domestic goose in October; of a *Taenia* from the intestine of *Gasterosteus pungitius* in June, and of a *Taenia nov. sp.,* different from the *Taenia pusilla,* in the house mouse in whose abnormally enlarged cholecystic duct I found that parasite frequently in winter in Berlin as well as in Heilsberg.

ALTERNATION OF GENERATIONS OF CESTODES WITH A REVIEW OF THE GENUS *TETRARHYNCHUS*

Ueber den generationswechsel der cestoden nebst einer revision der Gattung *Tetrarhynchus*. Zeitschrift für Wissenschaftliche Zoologie, 2: 198–253, 1850. Selections from pp. 200–202. Translated from the German.

Carl Theodor Ernst von Siebold
(1804–1885)

Siebold's biography will be found with the preceding article in this chapter.

Siebold made many significant contributions to our knowledge of cestodes. He points out in this paper how other parasitologists such as Blanchard, Beneden, and Dujardin had confused the classification of cysticercus. In this paper, he clearly offers the hypothesis that a tapeworm can develop directly from the cysticercus.

. . . In order not to repeat myself in the course of this treatise, I must mention here in a few words the position and classification of the tapeworms in the helminth system. Although the suggestion often has been made by zoologists to combine the order of the cysticerci with the order of the cestodes, several systematists have actually joined the bladder worms with the tapeworms without satisfying the rest of their colleagues who oppose such innovation. The order of bladder worms, up to the present time, has been repeatedly followed, in turn, by the order of tapeworms. The older scientists have outdone us, as R. Leuckart already emphasized, with their insight in the understanding of the bladder worms. This is proved by their designation *Taenia hydatigena, Taenia cellulosa, Taenia cerebralis, vesicularis,* and so on. Rudolphi's systematic work led helminthologists astray from the complete understanding of the bladder worms so that even such an excellent scientist as Nitzsch vainly called attention to the fact that the so-called bladder worms were nothing more than another species form of other helminths and consequently should not be separated as a special group.

Because of the striking similarity which the heads of the bladder worms have to the heads of certain tapeworms, I initially conjectured that the bladder worms were nothing more than underdeveloped or larvalike tapeworms. However, I later came to the definite conclusion that the bladder worms are actually only underdeveloped, residual, hydropically degenerated tapeworms, changed by their migrations. One can convince oneself of this most easily by comparing the *Cysticercus fasciolaris* with *Taenia crassicollis*.

It is now the task of the heminthologist to discover the completely developed and sexual cestode form from which bladder worms and other asexual tapeworms develop. I have been successful in the case of some of the bladder worms, as I shall show later; surely, the remaining gaps will be filled soon by the efforts of other helminthologists. To be sure, various experiments have already been made to study tapeworms on their migrations during which certain changes which the cestodes undergo were completely unrecognized. For that reason, I must warn, above all, those scientists who wish to pursue the tapeworms on their often wide and hidden migrations not to get lost; this can easily happen because one cannot study such migrating helminths step by step and, in these investigations, one can pick up the lost thread at the right place only by the help of very careful reflection. . . .

CHAPTER **33**

Taeniasis
Solium—Cysticercosis

THE ANATOMY OF *GLANDIA*

Miscellanea Curiosa Sive Ephemeridum Medico-Physicarum Germanicarum Academiae Imperialis Leopoldinae Naturae Curiosorum Decuriae II. Annus Septimus, Anni MDCLXXXVIII [1688] Observatio XXIV. Nuremberg: Literis Joannis Ernesti Adelbulneri, 1716. Pp. 58–59. Selection from page 58. Translated from the Latin.

Philip Jacob Hartmann
(1648–1707)

Hartmann's biography appears with his contribution on hydatids. Gesner (1558) usually is credited with the first description of Cysticercus cellulosae *in man. This is the first record of* Cysticercus cellulosae *in the pig.*

I. In the heart of a pig I noticed that there were very many cysts, over 20 in the parenchyma of each inner ventricle; each single white capsule had filled its own depression; when the capsules were cut open a peculiar skin of thin membrane could be removed. This covered both a clear liquid and a white filament coiled like a white thread—itself a small worm. . . .

EXPERIMENTAL PROOF THAT *CYSTICERCUS CELLULOSAE* CHANGES TO *TAENIA SOLIUM* WITHIN THE HUMAN INTESTINE

Experimenteller nachweis, dass Cysticercus cellulosae innerhalb des menschlichen darmkanales sich in Taenia solium umwandelt. Wiener Medizinische Wochenschrift, 5:1–4, 1855. Translated from the German.

Friedrich Küchenmeister
(1821–1890)

The son of a Protestant minister, Küchenmeister began his education by studying for the ministry; however, in 1840 he changed to medicine in Leipzig and later went to Prague. His investigations in parasitology started in 1846, when he began the private practice of obstetrics and gynecology in Zittau. A fierce and devastating debater of his experiments and of scripture, he gained few friends in the scientific world. His knowledge and exposition of scripture helped him convince Cobbold that Moses gave us the first description of Dracunculus medinensis *(''the fiery serpents''). His classic* Dit in und an dem Korper des Lebenden Menschen Vorkommenden Parasiten, *published in 1855–1856, gained him prompt recognition and translation into English by the Sydenham Society in 1857. In 1859 he moved to Dresden, where he continued to do research and to practice medicine. His work is proof that good research can be done apart from the university.*

His classic experiment demonstrating the development of cysticercus of Taenia solium *to the adult tapeworm in the human host is recorded here.*

Although it is the custom to acknowledge honors bestowed by a learned society or corporation in a private letter, nevertheless, I prefer to give my thanks for your sending my diploma as corresponding member of your society in this esteemed weekly and to combine it with a report of an experiment conducted by me a short time ago—administration of *Cysticercus cellulosae* to a human in food—to show you that, as far as I am able, I will gladly fulfill the obligations accruing to me because of my nomination.

In the beginning of 1853 I had already taken steps (see my small article on cestodes in general and those of man in particular) to be allowed to administer bladder worms to a murderess under sentence of death. All my endeavors at that time were in vain, in spite of the kind promises of physician colleagues. Some time ago, a convict was scheduled to be dispatched from this life to death by the guillotine several miles from my home. Through the mediation of colleagues, whose names, unfortunately, I am not allowed to mention, I was successful in actually carrying out what I had tried in vain in 1853, although the brief time at my disposal (six to eight days) gave me scant hope for success. About 130 hours before the hour of execution of the convict, because of lack of *C. cellulosae,* fresh *Cysticercus tenuicollis* from the pig mesentery was administered to him by a colleague and about 10 hours before that day six pieces of *Cysticerci pisiformis* from the rabbit. Since it is the custom to allow the convict certain extras in the way of food following official confirmation of the death sentence, the doctor in question then gave the convict, at my suggestion, good bouillon soups with noodles (star-shaped or triangle-form) or similar starches; after the soups were cooled to blood temperature, he added seven pieces of bladder worms whose tail vesicles had been partially opened or partially cut off, so that they were about the size of the noodles. Thus the convict received the bladder worms in the soup without knowing it.

About 84 hours before the convict's death, my wife found some bladder worms in our evening meal (which consisted of warm roast pork from a restaurant near my home in Zittau). I thought, "Where these bladder worms come from, there are still others," and I hurried to make further inquiries at this restaurant about uncooked, fresh pork.

After pleading for a while, I explained to the people that because of my research on worms I had been looking for a long time in vain for such meat because it was mostly kept a secret. Finally, I discovered that the pork came from a pig which had been slaughtered in this restaurant about 60 hours previously, and I received one pound of raw meat, which had been kept in the cellar, containing the greatest number of bladder worms. Since the evening had already progressed too far for me to get to the place where the convict was held, I kept the meat at a mild temperature in an unheated room over night and rode before daybreak on the fourth day before the execution to the place where the convict was staying, in the company of a physician attached to the court. Exactly 72 hours before the death of the convict, I had arrived at the convict's place of detention and, at once, the first-mentioned doctor prepared a breakfast for the convict with the bladder worms which I supplied. Since soup at this time might have been suspicious, I suggested a few slices of bread and butter with Cervelat sausage from which the peppercorns were removed and

peeled out and the holes filled with bladder worms. The doctor in question did not have Cervelat sausage at hand, so he took blood sausage and removed some of the fat pieces from it; in their place he inserted some of the bladder worms, and everything else was smoothed over from the side. Thus, 72 hours before his death, the convict received 12 pieces of *C. cellulosae*; 60 hours before death, 18 in a rice soup; 36 hours before death, 15 in noodle soup; 24 hours before death 12 in sausage; and 12 hours before death, in soup again, 18 pieces of the latter (altogether 75 pieces), which had been removed about 72, 84, 108, 120, and 132 hours after slaughtering of the animal.

The execution followed about 120 hours after administration of *C. tenuicollis,* 72 hours after the first, and 60 hours after the second administration of *C. cellulosae.* The sausage and soups had tasted so good to the convict that on the evening before his death he thought it necessary to express his warm thanks to the doctor concerned.

The day after execution I went to the Institute of Anatomy about 20 hours from here, where the cadaver had been delivered, but to my sorrow I could get to examine the intestine only 48 hours after the execution. The examination was undertaken in the presence of several professors by medical examiners, Dr. D., Dr. Z., and myself.

As little as was my hope of finding young *Taeniae,* in view of the brevity of the feeding periods, even under the most fortunate circumstances, I did not expect to find the hooklets of the young *Taeniae* again, since they fall off easily in the intestinal mucus when it begins to decompose; yet I had the good fortune, as we shall soon see, of finding a few young *Taeniae* with hooklets. While searching through the mucus deposited in another thick layer, it seemed unlikely that I would succeed in finding something that represented a young *Taenia;* yet I was successful in finding a small *Taenia* which was tightly attached with its projected proboscis to a piece of the duodenal mucosa which I had softened in water for a few minutes. The rest of the dissectors convinced themselves of this also. As can easily be imagined, I was somewhat happily excited by this finding and asked Dr. Z., therefore, to fix on a glass slide the small cestode plus the portion of the mucosa to which it was attached.

This worked out rather well, and we saw a

young *Taenia* with projected proboscis to which four hooklets pointing forward were loosely attached; these, when compared with other preparations of *Taenia solium, Taenia serrata vera,* and *Taenia cystic. tenuicolli,* proved clearly to be hooklets of the *T. solium.* In the meantime, while the gentlemen studied the *Taenia* more carefully, I had examined the duodenum further and found another three specimens, of which two showed one or two pairs of hooklets each and likewise belonged to *T. solium*; the third, which Dr. D. lifted out of the intestinal mucosa, contained, except for two hooklets of the first row, the undamaged hooklet circle, a total of 22 hooks of *T. solium.* At the present time, this preparation like the others is still at the Institute of Anatomy; as far as the latter preparation is concerned, it is to be deplored that a large number of the hooks of the first row on addition of liquid gelatin were displaced into the neighborhood of the *Taenia*'s proboscis; yet the hooklets of the second row are preserved in their place in complete number and order.

Anyone who has ever seen the hooklets of the *T. solium* will admit that there was no doubt that the four *Taeniae* provided with more or fewer hooklets belonged to the *T. solium* and the administered *C. cellulosae,* and not to the other cysticerci. In addition to these four *Taeniae,* we found in the rinse water of the intestinal mucosa six other young *Taeniae,* all without hooks. All ten *Taeniae,* with the exception of one which was about 6–8 mm long, and which had a nicely formed, hardly damaged appendage, measured 3–4 mm in length. All showed, posteriorly, the small, s-shaped, arched, notched contraction known to everyone who has ever tried to change second-stage cestodes with tail vesicles into *Taeniae* in feeding experiments.

No traces were found in the entire intestine of the last feedings, and I believe that only the first two feedings with *C. cellulosae* produced results, since probably most of the *C. cellulosae* were already dead at the time of entrance into the intestine of the convict. For up to now I have not been successful in raising *Taeniae* from bladder worms which were used later than three to four days after killing of their host.

If we again briefly look at the results obtained by this experiment, the following is established: (1) that the *C. cellulosae* is the scolex of the *T. solium hominis*; (2) that the mode of infection with *T. solium* is exactly the same as with all others originating from bladder worms and probably like that of most of the *Taeniae*; (3) that we, therefore, infect ourselves with *T. solium* since cysticercus is transmitted by those foods which we eat raw or which, already cooked, we eat cold and get in portions from butcher shops and other places; I proved this already as cited above; (4) that the existing health legislation of many states with regard to wormy pork is hardly justified, since it lets the butcher who sells much meat bear the loss. Public instruction and warning to be careful with infected pork would work better than such measures; (5) I am finally adding that according to the experiments of Beneden and the experiments carried out by Professor Haubner and me on the government commission, as a result of my proposal to the Royal Saxon Ministry of State, it has been proven again that *C. cellulosae* can be raised in the pig by feeding with mature segments of *T. solium* and in such amounts that in 4½ drachma of meat from a pig used for the experiment I counted 133 *C. cellulosae,* which for one stone of pork gives approximately 80,000 pieces of this cysticercus; (6) that we have not been successful in raising *C. cellulosae* either in the dog or in the sheep by feeding mature segments of *T. solium;* neither have we succeeded in raising *C. cellulosae* (a) from *Taenia serrata vera* (ex. *cystic. pisiformi*), (b) from *Taenia* ex *cysticerce tenuicolli,* (c) from *Taenia coenurus* (ex. *Coenuro cerebrali*), (d) from *Taenia echinococcus*; yet it is really very simple to produce with these *Taeniae* (a) *C. pisiformis,* (b) *C. tenuicollis,* and (c) *Coenurus cerebralis*; the autopsy, which unfortunately was undertaken too early, suggests that *Echinococcus* rises from *T. echinococcus.*

Accordingly, I leave it to everyone himself, even if he is unable to differentiate the hooklets of the various kinds of *Taenia,* to judge the book *On Tape and Bladder Worms, etc.,* by Th. v. Siebold which has recently been published by Engelmann in Leipzig.

While I hasten toward conclusion, I only regret that I am not permitted to thank openly those who helped me so kindly in the above experiment. Furthermore, I direct the plea to influential members of your society, alas to all friends of physiology and medical science who read these lines, that everyone in his own field work toward the end that the surely harmless experiment of bladder-worm feeding be allowed to be repeated on criminals under probable death sentence; so that the whole developmental cycle of *T. solium* could be observed by, for instance, feeding at four-week intervals very fresh *C. cellulosae* in regular amounts every time. My experiment has left undecided whether *C. pisiformis* and *tenuicollis* can develop in man. I do not believe that this occurs. In the case of a subsequent pardon of the convict, the tapeworms can easily be expelled; this will calm anxious souls and will serve science at the same time.

CHAPTER 34

Taeniasis saginata

THE IMPORTANCE OF FEEDING OF CATTLE
AND THE THOROUGH COOKING OF THE
MEAT AS THE BEST PRESERVATIVES
AGAINST TAPEWORMS

Seventh Annual Report of the Sanitary Commissioner (1870)
with the Government of India, Calcutta, pp. 82–83, 1871.

John Hamer Oliver
(1837–1873)

*After qualifying in medicine, Oliver was commissioned
as a staff assistant surgeon and assigned to the 20th
Hussars. He spent almost his entire career as a medical military officer in India, but was assigned to the
Dalhousie Convalescent Depot in England for a few
years before his early death.*

*The beef tapeworm was initially differentiated from
the pork tapeworm (*Taenia solium*) by J. A. E. Goeze
in 1782. The larval stage in cattle had been described
by J. J. Wepfer in 1675. Oliver recorded in this brief
note the development of the cysticercus of* Taenia
saginata *into the adult tapeworm in man.*

. . . The rejections of ration beef on account of
cystic disease in 1870 were very few, and were
chiefly confined to Rawul Pindee. In connection
with the appearance of these cysts, some interesting facts have been recorded by Dr. Oliver, of the
Royal Artillery, at Jullundur. It appears that at
one time cysts were very frequently met with at
this station, and that large quantities of beef were
in consequence destroyed. Dr. Oliver was led to
believe that the cattle were infected after their
purchase by the Commissariat, and that the
medium through which this took place was a
large dirty tank where they were taken to water.
The tank, besides being generally filthy, was
close to the huts of the camel drivers—men who
are notoriously dirty in their habits, and who are
not unfrequently affected with *Taenia
mediocanellata*. Human filth was often to be seen
on the banks of the tank, and the microscopic

examination of mud and stagnant water taken
from the margin exhibited taenia ova. The connection between the cysts and this tank was further supported by the fact that the cysticerci
found in the cattle were of very small size.
Whether Dr. Oliver's opinion is correct or not, it
is certainly remarkable that the "cysticercus entirely disappeared from amongst the cattle a few
months after means had been taken to secure
them a good supply of well water." The following facts are of interest:—"During 1868 and
1869," writes Dr. Oliver, "I from time to time
obtained pieces of beef badly infected with cysticercus, and made some experiments as to the
results of its consumption under different conditions.

"*1st*—After explaining to them the possible
consequences of eating it, a buttock of beef studded with cysticercus was given to three natives of
low caste. They all declared that they were free
from taenia. The meat they cooked in their own
way. These men were under my observation for
some six months. Two of them had no symptom
of taenia, but the third, who was a low class
Mahomedan syce, and had probably eaten the
meat in a very raw state, developed a *T.
mediocanellata* in about three months.

"*2nd*—My own sweeper ate this cyst-infected
beef regularly two or three times a week for some
months. He cooked it well, generally as an ordinary stew, and has never shown a sign of having
tape-worm.

"*3rd*—In the case of a Hindoo boy of low
caste, two scolices of cysticercus within three or
four months produced a *T. mediocanellata*."

From these and other cases, which were made
the subject of careful investigation, Dr. Oliver
concludes that "the safety or otherwise of eating
cyst-infected beef simply depends on the manner
in which it is cooked. If this meat is thoroughly

done, and presents no rawness when cut into, the measles appear like little nodules of coagulated albumen, are doubtless perfectly inert, and may be eaten with impunity.'' Special orders have been issued enjoining on all Commissariat Officers the great importance of the very careful watering and feeding of the cattle intended for slaughter, and attention has also been again drawn to perfect cleanliness in the cook-rooms and thorough cooking of the meat as the best preservatives against tape-worm. . . .

THE PARASITES OF MAN, AND THE DISEASES WHICH PROCEED FROM THEM

Die Menschlichen Parasiten und die von ihnen Herruhrenden Krankheiten. Ein Hand-und Lehrbuch für Naturforscher und Äerzte. 1st Ed. Leipzig und Heidelberg: C. F. Wintersche Verlagshandlung, 1863. 766 pp. Selections from 293–297. Translated from the German.

Friedrich Rudolf Leuckart
(1822–1898)

Leuckart's biography appears with his contribution on Fasciola hepatica.

This is the description of the life cycle of Taenia saginata *in the animal host from Leuckart's classic text. The illustrations come from the English translation of 1886 (Rudolf Leuckart,* The Parasites of Man and the Diseases which Proceed from Them. *Translated from the German by William E. Hoyle. Edinburgh: Young J. Pentland, 1886, +771 pp.).*

. . . On 13 November 1861, I fed a mature segment of *Taenia mediocanellata* about four feet long to a four-week-old calf. A week later, I repeated the feeding with smaller pieces of the same tapeworm.

The experimental animal was hardly affected by my experiment and remained healthy after these feedings. I was ready to excise a neck muscle as I was accustomed to doing with my pigs, in order to test the success of the experiment, when my servant brought me news, on 9 December, that the animal had died the previous night (that is, 25 and 17 days after the first and second feedings, respectively). The animal had been sick the day before and had not been able to stand any longer, but had taken its milk as usual.

The post-mortem examination which was undertaken immediately showed that the feeding had produced a rich result. All the muscles, especially the chest, neck and psoas muscles, were covered with cysts which were 1.5–3 mm wide and 2–4 mm in length. They had a whitish appearance as though filled with a chalky or caseous mass, as I had never observed in young cysts of the *Cysticercus cellulosae* in a similar way. Inside the exudative layer, which was surrounded by a firm connective tissue membrane, they contained a light, clear vesicle of 0.4–1.7 mm in diameter. On cutting into this cyst, this protruded and proved on closer examination to be a young cysticercus. . . .

At this stage of development no suckers could be found (Plate 103, Fig. 1). The inner parts of the head cone showed little enlargement of the end, and in the region of the smaller cysticerci it was a simple conical shape. . . .

Although these cysts were extremely numerous and in many places so tightly pressed together that they were estimated to number many thousand, the death of the experimental animal could hardly thus be explained. In spite of this, it probably was the cysticerci which had killed the calf. Further examination showed that the spread of the parasites was in no way limited to the peripheral body muscles. The internal organs also were infected by immense numbers. At first it was the heart which was conspicuous in this respect, for its walls were thickly permeated by large and small cysts, as though with tubercles. But even more striking was the appearance of the kidney capsule; thousands of little white nodules were intercalated between the swollen lymphatics. Each one of these nodules, in spite of the resemblance to a tubercle, contained one young cysticercus as described above. This group of cysts followed the course of the lymphatic vessels and lymph nodes into the inguinal region. The smaller nodes, rich in connective tissue, were particularly infected by cysts, while the larger nodes, in many cases swollen to the size of a walnut, were almost completely free from them. The appearance of the lymphatics in the neck was very similar but less striking, insofar as the number of cysts seemed smaller. Swelling and erythema were always present, so that the whole lymphatic system of our animal (with the exception of the thoracic duct) was abnormal. Some of the lymph nodes were not only congested, but also full of edema and infiltrated by blood

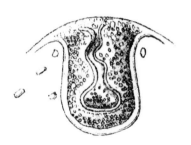 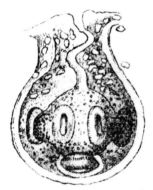

Plate 103. Fig. 1. Head rudiment of *Cysticercus Taeniae saginatae* before the development of suckers. *Fig. 2.* Head rudiment of *Cysticercus Taeniae saginatae* after development of the suckers. [The 1886 English translation dropped *Taenia mediocanellata* in favor of *Cysticercus Taeniae saginatae*—Eds.]

throughout the whole mass. These petechiae, some of which were bean-sized, were found in various places under the skin.

Since the rest of the viscera were comparatively though not completely free of cysticerci (in the brain I found perhaps about a dozen vesicles, most of which were lying free between the gyri of the hemispheres), I have few misgivings in attributing the cause of death of my experimental animal to the pathologic state of the lymphatic system and to relating the latter to the state of inflammation resulting from the migration and development of such a large number of parasites.

My honored colleagues, Professor Seitz and Dr. Mosler, to whom I communicated this case, were of exactly the same opinion and emphasized in this connection the resemblance of this disease to acute miliary tuberculosis. In this regard, I was also reminded of the mysterious ''bovine'' tuberculosis.

There is still the possibility that the death of the experimental animal occurred as the result of helminthiasis or on account of an accidental complication involving another disease. This much at least has been proven by my experiment—that the cysticercus of *T. mediocanellata,* as previously mentioned in the identification of the worm, lives in cattle and is found not only in the muscles, but also in considerable numbers in the internal organs, especially in the lymphatics. The position of the head proves that it is different from the *C. cellulosae.* How this difference further manifests itself we must, however, leave undecided for the time being; nevertheless, I hope to be able to report soon

on this matter as well, since I have just received new material from friends to repeat and expand my experiments.

At this time I will only remark that this new experiment was successful also. The calf, which had become quite sick in the third week after feeding, but had gradually recovered completely, after 48 days showed in the excised sternomastoid muscle about a dozen cysticerci cysts of the shape and appearance of the common hog cysticerci (Plate 104, Fig. 1 and 3). As in the latter, the head was attached to the central zone of the vesicle. But this head cone was without a bend and in spite of its small size (hardly 1 mm), also in spite of the small size of the vesicle (3–4 mm), was already provided with completely developed suckers (Plate 103, Fig. 2). Instead of the protruding hooks, there was on the bottom of the invagination, between the suckers, a tight circle of small rudiments (Plate 104, Fig. 2).

The larval stage of *T. mediocanellata* may lag behind that of *C. cellulosae* with respect to size and thus has escaped the helminthologist up to the present time. On the other hand, this fact could be explained by the assumption that the cysticercus in question usually lives alone; the way of life and feeding habits of cattle deviate significantly from those of the pig, which lends support to this hypothesis.

The specific nature of *T. mediocanellata* has been established by my experiments beyond any doubt. There are actually two species among the common human tapeworms, an armed variety which we get from the pig and an unarmed variety which is obtained from cattle and perhaps

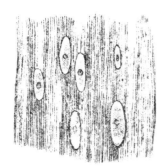 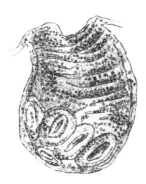 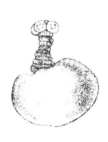

Plate 104. Fig. 1. Cysticercus Taeniae saginatae, embedded in the muscle. *Fig. 2.* Head rudiment of an adult *Cysticercus. Fig. 3. Cysticercus* with evaginated head.

other ruminants. With this consideration of peculiarities in the local and geographic behavior of both these species, we find a complete and sufficient explanation. Where pork is eaten predominantly, as in the northern sections, *T. solium* will occur more frequently; while, on the other hand, where beef is the main meat, *T.*

mediocanellata may be found more frequently. In all probability, the latter species has the greater region of distribution. It not only inhabits Europe and Africa, as we have seen above, but also the Orient (Davaine), America (Weinland), and probably is present everywhere to some extent. . . .

CHAPTER **35**

Hymenolepiasis

TAENIA NANA SIEB. A CONTRIBUTION TO HUMAN HELMINTHOLOGY

Ein beitrag zur helminthographia humana. Zeitschrift für Wissenschaftliche Zoologie, 4: 53–76, 1852. Selection from pp. 64–65. Translated from the German.

Theodore Bilharz
(1825–1862)

Bilharz' biography will be found in the chapter on Schistosomiasis.

   Bilharz' sojourn in Egypt not only resulted in a description of Schistosoma, *but he gave the original description of* Hymenolepis nana. *Grassi (1887) showed that the life cycle of* H. nana *did not require an intermediate host.*

   . . . It will not surprise us that there is a special tapeworm among the many helminths inhabiting man in the countries of the Nile. Bilharz has discovered such and wanted to call it, after its land of origin, *Taenia aegyptiaca,* but since it may be discovered later that this parasite is not limited to Egypt, I [Siebold was Bilharz' correspondent—Eds.] have suggested that it be named *Taenia nana* because this tapeworm differs by its smallness so greatly from the other two species of man. I can state with certainty that this small tapeworm is not a torn off or damaged fragment, since I found many undamaged specimens and was provided with a rounded terminal segment. I received the following first report of this parasite from Bilharz under the date of 1 May 1851:
   "The first incision into the intestine from the cadaver of a boy who died of meningitis disclosed immediately large numbers of a small tapeworm. The worm was a fully developed *Taenia* with broad segments; it was the width of a sewing thread and a length of hardly 10 mm. The head is large, its frontal surface plain and square; the corners formed by the round suckers are placed on spherical protuberances. The head gradually loses its width posteriorly and becomes the long, narrow neck. The segments behind the neck gradually widen until at the posterior end of the body, they attain three to four times the width of the head. This *Taenia* by the way, inhabited only a limited portion of the ileum.''

On 1 December Bilharz wrote further about this tapeworm:

   "*Taenia nana* certainly is a fully developed parasite. [See Plate 72, Fig. 18—Eds.]. I have observed eggs in the live animal which, unfortunately, I have not found again, and recognized them only in specimens preserved in alcohol. They are completely round, and seem to have a single, thick, yellowish shell; however, under the effect of the alcohol, the content of the eggs contracts into a ball and hence a thin vitelline membrane may still be present. The six hooklets of the *Taenia* embryos are clearly visible in the fresh eggs. As you have already mentioned, I find all cirri attached to one side. The eggs are [30 to 47 microns in diameter—Eds.]. . . .''

CHAPTER 36

Echinococcosis

TAENIA HYDATIGENA:
SIMILARITY OF HYDATIDS IN ANIMALS AND
MAN

Miscellanea Zoologica: Quibus Novae Imprimis Atque
Obscurae Animalium Species Describuntur et Obser-
vationibus Iconibusque Illustrantur. Hagae Comitum: Petrum
van Cleff, 1766, pp 219. Selections from pp. 173–174.
Translated from the Latin.

Peter Simon Pallas
(1741–1811)

*Pallas was born in Berlin, the son of a professor of
surgery. He was a brilliant student of languages and in
his spare time studied natural history. At the age of 19
he received his medical degree from Leyden; his thesis,*
De Infestis viventibus Intraviventia, *was his major
contribution to parasitology.*

*Elected to the Royal Society in 1764 for his contribu-
tions to entomology, he later published his monumental* Miscellanea Zoologia, *which included a remarkable section on the classification of tapeworms.*

*An invitation by Catherine The Great to the chair of
natural history at St. Petersburg in 1767 allowed him
to explore Russia until he returned to Germany in
1809. Among other accomplishments, his observations
on the sequence of rock formations in Siberia, according to Cuvier, gave birth to modern geology.*

*In the following article, Pallas pointed out the close
resemblance of the scolex of the encysted bladder
worm and the head of the tapeworm.*

. . . Our *Taenia hydatigena* from the mouse
liver has a head like that of *Taenia cucurbitina*
and *Taenia caninae*. Figures 12 and 13 (Plate
105) show the latter in natural size. Figure 11
(Plate 105) shows a superior and lateral view of
the head of *T. hydatigena* with the papilla (*b b*),
as described, and the rostellum (*a*) which is not
found in *Taenia lata* from man or horses described by Bonnet. . . .

These hydatids (cysts) are most commonly
found in the lungs and liver of sheep and oxen.
They are also found in man. Chirurgus tells of
having observed in the liver of a 40-year-old
woman a large cyst which had caused her severe
pain and finally death. From the cavity of the

Plate 105. Fig. 1. Taenia hydatigena, almost spherical, with a squat body resembling a round sac. A transparent cyst (chalaza)
appears clearly in the sketch. *Fig. 2.* Another, almost spherical, its sac is furnished with an attenuated neck. *Fig. 3.* Another
whose sac is oval in a transverse direction and is endowed with a long, rounded neck. *Fig. 4.* Another of oval shape, the neck of
whose unusual sac is relaxed and extended. *Fig. 5.* Another of oblong shape, with a somewhat larger body, but with its natural
thickness (*magnitudo*). *Fig. 6.* Another with the thin neck of the sac slightly rounded. A transparent coagulum, arising from the
thick lymph fluid (a) exudes from the protruding apex (b) of its body. *Fig. 7.* Another, longitudinally cut, on which the small
growth (*molecula*) (a) was found, and which was noteworthy especially for the tumor (b) added as if it were a secondary cyst
(chalaza). A gelatinous channel issuing from the body or cyst (c) appears clearly in this figure.
Fig. 8. Presents a view of the still contracted and bud-shaped (papilliformis) body of a taenia of this type. *Fig. 9.* Is the head of
the *hydatis* represented in Fig. 6. *Fig. 10.* A head of a taenia of this type from the mesentery of a pig, notable for its linear
elongated neck; (a) indicates the snout ringed with small spines, (b, b, b) buds (papillae) which surround the snout. *Fig. 11.* The
head of a *Taenia hydatigena* from a mouse's liver, drawn from the side and front. (a) again indicates the head ringed as it were
with scythes. (b's) four budlike (papillaria) mouths, which make the head almost square. *Fig. 12.* Taenia from the liver of a
mouse with its eyes (a) bared for seeing and with the bubble (bulla) (b) very small. *Fig. 13.* Another, smaller, on which likewise
the head (a) is very clearly apparent and the sac (b) is a little larger.

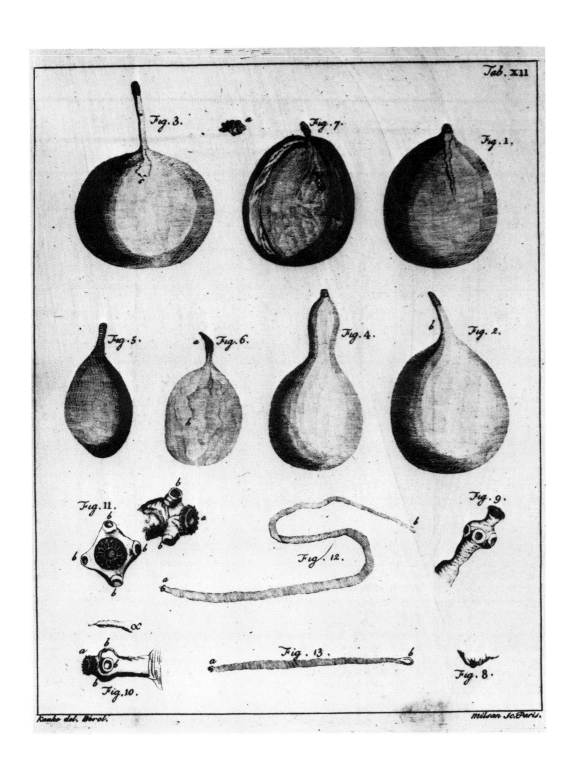

liver flowed four measures of clear water; the contracted membrane of its own unattached cyst, which previously had contained water and was dilatable, was found on the bottom.

Similar hydatids were found by De Haen in the liver of a 24-year-old youth who had suffered for four years with a tumor of the epigastrium. He compared the membrane of hydatids with the albumen of egg poured into a dish and heated. If he had seen our *T. hydatigena* alive in animals, considering his reputation for preciseness, he would not have delivered an opinion deriving hydatids from worms, which he actually did.

I cannot persist in denying that these hydatids derive their origin from *T. hydatigena*. However, they are so different in every respect from the latter's structure and nature that it seems to me not the slightest similarity exists among them. They are alike, however, in that each finds support in its own membrane. They are distinguished from hydatids accustomed to grow in many other parts of animals: hydatids of the brain, the ovaries, the placenta in the case of the vesicular mole, and so on.

Concerning hydatids in general, but particularly concerning those found free in the hollows of internal organs or in external tumors, sometimes hidden or excreted from the bowels or in urine, there exist many obscure facts. From those which I have reported, from the observations read here, in Bidloo, in Tulpius, and in the records of various societies, this at least is clear: multifarious is the origin and multifarious is the nature of lymphatic tumors which come under the general name of hydatids; and in certain internal organs and parts of the body, hydatids of only a particular species are known to be produced.

STUDY OF THE NATURAL HISTORY OF THE INTESTINAL WORMS OF ANIMALS

Versuch Einer Naturgeschichte der Eingeweiderwurmer Thierischer Korper. Blankenburg: P. A. Pape, 1782. 471 pp. Selections from pp. 258–260. Translated from the German.

Johann August Ephraim Goeze (1731–1793)

Goeze's biography will be found in the previous chapter on Taeniasis.

Rudolphi (1771–1832) first used the term "Echinococcus"*; however, the differentiation of* Echinococcus *into a separate class occurred much earlier in Goeze's text. He described the scolices of the hydatid and related it to tapeworms.*

The small social granular tapeworm (*Taenia visceralis socialis granulosa*)

This is almost an intermediate form between the large spherical-shaped tapeworm and the multiheaded one found in the brain matter of giddy sheep. . . .

On the first of November 1781 I received an extremely mutilated sheep liver which was so permeated and covered with large and small water vesicles (the former like hen eggs, the latter like hazel nuts) that from the outside practically nothing could be seen of the substance of the liver. The animal, by the way, was perfectly healthy. The whole size of this monstrous liver was two hands wide, almost half an ell [one ell = 45 inches—Eds.] long; the weight, however, was four pounds. I had to divide it into two pieces in order to put it into a sugar glass with spirits of wine. When I pricked the full vesicles with a needle, the water gushed out like a fountain. These full vesicles contained nothing but lymph and no particular inner vesicle. On separating one

Plate 106. Fig. 6. The entire compressed worm, from (a) the vesicle within which it grows; (b, b) the body with flattened granules; (c, d, e) the likewise flattened suckers; (f) the crown of hooklets on the surface of the invaginated head. *Fig. 7.* A detached and compressed worm. (a, b) the prominent folds of the body; (c, d) two suckers; (e) the prominent crown of hooks. *Fig. 8.* A somewhat compressed worm, without folds. (a, b) the body filled with innumerable atoms; (c, c) the caudal extremity which is attached to the capsule; (d, d, d, d) the suckers; (e, f) the double crown of hooklets.

Fig. 9. A leatherlike gristly vesicle from the liver of a sheep; inside the small granules lie by thousands on a delicate membrane. *Fig. 10.* The same granules in water. *Fig. 11.* The same granules still attached to the delicate membrane.

Fig. 12 Five granules of various sizes. (a) like a heart, on top a black line; (b) the retracted hook crown; (b) still contracted, somewhat flatter; (x, y) two suction vesicles; (z) the black center line or invaginated hook crown. (c) like a cup; on top (x, y) two suckers; (d) like a cone; on top (x, y) two suckers; (z) the third edge; (n) the extended hook crown; (o) lower end pointed without opening. (e) a cone-shaped one, dotted; (m, n) on the edge two suckers; (o) on top a black crown; (p) inferiorly an indented opening. *Fig. 13.* Granules, or a true tapeworm; under the compression slide. (a, b, a, b) the dotted body; (c, d, e, f) the four suckers lying in a row here; (g, g) the double hook crown; (h) posteriorly an opening. *Fig. 14,* (a, b, c) three detached hooks, like buttons.

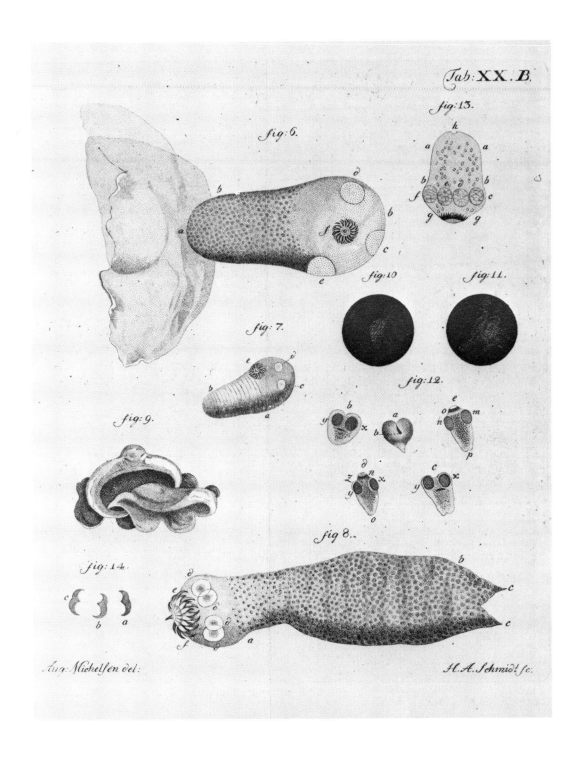

fig: 13.

fig: 6.

fig: 10.   fig: 11.

fig: 7.

fig: 12.

fig: 9.

fig 8.

fig: 14.

of the pieces of the liver, I had to damage some of the vesicles lying inside. From these rather hard, leatherlike, outer vesicles, bluish, callous inner vesicles fell out which were still closed. In substance, to be sure, they were somewhat softer than the outer capsule, but much more gristly than the vesicles of spherical or multiheaded tapeworms.

On opening them there was found, in various places, a whitish-gray granular matter, like the smallest fish roe, which was connected with a very delicate mucous membrane; this dropped off immediately in water so that the granules swam around individually. In one vesicle like a pigeon egg there were many thousand, so small that one could hardly discern them with the naked eye. Under No. 4, Tub. A, of my magnifying glass, I could observe the organized character of these bodies. They had very varied forms: some like a heart, on top, with a notch and a black line; some like a pitcher, on top, with two round buttons, one on each side; some like a horseshoe with a short, black center line; some like a round handle, on top an indentation with two side buttons and in front lopped off with a blackish crown. When I used No. 1, Tub. A, I saw plainly that they were true tapeworms (Plate 106). The bodies were flat and dotted black; in front four suckers and on the rounded foreshortened proboscis the exceedingly small double-hook crown; however, on each one, posteriorly, was a small, sloping indentation like an anus. The others were arranged in very special forms; the black center line was the hook crown. Under the compressing slide the four suckers, the hook crown, and the dots appeared even more plainly. In these worms I noticed something that I have never observed in any kind of tapeworm, namely, that on compression, the delicate hooks of the crown came off and flowed around freely.

Therefore, this is a kind of tapeworm which differs from those in the brain matter of giddy sheep in the following ways: (1) that these vesicles with the granular matter, or with many thousands of extremely small worms, are covered with a strong, leatherlike outer capsule in which they lie free; (2) that this roelike matter in the inside vesicle swims around in a clear lymph, the individual worms only connected with one another by a delicate mucous membrane, but not like the other attached to the capsule particularly

nor even to its own membrane; (3) that every granule, or worm, is a hundred times smaller than one of the white corpuscles or worms in the brain vesicle of giddy sheep.

This is the same phenomenon which the eagle-eyed Pallas already noticed but left unexplained.

ON THE TRANSFORMATION OF *ECHINOCOCCUS*-BROOD (CYSTS) TO *TAENIA*

Ueber die verwandlung der Echinococcus-brut in taenien. Zeitschrift für Wissenschaftliche Zoologie, 4: 409–425, 1853. Selections from pp. 409–411. Translated from the German.

Carl Theodor von Siebold (1804–1885)

The biography of Siebold appears in an earlier chapter on Taeniasis.

In this paper, Siebold first demonstrated that adult Echinococcus granulosa *could be obtained in dogs fed the hydatid brood.*

Since the transformation of the *Cysticercus pisiformis* into *Taenia serrata* succeeded so perfectly, my desire became particularly strong to discover what results would be obtained by feeding dogs with *Echinococcus* brood. *Echinococcus veterinorum,* which appears so often in our slaughter animals, seemed to me to be particularly well suited for such experiments, since I could obtain it fresh, with the assurance of having living brood for feedings.

I must start with the premise that the composition and organization of the *E. veterinorum,* as well as the relation of the broodless *Echinococcus* (formerly called *Acephalocystis*) to the *Echinococci* on the brood-covered inner surface of the abdominal wall, are known.

I need hardly mention that the *Echinococcus* cysts containing brood are easily recognized because upon damage to a mother cyst the brood is swept out in large number with the emerging liquid. In this condition, the content of a fertilized *Echinococcus* cyst forms a cloudy, milky liquid which clears as soon as it settles; thereby, the brood suspended in it sinks rapidly and forms an extremely fine granular precipitate. In some *Echinococcus* vesicles, larger or smaller numbers of *Echinococcus* larvae (nursing brood) are still attached with the posterior body end to the ruptured and shrunken cysts from whose inner surface they had grown prior to rupture. In this condition, such groups of *Echinococcus* brood appear to the unaided eye to be the size of a pinhead. Having let the brood flow out of the mother cyst, I poured it immediately into lukewarm milk and conducted feeding experiments at the Institute of Physiology during the summer of 1852. The milk, saturated with

Echinococcus brood, was poured in short sequential intervals down the throats of young dogs, most only a few weeks old, whose jaws were held apart by an assistant. After the dogs had thus swallowed a sufficient quantity of *Echinococcus* brood, pure lukewarm milk was set before them which they lapped up eagerly; this way, I was sure that after these many swallowing movements the small *Echinococcus* larvae had been washed down into the stomachs of the dogs. These dogs

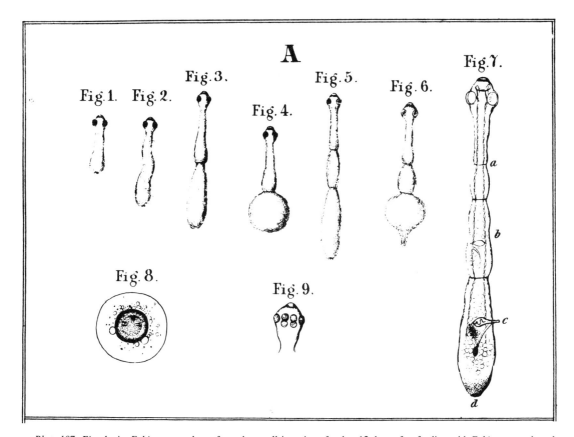

Plate 107. Fig. 1. An *Echinococcus* larva from the small intestine of a dog 12 days after feeding with *Echinococcus* brood. *Fig. 2.* A somewhat larger *Echinococcus* larva from the same site. *Fig. 3.* A two-segment *Taenia echinococcus* from the small intestine of a dog, 22 days after feeding with *Echinococcus* brood. *Fig. 4.* The same *Taenia* with rear segment shortened by contraction. *Fig. 5.* A three-segment *T. echinococcus* further advanced in growth, likewise from the small intestine of a dog, 22 days after feeding with *Echinococcus* brood.
Fig. 6. A completely grown three-segment *T. echinococcus* whose neck shows an indentation and whose last segment is in the contracted, shortened state. *Fig. 7.* A completely grown, sexually mature *T. echinococcus*. The excretory system is indicated in the head, neck, middle segment, and in the upper half of the rear segment by simple lines. (a) The indentation on the neck; (b) the middle body segment with the sexual organs not yet completely developed; (c) the rear body segment with the completely mature sexual organs; (d) sphincterlike opening on the posterior end of the body. The vitelline bodies have been omitted; the outlines of the immature and mature eggs gleam through from the two posterior body segments. The walls of the ovary also have not been included in this figure. *Fig. 8.* A mature egg from a *T. echinococcus* which contains the embryo provided with the six hooks. *Fig. 9.* Head of *T. echinococcus* with six suckers, which monstrosity I once saw.

were carefully tended and watched. After killing them, the dissection gave the following results.

On 22 May, a young dog of undetermined species received a large portion of *Echinococcus* brood in milk. On 3 June, 12 days after feeding, he was killed by chloroform and dissected immediately. The stomach contained no trace of helminths; however, in the mucosa of the entire small intestine innumerable *Echinococcus* larvae were found, all with extended heads. Usually they were lying with their heads deep between the villi. Because of their small size, they could be found only with the help of a magnifying glass in the mucosa which had been scraped off with the back of a scalpel and differentiated from the fragmented villi. Segmentation could not be discerned on any of these small larvae (Plate 107, Figs. 1 and 2); they showed the well-known scolex form and inside contained the evenly distributed characteristic calcium bodies whose number had remained unchanged since the feeding. No trace of sex organs could be discerned; however, on the posterior end of these larvae I noticed a sphincterlike opening which, on closer inspection, I recognized as the place from which the stemlike appendage had projected earlier by which the individual *Echinococcus* larvae were connected with the cyst from which they came. All these recovered larvae corresponded in their entirety, as well as in their individual characteristics, so completely with the brood of the *Echinococcus veterinorum* that there could be no doubt about their origin. However, it must be emphasized that their extended bodies were more slender than in those specimens of the *Echinococcus* brood which have everted their heads in the liquid of the mother cyst. This evidently stems from the fact that the latter are more puffed up by the thin, viscid liquid absorbed from their surroundings, while the specimens remaining for longer time already in the thick, viscid chyle of the small intestine have given off their excess moisture by exosmosis. In the light, the chalk-white posterior portion of most of these *Echinococcus* larvae contrasted with the remaining colorless, completely diaphanous body. Under the microscope, this difference stemmed from a very fine granulated mass lying embedded in the parenchyma at the posterior end of the body. . . .

I must add to these reports that in all these dissections I have always examined the contents of the large intestine of the dogs, but have never been able to discover in this portion of the digestive canal either *Echinococcus* larvae or *Echinococcus* tapeworms.

From these experiments one becomes convinced that the *Echinococcus* brood which reaches the intestinal tract of a dog fresh and alive is not always destroyed therein, but under certain favorable conditions, develops into odd, sexually mature tapeworms provided with a pair of segments.

Proof that the brood of the *E. veterinorum* must adapt well in the duodenum of the dog is the elongated state in which the *Echinococcus* larvae are seen there soon after feedings, the growth of the same which follows soon thereafter, and finally the production of eggs and embryos in those body segments having reached sexual maturity.

According to this, the same thing occurs in the intestinal tract of the dog with both the *Echinococcus* larvae and *C. pisiformis:* both grow into segmented and sexually mature tapeworms. This stage is the same for both helminths and hence they must be classified in the same helminth system. It has been known for a long time to the helminthologists that *C. pisiformis* is another developmental stage of *Taenia serrata*. However, that species of adult tapeworm to which the larval *Echinococcus* brood belongs seems to have escaped the eyes of the helminthologists until now. I suspect that this might be due in part to the small size of this species of tapeworm and in part to the short time span which is required for its sexual maturation.

The rapidity with which the *Echinococcus* larvae develop into sexually mature tapeworms can be seen from my earlier experiments. Fifteen to 22 days after being fed to dogs, these unsegmented larvae are found in the intestinal tract of the animal as two-segmented bodies. . . .

ON THE TAENIA BELONGING TO ECHINOCOCCUS HOMINIS

Ueber die zu Echinococcus hominis gehörige tänie. Archiv für Anatomie, Physiologie und Wissenschaftliche Medicin, 412–416 (one plate, not reproduced here), 1863. Translated from the German.

Bernhard Naunyn
(1839–1925)

The son of a Berlin burgomaster, and Prussian by training and by temperament, Naunyn was Frerich's clinical assistant for seven years and then served as professor of clinical medicine at Dorpat, Bern, and Königsberg before he finally succeeded Kussmaul at Strassburg. While his reputation rests primarily upon his work on the metabolism of diabetes (even Joslin came from Boston to study with him) and in diseases of the liver and the pancreas, early in his career he investigated the hydatids. He was one of the founders of a major German journal of pathology, the Archiv für Experimentelle Pathologie und Pharmakologie.

The relationship of human echinococcosis to animal infection had been suspected for many years. Naunyn succeeded in infecting dogs with fresh human Echinococcus *hydatid cysts; he reports the results in the following article.*

Since it has been proven by Siebold that the scolices of the *Echinococcus veterinorum* are capable of developing, in the intestine of the dog, into peculiar small *Taeniae* which he called *Taenia echinococcus*, the way was paved for concluding the long battle over the identity of the several *Echinococcus* species in the various animals. Other investigators, namely Küchenmeister, Beneden, and lately Leuckart, were also successful in raising the same *Taenia* described by Siebold from *Echinococcus* scolices of animals of various species, the lamb, the pig, and cattle.

For the *Echinococcus* of man, similar experiments have already been attempted several times but always with negative results. . . .

Through the kindness of Professor Frerich, who pursued this subject with great interest, in February of this year I received an invitation and the opportunity to repeat these experiments. On 17 February, at the University Medical Clinic here, which is under the direction of Frerich, a large tumor in the liver, considered to be hepatic *Echinococcus*, was punctured. The puncturing had to be carried out with the probing trocar and only a small amount, about 300 to 400 cc, of the completely clear, lightly yellow-colored liquid

contained in the sac could be drained. In it, a small number of brood capsules were swimming around, filled with very lively moving scolices, some still well preserved.

The patient died of typhus. Besides the characteristic findings of this disease, the autopsy showed that the left lobe of the liver was almost completely atrophic. It was displaced by a large *Echinococcus* sac about seven inches in diameter filled with bloody liquid. The capsule of the mother vesicle, preserved in its continuity, was in some areas three millimeters thick; in the liquid there were several well-preserved daughter cysts. It was concluded that this was a specimen of *Echinococcus altricipariens Küch*.

The liquid obtained from the living patient by aspiration contained, by rough estimate, a few hundred scolices; it was divided into two unequal portions and administered to two dogs held in readiness for this purpose for several days, while observing the necessary precautions. After the feeding, they were placed in a kennel and, as in the preceding five days, fed only with cooked foods. Of the two dogs, the one who had received the considerably smaller portion of the available scolices and who, following the feeding, seemed less lively was killed on the 28th day after feeding. The intestine was completely free from intestinal worms of any kind. Liver, lungs, and kidneys showed nothing abnormal. The second dog was killed on the 35th day after feeding. There could be no further delay since, as is known, the *T. echinococcus* reaches sexual maturity at this time, and soon after the onset of sexual maturity its migration was to be feared.

Lung, liver, and kidneys of the dog showed nothing abnormal. Small living *Taeniae*, 1 to 1½ *linien* long [1 *linien* = 1/12 inch—Eds.], completely similar to the known *T. echinococcus*, were located intermittently between the villi through the upper half of the intestine from the pylorus on. They had four segments. In the third segment the penis, cirrus pouch, and vulva were identified; in the fourth the sexual parts were completely developed and form entirely in the same way as Leuckart described in *T. echinococcus* after completed fertilization. The cirrus sac with the penis and the ball-shaped, coiled vas deferens, the vagina with the peculiar enlargement described by Leuckart, and the receptaculum were plainly recognizable; testicles, vitellaria, and ovary were not plainly visible; however, the uterus was distended with eggs. They did not yet possess a solid shell. Embryonic hooklets could not be found. Segmentation was in various stages.

The head showed four suckers, between them a bulging rostellum and on the root of it 36–44 hooks arranged in two rows. In front of the rostellum were found the peculiar dark spots mentioned by Siebold. The hooks have exactly the same form as those which the *T. echinococcus* show at five weeks of age. In comparison with those scolices they are already considerably larger and thicker. The course of the four vessels' walls was exactly the same as Siebold described years ago. Therefore, since these *Taeniae* in all known characteristics correspond to the *Taenia echinococcus von Siebold,* they must be considered identical.

It is highly probable that these *Taeniae* originated from the scolices of the human *Echinococcus* administered to the dog six weeks previously.

Apart from the fact that *T. echinococcus* is very rare in our city dogs (I never succeeded in finding any, although I examined about 20 dogs carefully for them), the result here is relatively reliable since we can determine fairly accurately the age of the *Taenia* from the data given by various investigators about the time in which the *Echinococcus* scolex introduced into the intestine of the dog reaches sexual maturity.

Siebold, in one case, found mature embryos of the same *Taenia* four weeks after feeding, Küchenmeister found them only in the eighth, and Leuckart not before the seventh week. I myself, in several feedings undertaken earlier, have never seen mature embryos of *Taenia* obtained before the end of the sixth week. After five weeks I found *Taeniae* with an already sexually mature fourth segment and very often with eggs at the point of development. The age of these *Taeniae* containing eggs, which were still in the first stages of embryonic formation, cannot in any case be estimated at more than six weeks. The dog in this experiment had been kept locked up for 41 days and fed with cooked foods; an autoinfection could therefore not have taken place during this time. According to the above data, the *Taeniae* could hardly have come from an infection occurring before this time. Therefore, it is highly probable that this *Taenia* originates from the scolices of the human *Echinococcus* intro-

duced on 17 February and that, therefore, the *Echinococcus* of man is the bladder-worm stage of *T. echinococcus* living in the intestine of the dog (the present experiment relates particularly to *Echinococcus altricipariens Küch.,* as well as to that of animals). It is, therefore, not proper to represent either the *Echinococcus hominis* or the *E. altricip. Küch.* as a separate species. . . .

ON *ECHINOCOCCUS* GRAFTS

Des greffes échinococciques. Comptes Rendus Hebdomadaires des Séances et Memoires de la Société de Biologie, 53: 115–116, 1901. Translated from the French.

Felix Dévé
(1872–1951)

Born in Beauvais, Dévé graduated from the Faculty of Medicine in Paris in 1901. He made his first observations on echinococcosis as a student, and in his last year of internship he began his classic experiments.

He became professor of clinical medicine in 1924 at Rouen and during his lifetime published numerous reports on echinococcosis. Dew in his text Hydatid Disease *referred to Dévé's status in this field of research as follows: "In this respect I must pay tribute to the remarkable contributions of F. Dévé of Rouen, to whose work I have alluded in many places in the text. This observer, although he has access only to a limited number of cases of hydatid disease annually has by accurate study added more to our knowledge than any other worker and has become the recognized world authority."*

In addition to studying the pathogenesis of secondary abdominal cysts, he performed many experiments including the successful establishment of Echinococcus *cysts of the brain and bone by the hematogenous route.*

Documentation of the dissemination of Echinococcus *hydatid cysts from brood capsules and scolices and their subsequent localization is found in these papers by Dévé.*

Even though it is well known, through numerous clinical observations and unchallengable experiments, that daughter cysts which fall in the peritoneal cavity can take a graft and continue their development, much debate continues concerning two other *Echinococcus* forms which have completely and significantly different structures: brood capsules and scolices. Two authors, Alexinsky and Riemann, recently have tried to reproduce the graft and development of those elements in the peritoneum of the rabbit; the former obtained four positive results in seven tests while the latter had only negative results in three cases.

We have been doing experimental research for a year, the results of which we shall give shortly. Now, we ask for permission to report on two experiments in which we achieved positive results.

Experiment I (Rabbit). On 21 September 1900, we injected intraperitoneally, brood capsules and scolices from a sheep liver cyst (it is known that in this animal *Echinococcus* never forms daughter cysts). The injection was given directly through the abdominal wall with a Debove syringe fitted with a needle whose internal diameter was 0.6 to 0.7 mm. The animal was sacrificed on 14 January 1901 (114 days later).

At the level of the anterior aspect of the cecum, a subperitoneal cyst 6 mm in diameter was found. Upon dissection, the abdominal cavity was found to contain 9 or 10 small cysts with transparent contents. The microscope showed the leaflike structures characteristic of hydatid cysts in their walls.

Experiment II (Rabbit). On 21 September 1900 we performed intraperitoneal injection of brood capsules and scolices originating from the liver cysts of a sheep. The injection, performed as in the previous experiment, was given exactly at the level of the *linea alba*. The animal was sacrificed on 11 January 1901 (after 111 days).

Findings. (1) Exactly at the site of the needle puncture where the inoculation was performed, on the anterior aspect of the *linea alba*, in the subcutaneous tissue, a group of four small, clustered cysts was found, forming a tumor 8 mm in diameter. (2) In the lesser omentum, a cystic mass, 11 mm in diameter when dissected, consisted of about 15 small, clustered cysts, polyhedral due to the contiguous pressure. The microscopic examination showed their undeniable *Echinococcus* nature.

These two experiments show that brood capsules and scolices can give rise to hydatid cysts and affirm that the formation of cysts results from a combination of brood capsules and scolices. What is the exact role of each entity?

This is a point to which we shall return again, but its interest is primarily academic. In any event, the results we obtained in these two cases confirm the conclusions reached in the work of Alexinsky, as well as the opinion recently given by Mr. Peyrot at the Surgical Society on the sub-

ject of the development of multiple cysts in the peritoneum.

It seems futile for us to insist on the significance of this concept, which modifies appreciably the ideas still classic in France on the biology of the *Echinococcus* parasite. Application of this concept to the natural history and pathological anatomy of hydatid cysts is very important. Our experiments demonstrate, in particular, the possibility, already suggested by Volkmann, of the development of cysts of the peritoneum following punctures (exploratory or aspiratory for therapeutic reasons) of abdominal cysts. Indeed, the opening left in these cases by a much larger needle than the one used for our inoculations easily permits the escape of brood capsules and, *a fortiori,* of scolices. On the other hand, the first cyst of our second experiment constitutes a perfect experimental reproduction of these grafts in the incisional scar reported by Billroth in Austria and, more recently, by Mr. Quenu in France.

These experiments demonstrate above all the need to protect all tissues during surgical procedures on hydatid cysts, especially in the peritoneal cavity, not only against daughter cysts, but also against microscopic brood capsules and invisible scolices.

We believe that the only prophylaxis for secondary postoperative echinococcosis would be to kill the infective *Echinococcus* parasites in the cyst by a taeniacide injection before opening the sac widely.

THE LOCATION OF SUBSEROSAL PERITONEAL *ECHINOCOCCUS* GRAFTS

Du siège sous-séreux des greffes echinococciques péritonéales. Comptes Rendus Hebdomadaires des Séances et Memoires de la Société de Biologie, 53: 117–118, 1901. Translated from the French.

Felix Dévé
(1872–1951)

Dévé's biography will be found with the preceding article in this chapter.

It is known that multiple hydatid cysts of the peritoneum are never located in the peritoneal cavity but in the subserosa. Since the report of Charcot and Davaine (1857) all authors have confirmed this fact.

This pathologic-anatomical concept has led them to conclude: (1) the extraperitoneal origin of causative hydatid organism (which could reach this site either through the circulation or by a direct approach); (2) primary multi-infestation by hexacanth embryos (which, according to classical opinion, are the only ones to give birth to hydatid cysts).

The experiments which we are going to describe demonstrate that subserosal cysts may come from *Echinococcus* products seeded into the peritoneal cavity, quite apart from the hexacanth embryos.

Experiment I (*Rabbit*). On 26 May 1900, at laparotomy, an inoculation was made into the peritoneal cavity from the wall of a hydatid cyst (3–4 sq. cm) which had been removed surgically from a man that morning. The inoculated cyst wall had its own germinative membrane to which there still adhered a certain number of brood capsules perfectly visible to the naked eye.

The animal was sacrificed 1 January 1901, eight months or 230 days after inoculation. In the thickness of the omentum we found an oblong, resistant, translucent mass, 2 cm thick and 5 cm in length, largely covered with fat. A puncture with a pipette produced three to four cm³ of crystal clear fluid. A cross-section showed that the cyst was well enclosed within the omentum and covered not only the peritoneal serosa, but also with fat in which many blood vessels were present. Microscopically we saw that, at its periphery, the adventitious fibrous membrane was continuous with the subserosa. Approximately 15 small cysts, with an average diameter of 8 mm were found all pressed together inside the large cyst. Microscopic examination revealed their *Echinococcus* nature (leaflike cyst walls). These cysts are sterile: the fluid collected did not contain scolices or hooks, nor could we find them on microscopic examination.

This experiment demonstrates (apart from the point we wish to establish in this paper) the possibility of recurrences of hydatid cysts originating from portions of the hydatid wall left in a wound. The actual source of the recurrences may have been either the cyst wall, that is, the germinative membrane, or, more likely, the brood capsules and the scolices which remained adherent.

Contrary to what was thought previously, this experiment demonstrates that a ruptured or punctured hydatid cyst does not die simply because its fluid is removed.

Experiment II (*Rabbit*). At laparotomy on 8 December 1900, two daughter cysts, the size of a large cherry, which had been taken from a liver cyst of a man operated on that morning, were inoculated into the peritoneal cavity. The animal died 25 December, 17 days after inoculation. At autopsy, we found that the two cysts were under tension and were transparent, having already been covered by omentum in spite of their size, as if enveloped in its thickness. Microscopic examination demonstrated that they were entirely covered by the peritoneum and were infiltrated with blood vessels at different points on their surface.

Experiments III and IV (described in a previous note). [In these experiments,] brood capsules and scolices were injected intraperitoneally. After three and one-half months, cysts developed in the gastrosplenic omentum, and subperitoneally, in the cecum.

In all these experiments, we can see that various *Echinococcus* products inoculated into the peritoneal cavity have been found after a variable period of time growing outside the cavity, but *under the serosa*. Similar findings have been reported by Bobrov and Alexinsky in Russia and Riemann in Germany. The importance of these findings has been well established by these authors.

Thus, the location of a cyst in the subserosa is not, as Freund and Ratimoff postulated, proof of the extraperitoneal and primary origin of such a cyst. . . .

These facts clarify the pathogenesis of multiple cysts of the peritoneum and of the numerous varieties of abdominal cysts which, thus far, have been studied separately (cysts of the omentum, mesentery, pelvis, and prostate, pedunculated visceral cysts, and cysts located near the liver, near the spleen, and the like). These cysts are, if not always, at least *more often secondary,* that is, consequent, to a rupture, either apparent or *latent,* traumatic or *spontaneous,* of a primary abdominal cyst (liver, spleen, and the like).

We may add that the same interpretation can be applied to *multiple subpleural cysts* (rupture into the pleural space of cysts of the lungs, liver, and spleen), some cases of which have been reported in the literature.

THE HISTOGENESIS OF THE HYDATID PARASITE (*TAENIA ECHINOCOCCUS*) IN THE PIG

Medical Journal of Australia, 1: 101–110, 1925. Selections from pp. 101–104, 106–109.

Harold Robert Dew
(1891–1962)

A native of Australia, Dew received his medical degree from Melbourne in 1914 and became a member of the Royal Army Medical Corps, serving in France and Palestine. He returned to Australia and became surgeon to outpatients at the University of Sydney from 1922 to 1930. Dew was appointed Bosch Professor of Surgery in 1930 at Sydney and maintained that position (as well as that of dean of the Faculty of Medicine) until his retirement in 1956. His contributions to our knowledge of hydatid disease are well recognized. His book Hydatid Disease *remains an authoritative source.*

We have reproduced in part his description of the development of the Echinococcus *hydatid cyst.*

The Development of the Taenia Echinococcus from Embryo to Hydatid Cyst

Introduction

We are indebted to Leuckart for the first true explanation of the life cycle of the hydatid parasite and as far as English literature is concerned, his description is still the only one followed. He infected four sucking pigs with ova of *Taenia echinococcus* and made careful observations on the resulting cysts in the liver. He noted that these were most frequently present in the interlobar spaces and particularly beneath the peritoneal coat. In one pig four weeks after feeding the liver was studded with small tubercular-like nodules which had a thick homogeneous capsule enclosing semi-solid granular contents. These had a diameter of 0.35 millimetre. At the end of eight weeks the parasite was a millimetre in diameter, showed slight lamination of the outer layer, possessed a well-marked inner germinal layer and contained fluid which escaped from it on puncture. Leuckart did not make use of serial miroscopical sections and consequently was not able to study the very early stages of the parasite.

The present investigation was undertaken particularly to investigate these earlier stages. The French literature contains the work of Dévé, but there is nothing in English concerning this phase of the development of the parasite. To some extent this work is a repetition of that of the French authority, but some new observations are added.

Material and Methods

A supply of mature taeniae and ova were obtained from artificially infected dogs. At first four dogs employed by drovers at the city abattoirs were obtained and given areca nut and castor oil in the hope that enough mature taeniae would be obtained for experimental purposes. This method proved very disappointing as only eight complete specimens were obtained. Resource was then had to puppies experimentally infected by feeding with mature scolices procured from the cysts of the lung and liver of the sheep. The scolices were collected by sedimentation from the fluid contents of the cysts and examined for viability under the low power of the microscope after warming with hot saline solution, which in living scolices causes active movement. In all six dogs were thus infested, each receiving half a test tube of hydatid "sand."

The first dog which was killed after a period of 36 days, was found to have a great number of *Taeniae echinococci* in the small intestine, but practically all these were immature and none contained mature ova. The remaining dogs were killed after a lapse of two months and in every case a plentiful supply of mature worms and ova was procured.

A series of sucking pigs, aged six weeks, were fed by means of a pipette with an emulsion of ripe proglottides warmed in milk. In all cases the presence of ova was determined microscopically and extremely heavy infestation was aimed at by giving many thousands of ova in each dose. These pigs were killed at varying times after infestation. The liver was examined, fixed in Zenker's fluid and serial sections were cut.

In this way sections of liver showing the hydatid parasite were obtained 12 and 28 hours and then three, seven, 14, 21, 28, 90 and 150 days after infestation. The pigs which were kept for the later stages, were also investigated by Dr. Kellaway with regard to the early immunological reactions.

Route Taken by the Embryo

The hexacanth embryo hatches in the stomach and by actively boring into the wall, makes its way into small radicles of the portal vein whence it is carried to the liver. In order to explain the peculiar examples of this disease in which the liver has escaped, many alternative routes have been supposed to exist. It has been suggested that the parasites pass through the biliary passages from the duodenum or through the subperitoneal tissues. The great frequency of extra-hepatic infestation in some animals, such as the squirrel, has led some investigators to postulate the existence of aberrant anastomotic veins leading from the stomach into the thoracic veins. All these hypotheses seem to be entirely unnecessary and rest on no direct observations and the evidence presented here makes it evident that in the pig at all events the parasite reaches the liver through the portal vein.

A pig, weighing nine kilograms, was given at 8 A.M. and at 10 A.M. extremely heavy doses of mature proglottides. The animal was killed by a blow on the head at 4:30 P.M. and was not bled in the usual way. The abdomen was rapidly opened, the portal vein was tied at the head of the pancreas and the inferior *vena cava* clamped. The liver was then removed and the portal vein milked of its contents into a large centrifuge tube containing distilled water. After haemolysis the fluid was centrifuged. The sediment was examined in the wet state and two hexacanth embryos were discovered. They were readily recognized by their size—30 μ × 25 μ—and by the presence of hooklets. In neither case were the hooklets complete and one embryo had only two left attached. It would appear that, unless the trauma of centrifugalization caused the separation, the useless hooklets are shed soon after piercing the stomach wall.

The direct evidence of the presence of parasites in the portal vein and the regular demonstration of the parasite in the liver within a few hours of feeding demand for their explanation a rapid means of entry which cannot be provided by any of the hypothetical alternate routes.

Site of Implantation in the Liver

The embryo is carried to the liver and may come to rest anywhere in the liver lobule. Leuckart stated that he found the favorite site to be the interlobar tissue, but as Dévé has pointed out he did not make any observations while the parasite was still of microscopic size. When this is done, as in the present investigation, it is found that the most frequent site is in the substance of the liver lobule about a third of the way towards the centre from the periphery. Very often the embryo is found much closer to the center of the lobule and Dévé has actually seen it in the central vein. There is no doubt that the parasite frequently passes the hepatic filter and enters the inferior *vena cava*. It appears to retain a fair degree of active mobility and, since the liver capillaries are readily distended, this hepatic "filter" may not be nearly so efficient as is usually supposed.

Great variation certainly exists in the diameter of the hepatic capillaries in different animals. This appears to be the only reasonable explanation of the fact that in the squirrel, for example, after infestation 98% of the resulting cysts appear in the lung.

In the pig the great proportion of the parasites come to rest in the substance of the hepatic lobule and show a striking predilection for those lobules situated close under the peritoneal coat of the organ.

Stages of Development in the Experimentally Infested Pig

The following is an account of the various stages of development in the liver of the experimentally infested pig. There are many factors which presumably influence the rate of development of the parasite. The age of the infested animal is obviously important. In a very young animal the times may be somewhat shortened, because the mere mechanical obstacles to the parasite, such as thickness of the stomach wall and the distance from stomach to liver *via* the portal vein, are very much less. The individual resistance of the pigs, varying vitality of the parasite, seasonal variations and variations in the state of the digestive organs of the pig may all be possible factors in inducing delay in the development in these early stages. That these various factors must be considered is apparent because even in the same infestation great variations in the stage of development are seen in different parasites. This description therefore, must be taken as referring to the above experiment only, that is experimental infestation of pigs, aged six weeks, of an average weight of 6.8 kilograms in mid-winter. In each case the most advanced follicle seen at the particular stage is described and regarded as the optimal development of the parasite in a given time.

The Twelfth Hour. The earliest stage observed in the liver was after a lapse of 12 hours. No doubt under ideal conditions the parasite may reach the liver earlier than this, because it can be discovered in the portal vein after six to eight hours. No definite parasite could be detected in the liver at the eighth hour.

At the twelfth hour stage (Plate 108) the parasite is hidden from view by a small accumulation of mononuclear cells. This accumulation of cells is the beginning of the hydatid follicle. The cellular reaction on the part of the host consists of mononuclear cells originating from the local connective tissue and the endothelial cells of the liver.

There are, however, a few cells of leucocyte type present. There is no indication as yet of polymorphonuclear eosinophile reaction which is such a feature in the later stages and which is typical of all helminthic lesions. There is evidence of the elaboration by the parasite of a diffusible toxin which manifests itself by cytolytic and karyolytic changes in the liver cells surrounding the follicle. These cells become opaque and non-granular and their staining reactions alter. The cytoplasm becomes much more acidophile and stains deeply with eosin. Iodine staining shows that the cell has become deprived of most of its glycogen. The nuclei show some breaking up of the chromatin network.

In the most advanced follicles there is a slight degree of vascular reaction and the neighbouring capillaries show increased numbers of corpuscles, but as yet there is little or no diapedesis.

At Twenty-eight Hours. In the stage of development at 28 hours the follicle has grown much larger by the accumulation of mononuclear cells and lymphocytes. The cells making up the follicle are a little more diffusely arranged, but still form a thick feltwork which effectually hides the small parasite from view.

The cells of the tubercle are still mainly fixed tissue mononuclear cells, but peripherally lymphocytes are seen and in some a few eosinophile cells, evidence of the reaction to the specific helminthic toxin. The liver cells in direct contact with the follicle often appear dissociated from each other, the hepatic columns are broken up and scattered and hepatic cells may be seen among the cells of the follicle. In addition these cells show distinct cytolytic and karyolytic changes which are, however, much more advanced than in preceding stages, although they rarely extend beyond two or three liver cells from the follicle.

Further from the centre there is a well marked vascular reaction. The capillaries are dilated and are filled with red blood corpuscles and lymphocytes. Sometimes extravasation of red blood corpuscles among the cells of the follicle may be observed. The periportal areas show much cellular accumulation of lymphocytes and some eosinophile cells which in some sections are quite numerous in this situation.

At Seventy Hours. In the third day, at 70 hours, the follicle has become much larger and all the preceding changes are much more advanced. In the case of more than one parasite occupying the same liver lobule, an event which can only occur with very heavy experimental infestation, the follicle may be very large and irregular. . . . The cells of the follicle are of the same type, but there is an increase of the oval nucleated endothelial cell and a great increase in the number of eosinophile polymorphonuclear leucocytes. These cells are mainly aggregated around the periphery of the follicle and from this stage are a striking feature of the reaction which in this respect resembles that of other helminthic lesions.

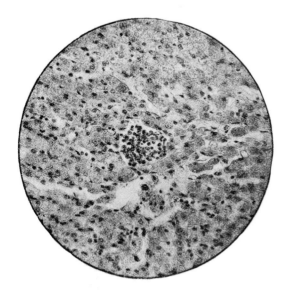

Plate 108. Hydatid follicle at 12 hours after infestation showing accumulation of mononuclear cells hiding the parasite.

At the end of the third day the parasite is usually completely hidden by the accumulation of cells, but a fortunate section may show it. It has increased in size, but still shows the peculiar helminthic arrangement of its chromatin which stains deeply but irregularly and appears to be diffusing through the whole cell preparatory to the vesicular change. Giant cells are commonly seen and take the form of typical foreign body giant cells. They appear to be formed by the fusion of endothelial cells. There is a definite vascular reaction around the follicle and extravasation of red blood corpuscles is commonly seen. The liver cells show the same degenerative changes as before, but the changes appear now to be delimited to the three or four rows of cells immediately around the follicle. The cellular activity in the periportal zones is striking; there is an increase of all cells, especially the eosinophile cells and the condition is reminiscent of that found in early cases of bilharziosis of the liver as described elsewhere by the writer. . . .

At Four Weeks. At the stage of development at four weeks but little further change can be noted. There is a great variation in the size of the follicles and cysts and it is very difficult in this set of experiments to detect any difference between many at this and at the previous stage. In the more advanced follicles the organization of the follicle wall is progressing and the wall is becoming more clearly marked off in layers. The laminated membrane of the cyst has developed and often during fixation reveals its elastic nature by curling up inside the cyst. The nuclear material which comprises the germinal layer of the hydatid cyst, is scattered irregularly in small masses on the inner aspect of this laminated membrane. The inner layer of the follicle is made up of radially arranged columns of endothelial cells with many giant cells. Between the columns can be seen very many eosinophile cells which are a characteristic feature of the tissue reaction. They may even be aggregated in direct contact with the laminated membrane of the parasite. Further out in the other layers of the follicle some little increase is seen in the process of the organization in the form of concentrically arranged fibroblasts and new blood vessels (Plate 109). As in the other stages the periportal cellular reaction is distinct. From this stage onwards the parasite grows steadily with the production of specific

fluid and the elaboration of a laminated cuticle and tends to assume a spherical shape, although even in these early stages there is evidence that the line of the least resistance may be followed, so that ovoid and even pouched cysts may be seen. In heavy infestations the aggregation of several parasites in one lobule leads to fusion of the follicular layers and varying types of cystic formation. The tissues of the host rapidly become organized with the formation of an adventitious cyst which encloses the parasite.

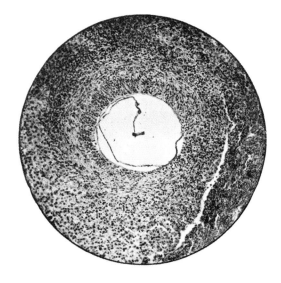

Plate 109. Stage of cyst at one month.

At Three Months. The parasite at three months may be from 40 to 50 millimetres in diameter. The laminated membrane is well developed and its characteristic elasticity is manifest by the ready stripping up when the cyst is punctured and the fluid withdrawn or during fixation. This property is a peculiar one and in microscopical sections the membrane is usually found retracted from the adventitious layer. The germinal layer is still thin and contains nuclear material scattered diffusely through it. There is as yet no sign of any production of brood capsules. Immediately external to the laminated membrane is a layer of endothelial and giant cells which in the main are arranged radially. This layer, however, is relatively much narrower than in the earlier stages. Between the columns of endothelial cells there are many granular eosinophile cells which have a tendency to clump together in close contact with the laminated membrane. Outside the endothelial cells is a thick layer of fibroblastic cells, arranged concentrically and enclosing spaces which contain blood vessels and young tissue cells of all types. The adventitia has become much more fibrous in structure and the fibrosis is more plentiful at the periphery where the layer merges into the zone of compressed liver cells which are undergoing atrophy. The eosinophile reaction in the periportal zones has quietened down and the reaction of the tissues of the host is mainly a local one which endeavours to keep the organization of the adventitious capsule in pace with the growth of the parasite. At this stage several small cysts were observed in very close contact with the large hepatic vein leading into the inferior *vena cava* and one actually projected into the lumen of the vein. It is easy to imagine the rupture at a later stage of a cyst containing brood capsules and the subsequent carriage of hydatid emboli to various parts of the body. . . .

Retrogression of the Cyst

In the later stages, namely from three to five months, of this set of experiments one could not help being struck by the evidence of retrogression of many of the cysts. Probably this is a more frequent occurrence than is usually believed. . . .

In one set of sections (three months) the laminated membrane had separated from the endothelial layer and there was no accumulation of eosinophile cells between it and the endothelial layer of the adventitia (Plate 110). The membrane appeared to be undergoing fragmentation and the eosinophile cells had actually invaded it. The appearances suggested phagocytosis of the membrane by the eosinophile cells. The inner portion of the adventitious layer showed the development of very large giant cells of a peculiar type with large pseudopodia, a finding which strengthens the belief that the cellular reaction of the host may at times overcome the parasite by phagocytosis, absorption and fibrosis.

In the fifth month retrogressive changes were even more marked and in some cases there had been absorption of the hydatid fluid, destruction of the hyaline laminated membrane and great thickening of the adventitia. The thickened adventitia had then somewhat irregularly contracted

on the collapsed cyst giving rise to a wrinkled thick-walled fibrotic sac enclosed in an area of dense fibrosis. In this way a peculiar multiloculated appearance may be produced or the cyst may be entirely replaced by a fibrous nodule. The deposition of calcium salts is not uncommon.

Summary

This short experimental study of the early stages of the development of the hydatid cyst leads to the following conclusions:

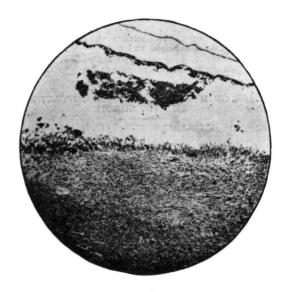

Plate 110. Section of the wall of a cyst at three months, showing separation of laminated membrane and accumulation of eosinophile cells between it and the adventitia.

(1) The hydatid hexacanth embryo finds its way to the liver by means of the portal vein and there is evidence to show that the liver barrier is by no means a perfect one.

(2) The time taken for the embryo to reach the liver is very short and sections show it in the liver lobules within 12 hours.

(3) The embryo tends to come to rest in the substance of the liver lobules and has a predilection for the subperitoneal lobules.

(4) By the local reaction of the liver tissue a hydatid follicle is rapidly produced. In the second week vesiculation commences.

(5) There is a very striking local eosinophile cellular accumulation and also much cellular

reaction in the periportal zone which brings this infestation into line with that of other helminths.

(6) There is evidence that in some cases the cellular reaction on the part of the host tissue overcomes the parasite in the earlier stages with the production of an aborted follicle.

(7) The adventitious capsule by organization becomes avascular and fuses intimately with the surrounding liver tissues. This fusion precludes any possibility of total enucleation of the whole cyst at operation.

(8) A remarkable feature is the persistency of patent biliary channels in the fibrous adventitia even close up to the parasite itself. This no doubt explains the frequency of complications in liver cysts due to the entry of bile and so forth.

(9) The cyst grows as a rule in a spherical form, but it also tends to take the line of least resistance, so that pouching is not uncommon. This pouching is determined by the local resistance of bands of fibrous tissue, large blood vessels or bile ducts.

(10) At the end of five months the cyst may reach a diameter of one hundred millimetres, but there is no trace of the formation of brood capsules at this stage.

CHAPTER **37**

Diphyllobothriasis

CONCERNING THOSE THINGS EXCRETED BY ANIMAL BEINGS

Praxeos Seu de Cognoscendis, Praedicendis Praecauendis Curandiso Affectibus Homini Incommodantibus Tractatus Tertius et Ultimus. De Vitiis, Libris Duobus Agens: Quorum. Primus Corpis: Secundus. Excretorum vitia Continet. Basel: Typis Conradi Waldkirchii, Chapter XIV, 1609. 1028 pp. Selection from pp. 992–993. Translated from the Latin.

Felix Plater
(1536–1614)

Plater was born at Basel and studied medicine at Montpellier and at Basel where he received his doctorate in 1557. He was appointed professor of medicine at Basel in 1571 and was city physician for 43 years, winning much praise for his management of affairs during five epidemics of plague (1563, 1576, 1582, 1593, and 1609). He performed the first autopsies in Basel since Vesalius' visit in 1543 and published a text of anatomy in 1583.

His Praxeos *is the first effort to introduce a system of nosology into medicine—an extremely important contribution, which was first published in 1602. He described cretinism, endemic goiter, and death in the newborn due to enlarged thymus.*

Although Thaddeus Dunus, also a Swiss, vaguely referred to Diphyllobothrium latum *in 1592, the following article, translated from the 1609 edition of* Praxeos, *is the first clear separation of the broad tapeworm,* D. latum, *from other genera of tapeworm. His clinical comments will be appreciated by those who have cared for patients with this infection.*

. . . Bodies are also passed through the anus, although rarely, and are of diverse types. Of these, one is characterized by a kind of membranous skin, similar to the fabric of the small intestines, equal to it in length but not at all empty inside as it, and about a finger's breadth wide. This they call the *Latum lumbricum* (the broad intestinal worm), but more correctly it should be called the *Taenia intestinorum* (the taenia of the intestines), since it has no likeness to the lumbricus; it is not alive, as is the lumbricus; nor is it stirred from its place, but remains fixed for a long time until it is finally passed, sometimes whole—to the great suffering or terror of the person enduring it since he thinks his intestines are being torn out—or it is passed in small pieces. On this fascia there are generally transverse black lines about a finger's breadth apart. They appear along its whole length and resemble vertebrae, swelling out in the intervals between them.

On another occasion, very long taenia of the same type were observed. However, they were shaped differently and appeared to be composed of many attached segments which could be separated from one another. These segments, since gourds sometimes bear square seeds, are called the *vermis cucurbitinus*. The worm is rarely passed whole, but generally in many pieces. Previously, each of these individual pieces was believed to have been an individual worm, called a *cucurbitinus*; however, they are only pieces broken off from the fascia.

In addition, there is another type of taeniae, resembling the former in length, but not very broad. It is completely rounded, like the intestinal worms and has little or no variation in structure throughout its length. This we call the little tongue. It, too, remains fixed in the intestine and is passed rarely by man, but rather frequently by dogs. At times, it is unbroken and at other times broken; even when it becomes weak, it is still able to cling to the anus so that it is not easily passed unless it is pulled.

While taeniae remain in the body, unless something else happens, few serious symptoms occur from which it can be perceived that an individual carries this foulness in his body before they pass unexpectedly, at which time they occasion great fright on being found. There is a pressing desire to take food much more often than was customary and a certain heaviness in the stomach. If anything is in the stomach, it is felt. The symptoms become worse when an intestinal worm dies or if a segment is broken off from the others and putrefies. . . .

TAENIA: WITH SINGLE LATERAL OSCULA

Taenia osculis lateralibus solitaris. Amoenitates Academicae. Holmiae: Laurentium Salvium. 2: 80–81, 1751. Translated from the Latin.

Carolus Linnaeus
(1707–1778)

Always primarily a naturalist, the great Swedish botanist Linnaeus also became a physician, but primarily to win the hand of the daughter of a wealthy practitioner, who refused to consent to the match unless his prospective son-in-law became a doctor. Linnaeus gave the most concise descriptions of plants and animals in all natural history and originated the binomial nomenclature in science, classifying man himself as Homo sapiens *in the order of primates. His medical writings include his materia medica, published between 1744 and 1752, and his scheme of nosology, which was described in a work called* Genera morborum, *which appeared in 1763. He seems to have had some notion of water-borne malarial fever and of the parasitic origin of disease, and he is said to have given good descriptions of peripheral embolism, hemicrania, and aphasia. When he was admitted to the nobility, he adopted the second name by which he is known, Carl von Linné.*

Linnaeus separated Diphyllobothrium latum *from other tapeworms on the basis of his knowledge of the difference in the* D. latum *scolex. This is the first accurate written description of* D. latum.

Description: It consists of a lined, flat, membranous body that is truncated anteriorly, gradually attenuated to a point posteriorly, with serrated sides corresponding to the segments. The sides are in folds, and both surfaces or flat sides are furrowed by five striae running lengthwise. In it the segments are by far the shortest of all *Taeniae,* so that the worm's width is often ten times the length of the segment. The osculum or single pore is seen only toward the base on the flat side. . . .

The worm dwells only very rarely in humans, but is very common in dogs. In both length and form it is similar to the former *Taenia,* yet is chiefly distinguished from it in that its segment makes up an eighteenth part of the width of the

worm itself; whereas, all the segments of the preceding *Taeniae* are for the most part as long as they are wide. In this type, no details of the internal structure are seen when it is held to the light, but merely two dark spots, or even none. Furthermore, in this one, we observe only one pore or osculum, unless our eyes, both naked and assisted, deceive us. The edges of this *Taenia* are also more undulating, for the segments are wider at the sides than in the middle. Finally, we always observe two dark spots at the truncated end; when the worm is begetting offspring, the segment is torn from it and there are present, so to speak, two nerves which break. At the more slender end there are transverse striae and articulations so small that they can barely be distinguished with the naked eye. While it is still living it stretches out and becomes, in one place or another, filiform; after its death, the segments become just as slender as they are wide. Furthermore, this worm is thicker throughout its length centrally than the preceding *Taenia,* so that a kind of backbone seems to run through it; but at the edges it is just as flat as the preceding one. Lastly, it must be observed that this species is the most widespread.

ON THE WORM CALLED IN LATIN *TAENIA* AND IN FRENCH *SOLITAIRE* [Plate only]

Sur le ver nommé en Latin *Taenia* et en françois *Solitaire.* Memoires de Mathematique et de Physique Présentés à l'Academie Royal des Sciences, par divers sçavans, & lus dans les assemblées, Paris, 1: 478–521, 1750.

Charles Bonnet
(1720–1793)

A native of Geneva and initially trained in law, Bonnet was profoundly influenced in his studies by La Pluche's Spectacle de la Nature *and Reanuir's* Memoirs of Insects. *He devoted himself to the study of insects and metaphysics, and in his* Treatise on Insectology *(1745) he was the first to record the phenomena of parthenogenesis. His works on plants were considered authoritative into the nineteenth century. Having allegedly ruined his eyesight by use of the microscope, his writings turned to metaphysical philosophy as he defended preconception and predestination in science. He died in Geneva at the age of 73.*

The plate reproduced here (Plate 111) is from his work of 1750, which described the body of Diphyllobothrium latum *with a* Taenia *scolex. This was corrected in 1777 (Plate 112) thus giving us the first accurate description of* D. latum. *Linnaeus' work was published a year later, in 1751.*

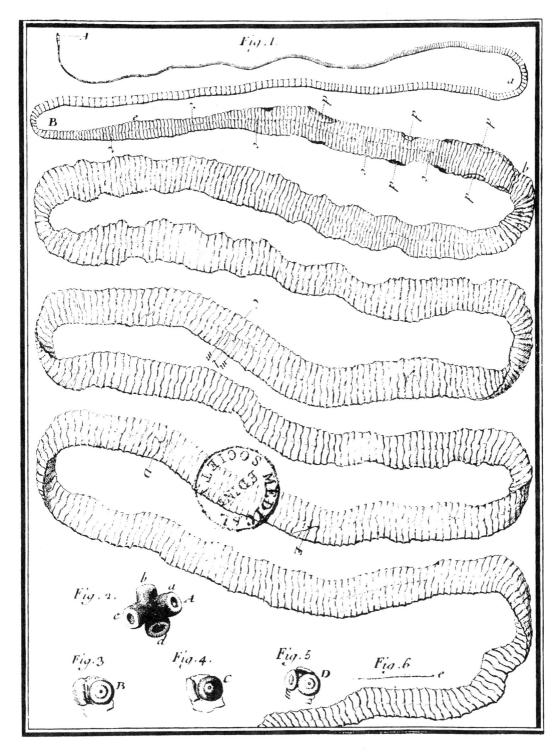

Plate 111.

NEW FINDINGS ON THE STRUCTURE OF *TAENIA*

Nouvelles recherches sur la structure du taenia. Observations sur la Physique sur l'Histoire Naturelle et Sur les Arts, IX. Paris: M. l'Abbé Rozier, 1777. Selections from pp. 243–267. Translated from the French.

Charles Bonnet
(1720–1793)

Explanatory Notes for Plate 112

The reader is advised to read the explanation of the illustrations if he wishes to acquire a clear idea of what has been discovered about the structure of the *Taenia*. The public has never before been offered figures conforming so closely to exact observations.

Figure 1 (Plate 112) represents, in the natural state, the anterior end of a short-ringed *Taenia*. This part has been named the frenulum, and at the end of it is the head. The rings are so short and so close together that one has difficulty distinguishing them at first sight. The artist has presented them in a manner to make them easily distinguishable. (t) is the head.

Figure 2 is the head of figure 1, enlarged with a magnifying lens. (t) is a small brown line that appears to be the end of a duct and indicates the mouth of the worm.

Figure 3 is the head of the preceding figures, as seen through the microscope: (b, b), the mouth, wide open, does not appear in its entirety; (l, l) the two lips, one overlapping the other a bit; (c, c) the uppermost part of the head, sufficiently raised and rounded.

Figure 4 is the head of another *Taenia* that had been preserved in a mixture of spirits for 15 years: (t) the head; (b, b) the mouth, which is short, but whose width is delineated by the brown line or shadow produced by the union of the two lips.

Figure 5 shows six rings of the short-ringed *Taenia*, viewed in the natural state. These six rings have been detached from the middle of the body or from that part of the *Taenia* which is widest. (c, c, c) the bodies, "in a flowerlike configuration," appear a little raised but are hardly noticeable because the rings have not been dried. On close inspection one discovers the stigma (s, s) placed in the middle of each ring and indicated here by a point. One can see that the rings are very short but are quite wide, with the junctions well demarcated.

Figure 6 is composed of the six preceding rings, again presented naturally, but after having been dried on a glass plate. The "flowerlike" bodies, which are some sort of little stomachs or intestines (c, c, c) are here much more discernible than in figure 5. The drying process has made them more visible. One sees again the stigmata (s, s) on three rings, although they are less easily seen on dry rings than on fresh ones.

Figure 7 shows the "flowerlike" bodies, enlarged with a magnifying glass and entirely separated from neighboring structures. (g, g) are two bodies larger than the others that are in adequate relief. They are full of a purple material, whose shades change during the drying process. Their form is not always constant, but usually approaches an oval shape. Their size does not vary much as is seen by inspecting figures 5 and 6 and those which I composed in 1743. (p, p, p) are other bodies of the same species, but smaller and full of less colorful material. . . .

Figure 8 is a fresh piece of a short-ringed *Taenia,* shown in its natural state. It is composed of 8 rings, which offer some irregularities that can be regarded, with basis, as some sort of anomaly. In the regular rings, one sees two stigmata, of which one (s, s) is more visible than the other (i, i). They appear as two very small dots and can only be perceived by close inspection. Lines have been drawn to show them better because points placed here would be confusing. (1, 2, 3, 4) are four stigmata which appear to belong to the same ring; there is reason to believe that two rings have been joined together by accident. Next to that one is another anomalous ring where one can see four stigmata.

Figure 9 shows the stigma most visible to the eye, enlarged by the microscope. One sees a fleshy nipple that juts out a little. The flesh appears a little elevated around the stigma.

Figure 10 is that of a similar stigma, again drawn from a microscopic view. (m) is the fleshy nipple that hangs at the entrance of the stigma and which appears to be as elongated as it can be.

Figure 11 represents a magnifying-glass view of a ring, in the middle of which are two "flowerlike" bodies, (g, g) full of a purplish-brown material. (s) is the large stigma; (m) the fleshy nipple that sticks out from that stigma and appears as a small white line; (i) the small stigma which appears as a brown point. The ring was freshly prepared.

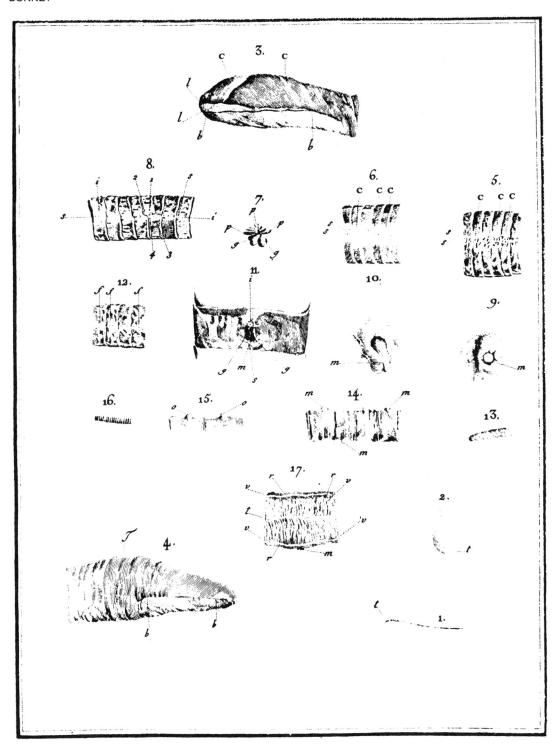

Plate 112.

Figure 12 shows, in the natural state, four rings in the midst of which are some white irregular spots (f, f, f), which are produced by the "flowerlike" bodies, which are viewed through the skin and a little in relief. These spots, or white elevations, are perceptible in different locations on the *Taenia*. One often sees on the same *Taenia* other places where purplish spots are found. These different appearances depend on the material filling the small intestines, or oral sacs.

Figure 13 represents, in the natural state, the anterior end of a yellow-colored *Taenia* with lateral nipples. This end appears to have been broken off; it ends in a blunt and rounded point. The rings are so short and so close that one cannot easily count them. The artist has represented them by very fine lines that demonstrate well the natural appearance. One should also notice in this figure that the anterior end is cylindrical instead of flattened as are most *Taenia*, especially the *Taenia* with umbilicated nipples or the *Taenia* with short rings.

In figure 14 the artist has represented in its natural state a fragment of a different *Taenia* with lateral nipples. This one is colored gray. This fragment is composed of four rings, whose articulations are easy to see. Three of these rings show a lateral nipple (m, m, m); the extent to which they protrude is easily discernible. Otherwise, the large rings of the *Taenia* are more flattened and more plump than the rings of the yellow *Taenia*.

Figure 15 shows, in the natural state, two rings of the *Taenia* in the preceding figure, where one can see distinctly the little opening (o, o) placed at the height of the lateral nipple. It is this opening that I have named the stigma.

Figure 16 represents, in the natural state, the anterior end of the same *Taenia*. One sees that it is flattened, and the rings are very close together.

Figure 17 is that of a ring of the same *Taenia* viewed with the light shining through it and the aid of a good magnifying glass. This ring was dried to make the interior easier to study. (r, r, r) are the ramifications, or rather the membranous sacs that constitute the stomach and intestines. They seem to branch off a common stem (t). Each branch has an irregular form and is twisted differently. (v, v, v, v) are two longitudinal vessels placed at the side of the rings. They are here more contracted and much less visible than they are in freshly expelled worms. The artist did not

wish to render them more perceptible than they naturally are. (m) is the lateral nipple. [Figures 13–17 probably refer to *T. saginata*—Eds.]

ON THE QUESTION OF THE INTERMEDIATE HOST OF *BOTHRIOCEPHALUS LATUS* BREMS

Zur frage des zwischenwirthes von Bothriocephalus latus Brems. Zoologischer Anzeiger, 5: 39–43, 1882. Selection from pp. 42–43. Translated from the German.

Maximilian Gustav Christian Carl Braun (1850–1930)

Braun was educated at Griswald and Würzburg in medicine and zoology, receiving his M.D. degree in 1874 and, three years later, a doctorate in zoology. Later he became professor of zoology. His final post was that of professor of zoology and comparative anatomy at Königsburg from 1891 until his retirement in 1922.

The reader may remember Hartmann's vague description of plerocercoids in an earlier chapter on cestodes. The following article contains the first recognition of the fact that the plerocercoid is an intermediate stage of Diphyllobothrium latum.

In connection with my first article in this journal, I am reporting on the results of further feeding experiments as well as the behavior of the scolex in pike meat. At first glance, such a scolex does not look at all like a bothriocephalus because the head is not noticeable; the latter is almost always drawn in, in which case—as I believe—an inversion of the head takes place as with the heads of cysticerci. If, however, the scolex taken from the muscles or the liver, the testes, ovary, and so on, of the pike is placed in warm water or egg white, the head unfolds and then one recognizes the suction grooves on it; the same thing occurs if a scolex remains for 24 hours in a ½ percent solution of sodium chloride with some intestinal mucus. I have had a similar experience with corresponding [parasites from] other native fish which I am not using for feeding experiments for the time being because they are only encapsulated in the intestine and for that reason will hardly reach man. I never find an appendage on the rounded rear end of the pike bothriocephalus; nor is segmentation present even in the largest specimens. The head is elongated, slightly pointed anteriorly, and usually separated from the neck by segmentation. In the body of the pike I have never found a capsule surrounding the scolex; even in sections I have not observed one.

Further experiments with native fish have shown me that the pike is not the only carrier of muscle bothriocephali. I found exactly the same forms in *Lota vulgaris*; therefore, it is possible that in Switzerland perhaps yet another fish might harbor corresponding forms in its muscle structure; I have examined tench, carp, roach, perch, and *Coreganus* sp. for muscle bothriocephali, but so far in vain; however, by these studies, the varieties of fish of this country are by no means exhausted.

Finally, I am going to report on the result of a feeding experiment with muscle bothriocephali from the pike on a puppy, an experiment which Professor E. Rosenberg suggested on the occasion of a lecture given by me regarding my findings. I was able to give to a three-week-old dog 17 pike bothriocephali in one day by force feeding. Up to that time, the animal had had only mother's milk; since the mother was absolutely not for sale, I had to accustom it to lapping up boiled cow's milk. The dog, which ingested only boiled cow's milk, thrived; but, because of his continual howling, had to be killed 10 days after infection. In the intestine, which was filled only with digested remains of milk of the known scrambled-egg color and consistency, I found sexually immature bothriocephali 14–15 cm long which matched, although not completely, corresponding initial parts of *B. latus*; they can only be attributed to the infection which took place.

Moreover, I had the same experiences as other researchers that the infection is not always successful; this happened to me with an experimental animal which I killed eight weeks after infection. There was no bothriocephalus in the intestine; the animal had lost its appetite because of long captivity in a small cage and was greatly emaciated. Certainly such conditions do not have a favorable influence on parasite growth and must be eliminated if possible.

Since, owing to the interest of the local medical faculty, there are now means at my disposal for continuation of my research, I shall repeat the experiments on a somewhat wider basis in order, if not otherwise possible, to eliminate the negative results by the larger number of favorable ones; this is not the place to point out the different variations of the experiments.

THE LIFE CYCLE OF *DIBOTHRIOCEPHALUS LATUS L.*

Le cycle évolutif du *Dibothriocephalus latus L.* Société Neuchâteloise des Sciences Naturelles–Bulletin, 42: 19–53, 1916–1917. Selections from pp. 22–32, 34–49. Translated from the French.

Constantin Janicki
(1876–1932)

The son of a famous engineer who had collaborated with De Lesseps, Janicki was born in Moscow and began his studies in Warsaw. The Russian domination of the University of Warsaw was so oppressive to Janicki that he went to Leipzig in 1894. He studied natural sciences for four years under Leuckart, then went on to Freiburg under Weismann. He continued his studies in Basel, earning his doctorate under Zschokke in 1906. He studied in Grassi's laboratory in Rome for five years and published works on protozoa. He returned to Professor Zschokke's laboratory in Basel as an assistant, then became privat *professor in 1911. The University of Warsaw, relieved of the Russian domination in 1919, appealed for Janicki's return, and he assumed the chair of professor of zoology.*

Felix Rosen

Felix Rosen was Janicki's co-worker and co-author; our efforts to obtain his biographical information were in vain.

Janicki worked in the Galli-Valerios Laboratories in Lausanne, and Rosen worked in the Zoological Laboratories in Neuchâtel. In this way they worked on different stages of the life cycle, confirming and completing their findings, including the first description of the procercoid of Diphyllobothrium latum. *Their monumental work was published in 1917. The importance of their work is accurately summarized by Janicki: "In the research which is the object of this work, the complete cycle of a representative of the family of dibothriocephalus is exposed for the first time. . . ." They established the existence of two intermediary hosts in this cestode.*

Observations on Several Species of Fish in Order to Arrive at a Deeper Knowledge of the Content of Their Stomachs and to Find the Stages Yet Unknown of the Plerocercoid (Janicki)

My observations of the summer of 1917 are all connected (with one exception mentioned further

660

on) with fish from the Leman and include the study of the following specimens (the research was pursued from the middle of April to the middle of August).

Specimens examined:
82 *Lota vulgaris*, average length of 24 cm.
138 *Perca fluviatilis*, average length of 15–20 cm.
690 *Perca fluviatilis*, average length of 7–12 cm.
70 *Perca fluviatilis*, average length of 6–7 cm.
3 *Esox lucius*, from 20 to 33 cm long.

The observations and research had a double purpose: (1) to seek indices in the stomachs of the fish which would give some idea of the nature of the primary intermediary host; (2) to pursue the study of the plerocercoid, tracing all the stages of its evolution until the moment, if possible, when it has just passed from the primary intermediary host into the fish.

Catching the little perches necessary to our study was specially authorized by the Department of the Interior of the canton of Vaud.

(1) I will not give here details on the subject of the content of the stomachs of the numerous fish examined. I will try only to show what these stomachs, for each species of fish, contained that was most characteristic.

Lota vulgaris of Vevey, from the market of Lausanne: The stomachs contained, above all, *Gammarus*, sometimes that exclusively, and in enormous quantities. One also found there larvae of chironomes and their nymphs; larvae of May flies and of coleopterae; remains of fish impossible to identify; more rarely *Asellus aquaticus*, *Lumbricus terrestris*, *Nephelis*, *Daphnies*, and larvae of *Liponeura*. The stomachs of these *Lotae* were examined from about the middle of April until 20 June.

Perca fluviatilis, from 15 to 20 cm, from Ouchy and the market of Lausanne: The stomachs contained in great majority water fleas and *Bythotrephes*, without any mixture of "copepodes" (selective appetite?). One also found some larvae of chironomes and some nymphs, remains of unidentifiable fish; rarely oligochetes, *Gammarus;* very rarely "copepodes."

The perch of the size indicated above were studied at the same time as the *Lotae*.

Perca fluviatilis, from 7 to 12 cm long: The stomachs contained water fleas and Bythotrephes, often without any mixture of "copepodes," sometimes exclusively *Diaptomus* and *Cyclops*, but always in much less quantity than the cladoceriae; larvae of chironomes (nymphs); remains of fish; very rarely *Nephelis* and *Gammarus*.

The perch of this size were studied in very great number during the period from 20 June to 7 August.

Perca fluviatilis, from 6 to 7 cm long (of about three months): The stomachs contained, especially, representatives of the group of *Cyclops* and of *Diaptomus*, sometimes exclusively; one also occasionally finds water fleas (7 August).

Esox lucius, of 20 and 33 cm long: A whitish pulp, stomach empty; in the second stomach some larvae of insects (25 April and 16 May).

(2) The research mentioned above is fully justified by two important observations, one of which is due to Max Braun (1883), made on the stomach of *Lota vulgaris*. Braun had found, in fact, in *Lota* stomach, five round holes, of which two still contained a larva of *Dibothriocephalus latus*, the head being turned toward the submucosa; the three other openings were empty, but not far from there, between the glands and the muscle wall of the stomach, Braun discovered three larvae. The length of these larvae exceeded 10 mm. The second observation was made by me in the summer of 1916. The stomach of a large *Lota* contained several encysted plerocercoids in its walls.

Max Braun had proposed a hypothesis based on his lone observation, and he arrived at this conclusion: "The cysticercus of the *B. latus* develops from the ciliated embryos in an as yet unknown intermediate host; together with this first intermediate host they reach the intestinal canal of the pike and the tadpole and there, following the process of digestion, they become free and penetrate the intestinal wall of the second intermediate host, migrating into its body wall." By saying "intestinal canal," Braun meant, in the first place, stomach. Later, it is true, Braun modified his observation and adopted the idea of a direct infection of the fish.

From the beginning of my observations (21 April 1917) I have had the opportunity to confirm the accuracy of the discovery made by Braun in

1883. When examining a burbot 33 cm long, I found on the external wall of the stomach a plerocercoid about 5 mm long which crawled freely and, not far from there, at only a few millimeters distance, was a very definite perforation of the wall, of a whitish appearance. Moreover, I found another plerocercoid between the pyloric appendages and a third on the liver. All three were approximately the same size. This finding soon led me to consider Braun's hypothesis as the leading thread of my future research and of all our work.

I became absolutely certain that the problem in question (to know the method of infection of the fish) could be resolved by a thorough study of the contents of the stomachs of numerous fish of very different ages; by this regressive method I arrived, as what follows will prove, very near the definitive solution.

Infection of the stomach wall is very frequent in burbots of the Leman. Out of 82 fish examined, 32 were infected by plerocercoids, of which 26 had stomach infection. . . . Infection of the musculature (remarkable fact) is extraordinarily rare in *Lota vulgaris*. Out of 32 fish infected, only three showed larvae in the musculature. My observations confirm, then, those conclusions of Mr. Schor. One finds free plerocercoids frequently enough in the body cavity, on the esophagus, the intestine, the liver, between the pyloric appendages, on the ovary, and especially on the stomach.

I have every reason to consider these plerocercoids as belonging to *Dibothriocephalus latus*; moreover, I recall that it is precisely by means of larvae obtained from *Lota vulgaris* of the Leman that Zschokke raised one of his bothriocephali of man.

The average size of the plerocercoids coiled in the musculature of the stomach wall is from three to five mm; I found a maximum of 8 mm, a minimum of 1 mm (I will speak later of a very young stage). The number of plerocercoids in a stomach varies from one to 18. Sometimes one finds them in the very outer musculature, making marked protrusions toward the exterior and covered only by a very thin layer of connective tissue. Passage to the exterior, which is probably made through a histolytic phenomenon, is easily accomplished. As a rule, the plerocercoids are quietly hidden in the muscular wall of the stomach. Slight movements are perceptible and visible only if one presses on the cyst by means of cover slips. But there is no doubt that these larvae can dig a canal in the wall of the stomach. I was able to affirm this directly with a plerocercoid of 2.5 mm in length, situated between the mucous membrane and the muscular layer; in this case the cyst formerly occupied by the worm is empty. I have had, besides, the opportunity to verify the tunnel itself, sometimes quite developed, ramified even, in the stomach wall of a *Perca fluviatilis* 16 cm long. The plerocercoid was 1.7 mm long. The free specimens in the body cavity are distinguishable in no way from the larger plerocercoids encysted in the stomach wall. . . .

It is remarkable to note that the infection of the stomach wall of the *Perca fluviatilis* of average size is an extremely rare phenomenon. In the 138 fish examined by me, I found only three cases of this infection. The infection of the musculature, on the other hand, is relatively frequent. Out of 100 *Perca fluviatilis* of average size (7 to 20 cm long), I found 26 with a muscular infection. In each individual fish the infection is not very great. One finds generally only one plerocercoid, sometimes two together. It is probable that the plerocercoids stay much less time in the walls of the stomach in *Perca fluviatilis* than in *Lota vulgaris*. They undoubtedly leave the stomach at a much earlier stage, which would also explain the much greater difficulty one has in finding them in the body cavity of *Perca fluviatilis*.

In my research on little perch of 7 to 8 cm long (end of April to end of May), I had the opportunity to discover some young stages of the larva of *Dibothriocephalus,* stages yet unknown until this day. Here it was a question of tiny worms measuring .49 to .76 mm in length, which were in the encysted state, slightly contracted, in the submucosa or the musculature. One of the cyst's own walls was not visible. The body of the little worm had an elongated oval shape. One of the ends of the body exhibited a cuticular differentiation in relation to the formation of the bothridiae. The finely granular parenchyma contained a very small number of calcareous corpuscles, compared with what we find later in the plerocercoid. Upon closer examination, one was able to distinguish already the excretory system. It was clearly a larva of *Dibothriocephalus* in a very young stage. The observations made on the larvae found in the burbot permit no doubt on this subject; the similarity of the larvae was striking. Max Braun was the first who succeeded in seeing a stage a little more advanced, about 1.6 mm long, in the wall of the stomach of a pike (*Esox lucius*).

I found similar stages afterward, one in an *Esox* of 33 cm long. The larva, bent in the shape of a knee, measured .56 mm long. Two other specimens were found in *Lota vulgaris* of 29 and 24 cm in length. The larvae measured .40 and .64 mm. It is important to note that in all these cases the worm outside of its cyst is always slightly longer than the cyst.

Encouraged by these discoveries, I applied myself to examining systematically even younger stages of plerocercoids, in little perch of the Leman.

On 25 June, I found in the free state, in mucus which fills the stomach of a tiny little perch (9.5 cm long), caught in my presence some hours before near Ouchy, two small worms of .68 mm in length which I soon recognized were the forms familiar to me from my research on the *Perca* cited above. The content of the stomach consisted of *Cyclops, Diaptomus,* and *Bosmina,* as well as of nymphs of *Chironomes.* On 29 June, I again found a similar worm of .59 mm in length by palpation; it was very lively, crawling on the internal wall of the stomach. The content of the stomach consisted solely of diverse species of *Cyclops* as well as of *Diaptomus.* (Several specimens of *Diaptomus* each contained, in their body cavity, a young larva of *Ichthyotaenia* of .5 mm in length with four suckers; this same larva was observed several times, free in the stomach.) Thanks to this evidence, I was able to formulate the idea that the primary intermediary host must be sought among the copepodae. At this moment, I received the news from my friend Rosen that his experiments at Neuchâtel had led to the result that a *Cyclops* and a *Diaptomus* were the primary intermediary hosts.

I no longer had any doubt whatsoever. I had before me a stage which had just left the *primary intermediary host* after its digestion and which was in the process of trying to pierce the stomach mucosa in order to penetrate the stomach wall. This early stage was a rapidly changing worm whose anterior end was a little enlarged, the posterior end contracted and narrower. The posterior end was clearly recognized by the presence of an excretory pore; a slight invagination at the anterior end was distinguished with some difficulty. The parenchyma, with calcareous corpuscles, presented the same general characteristics as in the encysted forms of the stomach wall. The cuticle of the whole anterior half of the body was covered by fine, silklike hairs, rigid, and directed toward the rear. . . .

In spite of the great number of fish (little perch) examined after this, I no longer had the luck to find this little worm again. The content of the stomachs (in all the fish examined and with only rare exceptions) was composed almost exclusively of *Daphnies* and *Bythotrephes.*

It was only on 6 August, after having had the opportunity to examine the preparations of my friend Rosen at Neuchâtel and having seen the young larva with the caudal appendage, that I found again the little worms in question, four specimens in young perch three months old. The content of the stomach was composed of *Cyclops* and *Diaptomus* with very few *Daphnies.*

One of the small worms which crawled freely in the content of the stomach still carried the spherical appendage, furnished with hooks, at its posterior end. While I observed this worm, the appendage detached itself. The isolated appendage continued to move very energetically, taking alternately an oblong or a spherical appearance. At the place from which the appendage was detached, there was a small, persisting stem. The caudal appendage did not contain any calcareous corpuscles. Without its appendage, the worm measured .76 mm long. It assumed a shape pointed at both extremities, a shape which alternated rapidly with the normal state (large in front, narrow in back). It may be that this spindlclikc form enables the worm easily to penetrate into the mucosa.

One sees, from the preceding description, that the wall of the stomach represents the portal of entry for the parasite into the secondary intermediary host (fish).

It appears doubtful to me that one can attribute the same importance to the rest of the intestinal tract, including the pyloric appendages, as to the stomach. Max Braun also, when he speaks of the intestinal tract, always seems to have the stomach in mind. Moreover, the observation of C. Ketchekian, made under the direction of M. Galli-Valerio, corresponds perfectly with what we are saying, since the plerocercoid observed in the musculature is never accompanied by bacteria. This can only be explained if one admits that the plerocercoid penetrates into the musculature coming directly from the acid milieu of the stomach. One would explain this absence of bacteria less easily by admitting a sojourn of the plerocercoid in the intestines.

It is not possible at the present time for us to give more precise indications on the relationships which may exist between the age of the fish and their predisposition to infection. At the moment, we do not have at our disposal sufficiently solid guidelines on the subject of the rapidity of plerocercoid growth. It seems to me, nevertheless (if I consider the relatively very advanced plerocercoids found in the stomachs of the burbots examined), that the infection must take place rather early. The little perch of 7–12 cm are already infected in the musculature (about 10 per cent). The presence of free plerocercoids in the stomachs of little perch of three months also speaks in favor of a very precocious infection. (It is true that in the 70 specimens of this age examined, I could find no plerocercoids in the musculature.) We can then admit that the method of infection known today can attack all the young fish of the species examined, but that does not mean, naturally, that the infection cannot take place later, since I have myself found a very early stage (.40 mm) in a burbot 29 cm long.

Concerning the questions of whether the infection takes place at any time in the year, and whether the intensity varies according to the season, I must wait to make new observations. In any case, infection is certain in the spring. My observations on this point coincide perfectly with the opinion expressed by Max Braun.

Experimental Research on the Life Cycle of *Dibothriocephalus Latus* (Rosen)

Following the kind invitation of Dr. C. Janicki, I began diverse experiments in October of 1916 destined to resolve if possible the problem of *Dibothriocephalus latus*.

In spite of the conviction of Dr. Janicki that a direct infection of the fish by ciliated larvae of the bothriocephalus does not take place, I could not resist repeating the experiments in direct infection, already made by Janicki, for the following reasons. The research done by Janicki was on

material fixed in formaldehyde and without the use of stains. It seemed to me that this method was not sufficient, especially since examination *in vivo* had taken place only occasionally. Also, I adopted in my experiments a very special method of infection which would cause the fish to become infected, assuming that direct infection took place. Here is the procedure:

Since the ciliated larvae always assemble and group themselves at the surface of little depressions in which they hatch, the young trout (5 to 8 cm long) were kept in small receptacles until the moment when the lack of oxygen obliged them to come to the surface to breathe. This surface contained enormous quantities of ciliated larvae, and the contact between the trout and larvae was thus surely established.

The experiments were made on the following fish: (1) *Trutta fario;* (2) *Trutta iridea;* (3) *Salmo salvelinus;* (4) *Lota vulgaris;* (5) *Perca fluviatilis;* (6) *Esox lucius.*

The specimens used measured from 5 to 15 cm in length and were from a few months to about one year in age. The fish were divided into 10 aquariums supplied with plants rich in the emission of oxygen, but without any equipment for the aeration of the water.

The diverse experiments were made from October 1916 to April 1917. The test of infection of the fish by ciliated larvae took place twice—in November and December, each time for ten consecutive days.

The investigation on the salmonidae and on the pikes was meticulous. The intestinal tract was the principal object of the investigation (during the test of infection and the following 20 days), first in the living state, then in the fixed and stained state. From time to time, the sectioning in paraffin blocks provided information that a magnifying glass or dissecting microscope could not furnish.

The whole musculature of the fish exposed to infection for more than three months was carefully examined in the fresh state, next mounted, sectioned, and stained.

But despite all the care taken in this research, despite the long duration of the experiments (six months), and despite the very special conditions which seemingly should have caused the fish to become infected, the results were absolutely negative.

At the same time, taking into consideration the equally negative results obtained previously by Janicki, nothing else remained except to consider the existence of a life cycle unknown until then in cestodes, a cycle with two intermediate hosts; that is to say, the existence of another group of animals into which the ciliated larva had to penetrate first, grow, and develop until the moment when it could in its turn infect the fish, as plerocercoid host.

Plerocercoids were found in carnivorous species, thus the idea arose that the primary intermediary host might very well be a white fish. Although the direct infection of the fish indicated above seemed less and less probable, in December 1916, I began tests of infection of various white fish (*Abramis brama, Alburnus lucidus, Leucicus rutilus*). But the same experiments ended again in a completely negative result.

These experiments being negative, it was necessary to search for the primary intermediary host among the diverse invertebrates serving as food for our fish.

Although the experiments and research on the invertebrates were simpler to conduct well, the considerable number of species to examine, which could all very well enter into account, made the task, at the onset, most arduous, and singularly complicated the problem.

Let us consider, in fact, the dimensions of the oncosphere. Let us remember that the larva possesses no offensive apparatus (as one finds in many of the larvae of trematodes); one would not expect a very strong infection; finally, let us take into consideration the uncertainty created by a negative result; and the reader will appreciate the complexity of this research.

Nevertheless, an important leading idea aided me. It is known that parasites, especially the intermediate stages, are organisms which are rarely encountered in different animal species. If this is the case, however, the diverse hosts generally belong to closely related species.

With this principle in mind, I sought to find the food common to all the fish infected by plerocercoids. But the data of the specialized literature and the personal information furnished me by Professor Fuhrmann quickly convinced me that gaps existed.

Let us add, moreover, that the food varies according to the age of the fish being considered,

and that one knew neither at what age the fish become infected, nor whether age has any influence whatsoever on the fish, but only, from the research of Mr. Braun, that one does not find plerocercoids of less than 6 mm in the adult fish. One could at most deduce that the infection must take place during the early age of the fish—a conclusion which leads us to affirm that it is precisely at that age that not a great deal is known about the nutrition of most of the fish in question.

The only thing to do then was to draw up a chart of the most well-known animal species serving as common food to our fish, a chart based on the current knowledge of nutrition of young fish.

This preliminary research finished, I finally arrived at the conclusion that the animals entering into account could be classed in four principal groups: (1) plankton; (2) different species of *Chironomus, Corethra,* and other insect larvae; (3) gammaridae; and (4) oligochetae.

To think of the first of these groups in advance was a little rash; in fact, the *Coregonae* are plankton-eaters par excellence and yet, in general, none of them is known as a carrier of plerocercoids, whereas the *Lota vulgaris,* fish of the deep, which does not seem to eat plankton, is one of the most often infected fish. The plankton was thus put in the background, and experiments were immediately undertaken on the other three groups. . . . [All experiments on these three groups were negative—Eds.]

It was then that I returned to the plankton, which I had reserved for the reasons explained above. Allow me to give further explanations on this subject.

If one considers the organization and the *modus vivendi* of a ciliated larva of *Dibothriocephalus latus*—a *modus vivendi* clearly planktonic—it is first of all plausible to consider the organisms of plankton as being the closest in biologic relationship with ciliated larvae. It was then natural to search for the primary intermediary host in the plankton, as soon as the hypothesis of *direct infection* of the fish by this larva had been discarded. But the *Coregonae,* plankton-eaters, are almost never infected, whereas the *Lota vulgaris* (species of the deep) is infected very often; this fact, I say, is so striking that in undertaking my experiments, I was skeptical in advance. However, after the negative results obtained with the three other groups of animals, the study of plankton returned to the forefront. Moreover, Professor Fuhrmann had indicated as intermediate hosts of many cestodes representatives of the family of *Copepodae* and had observed that the *Coregonae* (the palée in particular) are only slight eaters of these animals.

It is thus that, on 17 June, my research and experiments on plankton began, experiments which, this time, fortunately were crowned with success.

Experiments and Research on Plankton

General remarks: The embryos of the parasite are obtained by a complicated procedure of extraction of eggs from human stools. Once these eggs are isolated, they are placed in Petri jars, filled almost to the top with water. The time necessary for their development varies according to the atmospheric conditions and the height of the column of water. In the summer, at a water depth of one cm, about 20 days are sufficient to hatch the eggs and to obtain the ciliated larvae.

In nature, human stools containing eggs of *Dibothriocephalus latus* are carried away by sewers and streams to neighbouring lakes (in Switzerland, principally the lakes of Neuchâtel, Bienne, Morat, and Leman). It is not yet known how much time it takes for the eggs to hatch in the natural conditions of the environment, nor if there exists a certain periodicity in their development because most of the data which could elucidate these questions is absolutely lacking. Thus we have no indication of the distance which the eggs are carried in the lakes, which would be important to know because of the influence of the temperature. I can only state with certainty that the development is completely arrested as soon as the temperature nears 0°C.

The young larva (Plate 113, Fig. 1; Plate 114, upper left), from the time that it hatches, revolves slowly in the water, always in the plane of its axis, maintained in movement by its ciliary covering whose regular movements cause it to advance continuously. I warmly thank Mr. T. Delachaux who so graciously executed the two plates. The larva appears as a very regular sphere of variable size (from 42 to 48, attaining even sometimes 55 μ in diameter). It is composed of two parts, qualitatively and morphologically different: (1) the oncosphere, which alone possesses

the power of infection and later forms the plerocercoid, and (2) the embryonic envelope, which disappears quickly as soon as the larva has penetrated its host.

The oncosphere (also of variable size, 22–27, even 30 μ in diameter) is composed of quite a considerable number of cells (about 18 to 20 on a microscopic field), whose limits are indistinct *in vivo*. In one of the points of the oncosphere, which is characterized by a greater transparency of tissue, one notes three pairs of small hooks, each one of which measures half the diameter of the oncosphere. These hooks are attached to the internal wall of the sphere and are curved approximately like its surface. They move very energetically, and on first glance one thinks of the presence of muscular fibrillae. In examining the hooks more closely, one establishes that the movements of which they are capable are due to the extreme contractibility of the plasma of the oncosphere.

Attached directly to the oncosphere is the embryonic envelope. It has an epithelium formed of a single layer of alveolar cells, whose contours, the same as those of the nuclei, are only faintly visible.

Under a fine cuticle, which surrounds the whole ciliated larva, is found a bluish layer of homogeneous cytoplasm, which separates it from the embryonic envelope. The cuticle has ciliary hairs and is enveloped by a layer of refringent granulations, arranged like the meshes of a net.

The larva so summarily described—a real jewel—is obtained by thousands, thanks to the method developed by Janicki which was the *sine qua non* of the research undertaken on this vast scale.

The larvae, characterized by a negative heliotropism, all gather at the darkest spot of the receptacle in which they hatch and are then easily gathered by the thousands by means of a fine pipette and afterward distributed in the experimental aquariums.

Let us now examine the experiments themselves.

The necessary material was caught on 19 June in the lake of Neuchâtel, partly near the shore, not far from the drains, and partly in the pelagic region at the surface and to a depth of 70 m.

They were distributed in jars of from 2 to 4 liters. Some of these were placed at the tempera-

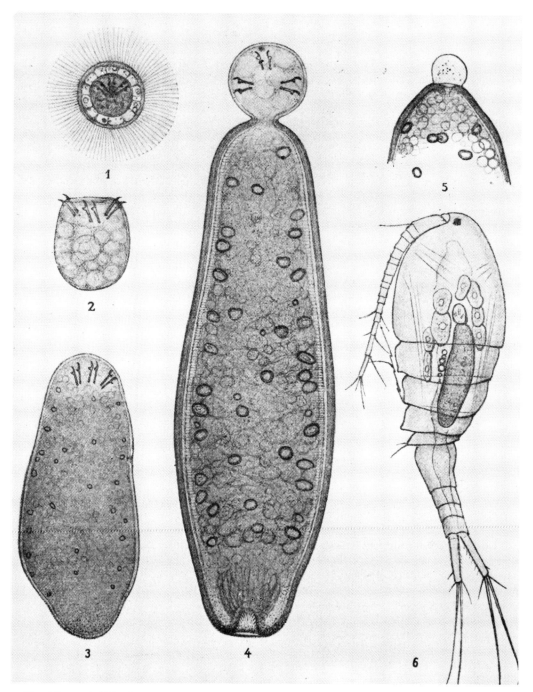

Plate 113. Fig. 1. Ciliated larva which has just hatched. *Fig. 2.* Oncosphere of the body cavity of the *Cyclops strenuus,* five days after the piercing of the digestive tube. *Fig. 3.* The same, 12 days old. *Fig. 4.* Free procercoid extracted from the cavity of *Cyclops str.* 20 days after infection. *Fig. 5.* The extremity of a procercoid, illustrating the disappearance of the spherical appendage, 40 days after infection. *Fig. 6. Cyclops strenuus* with a procercoid.

ture of the laboratory (20°, 25° C), others in running water (+12° C) in order to be able to make eventual observations on the influence of the temperature. From 19 to 25 June, all the plankton thus conserved were infected by a very large number of ciliated larvae. These, gathered by a pipette, kept together in watch glasses, were poured from there into the eight experimental jars, where they were left to themselves.

The research began on 20 June with *Daphnies*. Finding no trace of ciliated larvae either in the intestine or in any other part of the body, I tried placing a *Daphnie* in a watch glass in the presence of several ciliated larvae. Close observations through a microscope did not permit me to verify the absorption of a single larva, nor a diminution of their number.

The *Leptodora* behaved in a similar manner. Several *Bythothrephes* similarly gave a negative result.

Then I began to consider the copepodes, which caused a cruel deception at the beginning. An exclusively littoral species, the *Cyclops viridis,* which does not fear dirty waters and lives at the mouth of the drains of the lake, seemed definitely indicated to enter into contact with the ciliated larvae and "nourish" itself on them. The research, alas, gave a particularly negative result here. The ciliated larvae were indeed absorbed, but were found again a little later, half digested, in the intestine.

I must note that the experiments repeated later on *Cyclops oithonoides, Cyclops macrurus, Cyclops vernalis,* and others, and probably, *Cyclops Leuckarti,* gave a negative result.

Finally, on 24 June, I undertook the study of *Cyclops strenuus,* one of the most common and most widespread species in all the lakes.

At first, I did not observe anything special. The numerous fat droplets which filled the body of these crustaceans, moreover, prevented a very detailed observation. In rapidly draining the water from beneath the cover slip, so that the pressure of the latter lightly crushed the animal and removed the little fat droplets, the examination had no more obstacles. My astonishment was then immense. By examination of some of these fat droplets at a higher power (Apochr. 3 mm and Ocul. 8 Zeiss), I confirmed that several were nothing more than oncospheres which were already in the body cavity. One after the other, all the specimens examined were found infected, containing from one to eight or even ten oncospheres. There was no longer any doubt that we were in the presence of the primary intermediary host or in any case of a species very closely related to the true host. It was a question of being prudent before affirming too categorically to have found the definitive solution to the problem, for the *Diaptomus gracilis* also revealed themselves infected, less often, but quite as strongly as the *Cyclops strenuus.* Let us say from now on that these two species are indeed the primary intermediary hosts of *Dibothriocephalus latus,* and let us follow the development of the larva in one of them, the *Cyclops strenuus.*

After the ciliated larva has penetrated into the *Cyclops,* it loses its embryonic envelope, and the very contractile oncosphere seeks immediately to pierce the intestinal wall, entering the body cavity. The larva reaches its goal so rapidly that it is rarely found still in the intestine six hours after it has been ingested. Let us add that the oncosphere does not float freely in the body cavity as one might think, but stays a rather long time fixed by its hooks to the external wall of the intestine (10–15 days) where it almost loses it contractility.

The development consists first and especially of an increase in size during which the shape becomes more and more oval. The sixth or eighth day, the oncosphere which measured .024 mm originally has already attained .1 to .15 mm (Plate 113, Fig. 2).

As soon as the larva has attained .2 mm, which occurs from the eighth to the twelfth day, the rapidity of the development being rather irregular, one observes important differentiations in the structure. The whole body shows a characteristic young parenchymatous tissue formed of small cells with large nuclei. Some rare calcareous corpuscles appear here and there between the cells of the tissue. The longitudinal and transverse musculature begins to become visible, and the cuticle of the body is more strongly developed.

At the two extremities of the body appear different formations (Plate 113, Figs. 3 and 4).

One of the ends, which is characterized by the presence of the hooks, already possesses a clearer and more homogeneous tissue. In the course of subsequent development, this extremity detaches itself little by little from the rest of the body by a more and more accentuated strangulation, and, when the larva is from 12 to 15 days old and measures .35 to .40 mm, this end assumes a spherical shape united to the body by a narrow peduncle (Plate 113, Fig. 4). The spherical terminal appendage presents a shape almost identical to the final shape: the oncosphere. The only characteristics which distinguish it are: the cuticle of the body, already greatly thickened, covering also the spherical appendage, the already larger size, and the impression that one is dealing with a formation in the process of degeneration.

This spherical appendage remains a long time without changing, and it is only 15 to 20 days later, when the larva has attained .5 to .6 mm, that it is completely enveloped by the cuticle of the body. Thus separated from the rest of the body of the larva, it decomposes little by little, and the embryonic hooks, losing their support in this degenerated protoplasm, disappear (Plate 113, Fig. 5).

Let us examine now the other end of the larva, that which undergoes the most marked transformation.

When the spherical appendage is not yet developed, this end is already distinct from the rest of the body because of its more compact tissue and its more visible musculature. The cuticle is already covered, at this end by fine, silky hairs. Around the end, one begins to perceive longitudinal stripes, and the tissue in general becomes a little darker. The former quickly become distinct and permit one to distinguish their glandular character. The end as a whole differentiates itself much more slowly and little by little forms an invagination. Fourteen to sixteen days after infection, when the larva has attained a length of .4 mm, the longitudinal glandular stripes are very definite and, viewed from above, have the appearance of a rosette. The invagination is also now completely developed, in the shape of a cone, provided with silky hairs, and recognizable by an invaginated terminal indentation. The glandular formations of the rosette appear to come to a head in this indentation.

During the time when these transformations are being made at the two poles of the larva, the larva as a whole has undergone some rather important transformations. The whole tissue is impregnated with the young parenchyma characteristic of cestodes; the calcareous corpuscles

which are later so characteristic of the plerocercoid are already found in considerable number. The longitudinal and transverse musculature is already well-developed, and the cuticle has undergone a considerable reinforcement.

The larva is now nearly entirely covered with silky hairs which are especially well-developed in the terminal indentation. They are, on the contrary, very sparse toward the spherical appendage of the other extremity. (This appendage itself possesses neither silky hairs nor calcareous corpuscles.) These silky hairs are slightly curved and face toward the rear, but in the invaginated indentation they are facing anteriorly, that is to say, in harmony with the direction they have in the rest of the body. The entire organism is now free in the body cavity. If one makes it emerge from the *Cyclops* by as weak a pressure as possible in order not to damage it, one affirms that this larva executes strong peristaltic movements, as well as rather considerable movement in distance. It continually changes shape and becomes oval, sometimes spindle-shaped, or presents very bizarre contours. The cone-shaped indentation evaginates or invaginates itself alternately.

Whereas during the very early stages of the larva it was the part of the body carrying the hooks which represented the anterior part (that is to say, that which was found in front in the crawling movements), the reverse now takes place; it is the extremity supplied with the rosette of the invagination which is facing anteriorly.

Having arrived at this stage of development after two or three weeks of life, the larva now measures up to .5 mm. A more prolonged sojourn in the *Cyclops* does not seem to bring about any modification in the organization of the larva, except for the shedding of the spherical appendage and a slight increase in size up to .6 mm. For the larva that we have just described, we propose the name procercoid, a name which will become indispensable, doubtless due to its clarity.

Let us say now several words about the *Cyclops strenuus* itself. Of all the ciliated larvae which penetrate into the *Cyclops* or the *Diaptomus* at the time of a strong infection, at most two arrive at their complete development. They are then found still almost immobile and free in the cavity of the *Cyclops* along the digestive tube (Plate 113, Fig. 6). All the others are arrested in the primitive stage of an oncosphere of approximately .12 mm. It is extraordinary that these larvae are still living and fixed on the external wall of the digestive tube of the *Cyclops* three months after infection. Driven out of its body by pressure, they still execute swimming motions.

As soon as the procercoid has lost its spherical appendage in the body of the *Cyclops*, it initiates rather rapid movements in its host. The *Cyclops* seem very restricted in their habitual movements. One sees these little crustaceans, which usually execute very rapid, jerky movements, drag themselves slowly on the bottom of the receptacle.

From this fact one can explain the infection of the burbot by the intermediary of plankton. The fish which lives in the adult state at considerable depths is found in the young state in the littoral zone. The heavy, infected *Cyclops* which drag themselves on the bottom thus represent easy prey for this fish. I also hope to arrive at an explanation for the enigma of the *Coregonae* as soon as the material necessary for experimentation is at my disposal.

Infection of the Fish

After having pursued the development of the oncosphere up to the procercoid stage, it remained to infect one of the fish known to be a plerocercoid carrier, and thus to complete the life cycle of *Dibothriocephalus latus*.

The presence of the caudal appendage of the procercoid caused doubt as to whether the larva at this stage was already suitable for infecting the fish, or whether the ability to infect was acquired only after the disappearance of the appendage. It is true that, in this state, the procercoid already possessed the qualities required for a good infection: (1) it is completely covered with well-developed silky hairs; (2) the completely developed invaginated extremity was likewise covered with silky hairs; (3) the glands converged on the end of the larva; and (4) finally, it had the ability to move rather rapidly and, in particular, to execute peristaltic movements—all favoring the perforation of the intestinal wall. But here, likewise, only an experiment could bring about the definitive solution, and it was attempted for the first time on 6 August 1917.

Six small trout (*Trutta fario*) (7 cm long and 8 months old) were placed in an aquarium with quite a considerable number of *Cyclops* and *Diaptomus* (more than 100), which had been in-

fected with ciliated larvae for six weeks. It was necessary to wait for a good while before the young trout decided to capture the little crustaceans which surrounded them. (These fish came from the cantonal hatchery of Boudry and had been fed until then on *Daphnies* and *Chironomes*.) After several hours, however, the little aquarium was completely rid of all its little crustaceans. Five to six hours later a trout was opened, and the content of its stomach and intestines was examined. On examining very closely the stomach and the intestine where the pyloric appendages are located, the presence of free, transparent procercoids detaching themselves slightly from the stomach was noted. Some of them still carried the caudal appendage, while others had already lost it (in the *Cyclops*, probably). The former drew first attention, and I can indicate at this time that the procercoids with or without appendage seemed to present exactly the same potential of infection. It is thus of no consequence for the infection of the fish whether the appendage has already fallen off in the body of the *Cyclops* or whether it still exists at the moment of the ingestion of the crustacean by the fish.

The course of the experiments gave a complete description of the fate of the procercoid in the stomach of the fish. Liberated by the digestion of the *Cyclops*, the procercoids move into the stomach of the fish. Having arrived at a certain place, they stop and begin to execute strong peristaltic movements directed against the gastric mucosa. As soon as the attachment is effected, the larvae contract and take a stockier shape; the peristaltic movements become progressively weaker, slower, and less frequent in proportion as the larvae penetrate more deeply into the mucosa. This concludes the direct observations on the larvae's mode of penetration. In order to know what happens next, it is necessary to have recourse to maceration or paraffin blocks and sections.

The second day after infection, the procercoids, always very contracted, are found buried in the submucosa. Liberated by means of needle dissection, they no longer move actively as they do in the free state in the stomach of the fish or when extracted from the *Cyclops*. The terminal invagination is also immobile. Only infrequent and slow movements testify to the vitality of the

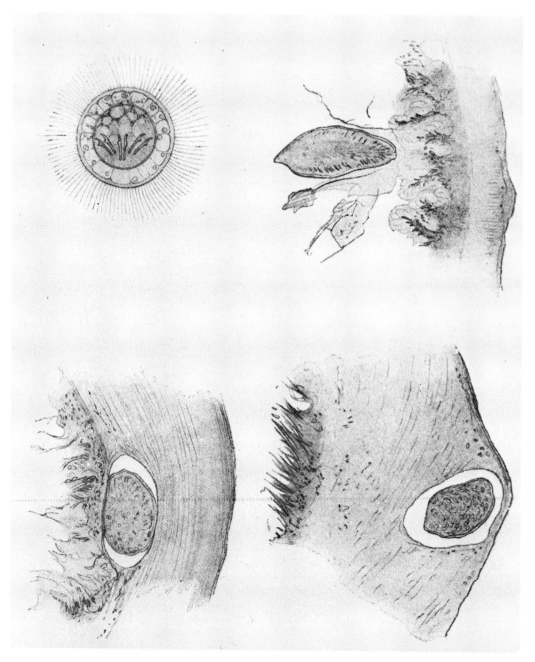

Plate 114. Upper left. A ciliated larva, showing all the details of its organization. *Upper right.* Transverse section of the stomach of the trout (*Trutta fario*) with a free procercoid. Six hours after infection. *Lower left.* Transverse section with a procercoid in the musculature of the stomach of the trout. Five days after infection. *Lower right.* Transverse section with the procercoid at the periphery of the musculature of the stomach of the trout. Twelve days after infection.

larva. The silky hairs of the cuticle seem to have disappeared.

The third or even fourth day after infection one still sees the larva, which can now be considered a plerocercoid, through the submucosa. Later they disappear into the parenchyma. Two of the three figures accompanying this text illustrate the continuation of the development of the larva (paraffin sections). The first of these figures shows the larva at the moment of its penetration into the musculature of the stomach (five to six days after infection); the second figure represents a larva at the moment when it is preparing to leave it (five to eight days later).

The procercoid does not seem to be surrounded by a capsule (see also Braun). On the contrary, it is probable that the musculature isolates the parasite. Thus the figures that Braun gives of the mode of migration of this parasite (particularly in the liver) are explained.

Having arrived at the periphery of the stomach, the larvae can now penetrate into the cavity and the musculature of the body, places where they have been found for a long time and [in which they have been] described by the name plerocercoids. The path traveled by the larva after infection indicates that this is the only possible route. It is evident that the procercoids can likewise pass directly from the intestine into the accessory organs (Plate 114).

It is thus that procercoids were in fact already found in the liver of *Trutta fario* six days after infection; that is to say, at a moment when the procercoids of the fish, infected at the same time, were found to be still in the muscular layer of the gastric wall.

These latter experimental results on the migration of the larva into the stomach of the trout were completely confirmed and pursued even further (penetration of the intestinal wall) by observations on fish (perch and burbots) made by Janicki, observations which are linked with the earlier ones of Max Braun.

Thus the experiments were terminated.

The life cycle of *Dibothriocephalus latus* is now completed: (1) by the negative result of the direct infection of fish by ciliated larvae; (2) by the positive result of a mode of development in cestodes unknown until now; that is, the existence of two intermediary hosts of which the first is revealed to be *Cyclops strenuus* and *Diaptomus gracilis*. The development passes from the oncosphere to the plerocercoid by an intermediary larva which develops in the *Cyclops* or the *Diaptomus*, namely the procercoid which units the characteristics of the initial and final stages: the oncosphere resides in the caudal appendage of the procercoid, the plerocercoid is preformed in its general appearance.

The procercoid presents the following characteristics: (1) a spherical caudal appendage with embryonic hooks, the appendage disappearing either in the *Cyclops*, in the *Diaptomus*, or in the intestinal tract of the fish; (2) a protractile terminal invagination, furnished with silky hairs and in which emerge (3) glandular formations; (4) a covering of silky hairs which disappear in the submucosa of the stomach of the fish; (5) a limited number of calcareous corpuscles dispersed in a finely granular parenchyma.

By the digestion of the infected *Cyclops* or the *Diaptomus,* the procercoids are liberated in the stomach or the intestine of certain fish, where they transform into plerocercoids, after penetrating the intestinal wall. By piercing the stomach, they enter the body cavity and from there migrate into the musculature or directly into the liver. . . .

Selected References

Anderson, Hamilton Holland, Warren L. Bostick, and Herbert G. Johnstone. *Amebiasis: Pathology, Diagnosis, and Chemotherapy*. Springfield, Ill.: Charles C Thomas, 1953. 431 pp.

Bacellar, Renato Clark. *Brazil's Contribution to Tropical Medicine and Malaria*. Rio de Janeiro: Gráfica Olímpica Editora, 1963. 379 pp.

Bulloch, William. *The History of Bacteriology*. London: Oxford University Press, 1938. 422 pp.

Dobell, Clifford. *Anthony Van Leeuwenhoek and His Little Animals. Being Some Account of the Father of Protozoology and Bacteriology and His Multifarious Discoveries in These Disciplines*. London: John Bale and Sons and Danielsson, 1932. 435 pp.

Foster, W. D. *A History of Parasitology*. Edinburgh: E. & S. Livingston, 1965. 202 pp.

Gould, Sylvester E. *Trichinosis*. Springfield, Ill.: Charles C Thomas, 1945. 290 pp.

Hirsch, August. *Handbook of Geographical and Historical Pathology. Vol. II: Chronic Infective, Toxic, Parasitic Septic and Constitutional Diseases*. Trans. from the 2nd German ed. by Charles Creighton. London: New Sydenham Society. Vol. 62, 1885. 681 pp.

Hoare, Cecil A. Early discoveries regarding the parasite of oriental sore. *Transactions of the Royal Society of Tropical Medicine and Hygiene*, 32: 67-92, 1938.

Hoeppli, R. *Parasites and Parasitic Infections in Early Medicine and Science*. Singapore: University of Malaya Press, 1959. 526 pp.

Inglis, V. A. and R. T. Leiper. Bibliography of Dracontiasis. *Journal of the London School of Tropical Medicine*, Supplements Nos. 1, 2: 1912.

Leiper, R. T., and V. A. Inglis. *Material for a Bibliography of the Trematode Infections of Man*. London: London School of Tropical Medicine, 1914. 53 pp.

Long, Esmond R. *Selected Readings in Pathology*. Springfield, Ill.: Charles C Thomas, 1961. 306 pp.

Major, Ralph H. *Classic Descriptions of Disease*. Springfield, Ill.: Charles C Thomas, 1965. 679 pp.

Marcial-Rojas, Raúl A. *Pathology of Protozoal and Helminthic Diseases*. Baltimore: Williams & Wilkins, 1971, 1010 pp.

Marroquín, Horacio Figueroa. *Historia de la Enfermedad de Robles en América y de su Descubrimiento en Guatemala*. Guatemala: Editorial Lux, 1963. 90 pp.

Morishita, Kadru, Yoshitaka Komiya, and Hisakichi Matsubayashi. *Progress of Medical Parasitology in Japan*. Tokyo: Meguro Parasitological Museum. Vol I, 1964, 753 pp.; Vol. II, 1965, 390 pp.; Vol. III, 1966, 644 pp.; Vol. IV, 1972, 604 pp.; Vol. V, 1973, 293 pp.

Mulligan, H. W., ed. *The African Trypanosomiases*. New York: Wiley-Interscience, 1970. 950 pp.

Rath, Gernoth. *Famous Tropical Physicians*. Leverkusen, Germany: Farben-fabriken Bayer A.G., 1963. 64 pp.

Reinhard, Edward G. Landmarks in Parasitology II. Demonstration of the life cycle and pathogenicity of the spiral threadworm. *Experimental Parasitology*, 7: 108–123, 1958.

———.Parasitological Reviews: Landmarks of Parasitology I. The discovery of the life cycle of the liver fluke. *Journal of Experimental Parasitology*, 6: 208–232, 1957.

Russell, Paul F. *Man's Mastery of Malaria*. London: Geoffrey Cumberlege, Oxford University Press, 1955. 308 pp.

Scott, H. Harold. *A History of Tropical Medicine*. London: Edward Arnold, 1939. Vol. I, 648 pp.; Vol. II, 571 pp.

Shelley, Walter B., and John T. Crissey. *Classics in Clinical Dermatology*. Springfield, Ill.: Charles C Thomas, 1953, 485 pp.

Singer, Charles, and E. Ashworth Underwood. *A Short History of Medicine*. London: Oxford University Press, 1962. 854 pp.

Symposium — A Bicentennial Sampler: Milestones in the History of Tropical Medicine and Hygiene, edited by Eli Chernin, in *The American Journal of Tropical Medicine and Hygiene*, 26, No. 5, Part 2, September, 1977.

Symposium — Fifty Years of American Parasitology: Some Fulgent Personalities in Helminthology (Donald V. Moore), Arthropodology (William E. Collins), Protozoology (Martin D. Young). *The Journal of Parasitology*, 62, No. 4, 497–514, 1976.

Trussell, Ray E. *Trichomonas vaginalis and Trichomoniasis*. Springfield, Ill.: Charles C Thomas, 1947. 231 pp.

Warren, Kenneth S. *Schistosomiasis: The Evolution of a Medical Literature, Selected Abstracts and Citations, 1852–1972*. Cambridge, Mass.: MIT Press, 1973, 1307 pp.

Index

Library of Congress Cataloging in Publication Data
(For library cataloging purposes only)
Main entry under title:

Tropical medicine and parasitology.

Bibliography: v. 2, p.
Includes index
1. Tropical medicine—Addresses, essays,
lectures. 2. Medical parasitology—Addresses,
essays, lectures. I. Kean, Benjamin Harrison,
1912–   II. Mott, Kenneth E. III. Russell,
Adair J.
RC961.5.T74   616.9′88′3   76-12908
ISBN 0-8014-0992-6 (v. 2)